SHORT LOAN.

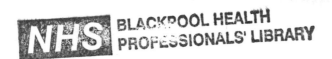

OBSTETRIC ANESTHESIA AND UNCOMMON DISORDERS

OBSTETRIC ANESTHESIA AND UNCOMMON DISORDERS

■ ■ ■ ■ ■ ■ ■ ■ ■ ■ ■

David R. Gambling, M.B., F.R.C.P.C.
Co-Director of Obstetric Anesthesia
Associate Clinical Professor
Department of Anesthesiology
University of California, San Diego, School of Medicine
San Diego, California, United States

M. Joanne Douglas, M.D., F.R.C.P.C.
Clinical Professor
Head, Division of Obstetric Anesthesia
University of British Columbia Faculty of Medicine
Department of Anesthesiology
British Columbia Women's Hospital
Vancouver, British Columbia, Canada

W.B. SAUNDERS COMPANY
A Division of Harcourt Brace & Company
Philadelphia London Toronto Montreal Sydney Tokyo

W.B. SAUNDERS COMPANY
A Division of Harcourt Brace & Company

The Curtis Center
Independence Square West
Philadelphia, Pennsylvania 19106

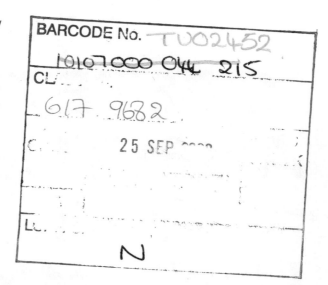
Library of Congress Cataloging-in-Publication Data

Obstetric anesthesia and uncommon disorders / [edited by] David R. Gambling,
M. Joanne Douglas

p.   cm.

ISBN 0–7216–6157–2

1. Anesthesia in obstetrics.   2. Anesthesia–Complications.   3. Pregnant
women—Surgery.   I. Gambling, David R.   II. Douglas, M. Joanne.
[DNLM: 1. Anesthesia, Obstetrical.   2. Pregnancy Complications.
WO 450 01425 1998]   RG732.02645 1998   617.9′682—dc21

DNLM/DLC   97-1435

Obstetric Anesthesia and Uncommon Disorders   ISBN 0–7216–6157–2

Printed in the United States of America.

Last digit is the print number: 9   8   7   6   5   4   3   2   1

To
Sadie, Gordon, Samantha, and Jake (DRG)
and
Bill, Matthew, and Mark (MJD)
for their love, humor, guidance, and support

CONTRIBUTORS

Penny J. Ballem, M.D., F.R.C.P.C.
Clinical Associate Professor of Medicine, University of British Columbia Faculty of Medicine; Vice President, British Columbia Women's Hospital and Health Center, Vancouver, British Columbia, Canada
Hematologic Disorders

Sheila E. Cohen, M.B., Ch.B., F.R.C.A.
Professor and Director of Obstetric Anesthesia, Stanford University School of Medicine, Stanford, California, United States
Parturients of Short Stature

Chantal Crochetière, M.D., F.R.C.P.C.
Assistant Professor, Université de Montréal Faculty of Medicine; Head, Obstetrical Anesthesia, Hôpital Sainte-Justine, Montreal, Quebec, Canada
Myopathies

Edward T. Crosby, M.D., F.R.C.P.C.
Associate Professor, University of Ottawa Faculty of Medicine; Director of Obstetrical Anesthesia, Ottawa General Hospital, Ottawa, Ontario, Canada
Scoliosis and Major Spinal Surgery • Spinal Cord Injury, Spina Bifida, Tethered Cord Syndrome, and Anterior Spinal Artery Syndrome

M. Joanne Douglas, M.D., F.R.C.P.C.
Clinical Professor and Head, Division of Obstetric Anesthesia, University of British Columbia Faculty of Medicine, Department of Anesthesiology, British Columbia Women's Hospital, Vancouver, British Columbia, Canada
Malignant Hyperthermia • Hematologic Disorders

David R. Gambling, M.B.B.S., D.R.C.O.G., F.R.C.P.C.
Co-Director of Obstetric Anesthesia and Associate Clinical Professor, Department of Anesthesiology, University of California, San Diego, School of Medicine, San Diego, California, United States
Structural Heart Disease • Vascular Diseases

Margaret Bunce Garahan, M.D., Dip.A.B.A.
Assistant Professor of Anesthesiology, University of Vermont College of Medicine; Attending Anesthesiologist, Fletcher Allen Health Care, Inc., Burlington, Vermont, United States
Dermatoses

Larry C. Gilstrap, III, M.D.
Emma Sue Hightower Professor and Chair,
Department of Obstetrics, Gynecology, and Reproductive Sciences, University of Texas Medical School at Houston, Houston, Texas, United States
Rare Endocrine Disorders

Beth Glosten, M.D.
Associate Professor, Department of Anesthesia, University of Washington School of Medicine, Seattle, Washington, United States
Osteogenesis Imperfecta • Unusual Maternal and Fetal Conditions

Caroline Grange, M.B.B.S., F.R.C.A.
Consultant Anesthetist, Oxford Radcliffe National Health Service Trust, Oxford, England, United Kingdom
Miscellaneous Conditions

Holly C. Gunn, M.D.
Acting Assistant Professor, Department of Anesthesiology, University of Washington School of Medicine, Seattle, Washington, United States
Unusual Maternal and Fetal Conditions

Paul R. Howell, B.Sc., M.B., Ch.B., F.R.C.A.
Consultant Anesthetist, St. Bartholomew's Hospital, London, England, United Kingdom
Adult Respiratory Distress Syndrome • Cystic Fibrosis • Acute Severe Asthma • Pneumothorax and Pneumomediastinum

Victor F. Huckell, M.D., F.R.C.P.C.
Clinical Professor of Medicine, University of British Columbia Faculty of Medicine; Staff Cardiologist, Vancouver Hospital and Health Sciences Centre, Vancouver, British Columbia, Canada
Structural Heart Disease • Disorders of Cardiac Conduction

Mark D. Johnson, M.D.
Chairman, Department of Anesthesiology; Director, Operating Rooms, Melrose-Wakefield Hospital, Melrose, Massachusetts, United States
Cardiopulmonary Resuscitation • Airway Obstruction and Difficult Tracheal Intubation • Intracranial Lesions

Girish P. Joshi, M.B.B.S., M.D., F.F.A.R.C.S.I.
Associate Professor, University of Texas Southwestern Medical Center at Dallas, Dallas, Texas, United States
Pulmonary Embolism

Gabriela Lauretti, M.D., Ph.D.
Assistant Professor, Discipline of Anesthesiology of the Department of Surgery, Orthopedics and Traumatology, Faculty of Medicine of Ribeirõo Preto, University of São Paulo, São Paulo, Brazil
Infectious Diseases

Anita Licata, M.D.
Assistant Professor of Medicine, Dermatology Division, University of Vermont College of Medicine; Attending in Medicine, Fletcher Allen Health Care, Inc., Burlington, Vermont, United States
Dermatoses

Stephen Longmire, M.D.
Associate Professor of Anesthesiology and Obstetrics, Department of Anesthesiology, Baylor College of Medicine, Houston, Texas, United States
Autoimmune Diseases

Carol J. Luppi, R.N.C., B.S.N.
Co-Chair of Critical Care Obstetric Nursing Team, Brigham and Women's Hospital, Boston, Massachusetts, United States
Cardiopulmonary Resuscitation

Ann E. Newton, M.B.B.S., F.A.N.Z.C.A.
Clinical Senior Lecturer, University of Queensland Medical School; Anesthesia Staff Specialist, Mater Misericordiae Hospital, Brisbane, Queensland, Australia
Seizures and Coma ■ *Peripheral Neuropathies*

Dawn C. Over, M.B., B.S., F.R.C.A.
Consultant Anesthetist, Southmead Hospital, Bristol, England, United Kingdom
Cardiopulmonary Resuscitation

Michael J. Paech, M.B.B.S., D.R.C.O.G., F.R.C.A., F.A.N.Z.C.A.
Clinical Lecturer in Anesthesia, University of Western Australia School of Medicine; Staff Anesthetist, King Edward Memorial Hospital for Women, Perth, Western Australia
Metabolic and Liver Disease

Timothy J.G. Pavy, M.B., B.S., D.A., Dip. Mid. C.O.G., F.A.N.Z.A., F.R.C.A.
Clinical Instructor, Department of Anesthesia, University of Western Australia; Head, Department of Anesthesia, King Edward Memorial Hospital, Subiaco, Western Australia
Psychiatric Disorders

Roanne Preston, M.D., F.R.C.P.C.
Assistant Professor, University of Ottawa Faculty of Medicine; Staff Anesthetist, Ottawa General Hospital, Ottawa, Ontario, Canada
Spinal Cord Injury, Spina Bifida, Tethered Cord Syndrome, and Anterior Spinal Artery Syndrome

Emily F. Ratner, M.D.
Assistant Professor, Department of Anesthesiology, Stanford University School of Medicine, Stanford, California, United States
Parturients of Short Stature

Kerri Robertson, M.D.
Associate Clinical Professor of Anesthesiology, Duke University School of Medicine; Chief of Transplant Services, Department of Anesthesiology, Duke University Medical Center, Durham, North Carolina, United States
Transplantation

Shiv K. Sharma, M.B.B.S., M.D., F.R.C.A.
Assistant Professor, University of Texas Southwestern Medical Center at Dallas, Dallas, Texas, United States
Pulmonary Embolism

Glenn K. Shopper, M.D.
Assistant Professor, University of Missouri, Kansas City School of Medicine and Director of Obstetric Anesthesia, Truman Medical Center, Kansas City, Missouri, United States
Airway Obstruction and Difficult Tracheal Intubation

Jack A. Stecher, M.D.
Instructor, University of Texas Southwestern Medical Center at Dallas; Staff Physician, Baylor University Medical Center, Dallas, Texas, United States
Vascular Diseases

Jean E. Swenerton, M.D., F.R.C.P.C.
Clinical Associate Professor, Division of Obstetric Anesthesia, Department of Anesthesia, University of British Columbia Faculty of Medicine; Staff Anesthesiologist, British Columbia Women's Hospital and Health Centre, Vancouver, British Columbia, Canada
Disorders of Cardiac Conduction

Donald H. Wallace, M.D., F.F.A.R.C.S.
Professor, Department of Anesthesiology and Pain Management, University of Texas Southwestern Medical Center; Attending Anesthesiologist, Parkland Memorial Hospital, Dallas, Texas, United States
Rare Endocrine Disorders

Frank G. Zavisca, M.D., Ph.D.
Associate Professor of Anesthesiology, Louisiana State University School of Medicine in Shreveport; Director, Obstetric Anesthesiology, Department of Anesthesiology, Louisiana State Hospital-Shreveport, Shreveport, Louisiana, United States
Intracranial Lesions

PREFACE

The stimulus for this textbook was the number of occasions, often at night, when we were asked to provide anesthetic care to a parturient with an uncommon medical or surgical condition. Some textbooks of obstetric anesthesia touch briefly on a few of these conditions, but often the emphasis is on common disorders and pregnancy-related complex conditions, such as pre-eclampsia. Although textbooks cover anesthesia in nonpregnant patients with uncommon disorders, they do not emphasize those issues of importance to the parturients, such as the impact of the disorder on the pregnancy, the impact of the pregnancy on the disorder, and the effect of therapy for the disorder on the fetus and neonate. The obstetric and anesthetic literature has contained a number of case reports describing the management of a parturient with a particularly unusual syndrome. Unfortunately, access to these reports is usually limited, especially at night or in an emergency, and the principles of management have not been outlined in a convenient resource.

This text is about uncommon conditions that have the potential to have an impact on the parturient and is organized on a systems basis. Not all unusual conditions are discussed. Even during the writing of this text, case reports were published of rare conditions in which pregnancy had not been previously described. This text covers some slightly more common conditions, such as muscular dystrophy, and some extremely rare conditions, such as Gorlin's syndrome. Other acute complications of common medical disorders, such as status asthmaticus, are also included, as their management may be made more difficult by pregnancy. Cardiorespiratory arrest and cardiopulmonary resuscitation in pregnancy are reviewed with useful protocols provided.

The contributors are obstetric anesthesiologists and medical specialists from many countries who have an interest, or expertise, in the area discussed. Tables, figures, and illustrations have been added as aids to the understanding of complex concepts and unusual clinical presentations. The references are as current as possible, and the management guidelines are often based on a common-sense approach, as the literature may not describe the anesthetic technique. The management approach may be different in the future as more cases are reported and a greater understanding of the pathophysiology of each disorder is obtained. A good example is the current use of regional anesthesia for delivery in parturients with certain cardiac conditions, whereas 10 years ago it was contraindicated.

This text should prove useful to the practicing anesthesiologist, in both the tertiary referral center and community hospital, who may have a parturient with an unusual syndrome suddenly present for care. A multidisciplinary team approach is emphasized, and other members of the team (perinatologists, obstetricians, midwives) will also find it useful as a reference for case reports and for understanding implications of anesthetic care.

In summary, *Obstetric Anesthesia and Uncommon Disorders* provides in a single source a ready reference for the majority of unusual conditions that are of relevance to obstetric anesthesiologists. It will assist the clinician in patient management when caring for a patient with an unusual disorder in an urgent or emergency situation.

David R. Gambling, M.B., F.R.C.P.C.
M. Joanne Douglas, M.D., F.R.C.P.C.

ACKNOWLEDGMENTS

We would like to thank the contributors of each chapter for their hard work and for spending time during their busy professional schedules to produce a thorough and clinically relevant document. We also would like to acknowledge our former mentor and colleague, Professor Graham McMorland, who always encouraged us, by his example, to be academically productive and clinically inquisitive.

We would also like to thank various people for their administrative and secretarial assistance, namely, Lois Obenhauer (Vancouver); Debby Rodi, Linda Sutherland, and Kimberley Herring (San Diego); and Lesley Day and Amelia Nicholas (W.B. Saunders, Philadelphia).

CONTENTS

STRUCTURAL HEART DISEASE

David R. Gambling, M.B., and Victor F. Huckell, M.D.

The aim of this chapter is to describe the pathology and pathophysiology of various uncommon cardiac lesions that are occasionally present in pregnant women. A structural defect may involve the myocardium or the heart valves, or it may be a complex congenital lesion. Other cardiologic problems are discussed elsewhere—disorders of cardiac conduction in Chapter 2, myocardial infarction and cardiopulmonary resuscitation in Chapter 3.

A structural lesion may be associated with few symptoms in the nonpregnant state, but it becomes apparent for the first time in mid- to late pregnancy as a result of the physiologic hemodynamic stresses that develop (see later). More often, patients with significant heart disease present electively in early pregnancy (with substantial files from cardiologists and cardiac surgeons). Increasing numbers of case reports are appearing in the anesthetic literature concerning the obstetric and anesthetic management of pregnant women with complex congenital heart disease. These complex lesions are uncorrected, fully corrected, or partially corrected (palliated). This chapter outlines the various surgical procedures that are performed, hemodynamic goals, and anticipated hemodynamic emergencies during labor and delivery. We also delineate the problems associated with prosthetic heart valves and cardiopulmonary bypasses during pregnancy. The management of pregnant women with mixed or severe valvular lesions and with cardiomyopathy is also presented.

In many cases there is no consensus as to the optimal anesthetic technique for the conditions being discussed, and therefore there is no cookbook–like approach to management. We describe case reports and point out the advantages and disadvantages of one technique over another. Although general and regional anesthesia significantly affect the hemodynamic changes that occur during labor and delivery, *the choice of technique is often immaterial if appropriate hemodynamic goals are considered and invasive monitoring is used to attain them.* The most likely cardiovascular effects of commonly utilized anesthetic and obstetric drugs are shown in Table 1–1.

SCOPE OF THE PROBLEM

Whereas there has been a drastic decline in the incidence of rheumatic heart disease among women of childbearing age over the last two to three decades, more women with congenital heart disease are living to reproductive age because of improved surgical techniques. In the last 25 years there has been a decline in overall maternal and fetal morbidity and mortality from cardiac disease; however, heart disease remains the leading cause of indirect maternal mortality.[1-4] Maternal mortality ranges from 0.4% in the New York Heart Association (NYHA) class I to II disease to 6.8% in class III to IV disease (Table 1–2). The risk to the mother with congenital heart disease depends on the type of malformation and the functional impairment it produces (Table 1–3).

The overall incidence of congenital heart disease in pregnancy remains relatively stable at 0.4% to 4.1%. Improved medical management and early surgical correction have resulted in greater numbers of patients with congenital heart disease becoming pregnant. Many of those affected lead active and productive lives, but many present to the obstetrician with only partial repairs or complex palliations of the heart lesions.

The principal danger for a pregnant woman with a complex heart lesion is cardiac decompensation because of the inability to meet the additional demands imposed by the physiologic changes of pregnancy and parturition. If present, infection, hemorrhage, and thromboembolism compound the risk, but with meticulous peripartum care many women deliver healthy neonates without adverse sequelae. Despite optimal care, however, some women with cardiac disease continue to suffer significant morbidity and mortality.[2, 3]

It is essential to understand the impact of the physiologic changes of pregnancy upon the specific heart lesion to properly counsel and manage these patients. Pregnant women with complex heart disease should be managed by a team.[4] This team should include representatives from obstetrics and perinatology, anesthesiology, neonatology, cardiology, intensive care,

TABLE 1–1. CARDIOVASCULAR EFFECTS OF COMMONLY USED ANESTHETIC AND OBSTETRIC DRUGS

	Heart Rate	Blood Pressure	Systemic Vascular Resistance	Cardiac Output	Myocardial Contractility	Venodilation
Etomidate	0	0/↓	0/↓	0	0	0
Ketamine	↑↑	↑	0/↑	↑	↑*	0
Thiopental	↑	↓↓	0 or ↑†	↓	↓	↑
Propofol	0/↑	↓	↓↓	0 to ↓	↓	↑
Succinylcholine	0 to ↓ with repeat doses	0 to ↑	0 to ↑	0	0	0 to ↓
Atracurium	0 to ↑	0 to ↓	0	0	0	0 to ↑
d-Tubocurare	0 to ↑	↓	↓	↓	0	0
Pancuronium	↑	↑	0 to ↑	↑	↑	0
Rocuronium	0 to ↑	0	0	0	0	0
Vecuronium	0	0	0	0	0	0
Fentanyl	↓	0 to ↓	0	0	0	0
Meperidine	0 to ↑	↓	↓	↓	↓	↑
Morphine	0	↓	↓	↓	↓	↑
Halothane	0 to ↑	↓	↓	0 to ↓	↓↓	↓
Isoflurane	↑↑	↓	↓↓	0 to ↑	↓	↓
Sevoflurane	↑	↓	↓	0 to ↓?	↓	0
Nitrous oxide	0 to ↑	0 to ↑	0 to ↑	↓/↑	0	0 to ↓
Lidocaine	0	0	0	↑	↑	↑ if used for regional anesthesia
Lidocaine toxicity	↓	↓	↑	↓	↓	↑
Midazolam	0 to ↑	↓	0/↓	0	0/↓	0
Ergometrine	↑	↑↑	↑	↑	↑	↓
Oxytocin	0 to ↑	0 to ↑ —<10 u ↓ >10 u bolus dose	0 to ↓	0	0	0 to ↑
Magnesium sulfate	0 to ↓	↓	↓	0	0	↑
Nitroglycerin	0	↓↓	0 to ↓	↓	0	↑↑
Terbutaline	↑	0 to ↓	0 to ↓	↑	0 to ↑	↑

The response is represented by a 5-point scale from a marked increase (↑↑) to marked decrease (↓↓). 0 is no effect, ↑ is a slight increase, ↓ is a slight decrease.
*Secondary effect from endogenous catecholamine release.
†May ↓ from histamine release.
There are various caveats in the interpretation of these data. Some values are derived from animal studies only, some from human volunteers, and some from patients. Values may vary depending on whether a patient is ventilated mechanically or breathing spontaneously. In addition, the hemodynamic effects of these agents may change in the presence of other anesthetic agents. Furthermore, the hemodynamic response may be different in patients who are hypovolemic or in those who have sympathetic overactivity or sympathectomy. The values and ranges indicated in this table are the authors' opinion of the most likely clinical response for most patients and have been taken in part from Bowdle TA, Horita A, Kharasch ED (eds). The Pharmacologic Basis of Anesthesiology: Basic science and practical applications. New York, Churchill Livingstone, 1994; and Norris MC (ed). Obstetric Anesthesia. Philadelphia, JB Lippincott, 1993.

nursing, and social work. Pediatrician involvement is pertinent, in that the offspring of patients with congenital heart disease have a 5 to 15% likelihood of being affected by the same defect due to inheritance.[5] In addition, the fetus can be compromised because its nutrient and oxygen supply can be impaired by the mother's cardiopulmonary insufficiency.[6] It is also important to use in utero echocardiography and provide the mother with genetic counseling.[7] Almost all cardiac defects can be detected in the fetus at 18 weeks of gestation.[8]

PHYSIOLOGY OF PREGNANCY

This topic is discussed in standard texts, but it is important to briefly review how the cardiorespiratory changes, which occur throughout the pregnancy and peripartum period, may affect the well-being of women with heart disease. A comparison of normal cardiorespiratory parameters between the pregnant and nonpregnant states is shown in Table 1–4.

1. Respiratory. Minute ventilation and oxygen consumption increase during pregnancy, with a state of mild hyperventilation caused by the central action of progesterone. Increased minute ventilation results in a mild respiratory alkalosis.
2. Blood volume. By term, plasma volume is 40 to 50% higher than prepregnant levels, with increases in plasma volume exceeding those of red blood cell mass. (This increases by 20–30%.) This disproportion produces a dilutional or physiologic anemia, which is treatable with supplements of oral iron.

TABLE I–2. NYHA FUNCTIONAL CAPACITY AND OBJECTIVE ASSESSMENT*

Functional Capacity	Objective Assessment
Class I. Patients with cardiac disease but without limitation of physical activity. Ordinary physical activity does not cause undue fatigue, palpitations, dyspnea, or angina.	No objective evidence of cardiovascular disease.
Class II. Patients with cardiac disease resulting in slight limitation of physical activity. They are comfortable at rest. Ordinary physical activity results in fatigue, palpitation, dyspnea or angina.	Objective evidence of minimal cardiovascular disease.
Class III. Patient with cardiac disease resulting in marked limitation of physical activity. They are comfortable at rest. Less than ordinary activity causes fatigue, palpitation, dyspnea, or angina.	Objective evidence of moderately severe cardiovascular disease.
Class IV. Patients with cardiac disease resulting in inability to carry on any physical activity without discomfort. Symptoms of heart failure or the anginal syndrome may be present even at rest. If any physical activity is undertaken, discomfort is increased.	Objective evidence of severe cardiovascular disease.

*AHA Medical/Scientific Statement: 1994 Revisions to Classifications of Functional Capacity and Objective Assessment of Patients with Diseases of the Heart. Circulation 1994; 90:644.

3. Cardiac output. Cardiac output (CO) starts to increase by the 10th week of gestation and continues to rise to a peak of 30 to 50% above baseline at 32 weeks' gestation. Studies suggesting significant decreases in CO during the latter half of pregnancy were performed with patients supine—a position

TABLE I–3. MATERNAL MORTALITY ASSOCIATED WITH HEART DISEASE IN PREGNANCY*

Group 1—Mortality <1%

Atrial septal defect
Ventricular septal defect
Patent ductus arteriosus
Pulmonary/tricuspid disease
Tetralogy of Fallot, corrected
Bioprosthetic valve
Mitral stenosis, NYHA class I and II

Group 2—Mortality 5–15%

2A Mitral stenosis NYHA class III–IV
    Aortic stenosis
    Coarctation of aorta, without valvular involvement
    Uncorrected tetralogy of Fallot
    Previous myocardial infarction
    Marfan syndrome with normal aorta
2B Mitral stenosis with atrial fibrillation
    Artificial valve

Group 3—Mortality 25–50%

Primary pulmonary hypertension or Eisenmenger reaction
Coarctation of aorta, with valvular involvement
Marfan syndrome with aortic involvement

*From Clark SL. Structural cardiac disease in pregnancy. In Clark SL, Cotton DB, Phelan JP (eds): Critical Care Obstetrics. Oradell, NJ, Medical Economics Books, 1987; p 92.

TABLE I–4. NORMAL HEMODYNAMIC AND VENTILATORY PARAMETERS IN THE NONPREGNANT AND PREGNANT PATIENT

	Nonpregnant	Pregnant
Central venous pressure (mm Hg)	1–10	Unchanged
Pulmonary artery pressure (mean) (mm Hg)	9–16	Unchanged
Pulmonary capillary wedge pressure (mm Hg)	3–10	Unchanged
Cardiac output (L/min)	4–7	↑ 30–45%
Systemic vascular resistance (dyne-sec•cm^{-5})	770–1500	↓ 25%
Pulmonary vascular resistance (dyne-sec•cm^{-5})	20–120	↓ 25%
Arterial P_{O_2} (mm Hg)	90–95	104–108
Arterial P_{CO_2} (mm Hg)	38–40	27–32
Arterial pH	7.35–7.40	7.40–7.45
A-V oxygen difference (ml per dl)	4–5.5	↓ or normal
Oxygen consumption (ml/min)	173–311	249–331

From Gonik B. Intensive care monitoring of the critically ill pregnant patient. In Creasy RK, Resnick R (eds): Maternal-fetal Medicine: Principles and Practice. Philadelphia, WB Saunders, 1989, p 850.

associated with aortocaval compression. There is a less significant fall in CO at this time if measurements are made in the left lateral decubitus position, because venous return is maintained. The increase in CO is due to greater stroke volume in the first half of pregnancy, in contrast to the latter half when CO is maintained by an increase in heart rate superimposed on an increase in stroke volume. There is a rise in endogenous circulating catecholamines during labor, which produces a positive inotropic and chronotropic myocardial response. Left ventricular end-diastolic volume rises as a result of an expanded plasma volume, and this leads to an increase in myocardial contractility and stroke volume. Cardiac output and changes in cardiac function can be readily assessed by echocardiography in women with congenital heart disease. Echocardiography is often very helpful in early pregnancy because it serves to provide baseline hemodynamic values with which to guide therapy in late pregnancy.

4. Blood pressure. The placental bed acts as a low-resistance arteriovenous shunt and, in addition, there is physiologic vasodilatation in the arterial vascular bed due to the hormonal influence of endothelial prostacyclin and circulating progesterone. As a result, blood pressure usually falls during pregnancy, with an increase in pulse pressure due to a greater decrease in diastolic pressure.

5. Labor and delivery. Pain from labor and increased venous return, from the contracting uterus, raise CO by 20 to 50%. Heart rate decreases, and stroke volume increases. These changes are less pronounced in the lateral decubitus position. The mode of anesthesia influences the hemodynamic changes during labor and delivery in a significant manner.

SYMPTOMS AND SIGNS OF NORMAL PREGNANCY

Cardiopulmonary symptoms and signs of normal pregnancy may simulate heart disease. These include easy fatiguability and dyspnea. Dyspnea is almost always limited to the awareness of breathing, however, rather than the uncomfortable awareness of the necessity of breathing. Hyperventilation is caused by the stimulating effects of progesterone. Hyperventilation, together with an increased work of ventilation, makes many women aware of their breathing. It is also partially responsible for compensated respiratory alkalosis. Tiring easily may be due to the soporific effects of progesterone and its effects on smooth muscle. Orthopnea is more common in obese women and may be due to limitation of diaphragmatic motion. Chest pain during pregnancy is most commonly due to hiatus hernia, esophageal reflux, or ribcage distension. Tachycardia is normal in pregnancy, as are premature depolarizations of either atrial or ventricular origin. Syncope in later pregnancy, when the patient is supine, is usually caused by inferior vena caval compression. Syncope sometimes occurs with the sudden assumption of the upright position, based on orthostasis.

Some cardiovascular findings on physical examination may be confusing. Peripheral edema occurs in 60 to 80% of pregnant women, and is attributed in part to hemodilution, causing a fall in protein oncotic pressure and an elevation of capillary pressure as a consequence of elevated venous pressure in the legs. This peripheral edema is not associated with hepatomegaly. Pulmonary crackles are likely to be the result of upward displacement of the diaphragm. Prominent neck veins are related to a hyperactive cardiac state. Mean right atrial pressure is not elevated, however; neither is the hepatojugular reflex positive. Pseudocardiomegaly is related to displacement of the apex. Heart sounds normally become increased. There is often a third heart sound due to volume loading. In addition, right ventricular outflow tract murmurs are common.

SYMPTOMS AND SIGNS OF HEART DISEASE IN PREGNANCY

Certain symptoms and signs suggest the presence of heart disease.[9, 10] These include severe or progressive dyspnea, progressive orthopnea, paroxysmal nocturnal dyspnea, hemoptysis, exertion syncope, and chest pain related to effort or emotion. Physical findings strongly suggesting the presence of heart disease include cyanosis, clubbing, persistent neck vein distension, palpable thrill, diastolic murmurs, true cardiomegaly, documented sustained dysrhythmias, and pulmonary hypertension.

TABLE 1–5. FACTORS TO AVOID IN PARTURIENTS WITH CONGENITAL HEART DISEASE

1. Anxiety/pain	5. Anemia
2. Salt and water retention	6. Infection
3. Sudden stress or exercise	7. Dysrhythmias
4. Heat and humidity	8. Thromboembolism

GENERAL PRINCIPLES OF MANAGEMENT OF THE PARTURIENT WITH HEART DISEASE

Most women with cardiac disease who remain asymptomatic throughout pregnancy tolerate labor and delivery well. This is not too surprising in that the hemodynamic changes that occur in pregnancy represent a significant stress test. Conversely, women who are breathless at rest (i.e., NYHA class IV, and groups 2 and 3 listed in Table 1–3) usually tolerate pregnancy poorly. Factors that have an adverse affect on outcome in these cases, regardless of functional status, are listed in Table 1–5.

Patients in functional class III to IV categories with surgically correctable lesions should undergo surgery before pregnancy. If the woman is pregnant when first seen, conservative therapy includes bed rest in the left lateral position, prudent use of diuretics or volume loading, and infective endocarditis antibiotic prophylaxis (Table 1–6). Doses of gentamicin or vancomycin should be modified, or second doses omitted, in women with renal dysfunction.[11] Digoxin treatment is

TABLE 1–6. ANTIBIOTIC PROPHYLAXIS FOR GENITOURINARY/GASTROINTESTINAL PROCEDURES*

Drug	Dosage Regimen
Standard Regimen	
Ampicillin, gentamicin, and amoxicillin	Intravenous or intramuscular administration of ampicillin, 2 g plus gentamicin 1.5 mg/kg (not to exceed 80 mg), 30 min before procedure; followed by amoxicillin, 1.5 g orally 6 h after initial dose; alternatively the parenteral regimen may be repeated once 8 h after initial dose
Ampicillin/Amoxicillin/Penicillin Allergic Patient Regimen	
Vancomycin and gentamicin	Intravenous administration of vancomycin, 1 g over 1 h plus intravenous or intramuscular administration of gentamicin 1.5 mg/ kg (not to exceed 80 mg), 1 h before procedure; may be repeated once 8 h after initial dose
Alternative Low-risk Patient Regimen	
Amoxicillin	3 g orally 1 h before procedure; then 1.5 g 6 h after initial dose

*From Dajani AS, Bisno AL, Chung KJ, et al. Prevention of bacterial endocarditis: Recommendations of the American Heart Association. JAMA 1990; 264:2919. Copyright 1990, American Medical Association.

only given where there is indication (e.g., atrial fibrillation) or heart failure with documented ventricular dysfunction. No evidence exists that digoxin helps this class of patients if they are in sinus rhythm or have normal systemic ventricular function.

The immediate postpartum period is critical, especially if pulmonary hypertension is present. Most fatalities occur in the first week after delivery, but others occur as late as 3 to 4 weeks after delivery. For this reason invasive monitoring should not be discontinued immediately after delivery, and full therapeutic and monitoring support in a critical care area should be provided. The anesthesiologist has a role in assisting with postoperative pain management. In particular, epidural analgesia may be helpful in reducing the stress response as well as inducing favorable rheologic changes. Sympathectomy generally improves microvascular flow, and regional anesthesia decreases the risk of perioperative deep vein thrombosis (DVT) in surgical patients.[12]

Anticoagulation in Pregnancy

Anticoagulant therapy is provided in pregnancy as long-term thrombolysis in patients with a history of thromboembolism or as prophylaxis in patients with valvular heart disease or prosthetic heart valves. Oral anticoagulant therapy during pregnancy is contraindicated. Warfarin therapy in the first trimester is associated with an increased incidence of fetal death and birth defects (warfarin embryopathy), and there are reports of neonatal central nervous system (CNS) abnormalities from warfarin later in pregnancy.[13] In addition, prematurity and low birth weight are more frequent in pregnancies when the mother has received oral anticoagulants during the gestational period.[14] Many have abandoned the concept of reinstituting oral anticoagulation for the mid-trimester.[15] The exception is the patient with mechanical valves in whom some recommend warfarin after 13 weeks' gestation, in combination with low-dose aspirin (60–80 mg/day), because of concerns about the efficacy of heparin in preventing systemic embolism.[16] Warfarin is given in the postpartum period and appears safe in women who breast-feed. No active drug has been found in breast milk or the blood stream of breast-fed infants.[15, 17]

Heparin is the drug of choice during pregnancy because it is a large molecule that does not cross the placenta. Numerous regimens for heparin administration have been devised. The activated partial thromboplastin time (APTT) is monitored closely because heparin requirements increase as pregnancy progresses.[16] Most physicians now recommend subcutaneous heparin q12h throughout the entire pregnancy, maintaining APTT at 1.5 to 2 times control levels. Adverse pregnancy outcomes are less with heparin compared with warfarin. Complications such as heparin-induced osteoporosis or thrombocytopenia are rare.

There is interest in using low-molecular-weight heparin during pregnancy because it has a long half-life, allowing once-a-day dosing, and it is more bioavailable after subcutaneous injection. With a molecular weight of 4000 to 5000, it does not enter the fetal circulation. Low-molecular-weight heparin may be associated with fewer maternal side-effects, but more studies in pregnancy are still required before it gains widespread use, as it probably will.[17]

When valvular surgery is required, tissue valves (bioprostheses) should be considered in women of childbearing age. The valves are associated with improved pregnancy outcome, and they help to avoid the problem of anticoagulation during pregnancy.[18, 19] Thromboembolic phenomena can still occur, however, and the bioprostheses' long-term durability is poor, with an increased need for subsequent valve replacement (35% patients in one series).[20] This finding helps explain why some physicians believe that a mechanical valve (especially the newer, less thrombogenic valves), with aggressive heparinization throughout pregnancy, is appropriate.[21]

Other treatments such as streptokinase and urokinase are relatively contraindicated in pregnancy because of reports of placental abruption and postpartum hemorrhage.[21] Streptokinase has been given with success to treat prosthetic mitral valve thrombosis during pregnancy.[22] The thrombosis was confirmed by echocardiography and cinefluoroscopy at 28 weeks' gestation in a woman with a history of progressive exertional dyspnea. Streptokinase, 250,000 IU, was administered as an intravenous (IV) infusion over 30 minutes followed by 100,000 IU/hr for 24 hours. Valve function returned to normal within 18 hours of commencing treatment.

Pregnancy and successful delivery have been described in a woman with triple heart valve prostheses (aortic, mitral, and tricuspid).[23] The patient was on oral warfarin therapy throughout her pregnancy until 32 weeks, when it was discontinued and intravenous heparin commenced. At 34 weeks, a cesarean section was performed using general anesthesia. The only adverse sequelae were frequent maternal cardiac dysrhythmias that were treated with verapamil and mexiletine. Follow-up revealed no neonatal complications.[23]

Intracardiac Shunts

Congenital heart disease with intracardiac shunts falls into two main categories, cyanotic and acyanotic lesions. A simple classification of congenital heart disease with and without shunts is shown in Table 1–7. It is the impact of the shunts on cardiac chambers that is often evaluated to determine clinical significance and

TABLE 1–7. CLASSIFICATION OF CONGENITAL HEART DISEASE

Congenital Heart Disease Without Shunt

General	*Left-sided*	*Right-sided*
Dextrocardia	Aortic stenosis	Pulmonary stenosis
Cardiomyopathy	Coarctation of aorta	Ebstein's complex
Heart block	Mitral stenosis	Idiopathic dilatation of pulmonary artery

Congenital Heart Disease With Shunt

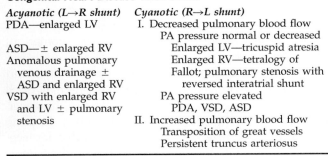

Acyanotic (L→R shunt)
PDA—enlarged LV

ASD—± enlarged RV
Anomalous pulmonary venous drainage ± ASD and enlarged RV
VSD with enlarged RV and LV ± pulmonary stenosis

Cyanotic (R→L shunt)
I. Decreased pulmonary blood flow
    PA pressure normal or decreased
        Enlarged LV—tricuspid atresia
        Enlarged RV—tetralogy of Fallot; pulmonary stenosis with reversed interatrial shunt
    PA pressure elevated
        PDA, VSD, ASD
II. Increased pulmonary blood flow
    Transposition of great vessels
    Persistent truncus arteriosus

prognosis (e.g., does the patient with an atrial septal defect [ASD] have right ventricular hypertrophy or not?). The optimal cardiovascular parameters required in parturients with intracardiac shunts during induction and maintenance of anesthesia are listed in Table 1–8.

Acyanotic Heart Lesions

Examples of acyanotic lesions (left-to-right [L-to-R] shunt) include:

1. Patent ductus arteriosus with left ventricular (LV) hypertrophy

TABLE 1–8. OPTIMAL CARDIOVASCULAR PARAMETERS FOR THE PARTURIENT WITH AN INTRACARDIAC SHUNT

Cardiovascular Parameter	R→L Shunt	L→R Shunt
Heart rate	↔	↔
Heart rhythm	Sinus	Sinus
Preload	Maintain	Maintain
Contractility	↔	↔ to ↑
SVR (afterload)	⇑	⇓
PVR	⇓⇓	⇑⇑
Anesthetic considerations	Avoid large falls in SVR from high-dose Pentothal, abrupt sympathectomy, etc. Use oxytocin cautiously Avoid increases in PVR from hypoxemia, acidemia, hypoventilation, or excessive IPPV Use prostaglandin $F_{2\alpha}$ cautiously, if at all	Avoid pulmonary artery vasodilators and myocardial depressants Avoid increases in SVR from cold, anxiety, or pain

↔ keep in the normal range; ↑ slightly above normal; ⇑ increase and avoid a drop; ⇓ decrease and avoid an increase.

2. Atrial septal defect
3. Anomalous partial venous drainage (with or without ASD) with right ventricular (RV) hypertrophy
4. Ventriculoseptal defect (VSD) with biventricular hypertrophy, with or without pulmonary stenosis.

Atrial septal defect is the most common acyanotic heart lesion and the one most likely to be missed on screening. Women with left-to-right shunts, without pulmonary hypertension, can tolerate pregnancy well because of the associated physiologic decrease in systemic vascular resistance (SVR). In one series, 19% of pregnancies in women with L-to-R shunts were complicated by congestive heart failure (CHF). This rate of heart failure (usually right ventricular failure) was reduced to 1% in similar patients after surgical correction of the lesion.[24] The success in reducing CHF, however, depends on the size of the shunt both before and after surgical correction.

Cyanotic Heart Lesions

A congenital heart lesion characterized by right-to-left (R-to-L) shunt is associated with recirculation of desaturated blood. Peripheral cyanosis occurs when more than 5 g/dl of unsaturated hemoglobin is present. Cyanosis varies directly with hematocrit level. An anemic parturient woman with poor oxygen saturation may not manifest cyanosis, whereas a woman with polycythemia may appear cyanotic at higher oxygen saturations.[25]

Cyanotic lesions are more likely to be associated with the following:

- Congestive heart failure
- Worsening of functional status
- Preterm labor
- Fewer live births
- Small-for-dates neonates.

Overt maternal cyanosis is associated with fetal wastage of about 50%. In one series a deterioration of fetal, but not maternal, condition was the factor that limited continuation of the pregnancy.[26]

A further categorization of cyanotic lesions can be made based on the amount of blood flow to the pulmonary circulation and the presence or absence of elevated pulmonary artery pressure.

I. Low pulmonary blood flow
  A. Pulmonary artery pressure normal or reduced
    1. Tricuspid valve atresia
    2. Pulmonary valve stenosis/atresia with ASD or VSD
    3. Tetralogy of Fallot (i.e., VSD, right ventricular hypertrophy (RVH), aorta overriding septum, RV infundibular stenosis, pulmonary valve or pulmonary artery stenosis)
    4. Single ventricle, cyanotic (pulmonary artery

[PA] pressures may be normal, decreased, or increased, depending on the degree of pulmonary stenosis)

5. Double-outlet RV with pulmonary stenosis or subaortic VSD (with preferential systemic blood flow)
6. Outgrown or insufficient palliative anastomosis for cyanotic heart disease

In tetralogy of Fallot, and similar lesions with obstructed pulmonary outflow tracts, a reduction in SVR and blood pressure (BP) is best treated with a pure α-agonist such as phenylephrine. If there is obstruction of the RV outflow tract, catecholamine release from inadequate pain relief, light general anesthesia, and/or exogenous catecholamine release associated with stress or anxiety should be avoided. Infundibular obstruction can be relieved by inhalation anesthetics, short-acting β-blockers (e.g., esmolol), volume load, and peripheral vasoconstrictors.

B. Pulmonary artery pressure increased
1. Patent ductus arteriosus (PDA)
2. VSD
3. ASD

II. Normal or high pulmonary blood flow
A. Transposition of the great arteries
B. Persistent truncus arteriosus (large communication between aorta and PA)
C. Taussig-Bing double-outlet RV, subpulmonic VSD (with preferential pulmonary blood flow).

Eisenmenger Syndrome

This is any condition in which there is a large communication between the systemic and pulmonary circulations with pulmonary hypertension, bidirectional shunt, and cyanosis. Over time those lesions with large L-to-R shunts, high pulmonary blood flow, and normal pulmonary vascular resistance (PVR) may develop R-to-L or bidirectional flow (shunt reversal). Currently, there is no way of predicting who will develop this Eisenmenger reaction. Such lesions include large ASDs or VSDs, large PDAs, and excessively large surgical systemic-pulmonary anastomoses, either from palliation or definitive repair. When shunt reversal occurs, there is an increase in PVR resulting from structural changes in the pulmonary vasculature. These changes lead to an increase in PVR until pulmonary artery pressures finally exceed systemic pressures.

For patients with congenital heart disease, Eisenmenger syndrome represents an end-stage for which the only treatment is heart-lung transplantation. Avoiding further increases in PA pressures in such patients is therefore of critical importance. If BP and oxyhemoglobin saturation (SaO$_2$) fall despite volume replacement, titration of drugs with predominantly chronotropic and inotropic effects is preferable to drugs with peripheral vascular effects (e.g., dopamine rather than phenylephrine), because the latter may increase PVR. In an emergency, phenylephrine can be given to increase pulmonary blood flow because the elevation in PVR is usually small and the direction of the shunt is dependent on the ratio of PVR to SVR.

Women with primary pulmonary hypertension should not become pregnant because the mortality rate is extremely high. This idiopathic condition affects mostly young females, and pregnancy causes a marked increase in already elevated PA pressures, which worsens as pregnancy advances. The RV pressure increases and volume overload occur with RV dilatation and tricuspid regurgitation. Consequent to these changes, the interventricular septum may shift to the left, resulting in a reduction in LV function and CO. Epidural analgesia is often administered in the intrapartum management of such patients.[27–32]

Hematologic Changes

A physiologic response to hypoxemia in a woman with a cyanotic lesion is polycythemia, which is *a useful compensation up to a hematocrit level of 60%*. An increase in blood viscosity beyond this level negates any advantages that an increase in hematocrit brings in terms of oxygen delivery. Symptoms of hyperviscosity include headache, sluggish mentation, disorientation, double vision, fatigue, muscle weakness, myalgia, and paresthesias.[33] Polycythemia contributes to tissue ischemia in low-flow states because of the greater blood viscosity, and this can lead to thrombosis in situ. A maternal hematocrit level greater than 60%, SaO$_2$ less than 80%, RV hypertension, and syncopal episodes are all poor prognostic signs in pregnant women with congenital heart disease.[34]

Patient Monitoring

Patients with congenital heart disease present with a range of clinical symptoms, and the natural history of each lesion varies. Severity is not based solely on NYHA classification because exercise intolerance may not be related to heart failure; neither can it predict the ability to tolerate pregnancy. An understanding of the pathophysiology of a particular lesion is required because significant variations in morphology among patients may exist. Echocardiography is helpful in assessing the functional characteristics of the anomaly at the time of admission. It also provides an accurate assessment of ventricular function and a comparison of the relative systemic and pulmonary blood flows.

All catheter and infusion systems should be air-free.

This is especially critical in cyanotic patients, in whom *entrainment of even small amounts of air can be disastrous.* For labor and delivery, a right radial artery catheter, double-lumen central venous pressure (CVP) catheter, electrocardiogram (ECG), and pulse oximeter are mandatory for symptomatic parturient women and those with known borderline myocardial or valvular function. Pulse oximetry can be inaccurate as an absolute value in cyanotic lesions. Changes in SaO_2 over time, however, are accurate.

The diagnosis of a right-sided lesion does not always preclude the use of a Swan-Ganz catheter (SGC). Indeed, the measurement of filling pressures in the systemic ventricle can provide good information throughout labor and delivery. The SGC can be utilized in women with Ebstein's anomaly or pulmonary stenosis versions of transposition. Its value is questionable, however, when the right heart is atretic because of difficulty associated with insertion and removal. In some centers the SGC is placed with fluoroscopy (with appropriate lead shielding). End-tidal carbon dioxide (CO_2) level recording is a rough but continuous monitor of ventilation-perfusion ($\dot{V}/\dot{Q}$) matching. Transesophageal echocardiography is a helpful monitor when available.[35]

Anesthetic Options

General and regional anesthetic techniques have been employed successfully in parturients with congenital heart disease.[28, 36, 37] The number of published cases is small, however, and one must consider the possibility that cases with adverse outcomes are rarely reported.

General anesthesia (GA), with endotracheal intubation, provides airway protection. Mechanical ventilation eliminates the work of breathing and may reduce oxygen consumption, thereby improving arterial oxygen content. The complications of controlled mechanical ventilation include decreased venous return as well as ventricular dysfunction, compression of pulmonary vessels, hypoxemia, hypo- or hypercarbia, and acidemia. Critical issues, such as mode and frequency of ventilation, peak inspiratory pressure. FiO_2, end-tidal (ET) CO_2, and blood gas analysis, are seldom reported in published cases describing the anesthetic management of parturient women with congenital heart disease. The choice of anesthetic drugs may not be of primary importance. If the hemodynamic effect of the lesion is worsened by tachycardia, anesthetic drugs that are known to cause an increase in heart rate (HR) through vagolysis (e.g., pancuronium) should not be administered (see Table 1–1). Intravenous drugs administered to patients with R-to-L shunt have a more immediate and pronounced effect because they reach the circulation sooner. Inhaled anesthetics, however, have a delayed onset in patients with R-to-L shunt.

Regional anesthesia (RA) allows spontaneous respiration with little disruption of $\dot{V}/\dot{Q}$ relationships, which may be critical in parturient women with complex heart lesions. Epidural catheter techniques offer continuous, titrated anesthesia or analgesia, and double catheters (one directed cephalad, the other caudad) offer versatility at the time of delivery. Saline should be used to determine loss of resistance when locating the epidural space, to avoid accidental intravenous injection of air and paradoxical systemic air embolism. Some investigators use epinephrine in the test dose, whereas others avoid it. Patients with congenital heart lesions may have an increased sensitivity to the neurotoxic effects of local anesthetics. There has been some argument in the past about the suitability of subarachnoid (spinal) anesthesia in patients with severe cardiac disease.[38, 39] Most consider that it should rarely, if ever, be given to parturients with intracardiac shunts because a sudden decrease in SVR worsens cyanosis by increasing R-to-L shunt. The decrease in venous return further reduces pulmonary blood flow and promotes preferential flow to the systemic circulation, which also worsens cyanosis. Mean BP is decreased, and myocardial oxygen supply is reduced. The tendency is to add oxygen at this time, whereas an increase in SVR is much more appropriate. Administration of oxygen to patients with fixed pulmonary hypertension and R-to-L shunt is irrelevant, in that it does not improve systemic oxygen saturation.

In women with valvular stenotic lesions and fixed stroke volumes, a sudden drop in SVR may be harmful as a result of increasing the gradient and impairing the myocardial blood flow. Subarachnoid opioids have been given successfully in women with complex heart lesions during labor, however, because they produce effective analgesia with minimal sympathetic block.[40–42] This may not be the case with intrathecal meperidine because it can exhibit a local anesthetic effect in higher doses. Sufentanil should be administered with some caution because a number of parturients exhibit a fall in BP after a 10-μg intrathecal dose, although the fall is not usually profound. Intrathecal morphine combined with pudendal block has been given successfully for vaginal delivery in a parturient with Eisenmenger syndrome.[43] In her case, peripheral SaO_2 was improved by the analgesic technique.

Maternal pushing, compression and decompression of the inferior vena cava (IVC), delivery, placenta removal, hemorrhage, and autotransfusion all have unpredictable effects on intravascular volume and overall hemodynamic status, independent of the anesthetic technique.

Cardiopulmonary Bypass

Leyse and coworkers were the first to employ extracorporeal circulation during open-heart surgery in a woman at 18 weeks' gestation with congenital aortic stenosis.[44] The woman did well, but she delivered an abnormal fetus with multiple congenital anomalies near term. Currently, cardiac operations with cardiopulmonary bypass (CPB) during pregnancy can be performed with reasonable safety for both mother and fetus,[45, 46] a fact that is supported in a survey by the Society of Thoracic Surgeons. They reported only one maternal death from 68 procedures requiring CPB and a fetal survival rate higher than 80%.[47] The well-being of the mother and fetus must be considered, although the best interests of the two may not always coincide. Optimal therapy for one may be inappropriate for the other. As a general principle, surgery requiring CPB should be delayed until the second trimester or later.[48, 49] Continuous intraoperative fetal monitoring is required to detect fetal bradycardia on bypass. One review describes a case in which successful treatment of fetal bradycardia on bypass was obtained by increasing the perfusion rate.[50] High normal range perfusion pressures during CPB should be kept at 60 mm Hg or more to compensate for the lack of autoregulation in the uteroplacental unit.[49] Hypothermia to 32°C is usual because lower temperatures have the potential to cause fetal dysrhythmias and cardiac arrest.[49]

Another problem associated with CPB during pregnancy is severe postpartum hemorrhage. This was described in a report of an emergency mitral valve replacement immediately after cesarean section.[51] Lamarra and coworkers described the use of aprotinin, a protease inhibitor, in a similar situation. They claimed that the surgical procedure was greatly simplified, and aprotoinin was an important factor in an uncomplicated outcome.[52] For a comprehensive review of CPB and pregnancy, we recommend the article by Strickland and coworkers.[53]

SPECIFIC CARDIAC LESIONS

The following are brief descriptions of some uncommon congenital heart defects reported during pregnancy, with recommendations for anesthetic and analgesic techniques based on the expected pathophysiologic changes.

Transposition of the Great Vessels and Single Ventricle

Single-ventricle anomalies are found in only 1.5% of patients with congenital heart disease, and 80% of these have transposition of the great arteries with an equal incidence of dextro- and levo-malpositions. There are at least 10 reports in the literature that describe this condition in pregnancy. Two of the reports describe epidural anesthetic management for labor and cesarean

delivery with successful outcomes.[54, 55] The Mustard operation has been done to treat transposition since the 1960s, and this has led to a major improvement in outcome beyond infancy. In a report from New Zealand, nine women with good-quality late survival after a Mustard operation remained asymptomatic during a total of 15 pregnancies, and there were 12 live births.[56] Unfortunately, no comments were made about analgesic or anesthetic methods.

The Mustard operation consists of creating an atrial baffle that directs pulmonary venous return to the right ventricle and the transposed aorta (Table 1–9). Systemic venous blood is directed to the left ventricle. Despite the hemodynamic stresses of volume loading in these patients, most do well, but some exhibit atrial flutter and occasionally develop congestive heart failure. Poorer outcome is more likely in women who show evidence of RV impairment before pregnancy. Even the asymptomatic parturient with a Mustard repair should be managed with early epidural analgesia, to avoid the adverse sequelae of high levels of circulating catecholamines.

Congenital Absence of the Inferior Vena Cava

In these rare cases, venous drainage from structures below the diaphragm is diverted via collateral channels back to the heart.[57] The collaterals include the azygous system of veins, vertebral veins, and superficial veins in the abdominal wall. Coexisting anomalies influence the management of affected patients. For example, pulmonary arteriovenous (AV) malformations and bronchial dysgenesis may affect oxygenation during intermittent positive-pressure ventilation (IPPV). Specifically, IPPV increases dead space ventilation in atretic bronchi and may cause rupture of pulmonary vascular anomalies. Regional anesthetic techniques may be influenced by circulatory changes around the vertebral column, and superficial dilated veins in the dorsolumbar area may hinder insertion of the epidural or spinal needle. Epidural doses should be fractionated and administered carefully because of the increased risk of intravascular injection. Other anomalies that are associated with this condition include esophageal varices and leg stasis ulcerations from venous congestion. The anesthetic management of a parturient with esophageal varices from portal hypertension has been described.[58]

Venous return is especially critical in these cases, and aortocaval compression should be avoided at all times. Pre-epidural fluid load is important. Epidural analgesia may be administered more safely while monitoring central venous pressure. Assisted vaginal delivery to avoid the Valsalva effect is recommended, especially if there are esophageal varices and portal hypertension.[58]

TABLE 1–9. **A LEXICON OF COMMON SURGICAL PROCEDURES FOR CONGENITAL HEART DISEASE**

Procedure	Description	Intent	Result
Blalock-Taussig	Subclavian artery to pulmonary artery anastomosis	PAL	Increases pulmonary blood flow
Central shunt	Conduit or anastomosis between aorta and pulmonary artery	PAL	Increases pulmonary blood flow
Damus-Kaye-Stansel	Pulmonary artery end-to-side anastomosis to aorta, valved conduit between RV and main pulmonary artery	COR	Increases blood flow to aorta and pulmonary artery when there is aortic stenosis and two ventricles; reestablishes RV to PA continuity
Fontan	Anastomosis or conduit between right atrium and pulmonary artery	PAL	Increases pulmonary blood flow in cases of univentricular heart or tricuspid atresia
Glenn (bidirectional Glenn)	SVC to pulmonary artery anastomosis	PAL	Increases pulmonary blood flow
Arterial switch or Jatene	Transection of aorta and pulmonary artery with reimplantation onto the proper ventricles, coronary arteries reimplanted	COR	Creates normal relationship between the ventricles and great arteries in transposition
Hemi-Fontan	SVC to pulmonary artery anastomosis with baffle placed in right atrium so that IVC blood flow goes across ASD to left heart	PAL	Increases pulmonary blood flow and sets the stage for eventual complete Fontan
Konno	Replacement of aortic valve with aortic valve annular enlargement	COR	Alleviates subaortic obstruction and replaces abnormal aortic valve
Mustard	Atrial switch with intraatrial baffle made of pericardium	COR	Reestablishes proper flow sequence to pulmonary artery and aorta in D-transposition of the great arteries
Norwood (first stage)	Pulmonary artery anastomosis to aorta, conduit from aorta to main pulmonary artery	PAL	Increases flow to aorta for subaortic obstruction with single ventricle
Potts	Descending aorta to pulmonary artery shunt	PAL	Increases pulmonary flow (rarely done anymore)
PA band	Constrictive band around main pulmonary artery	PAL	Decreases pulmonary flow
Rashkind	Atrial septostomy with catheter balloon	PAL	Increases mixing of blood for transposition of the great arteries or tricuspid atresia
Rastelli	Valved conduit from RV to PA, closure of VSD	COR	Increases pulmonary flow, may reestablish proper sequence of flow to aorta and pulmonary artery
Ross	Pulmonary autograft to aorta. Pulmonary homograft	COR	Correction for aortic stenosis. Avoids mechanical and bioprosthetic valve
Senning	Atrial switch with intraatrial baffle made of atrial wall flaps	COR	Reestablishes proper flow sequence to pulmonary artery and aorta in transposition of the great arteries
Waterston	Ascending aorta to right pulmonary anastomosis	PAL	Increases pulmonary blood flow (rarely done anymore)

From Segar DS. Common Surgical Procedures for Congenital Heart Disease. ACC Current Journal Review 1996; 5:46. With permission from the American College of Cardiology.

ASD = artrial septal defect; COR = total correction; PA = pulmonary artery; PAL = palliation; RV = right ventricle; SVC = superior vena cava; VSD = ventricular septal defect.

Epidural anesthesia is probably the better option for cesarean delivery, because subarachnoid block may diminish venous return excessively. General anesthesia may adversely affect associated intrathoracic vascular anomalies.

Truncus Arteriosus

Truncus arteriosus (TA) is a rare congenital malformation in which only one artery arises from the heart and it gives rise to the systemic, pulmonary, and coronary arteries. The prognosis from TA is usually poor if untreated, because CHF develops in infancy from excessive blood flow. Occasionally, survival to the reproductive years is seen. One case report describes maternal survival following cesarean birth using general anesthesia.[59] Truncus arteriosus represents a severe form of Eisenmenger reaction, because the pulmonary vessels are generally subjected to systemic pressures. Rare variations of truncus arteriosus exist, however, which have protected pulmonary vasculature with "pulmonary stenosis." In TA, systemic blood is desaturated, and compensatory polycythemia is present. Most recommend general anesthesia for cesarean delivery to avoid a decrease in SVR associated with regional anesthesia. A fall in SVR may lead to worsening cyanosis by increasing R-to-L shunt. Because invasive monitoring with a SGC is not possible, pulse oximetry can be utilized as a guide to patient well-being. An oxygen saturation of 75 to 85% represents approximately balanced systemic and pulmonary blood flows.[59] A fall in

SaO$_2$ is indicative of inadequate pulmonary blood flow, whereas a persistent rise in SaO$_2$ indicates excessive pulmonary blood flow.

Double-outlet Right Ventricle, Large VSD, Pulmonary Stenosis, Dextrocardia

The principles of managing patients with bidirectional intracardiac shunts and fixed pulmonary valvular resistance are to maintain preload and afterload to both ventricles and to maintain sinus rhythm. Increases in R-to-L shunting occur not only from a decrease in SVR, but also from an increase in PVR or intrathoracic pressure. Direct monitoring of arterial and central venous pressures is therefore important. Insertion of a SGC is often avoided in these cases for the following reasons:

- Interpretation of data and pressure waves may be difficult in the presence of a large VSD.
- Cardiac output changes may arise from a true change in cardiac output, shunting, or both.
- Potential for dysrhythmias and thromboembolic phenomena exists.
- Technical difficulty occurs in the presence of pulmonary stenosis or, if successful, the SGC may impinge on the already narrowed pulmonary outflow tract.

One case report describes successful general anesthesia for cesarean birth with ketamine, alfentanil, and vecuronium given slowly for induction.[60] Postoperative analgesia was provided with an epidural fentanyl infusion for 3 days, despite the administration of low-dose heparin. It was believed, quite rationally, that the advantages of adequate analgesia in this woman outweighed the risks of epidural catheterization in the presence of anticoagulation.[60]

Another case report, describing successful outcome in a woman with a similar lesion (pulmonary atresia, VSD, and PDA), rationalizes epidural anesthesia for cesarean birth.[61] Most *infants* with this condition require early surgical correction because a tendency for the ductus to close at birth leads to cyanosis and hypoxemia. Some patients survive without treatment because the PDA remains dilated, thus providing the pulmonary vascular beds with high flow rates. Changes in PVR, SVR, myocardial contractility, and venous return are less likely to occur with a well-controlled epidural anesthetic. There is concern that coughing and straining at induction and emergence from GA increase PVR. Of concern is the possibility that the decrease in pulmonary blood flow occurring with IPPV would be detrimental. The unwanted hemodynamic responses to induction and laryngoscopy, such as hypertension and dysrhythmias, are avoided when regional techniques are employed. Anesthetic induction agents may cause myocardial depression, and nitrous oxide has been shown to increase PVR.[62] It is essential, however, to prevent maternal hypotension when epidural anesthesia is induced. Hence, local anesthetic solutions must be administered in small increments until the desired level of anesthesia is achieved. Direct measurement of arterial and central venous pressures before initiating the epidural anesthetic contribute to patient safety in this situation.

Ebstein's Anomaly

This rare anomaly represents 1% of all congenital heart defects. The characteristic lesion is downward displacement and elongation of the septal cusp of the tricuspid valve. As a result, the proximal part of the right ventricle becomes thin-walled and poorly contractile ("atrialized"). There are varying degrees of severity based on the amount of tricuspid regurgitation, presence of an ASD with intracardiac shunting, extent of pulmonary hypertension, and presence of cardiac dysrhythmias such as supraventricular tachycardia. Wolff-Parkinson-White syndrome can be problematic in approximately 50% of these so-affected women.[63]

General and epidural anesthetics have been administered successfully in patients with Ebstein's anomaly,[63–66] and the arguments for and against general anesthesia are the same as those stated earlier. The patients have a markedly enlarged right atrium, and as a result there may be a prolongation of induction time with general anesthesia increasing the risk of aspiration of gastric contents. The prolonged induction occurs from pooling of drugs in the right atrium. To speed induction, a larger dose may be required, which may be detrimental by causing myocardial depression and systemic hypotension. An anesthetic induction agent that does not depress the myocardium, such as etomidate (maximum dose 0.3 mg/kg), is the best option.

Pulmonary and systemic emboli are a constant hazard during the later stages of pregnancy in these patients. Pulmonary emboli further increase PVR, promoting R-to-L shunt and arterial desaturation. Systemic emboli may occur via an atrial septal defect. Low-dose subcutaneous heparin is often given for prophylaxis. Phenylephrine, a predominant α-adrenoreceptor agonist, is the agent of choice in the treatment of hypotension in this situation. Hemorrhage is not tolerated, because RV dysfunction impairs the ability to cope with large volume shifts associated with blood loss and fluid replacement.

Cor Triatriatum Sinistrum

Unlike the right-sided lesions described earlier, this is an anomaly of the left atrium. A case report describes a previously healthy woman presenting with acute pulmonary edema in the early postpartum period.[67] Echocardiography demonstrated that she had cor triatriatum sinistrum, a rare anomaly comprising 0.1% of all congenital heart diseases. It is often associated with an ASD. A fibromuscular membrane divides the left atrium into a proximal chamber receiving pulmonary veins and, distally, a true chamber containing the appendage. Communication between the two chambers occurs via single or multiple fenestrations in the membrane. Depending on the size of these communications, the hemodynamics may be normal or may mimic mitral stenosis. Pressure in the distal chamber is usually normal, and the orifice remains patent throughout the cardiac cycle. Often, severe forms are manifested early on with pulmonary hypertension due to obstruction of left atrial flow. Milder forms may remain unrecognized if the communications between the two atrial chambers are wide. As in this case, the lesion can be unmasked by the hemodynamic stresses that occur throughout pregnancy and the peripartum period, because tachycardia and increased blood volume contribute to cardiac decompensation.[67] Mild pregnancy-induced hypertension (PIH) and colloid oncotic pressure reduction after delivery may have contributed to the development of pulmonary edema. Following treatment with oxygen, furosemide, and dopamine her condition improved rapidly.

Two-chambered Heart

A two-chambered heart has been described in pregnancy[68] in a woman who had previously undergone a Pott's anastomosis (see Table 1–9). At 25 weeks' gestation, having been asymptomatic, she developed acute, painless hemoptysis totaling 1400 ml in 48 hours. Cardiac catheterization revealed a heart that consisted of a single atrium, a single ventricle, and one AV valve. No information was provided about analgesic and anesthetic techniques or mode of delivery. Analgesic and anesthetic options in this situation are influenced by the functional status and ventricular function of the parturient.

Uhl Anomaly

This congenital anomaly, first described by Uhl in 1952, consists of arrhythmogenic RV dysplasia (almost total absence of RV myocardium). Some physicians make a distinction between Uhl anomaly and classic ventricular dysplasia. In Uhl anomaly, the right ventricle is enlarged and hypokinetic; there is tricuspid insufficiency and mild pulmonary insufficiency. A chest radiograph demonstrates an enlarged heart and hypoplastic pulmonary arteries. Unlike Ebstein's anomaly, the position of the tricuspid valve is normal. A familial

occurrence has been described, and autosomal recessive inheritance has been suggested.[69] Some 70 to 80 cases have appeared in the literature, but only one during pregnancy has been described.[70] In the discussion of this case, the investigators concede that vaginal delivery under epidural analgesia would have been suitable for peripartum management, but they chose general anesthesia for elective cesarean delivery, with arterial and central venous catheters placed for monitoring. Anesthetic induction was achieved with fentanyl 250 μg, etomidate 30 mg, and vecuronium (dose unspecified). A healthy baby was delivered (estimated gestational age [EGA] 37 weeks), and the mother did well despite a fall in BP shortly after delivery, which responded to intravenous fluids. She was discharged from the intensive care unit (ICU) on the first postoperative day.[70]

Severe Pulmonary Stenosis

Pulmonary valvular stenosis is one of the more common congenital cardiac anomalies seen in young adults of reproductive age. Faulty embryogenesis at 4 to 6 weeks leads to pulmonary valvular or infundibular stenosis. The right outflow tract obstruction can cause a pressure overload on the RV with resultant ventricular hypertrophy. Patients may be asymptomatic in childhood, but they develop syncope, dyspnea, palpitations, and fatigue with mild exercise as the subvalvular obstruction progresses. A high-grade systolic ejection murmur can be heard over the entire precordium with a systolic ejection click heard at the left upper sternal border.

A case report[40] describes a patient who underwent percutaneous balloon valvuloplasty (PBV) of the pulmonary valve at 10 weeks' gestation with a reduction in RV pressure (from 177/6 to 120/4). Although PBV has been effective during pregnancy in cases of pulmonary and mitral stenosis, it may unmask infundibular obstruction that necessitates further treatment with fluids and β blockade. This woman was maintained on aspirin, and atenolol for β blockade, throughout her pregnancy. At 39 weeks' gestation, labor was induced after placement of arterial and central venous lines. Analgesia was provided with sufentanil, which was infused through an indwelling subarachnoid catheter. The patient was comfortable after a 10-μg sufentanil loading dose and a 5 μg/hr infusion during the 5-hour labor. A ventouse-assisted vaginal delivery was performed following an intrathecal injection of 15 mg 1% plain lidocaine in divided doses for perineal pain. A fall in arterial blood pressure 45 minutes post-delivery was treated with two intravenous fluid loads, which improved CVP to 8 mm Hg from 3 mm Hg.[40] The goals of hemodynamic management in a patient with pulmonary stenosis are maintenance of adequate preload and normal heart rate and avoidance of reduction in myocardial contractility and afterload.

Other Reports

A rare presentation of pulmonary valvular stenosis occurs in *Watson syndrome*. This syndrome was first described in 1967 and is characterized by pulmonary valvular stenosis, café-au-lait spots, and mental retardation.[71] The phenotype also includes short stature, relative macrocephaly, Lisch nodules, and neurofibromas. The genetic defect responsible for this autosomal dominant condition may lie in the long arm of chromosome 17. One case report[72] of an uncooperative parturient with this disorder describes the successful use of incremental epidural anesthesia for cesarean birth. It was supplemented with boluses of ketamine to a total of 4.5 mg/kg over a 90-min period, to assure patient cooperation during insertion of invasive monitors. Ketamine was utilized to elevate systemic and pulmonary vascular tone, maintain heart rate, and provide an advantageous intropic effect.

Another rare presentation of pulmonary stenosis was in a woman with *Noonan syndrome*. This condition has all the clinical findings of Turner syndrome, but the karyotype is 46 XX with only 6% of cells on a chromosome culture having 45 or less chromosomes. These women are often mentally retarded and have pulmonary stenosis. In one report, a woman with untreated cyanotic heart disease from infancy presented at 24 weeks' gestation with a high-arched palate, low-set ears, small mandible, marked webbing of the neck, cubitus valgus, pectus excavatum, and short stature.[73] A heart catheterization revealed pulmonary artery infundibular stenosis, high VSD, and R-to-L shunt. The details of her labor and delivery were not mentioned but her newborn was developmentally normal at 7 months of age.

Potential anesthetic problems in patients with Noonan syndrome include difficult tracheal intubation and technical problems in performing regional anesthesia due to short stature and skeletal anomalies, such as lumbar lordosis, kyphoscoliosis, and narrow spinal canal. The decrease in functional residual capacity associated with pregnancy is exacerbated by pectus deformity and kyphoscoliosis (see Chapter 14), and these patients can rapidly become hypoxemic. The presence of pulmonary stenosis makes underhydration undesirable, especially before sympathetic block associated with epidural anesthesia, because sympathetic block leading to hypotension may reduce RV stroke volume. Conversely, overhydration, before inducing regional anesthesia, can be detrimental. Central venous catheters should be in place to guide fluid administration.[74]

PARTURIENTS WITH SURGICALLY CORRECTED CONGENITAL HEART DISEASE

Successful surgical repair of a heart lesion before pregnancy results in a significant improvement in maternal and neonatal outcomes. Palliated lesions, however, are still associated with an increased risk to mother and fetus during pregnancy.[75] In one series of women with unrelieved cyanosis, only 42% of pregnancies resulted in a live-born child. This compares with 72% live births in women whose cyanosis was relieved by palliative surgery.[76] In all cyanotic women, however, the babies were usually small for gestational age and immature. In mothers made acyanotic by surgery, the rate of successful pregnancies is comparable to that of all groups of mothers with congenital heart disease, and babies are of normal size.[76] A significant difference in pregnancy outcome is seen in women with poor cardiac status, regardless of whether palliation has occurred. Asymptomatic women have more successful outcomes with fewer cardiac or obstetric complications.

Surgical shunts can overcome severe obstruction to pulmonary blood flow. The goal is to maintain adequate arterial oxygen content when oxygenated pulmonary venous blood returns to the heart and mixes with systemic venous blood. The problem is in creating a shunt that does not produce excessive pulmonary blood flow. A lexicon of common surgical procedures for congenital heart disease is reproduced in Table 1–9. The following case reports describe the anesthetic management of parturients with surgically corrected heart lesions.

General anesthesia was recommended for cesarean birth in one case report of a woman with a single ventricle and pulmonary atresia who had undergone multiple palliative surgical repairs.[77] At 7 months of age, she received a *Blalock-Taussig shunt* (subclavian artery to PA) (Fig. 1–1) for an apparent tetralogy of Fallot. This shunt is preferentially performed on the side opposite the aortic arch to prevent kinking, but it can be created on either side. The shunt overcomes severe obstruction to the pulmonary circulation. At 11 years of age, she developed worsening cyanosis and fatigue. Cardiac catheterization at that time showed a closed shunt, pulmonary atresia, ductal stenosis, reduced pulmonary blood flow, double-outlet RV, and severe hypoplastic left heart. A successful *Pott's anastomosis* (left descending aorta to left PA) (see Fig. 1–1) was performed. She presented 12 years later, at 28 weeks' gestation, with severe CHF. She improved with conservative therapy (bed rest, oxygen, digoxin, and diuretics), but her condition worsened at 32 weeks' gestation. An opioid-based general anesthetic was given for cesarean delivery, and both mother and baby did well. Because pulmonary circulation was supplied

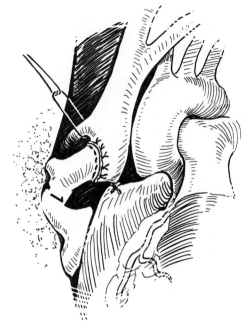

Glenn procedure

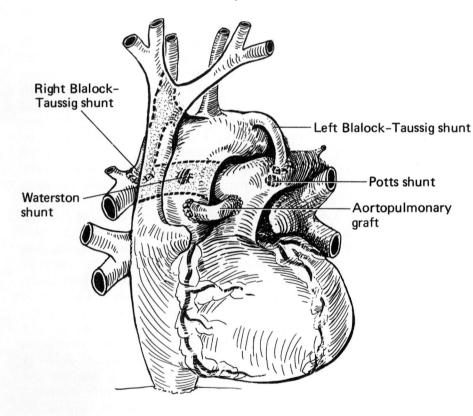

Right Blalock-Taussig shunt

Waterston shunt

Left Blalock-Taussig shunt

Potts shunt

Aortopulmonary graft

Figure 1–1. Surgical shunts between the systemic and pulmonary circulations. The original Glen procedure was a direct anastomosis between the azygous vein and pulmonary artery. It is presently modified *(top)* by creating an anastomosis between the superior vena cava and the transected distal end of the right pulmonary artery. *Bottom,* Other commonly used systemic to pulmonary artery shunts used as palliative procedures in patients with congenital heart disease. (From Dillard DH, Miller DW (eds). Atlas of Cardiac Surgery. New York, Macmillan, 1983.)

almost entirely through a shunt of fixed diameter, it was thought that avoiding a fall in SVR and maintaining an adequate preload were paramount. Increases in PVR from acidosis, pain, anxiety, high inspiratory pressure and positive end-expiratory pressure are best avoided.

Fontan procedure has been employed in patients with congenital tricuspid atresias and a wide range of congenital lesions that are associated with a single func-

tional ventricle. The procedure consists of connecting the right atrium with the pulmonary trunk, directly or via a synthetic, valved, or nonvalved conduit. Fontan reported the first atrial pulmonary connection for tricuspid atresia in 1971.[80] The right atrium was used as a pumping chamber. The right side of the heart can be bypassed utilizing cavopulmonary connections. Fontan procedure is often preceded by some form of palliative surgery. The main pathophysiologic consideration in these patients is that systemic venous return reaches the pulmonary circulation without ventricular augmentation (i.e., Fontan's circulation represents a passive conduit). Hence, adequate central blood volume and pressure are necessary to perfuse the pulmonary circulation. PVR and SVR are other critical determinants of patient well-being. It can be argued that general anesthetic techniques should be avoided for such cases, because they use potential myocardial depressants that may adversely affect PVR. A further consideration is that atrial fibrillation can be present and may be difficult to treat. Instrumentation of the right heart may trigger atrial fibrillation, which is a true emergency in these patients. Cardioversion equipment and antiarrhythmic drugs should be immediately available, therefore (see Chapter 2).

Two publications report the anesthetic management of three pregnant women who had previously undergone Fontan repairs.[78, 79] These reports describe epidural anesthesia and continuous intrathecal anesthesia employing a microcatheter, for cesarean birth, and successful epidural analgesia for labor and vaginal delivery. Regional techniques avoid deleterious increases in PVR that can be associated with intubation of the trachea, IPPV, and general anesthesia. Ensuring adequate preload, uterine displacement, and slow titration of local anesthetics compensate for the potentially deleterious effects of venodilatation from regional anesthesia. The rate of lowering of SVR is important. Gradual induction of epidural anesthesia is associated with slower rates of decline in SVR. Cautious volume replacement can compensate for the vasodilatation associated with a reduction in afterload. Conversely, a sudden profound sympathectomy from single-dose intrathecal anesthesia is contraindicated in this situation.

Other forms of complex malformations that are palliated with Fontan circulation include left AV valve atresia; double-inlet left and right ventricles; pulmonary atresia; intact ventricular septum and hypoplastic RV; and hypoplastic right or left ventricle in biventricular hearts with VSD (with or without straddling AV valve).[81] It is likely that more parturients with Fontan repairs will be seen over the next 10 years.

VALVULAR LESIONS

Chronic mitral or aortic regurgitations (volume lesions) are usually well tolerated during pregnancy if the patients remain asymptomatic or only mildly symptomatic. Parturients with severe valvular regurgitation or stenosis do not tolerate the changes in heart rate or increases in cardiac output that occur during pregnancy. Any woman with a symptomatic stenotic lesion warrants very close attention and possible surgical correction during pregnancy.

Mitral Stenosis. MS accounts for 90% of rheumatic

heart disease in pregnancy, with 25% of patients first developing symptoms during late pregnancy. Relative obstruction across the valve increases as pregnancy advances because of the greater blood volume, heart rate, and cardiac output. Increased obstruction leads to pulmonary venous congestion; it may produce pulmonary edema. Pure or dominant mitral stenosis is the most common pathology associated with acute pulmonary edema in pregnancy, followed by aortic valve disease and/or primary myocardial disease. Thrombi within the enlarged left atrium represent a major therapeutic challenge because of the risks and side effects of anticoagulation. Affected women require bed rest, careful diuresis, and immediate correction of dysrhythmia. Heparin administration throughout pregnancy should be considered in those with chronic or paroxysmal atrial fibrillation, left atrial thrombus, or prior embolic history. Intractable heart failure or hemoptysis is an indicator for urgent surgical intervention, which includes balloon valvuloplasty. During delivery and the immediate postpartum period the pulmonary capillary wedge pressure (PCWP) may increase by as much as 10 mm Hg and thus is a critical time for such patients. A postpartum increase in PCWP is most likely in the presence of severe MS (i.e., functional class III and IV).[82] The principal anesthetic considerations for mitral stenosis[83] are the following:

1. Prevent rapid ventricular rates
2. Maintain sinus rhythm
3. Avoid large, rapid falls in SVR
4. Prevent increases in central blood volume
5. Avoid hypoxemia and/or hypoventilation both of which may increase pulmonary artery pressures and cause RV failure.

Carefully titrated epidural analgesia for labor and delivery addresses the principal anesthetic issues. The concomitant use of invasive hemodynamic monitors is to be recommended in symptomatic parturients or in those with a critical stenosis.[84, 85] Hemmings and coworkers found that epidural analgesia during the first stage of labor caused a beneficial reduction of PVR and SVR, lowered pulmonary artery pressures, and returned CO to baseline levels.[84] Both epidural and general anesthesia have been described for cesarean delivery, however. In one case report alfentanil provided hemodynamic stability and allowed for immediate postoperative extubation but caused neonatal respiratory depression.[83] Epidural anesthesia with 0.5% bupivacaine has been given successfully in women undergoing urgent cesarean delivery for hemodynamic deterioration from severe MS.[86] Each patient was placed in 15° head-down position to maintain the PCWP at 25 mm Hg.

Aortic Stenosis. AS is found rarely in women of childbearing age and, when present in a moderately severe form, has been associated with high fetal and maternal mortality.[87] A reappraisal of congenital AS in pregnancy, however, demonstrated satisfactory outcomes in 25 pregnancies with no mortality in any of the 13 women concerned.[88] Almost 25% of the women were classified as having severe stenosis (<0.7 cm²), and deterioration in cardiac status occurred in 27% of the group studied. All patients were offered epidural anesthesia for pain relief or operative delivery. The cesarean section rate was 30%. Pulse oximetry, peripheral arterial and venous lines, and antibiotic prophylaxis were utilized in all patients. Transvalvular gradients increase progressively throughout pregnancy, as a consequence of more blood volume and less SVR. Such increases can result in syncope, angina, and reduced perfusion to the placenta and fetus. Bed rest in the left lateral decubitus position and avoidance of negative inotropes are recommended.

Augmented preload with intravenous fluids may be of benefit in maintaining a fixed stroke volume. Pulmonary congestion consequent to LV failure, however, may be exacerbated by fluid loads in the presence of hypervolemia of pregnancy. Other anesthetic considerations in the parturient with AS include maintaining sinus rhythm and avoiding bradycardia and sudden changes to the SVR.

In some cases percutaneous balloon aortic valvuloplasty is performed during pregnancy and is reported to be associated with good maternal and fetal outcomes.[89] Valvuloplasty is usually reserved for cases in which the aortic valve area is 0.3 cm² or less; valvuloplasty can usually increase the area to about 1.0 cm².

Case reports have advocated carefully titrated epidural anesthesia for labor and delivery in parturient women with severe AS.[90–92] These reports argue against general anesthesia for women with severe AS because of concern that induction of GA and tracheal intubation may result in hypertension and tachycardia, which decrease CO and coronary blood flow. In some cases the CO is low because of a high SVR associated with pain and anxiety. A gradual reduction in SVR associated with induction of epidural anesthesia serves to improve CO in the presence of a fixed stroke volume, assuming that the filling pressures are adequate. Some rationalize not using epinephrine with the epidural local anesthetic solution,[72, 86, 90] whereas others have used it in the test dose in parturients with cardiac disease.[61, 91]

Care should be exercised when administering oxytocin to these patients because a large bolus can cause hypotension and tachycardia and increases in pulmonary arterial pressure.[91] Slow infusion of a dilute oxytocin solution is usually well tolerated. As a general rule, care should be exercised in parturients with cardiac disease when administering other uterotonic agents such as ergometrine, which can induce systemic hypertension, and prostaglandin $F_2\alpha$, which has the potential to cause severe pulmonary hypertension if injected directly into the circulation in a large dose.[93]

If a general anesthetic technique is employed, an opioid-based anesthetic is useful when LV function is compromised.[94] There is a concern, however, that the slow induction period associated with this technique increases the risk of pulmonary aspiration. Any well-managed anesthetic technique is suitable if the risks and benefits are acknowledged, drugs are titrated carefully, and invasive monitoring is employed as a guide to appropriate therapy in the event of adverse hemodynamic changes.

Mixed Valvular Lesions. These present the dilemma of which lesion to treat. As a rule, therapy should be directed to the management of the dominant lesion (i.e., that with the most significant hemodynamic consequences). For example, if a woman presents with moderate to severe mitral regurgitation with mild mitral stenosis management should be designed to treat the regurgitant lesion even if this conflicts with the usual management of the mitral stenosis.

In a case report, a woman with moderate to severe mitral regurgitation and mild mitral stenosis was successfully managed with epidural analgesia for induced labor and ventouse-assisted vaginal delivery.[95] Invasive monitoring of radial artery pressure and PCWP allowed precise, continuous measurement of hemodynamic variables and appropriate fluid and drug therapy. Similar reports have described the successful use of epidural analgesia for labor and delivery in women with combined mitral and aortic regurgitation[96] and combined mitral and aortic stenosis.[97]

CARDIOMYOPATHIES

Cardiomyopathy can be classified as hypertrophic, restrictive, or dilated.

Hypertrophic Cardiomyopathies With or Without Obstruction

Idiopathic hypertrophic subvalvular stenosis (IHSS) requires maintenance of SVR to prevent cavity collapse and outflow tract obstruction. Obstruction to LV outflow is caused by a hypertrophic muscle mass at the base of the interventricular septum and a systolic anterior motion of the anterior leaflet of the mitral valve. This condition is intriguing in that there may not be a resting obstruction but only a potential obstruction, given the right conditions. In addition, there is an apical obliterative variety that does not have a subaortic pressure gradient. If, as usually occurs, a subaortic pressure gradient is present, the ventricle is less compliant and passive ventricular filling during diastole is reduced. It follows that atrial contraction becomes an important factor in increasing ventricular end-diastolic volume. Factors that affect the degree of obstruction include systolic volume of the ventricle (preload), force of the ventricular contraction, and transmural pressure distending the outflow tract. The obstruction is decreased by large systolic volumes, which distend the outflow tract, reduced ventricular contractility, and high aortic pressure. Conversely, the obstruction is increased by small systolic volumes, which are associated with reduced preload; high ventricular contractility; and low aortic pressure associated with a decrease in afterload.

When the LV outflow tract is narrowed, CO falls and mitral regurgitation may occur because the mitral valve becomes the point of relief for the build-up of ventricular pressure. Mild to moderate IHSS is usually well tolerated because the increase in LV end-diastolic volumes associated with pregnancy reduces outflow tract obstruction. Increases in heart rate and decreases in SVR counteract this effect. Outflow obstruction is exacerbated during the third trimester in the supine position and during labor, delivery, and early puerperium. Adverse effects during labor and delivery include increases in heart rate and contractility from endogenous catecholamines (pain and anxiety). Tachycardia limits diastolic filling, which decreases LV end-diastolic volumes. Increased contractility raises LV outflow tract obstruction. A decrease in venous return from the Valsalva maneuver can occur with pushing. The benefits of an epidural infusion of dilute local anesthetic with opioid for labor are clear.

β-Blockade is given to treat LV outflow obstruction by reducing cardiac contractility and heart rate. The anesthetic management of labor and delivery can be complex because β-blocker therapy may have been discontinued during pregnancy owing to concern that it may cause fetal bradycardia and intrauterine growth retardation. A case report described esmolol in a parturient with IHSS at term gestation.[98] Esmolol is a short-acting agent that can have an adverse impact on the fetus. In this case, it caused persistent neonatal hypotonia, hypotension, hypoglycemia, and bradycardia. Another report described a case of fetal bradycardia following maternal administration of esmolol that required an emergency cesarean section.[99] Labetalol in 0.25 mg/kg increments, up to a total dose of 1 mg/kg, may be preferable.

Spinal and epidural anesthesia cause a reduction in SVR, which has the potential to increase the outflow obstruction; therefore, they are relatively contraindicated. One report describes the adverse impact on the left ventriculoaortic gradient, and hence coronary perfusion, in a woman with IHSS who received a subarachnoid anesthetic for an orthopedic procedure.[100] The successful administration of general anesthesia for cesarean section has been described in women with IHSS.[101] Although volatile anesthetic agents are beneficial in that they produce a reduction in myocardial contractility, they should be administered cautiously to avoid a marked fall in SVR. (Halothane is superior to isoflurane, because it has less impact on SVR.) General anesthesia, for cesarean section, and lumbar epidural analgesia, for vaginal delivery, have both been associated with postpartum pulmonary edema in parturients with IHSS who did not receive invasive hemodynamic monitoring.[102] These patients should be closely monitored with a SGC for worsening outflow obstruction resulting from the diuresis that occurs in the first 48 hours postpartum.

The critical determinants of a good outcome are careful titration of anesthetic agents, adequate volume loading, and prompt replacement of blood loss guided by invasive hemodynamic monitors. Ephedrine is contraindicated in the treatment of hypotension associated with IHSS due to the risk of tachycardia and increased inotropy. Phenylephrine in 50-μg increments is the treatment of choice for hypotension following sympathetic blockade. Large doses of phenylephrine should be avoided to prevent reduction in placental perfusion. Although some believe that oxytocin is relatively contraindicated in parturients with IHSS, a dilute oxytocin infusion will likely be well tolerated.[101]

Restrictive Cardiomyopathies

Restrictive cardiomyopathy is a rare entity representing the end stage of myocarditis or an infiltrative process of the myocardium, such as amyloidosis or hemochromatosis. Restrictive cardiomyopathy mimics constrictive pericarditis and is characterized by impaired ventricular filling and poor contractility. CO is maintained initially by an increase in heart rate and filling pressure, but not by an increase in myocardial contractility. The anesthetic management depends on whether the dominant feature of the disease is restrictive ventricular filling or impaired ventricular function. Monitoring includes ECG for heart rate and ischemic changes and SGC to record filling pressures and CO. Transesophageal echocardiography should be employed when available. Therapy is directed toward providing adequate ventricular filling, heart rate, and myocardial contractility. β-agonists such as isoproterenol or dobutamine are the inotropic agents of choice, because in addition to increasing the ejection fraction, they raise heart rate and usually decrease SVR. Epidural anesthesia is preferred over general anesthesia because myocardial depressants can be avoided and positive-pressure ventilation can decrease venous return.

Dilated Cardiomyopathies

Unexplained dilated cardiomyopathy should be treated as heart failure, with or without congestion.

The onset occurs during the last month of pregnancy or within 5 months of delivery, and the condition is known as *cardiomyopathy of pregnancy.*[103–106] The incidence is unknown but is estimated to be between 1 in 3000 and 1 in 4000 pregnancies. Other etiologies, such as alcoholism, protein deficiency, or acute viremia, must be ruled out. Symptoms may occur suddenly, but often cardiac failure develops insidiously. Symptoms may resolve spontaneously in 20 to 40% of cases with little or no treatment. Peripartum cardiomyopathy can be associated with pulmonary hypertension, however, and may result in multi-organ failure.[107, 108] Women present with fatigue, dyspnea, edema, and occasionally chest pain with hemoptysis. They often have a raised jugular venous pressure (JVP), cardiomegaly, and gallop rhythm. Echocardiography reveals hypokinetic ventricles with normal valves. Serial echocardiography to monitor LV function throughout the pregnancy and postpartum period is recommended.[109] Postmortem studies show enlarged hearts that are soft and flabby with a dilated myocardium and variable endocardial thickening or areas of myocardial necrosis.

Treatment is empirical with diuretics, inotropes, afterload reducers, and anticoagulants. In one series, 78% of women with peripartum cardiomyopathy had evidence of myocarditis.[110] Resolution of the myocarditis was associated with a significant improvement in LV function. Resolution can occur spontaneously without loss of cardiac function. Immunosuppressive therapy with oral prednisone and azathioprine for 6 to 8 weeks has improved LV function and prognosis in women with myocarditis and LV dysfunction.[110]

Continuous venovenous hemofiltration has been successful in treating severe cardiomyopathy after failure of conventional therapy.[111] It is achieved by circulating blood over a highly permeable hemodialysis membrane but without exposure to an osmotic dialysis gradient. Serum is filtered across the membrane by hydrostatic pressure. The membrane allows passage of fluids and solutes with a molecular weight of less than 20,000 and so produces a filtrate with a composition approximating serum. Heart transplantation is reserved for severe cases unresponsive to all medical therapy (see Chapter 11).[112]

Mortality can range from 30 to 60%, but the prognosis is more grave if the cardiac size has not returned to normal within 6 months of delivery. Death results from failure to improve cardiac function or from cerebral or pulmonary embolism. The rate of recurrence is uncertain but is more likely if the cardiac size is slow to return to normal. The mortality rate associated with a recurrence is higher than from the first occurrence.[113]

Anesthetic management depends on the clinical status of the parturient and the mode of delivery. In one report of a woman who had pulmonary edema in an earlier pregnancy, serial echocardiography revealed persistent cardiomegaly in the next confinement. Successful outcome was achieved with epidural anesthesia and noninvasive hemodynamic monitoring for cesarean delivery.[114] In another report wherein cardiomyopathy presented atypically, a parturient with no history or physical signs of heart disease suffered a cardiac arrest at induction of general anesthesia for emergency cesarean delivery.[115] After resuscitation and delivery of the baby, the diagnosis was confirmed by echocardiography, but no etiology for the cardiomyopathy was determined.

CONCLUSION

The obstetric anesthesiologist should not be dogmatic about the choice of anesthetic for parturients with heart disease. Each case should be assessed individually, with special attention paid to the functional impairment. An understanding of the hemodynamics associated with the structural lesion and the appropriate use of invasive monitors are most important in providing optimal conditions for labor and delivery.

References

1. Mogensen L. Cardiac considerations related to pregnancy (editorial). J Intern Med 1994;235:383.
2. Anonymous. Cardiac disease in pregnancy. ACOG Technical Bulletin No. 168, June 1992. Int J Gynaecol Obstet 1993;41:298.
3. Clark SL. Cardiac disease in pregnancy (review). Obstet Gynecol Clin North Amer 1991;18:237.
4. Ramin SM, Maberry MC, Gilstrap LC. Congenital heart disease. Clin Obstet Gynecol 1989;32:41.
5. Rose V, Gold RJ, Lindsay G, Allen M. A possible increase in the incidence of congenital heart defects among the offspring of affected parents. J Am Coll Cardiol 1985;6:376.
6. Presbitero P, Somerville J, Stone S, et al. Pregnancy in cyanotic heart disease: Outcome of mother and fetus. Circulation 1994;89:2673.
7. Pitkin RM, Perloff JK, Koos BJ, Beall MH. Pregnancy and congenital heart disease. Ann Intern Med 1990;112:445.
8. Allan LD, Crawford DC, Chita SR, et al. Familial recurrence of congenital heart disease in the prospective series of mothers referred for fetal echocardiography. Am J Cardiol 1986; 58:334.
9. Elkayam U, Gleischer N. Changes in cardiac findings during normal pregnancy. In Elkayam U, Gleischer N (eds): Cardiac problems in pregnancy, 2nd ed. New York, Alan R. Liss, 1990, p 31.
10. Burrow GN, Ferris T. Medical complications during pregnancy, 3rd ed. Philadelphia, WB Saunders, 1988.
11. Dajani AS, Bisno AL, Chung KJ, et al. Prevention of bacterial endocarditis. Recommendations by the American Heart Association. JAMA 1990;264:2919.
12. Modig J. Influences of regional anesthesia, local anesthetics and sympathomimetics on the pathophysiology of deep vein thrombosis. Acta Chir Scand 1989 [Suppl];55:119.
13. Wong V, Chen CH, Chan KC. Fetal and neonatal outcome of exposure to anticoagulants during pregnancy. Am J Med Genet 1993;45:17.
14. Born D, Martinez EE, Almeida PAM, et al. Pregnancy in patients with prosthetic heart valves: The effects of anticoagulation on mother, fetus and neonate. Am Heart J 1992;124:413.
15. Toglia MR, Weg JG. Venous thromboembolism during pregnancy. N Engl J Med 1996;335:108.
16. Ginsberg JS, Hirsh J. Use of antithrombotic agents during pregnancy. Chest 1995 [Suppl] 108:305S.

17. McKenna R, Cole E, Vasan U. Is warfarin sodium contraindicated in the lactating mother? J Pediatr 1983;103:325.

18. Lee C-N, Wu C-C, Lin P-Y, et al. Pregnancy following cardiac prosthetic valve replacement. Obstet Gynecol 1994;83;353.

19. Badduke BR, Jamieson WRE, Miyagishima RT, et al. Pregnancy and childbearing in a population with biological valvular prostheses. J Thorac Cardiovasc Surg 1991;102:179.

20. Sbarouni E, Oakley C. Outcome of pregnancy in women with valve prostheses. Br Heart J 1994;71:196.

21. Barbour LA, Pickard J. Controversies in thromboembolic disease during pregnancy: A critical review. Obstet Gynecol 1995;86:621.

22. Ramamurthy S, Talwar KK, Saxena A, et al. Prosthetic mitral valve thrombosis in pregnancy successfully treated with streptokinase. Am Heart J 1994;127:446.

23. Furui T, Kurauchi O, Oguchi H, et al. Pregnancy and successful delivery in a patient with triple heart valve prosthesis. Int J Gynecol Obstet 1993;41:89.

24. Mortensen JD, Ellsworth HS. Pregnancy before and after surgical correction of left-to-right cardiovascular shunts. Obstet Gynecol 1967;29:241.

25. Patton DE, Lee W, Cotton DB, et al. Cyanotic maternal heart disease in pregnancy. Obstet Gynecol Survey 1990;45:594.

26. Burn J. 'The next lady has a heart defect.' Br J Obstet Gynaecol 1987;94:97.

27. Slomka F, Salmeron S, Zetlaoui P, et al. Primary pulmonary hypertension and pregnancy: Anesthetic management for delivery. Anesthesiology 1988;69:959.

28. Robinson DE, Leicht CH. Epidural analgesia with low-dose bupivacaine and fentanyl for labor and delivery in a parturient with severe pulmonary hypertension. Anesthesiology 1988;68:285.

29. Kasai H, Gohda Y, Sasaki K, Kemmotsu O. Anesthetic management of Caesarean section in a patient with primary pulmonary hypertension. Masui (Jpn J Anesthiol) 1988;37:476.

30. Spinnato JA, Kraynack BJ, Cooper MW. Eisenmenger's syndrome in pregnancy: Epidural anesthesia for elective cesarean section. N Engl J Med 1981;804:1215.

31. Tibaldi G, Marchi L, Huscher M, Forlini G. Anesthesia for cesarean section in a pregnant woman with Eisenmenger's syndrome. Description of a clinical case. Minerva Ginecol 1988;40:145.

32. Power KJ, Avery AF. Extradural analgesia in the intrapartum management of a patient with pulmonary hypertension. Br J Anaesth 1989;63:116.

33. Baum VC. The adult patient with congenital heart disease. J Cardiothorac Vasc Anesth 1996;10:261.

34. Weiss BM, Atanassoff PG. Cyanotic congenital heart disease and pregnancy: Natural selection, pulmonary hypertension and anesthesia. J Clin Anesth 1993;5:332.

35. Oxorn D, Edelist G, Smith MS. An introduction to transoesophageal echocardiography: II. Clinical applications. Can J Anaesth 1996;43:278.

36. Roberts SL, Chestnut DH. Anesthesia for the obstetric patient with cardiac disease. Clin Obstet Gynecol 1987;30:601.

37. Spielman FJ. Anaesthetic management of the obstetric patient with cardiac disease. Clin Anaesthesiol 1986;4:247.

38. Mostafa SM. Spinal anaesthesia for Caesarean section. Management of a parturient with severe cardiovascular disease. Br J Anaesth 1984;56:1275.

39. Prince GD. Spinal anaesthesia and cardiac disease (letter). Br J Anaesth 1986;58:683.

40. Ransom DM, Leicht CH. Continuous spinal analgesia with sufentanil for labor and delivery in a parturient with severe pulmonary stenosis. Anesth Analg 1995;80:418.

41. Ahmad S, Hawes D, Dooley S, et al. Intrathecal morphine in a parturient with a single ventricle. Anesthesiology 1981;54:515.

42. Abboud TK, Raya J, Noueihed R, Daniel J. Intrathecal morphine for relief of labor pain in a parturient with severe pulmonary hypertension. Anesthesiology 1983;59:477.

43. Pollack KL, Chestnut DH, Wenstrom KD. Anesthetic management of a parturient with Eisenmenger's syndrome. Anesth Analg 1990;70:212.

44. Leyse R, Ofstun M, Dillard DH, Merendino KA. Congenital aortic stenosis in pregnancy, corrected by extracorporeal circulation. JAMA 1961;1009.

45. Rossouw GJ, Knott-Craig CJ, Barnard PM, et al. Intracardiac operation in seven pregnant women. Ann Thorac Surg 1993;55:1172.

46. Ben-Ami M, Battino S, Rosenfeld T, et al. Aortic valve replacement during pregnancy. Acta Obstet Gynecol Scand 1990;69:651.

47. Becker RM. Intracardiac surgery in pregnant women. Ann Thorac Surg 1983;36:453.

48. Eilen B, Kaiser IH, Becker RM, et al. Aortic valve replacement in the third trimester of pregnancy: Case report and review of the literature. Obstet Gynecol 1981;57:119.

49. Paulus DA, Layon AJ, Mayfield WR, et al. Intrauterine pregnancy and aortic valve replacement. J Clin Anesth 1995;7:338.

50. Bernal MJ, Miralles JP. Cardiac surgery with cardiopulmonary bypass during pregnancy. Obstet Gynecol Surv 1986;41:1.

51. Shah AM, Ikram S, Kulatilake ENP, et al. Emergency mitral valve replacement immediately following Caesarean section. Eur Heart J 1992;13:847.

52. Lamarra M, Ahmed AA, Kulatilake ENP. Cardiopulmonary bypass in the early puerperium: Possible new role for aprotinin. Ann Thorac Surg 1992;54:361.

53. Strickland RA, Oliver WC, Chantigan RC, et al. Anesthesia, cardiopulmonary bypass and the pregnant patient. Mayo Clin Proc 1991;66:411.

54. Fong J, Druzin M, Gimbel AA, Fisher J. Epidural anaesthesia for labour and Caesarean section in a parturient with a single ventricle and transposition of the great arteries. Can J Anaesth 1990;37:680.

55. Alon E, Baumann H. Anesthesiologic management of cesarean section in a patient with transposition of the great vessels [German]. Reg Anaesth 1988;11:28.

56. Clarkson PM, Wilson NJ, Neutze JM, et al. Outcome of pregnancy after the Mustard operation for transposition of the great arteries with intact ventricular septum. J Am Coll Cardiol 1994;24:190.

57. Marsh NJ, Dorian RS. Epidural anesthesia in a parturient with congenital absence of the inferior vena cava. Anesth Analg 1992;75:1033.

58. Heriot JA, Steven CM, Sattin RS. Elective forceps delivery and extradural anaesthesia in a primigravida with portal hypertension and oesophageal varices. Br J Anaesth 1996;76:325.

59. Wilton NC, Traber KB, Deschner LS. Anaesthetic management for Caesarean section in a patient with uncorrected truncus arteriosus. Br J Anaesth 1989;62:434.

60. Rowbottom SJ, Gin T, Cheung LP. General anaesthesia for Caesarean section in a patient with uncorrected complex cyanotic heart disease. Anaesth Intensive Care 1994;22:74.

61. Atanassoff PG, Schmid ER, Jenni R, et al. Epidural anesthesia for a cesarean section in a patient with pulmonary atresia and ventricular septal defect. J Clin Anesth 1991;3:399.

62. Schulte-Sasse U, Hess W, Tarnow J. Pulmonary vascular responses to nitrous oxide in patients with normal and high pulmonary vascular resistance. Anesthesiology 1982;57:9.

63. Halpern S, Gidwaney A, Gates B. Anaesthesia for Caesarean section in a pre-eclamptic patient with Ebstein's anomaly. Can Anaesth Soc J 1985;32:244.

64. Linter SPK, Clarke K. Caesarean section under extradural analgesia in a patient with Ebstein's anomaly. Br J Anaesth 1984;56:203.

65. Krcilkova M, Kobilova J, Cech E. A successful delivery using epidural anesthesia in a woman with Ebstein's malformation [Czech]. Sbornik Lekarsky 1988;90:354.

66. Donnelly JE, Brown JM, Radford DJ. Pregnancy outcome and Ebstein's anomaly. Br Heart J 1991;66:368.

67. Thorin D, Aebischer N, Landolt J, et al. Acute pulmonary edema in the post partum and cor triatriatum sinistrum. Int J Obstet Anesth 1995;4:113.

68. Seeds JW, Cefalo RC. Pregnancy with congenital heart disease: A two chambered heart. Am J Obstet Gynecol 1977;127:213.

69. Hoback J, Adicoff A, From AH, et al. A report of Uhl's disease in identical adult twins. Evaluation of right ventricular dysfunction with echocardiography and nuclear angiography. Chest 1981;79:306.

70. Koenig C, Katz M, Gertsch M, et al. Pregnancy and delivery in the patient with UHL anomaly. Obstet Gynecol 1991;78:932.

71. Watson GH. Pulmonary stenosis, café-au-lait spots, and dull intelligence. Arch Dis Child 1967;42:303.

72. Conway JB, Posner M. Anaesthesia for Caesarean section in a patient with Watson's syndrome. Can J Anaesth 1994;41:1113.
73. Miller AP, Stonechipher HK, Boyd B. Turner's phenotype: Pregnancy and cyanotic congenital heart disease (letter). JAMA 1970;214:2337.
74. Dadabhoy ZP, Winnie AP. Regional anesthesia for cesarean section in a parturient with Noonan's syndrome. Anesthesiology 1988;68:636.
75. Holzman RS, Nargozian CD, Marnach R, McMillan CO. Epidural anesthesia in patients with palliated cyanotic congenital heart disease. J Cardiothorac Vasc Anesth 1992;6:340.
76. Whittemore R, Hobbins JC, Engle MA. Pregnancy and its outcome in women with and without surgical treatment of congenital heart disease. Am J Cardiol 1982;50:641.
77. Zavisca FG, Johnson MD, Holubec JT, et al. General anesthesia for cesarean section in a parturient with a single ventricle and pulmonary atresia. J Clin Anesth 1993;5:315.
78. Carp H, Jayaram A, Vadhera R, et al. Epidural anesthesia for cesarean delivery and vaginal birth after maternal Fontan repair: Report of two cases. Anesth Analg 1994;78:1190.
79. Cohen AM, Mulvein J. Obstetric anaesthetic management in a patient with the Fontan circulation. Br J Anaesth 1994;73:252.
80. Fontan F, Baudet D. Surgical repair of tricuspid atresia. Thorax 1971;26:240.
81. de Leval MR. Right heart bypass operations. In Stark J, de Leval MR (eds): Surgery for Congenital Heart Defects. Philadelphia, WB Saunders, 1994, p 565.
82. Clark SL. Monitoring and anaesthetic management of parturients with mitral stenosis (letter). Can J Anaesth 1987;34:654.
83. Batson MA, Longmire S, Csontos E. Alfentanil for urgent Caesarean section in a patient with severe mitral stenosis and pulmonary hypertension. Can J Anaesth 1990;37:685.
84. Hemmings GT, Whalley DG, O'Connor PJ, et al. Invasive monitoring and anaesthetic management of a parturient with mitral stenosis. Can J Anaesth 1987;34:182.
85. Clark SL, Phelan JP, Greenspoon J. Labor and delivery in the presence of mitral stenosis: Central hemodynamic observations. Am J Obstet Gynecol 1985;152:984.
86. Ziskind Z, Etchin A, Frenkel Y, et al. Epidural anesthesia with the Trendelenburg position for cesarean section with or without cardiac surgical procedure in patients with severe mitral stenosis: A hemodynamic study. J Cardiothorac Anesth 1990;4:354.
87. Easterling TR, Chadwick HS, Otto CM, et al. Aortic stenosis in pregnancy. Obstet Gynecol 1988;72:113.
88. Lao TT, Sermer M, MaGee L, et al. Congenital aortic stenosis and pregnancy—a reappraisal. Am J Obstet Gynecol 1993;169:540.
89. McIvor RA. Percutaneous balloon aortic valvuloplasty during pregnancy. Int J Cardiol 1991;32:1.
90. Choi HJ, Chui L, Hurd JM, Tremper KK. Epidural anesthesia for a woman with severe aortic stenosis undergoing a cesarean section. Anesth Rev 1992;19:61.
91. Brian JE Jr, Seifen AB, Clark RB, et al. Aortic stenosis, cesarean delivery, and epidural anesthesia. J Clin Anesth 1993;5:154.
92. Colclough GW, Ackerman WE, Walmsley PN, Hessel EA. Epidural anesthesia for a parturient with critical aortic stenosis. J Clin Anesth 1995;7:264.
93. Douglas MJ, Farquharson DF, Ross PLE, Renwick JE. Cardiovascular collapse following an overdose of prostaglandin F2-alpha. Can J Anaesth 1989;36:466.
94. Redfern N, Bower S, Bullock RE, Hull CJ. Alfentanil for Caesarean section complicated by severe aortic stenosis. A case report. Br J Anaesth 1988;60:477.
95. Sharma SK, Gambling DR, Gajraj NM, et al. Anesthetic management of a parturient with mixed mitral valve disease and uncontrolled atrial fibrillation. Int J Obstet Gynecol 1994;3:157.
96. Lynch III C, Rizor RF. Anesthetic management and monitoring of a parturient with mitral and aortic valvular disease. Anesth Analg 1982;61:788.
97. Shin YK, King JC. Combined mitral and aortic stenosis in a parturient: Epidural anesthesia for labor and delivery (letter). Anesth Analg 1993;76:682.
98. Fairley CJ, Clarke JT. Use of esmolol in a parturient with hypertrophic obstructive cardiomyopathy. Br J Anaesth 1995;75:801.
99. Ducey JP, Knape KG. Maternal esmolol administration resulting in fetal distress and cesarean section in a term pregnancy. Anesthesiology 1992;77:829.
100. Loubser P, Suh K, Cohen S. Adverse effects of spinal anesthesia in a patient with idiopathic hypertrophic subaortic stenosis. Anesthesiology 1984;60:228.
101. Boccio RV, Chung IH, Harrison DM. Anesthetic management of cesarean section in a patient with idiopathic hypertrophic subaortic stenosis. Anesthesiology 1986;65:663.
102. Tessler MJ, Hudson R, Naugler-Colville MA, Biehl DR. Pulmonary edema in two parturients with hypertrophic obstructive cardiomyopathy. Can J Anaesth 1990;37:469.
103. Nwosu EC, Burke MF. Cardiomyopathy of pregnancy. Br J Obstet Gynaecol 1993;100:1145.
104. van Hoeven KH, Kitsis RN, Katz SD, Factor SM. Peripartum versus idiopathic dilated cardiomyopathy in young women—a comparison of clinical, pathological and prognostic features. Int J Cardiol 1993;40:57.
105. Hoffmann, AC, Masouyé P, Rifat K, Suter PM. Peripartum cardiomyopathy: A case report. Acta Anaesth Scand 1991;35:784.
106. Brown G, O'Leary M, Douglas I, Herkes R. Perioperative management of a case of severe peripartum cardiomyopathy. Anaesth Intensive Care 1992;20:80.
107. Breen TW, Janzen JA. Pulmonary hypertension and cardiomyopathy: Anaesthetic management for Caesarean section. Can J Anaesth 1991;38:895.
108. Kluger MT, Bersten AD. Multi-organ failure in peripartum cardiomyopathy. Anaesth Intensive Care 1991;19:450.
109. Lee W, Cotton DB. Peripartum cardiomyopathy: Current concepts and clinical management. Clin Obstet Gynecol 1989;32:54.
110. Midei MG, DeMent SH, Feldman AM, et al. Peripartum myocarditis and cardiomyopathy. Circulation 1990;81:922.
111. Beards SC, Freebairn RC, Lipman J. Successful use of continuous veno-venous haemofiltration to treat profound fluid retention in severe peripartum cardiomyopathy. Anaesthesia 1993;48:1065.
112. Aravot DJ, Banner NR, Ohalia N. Heart transplantation for peripartum cardiomyopathy. Lancet 1987;2:1024.
113. Sutton MSJ, Cole P, Plappert M, et al. Effects of subsequent pregnancy on left ventricular function in peripartum cardiomyopathy. Am Heart J 1991;121:1776.
114. Gambling DR, Flanagan ML, Huckell VF, et al. Anaesthetic management and non-invasive monitoring for Caesarean section in a patient with cardiomyopathy. Can J Anaesth 1987;34:505.
115. McIndoe AK, Hammond EJ, Babington PCB. Peripartum cardiomyopathy presenting as a cardiac arrest at induction of anaesthesia for emergency Caesarean section. Br J Anaesth 1995;75:97.

DISORDERS OF CARDIAC CONDUCTION

Jean E. Swenerton, M.D., and Victor F. Huckell, M.D.

Disorders of cardiac conduction seen in pregnancy include those involving abnormal impulse generation or propagation (supraventricular and ventricular dysrhythmias, heart block) and specific disorders (pre-excitation syndrome, long QT syndrome). The clinical implications and current management of some of the more familiar disorders of conduction during pregnancy are discussed briefly. Emphasis is placed on the more uncommon disorders of cardiac conduction. For a review of normal cardiac conduction, the reader is referred to standard texts of cardiology.

PHYSIOLOGIC CARDIOVASCULAR CHANGES IN PREGNANCY

Blood Volume

The cardiovascular system undergoes considerable change during pregnancy, especially during labor, delivery, and postpartum (Table 2–1). Antepartum changes in cardiovascular adaptation facilitate perfusion of the developing fetoplacental unit. Circulating

blood volume increases and the peripheral vascular bed dilates, owing to the relaxing influence of estrogen and progesterone. During the first and second trimesters circulating blood volume increases to 75 ml/kg, which is an increase of approximately 10%. In the third trimester, total circulating blood volume increases by approximately 2 L. Plasma volume increases of approximately 50%, with a corresponding increase in body water, are largely adaptive responses to the expanded size of the vascular bed. Red blood cell volume increases, but to a lesser extent (20–30%) and at a slower pace. Interstitial volume also expands. Circulating blood volume decreases significantly immediately post partum, primarily because of blood loss associated with delivery. To maintain stable blood pressure at this time, total peripheral resistance rises, largely as a result of higher precapillary resistance.

Heart Rate

In conjunction with the antepartum rise in blood volume, resting heart rate (HR) increases steadily by 10 to 15% throughout pregnancy, reaching a peak of 10 to 20 beats above baseline during the third trimester. During labor and delivery sinus tachycardia is seen, with maximal HR occurring peripartum. Parturients who experience a greater degree of labor pain may maintain a higher sympathetic tone, which may contribute to a higher peripartum HR.

Palmer[1] studied 22 healthy parturients with or without epidural analgesia and with or without oxytocin augmentation. The baseline rhythm in all was sinus tachycardia (108–172 beats per minute [bpm]). The mean maximal HR (138 bpm) occurred within 30 minutes of delivery in 60% of the parturients. In the remaining 40%, the mean maximal HR occurred later, 0.5 to 5 hours post partum.

Cardiac Output

Increases in blood volume and HR produce a significant rise in cardiac output, which may vary in ex-

TABLE 2–1. PHYSIOLOGIC CHANGES IN CARDIOVASCULAR PARAMETERS DURING PREGNANCY

Cardiac output	Begins early pregnancy
	↑ 2nd and 3rd trimesters
	Inter-individual variability*
	Further ↑ during labor and delivery†
Heart rate	↑ steadily throughout pregnancy
	Peak 10–20 bpm above baseline 3rd trimester
	↑ with pain and stress
Rhythm	PADs and PVDs common
ECG	Shift of QRS axis in any direction
	Small rightward deviation of average QRS axis (1st trimester)
	Small leftward deviation due to progressive elevation of left hemidiaphragm (3rd trimester)
	Lead III: small Q; T wave inversion
	Transient ST-T changes common

*See text
†May vary with disease, use of medications, blood loss and stress of delivery
PADs = Premature atrial depolarizations
PVDs = Premature ventricular depolarizations

tent and timing. Cardiac output begins to rise early in pregnancy with a recorded increase of 500 ml/min (10% above prepregnancy control) by 5 weeks' gestation. Cardiac output continues to increase throughout the first and second trimesters (37% at 25 weeks) and reaches a plateau in the third trimester (53% at 36–40 weeks).

Van Oppen[2] and coworkers reviewed the literature, published between 1955 and 1994, on the effect of normal pregnancy on cardiac output, paying special attention to study design (cross-sectional/longitudinal), measurement technique, position of the subject, and parity. They challenged the validity of the commonly held belief that cardiac output and ventricular performance increase in the third trimester in normal pregnancies. Their analysis found cardiac output to be widely divergent (rose, fell, plateaued) during the third trimester, regardless of the method of measurement or conditions during measurement. They concluded that the tendency to report cardiac output as an average value negates differences among individual cases. This important information must be kept in mind when making management decisions for individual patients.

During labor and delivery, the combination of increased preload (increased venous return from the contracting uterus), decreased afterload, and increased HR results in a further 20% rise in cardiac output and heightened ventricular performance. In the majority of parturients, stroke volume and HR rise by 50% during labor, compared with prepregnancy values. Additional stresses that affect cardiac output include peripartum blood loss, postpartum reabsorption and excretion of the expanded extravascular volume, and lactation.

Electrocardiogram and Cardiac Conduction

Electrocardiogram (ECG) changes during pregnancy include shift of the QRS axis in any direction, the appearance of small q waves in lead III, T wave inversion and, commonly, ST-T changes. ST segment depression, coinciding with maximum HR, and most often asymptomatic, has been reported in the peripartum period during nonoperative and operative deliveries. ST changes are the result of multiple factors including tachycardia, hormonal milieu, and heart position changes. Venous air emboli, hypokalemia, and hyperventilation can also affect the ST segment during pregnancy.[3] It is unclear whether the sympathectomy produced by regional analgesia affects the ECG. In one study, 93 healthy parturients undergoing elective cesarean section using epidural or spinal anesthesia had a 37% incidence of ST depression (>1 mm) or ST elevation.[1] Although there is some evidence that myocardial dysfunction occurs during these ST changes, overt morbidity is rarely reported, and the clinical significance of the changes remains uncertain.

DYSRHYTHMIAS DURING PREGNANCY

Individual case reports suggest that there may be an increased propensity for tachydysrhythmias (mainly supraventricular) during pregnancy.[4] Proposed hypothetical mechanisms include hormonal, autonomic, and hemodynamic changes. As the circulation becomes more hyperdynamic, some women become more aware of the heart beat, changes in HR, and skipped beats. Premature ectopic atrial or ventricular depolarizations (PAD, PVD) and sinus tachycardia are usually the underlying causes. Palpitations, dizziness, dyspnea, presyncope and syncope, and chest pain are presenting complaints of a cardiac dysrhythmia (in descending order of frequency). Although these symptoms can accompany the normal cardiovascular changes associated with pregnancy, dyspnea, severe enough to limit activity, and syncope, with exertion, warrant evaluation.

Approach to Diagnosis and Management

The majority of cardiac dysrhythmias in pregnancy are benign, and hemodynamically significant dysrhythmias are uncommon (Fig. 2–1). If the possibility of a cardiac dysrhythmia exists, it is important to *establish the presence and nature of the dysrhythmia* by obtaining ECG documentation, and to ask three critical questions that have important management implications: *(1) Is there an identifiable precipitating factor? (2) Is there underlying structural heart disease? (3) Is there hemodynamic compromise?*

General Principles

1. When there is no identifiable precipitating factor, no underlying heart disease, and no hemodynamic compromise, reassurance is most often the appropriate management.
2. Successful management of a dysrhythmia may simply involve *identification and elimination of precipitating factors* (Table 2–2).
3. Clinically significant dysrhythmias that require treatment most often occur in those who have *underlying structural heart disease* and/or a history of a *preexisting dysrhythmia*. In the absence of clinically overt cardiac disease, a cardiac dysrhythmia may be the initial manifestation of congenital or acquired structural heart abnormalities that provide the substrate for abnormal cardiac impulse generation, conduction, or both. Structural heart disease has important implications (see Chapter 1). Fewer implications exist for dysrhythmias occurring in the absence of structural heart disease.
4. Identification and evaluation of underlying heart disease (Table 2–3) and choice of the most appro-

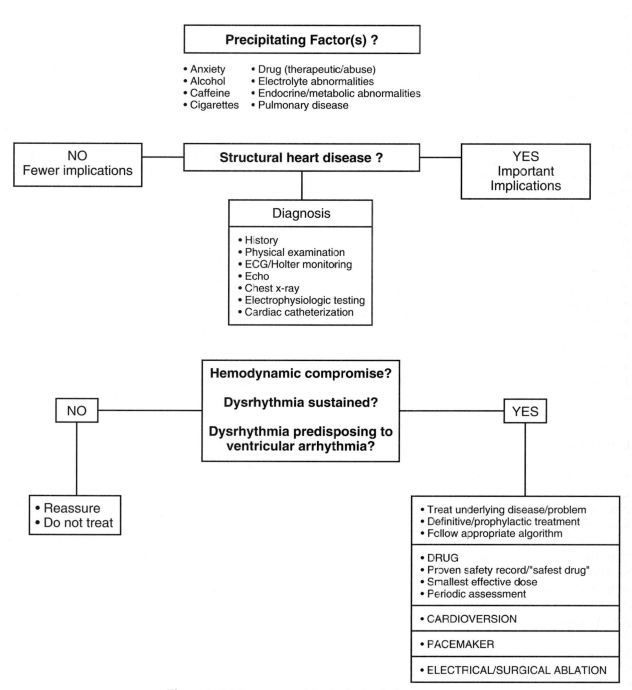

Figure 2–1. Management of dysrhythmias during pregnancy.

TABLE 2–2. CARDIAC DYSRHYTHMIAS: PRECIPITATING FACTORS

Anxiety
Structural heart disease: Corrected, uncorrected
Systemic disease: Endocrine, metabolic, pulmonary
Electrolyte abnormalities
Drugs of abuse: Alcohol, cocaine, caffeine, nicotine
  (cigarettes)
Therapeutic drugs: Beta-sympathomimetics, magnesium
Anesthesia-related
  Drugs: Atropine, ephedrine, epinephrine, neostigmine,
    volatile anesthetics
  Technique: Regional anesthesia; general anesthesia

priate treatment strategies are critical for producing a normal outcome for mother and baby.

5. In the presence of hemodynamic compromise, a sustained dysrhythmia or one predisposing to a ventricular dysrhythmia, definitive and prophylactic treatment in the form of drug therapy, cardioversion, or pacemaker therapy (temporary or permanent) is required. Treatment should take place in a setting where the *mother* and *fetus* can be *monitored closely* and the effects of treatment followed. Oxygen should be administered to the mother by face mask or nasal prongs, and left uterine displacement should be ensured.

6. It is important to minimize the risk for embolic events, which are associated with sustained cardiac dysrhythmias, by diagnosing and treating serious dysrhythmias promptly and appropriately.

7. Avoiding myocardial ischemia and electrolyte imbalance is crucial in women susceptible to dysrhythmias.

Cardiac Assessment of Conduction Disorders During Pregnancy

Cardiology consultation is requested frequently when the pregnant patient has palpitations of uncertain etiology or significance. Special consideration should be given to which diagnostic and therapeutic investigations are undertaken during pregnancy, weighing the potential benefits against the risks to mother and fetus. This determination calls for an assessment of the severity, anticipated course of the dysrhythmia during pregnancy, and appropriate therapy (Table 2–4).

Noninvasive diagnostic investigations (history, physical examination, ECG, Holter monitor, and echocardiography studies) are preferred over chest radiographic

TABLE 2–3. CARDIAC ASSESSMENT DURING PREGNANCY

History	Chest radiograph
Physical examination	Electrophysiologic testing
ECG/Holter monitoring	Cardiac catheterization
Echocardiography	

TABLE 2–4. QUESTIONS FOR THE CARDIOLOGIST

1. What are the risks of this woman developing a dysrhythmia during the increased sympathetic stress of the labor/delivery period?
2. What antiarrhythmic or other therapy do you recommend if she develops a dysrhythmia during pregnancy—antepartum, labor, and delivery?
3. Is prophylactic therapy indicated?
4. What is the risk-benefit ratio of any given investigation or therapy for mother and fetus?

studies, cardiac catheterization, and electrophysiologic investigations. The former studies avoid ionizing radiation exposure (chest radiograph, fluoroscopy), procedure-induced dysrhythmias, and/or hemodynamic compromise after administration of sedatives and anesthetics. Some radiographic procedures, especially in early pregnancy, have the potential to cause abnormal fetal organogenesis and increased incidence of childhood malignancy, particularly leukemia. Serial echocardiography assessments are useful and incur minimal risk to mother and fetus (Table 2–5). Chest radiographs are not ordered routinely but, if they are considered important to maternal evaluation and treatment, appropriate pelvic shielding keeps fetal radiation below minimally acceptable levels. When necessary, right heart catheterization can be performed successfully, without fluoroscopy, using a flow-directed catheter. Nuclear studies have little place in the diagnosis of valvular or coronary artery disease in pregnant women.

Sinus Node Dysrhythmias

1. Normal sinus rhythm: At rest, the normal heart rate is between 60 and 100 bpm. The sinus node rate is the result of opposing sympathetic and parasympathetic autonomic influences on the intrinsic discharge rate of the sinus node pacemaker cells. HR is influenced by age, physical activity, endocrine status, and respiration. HR steadily increases by 10 to 15% during pregnancy, reaching a peak of 10 to

TABLE 2–5. NONINVASIVE ECHOCARDIOGRAPHY ASSESSMENT DURING PREGNANCY

Two-dimensional echocardiography	Evaluation of LA dilation or thrombus
Doppler echocardiography	Transmitral gradient
	Mitral valve area
	Two dimensional exam technically inadequate
	Previous commissurotomy
	Densely calcified leaflets
	Intracardiac pressures (RV + PAP) if tricuspid regurgitation
Transesophageal echocardiography	Visualization of thrombi (usually in LA appendage)

LA = left atrium; RV = right ventricle; PAP = pulmonary artery pressures

20 beats above baseline during the third trimester. *Sinus arrhythmia*, in which the HR accelerates with inspiration and slows with expiration, is also seen commonly during pregnancy.

2. Sinus tachycardia is defined as a rate of 100 to 200 bpm. Sinus tachycardia is characterized by a gradual onset and offset and is due to acceleration of phase 4 diastolic depolarization of the sinus node pacemaker cells. Sinus tachycardia may be seen during pregnancy, especially in the third trimester (earlier in twin pregnancy) and at delivery, without any pathologic significance. Persistent sinus tachycardia may be associated with various pathologic states (fever, congestive heart failure, myocardial disease, endocrine or metabolic abnormalities) or intake of stimulants (caffeine, nicotine, cocaine, asthma medications, other drugs), which may warrant correction or treatment.[4]

3. Sinus bradycardia is defined as a sinus node rate below 60 bpm. It may occur normally, especially in the physically fit parturient. If symptoms due to hemodynamic impairment are present, atropine 0.5 to 1 mg q3 to 5 minutes intravenously (IV) to a total dose of 0.03 to 0.04 mg/kg is administered. Severe symptomatic bradycardia, with hypotension, may require treatment with transcutaneous pacing (if available) or a catecholamine infusion (dopamine, epinephrine, isoproterenol) according to Advanced Cardiac Life Support (ACLS) protocols. Rarely, permanent pacing is necessary for long-term management (atrial pacing to maintain A-V synchrony).

Parturients receiving spinal anesthesia for cesarean section may develop sudden, severe bradycardia and hypotension if the sensory level ascends very rapidly to a high level (>T2), with concomitant blockade of cardioaccelerator fibers.

4. Wandering pacemaker is the result of shift in the dominant pacemaker from the sinus node to latent pacemakers in the atria or atrioventricular junction. It rarely requires treatment.

5. Sinus node dysfunction or sick sinus syndrome (SSS) incorporates a range of abnormalities of sinus node impulse formation and conduction. These abnormalities include sinus bradycardia, sinus arrest, sinus exit block, sinoatrial and atrioventricular conduction disorders, and paroxysms of alternating, rapid, regular, or irregular atrial tachyarrhythmias with bradyarrhythmias. Although more usual in the elderly, SSS may occur in the under-30-year age group.[4] Its incidence during pregnancy is unknown, however. Treatment depends on the type of rhythm disturbance. Permanent pacing may be necessary for bradyarrhythmias, and drug therapy may be necessary for tachyarrhythmias.[4]

Schatz and coworkers[5] have described a 21-year-old primigravida with Ebstein's anomaly who had a severe bradycardia-junctional tachycardia syndrome. She required multiple drug treatments and temporary transvenous pacing during delivery. Mendelson[6] described a 32-year-old pregnant woman who had occasional fainting associated with sinus exit block. Pregnancy did not affect the frequency of syncopal episodes, and no therapy was required. She had three normal term deliveries.

Premature Atrial and Ventricular Depolarizations

Premature Atrial Depolarizations

ECG diagnosis of PAD is made when a premature P wave is noted with a P-R interval longer than 120 msec. Usually a difference occurs in the contour of the premature P wave, indicating a different focus of origin.[7] Premature atrial depolarizations are very common in the young, with a 64% incidence rate reported in a study of 50 healthy young women using 24-hour Holter monitors.[4] Most often PAD are identified during routine prenatal examination or evaluation of "palpitations" during pregnancy.

Contributing factors include stress, anxiety, infection, nicotine (cigarette smoking), caffeine (tea, coffee, cola), alcohol, and stimulatory drugs such as sympathomimetic asthma preparations or decongestants. Normally, premature atrial complexes do not require therapy. Avoidance or removal of precipitating factors may be therapeutic. Occasionally, PAD are a manifestation of occult heart failure or excessive adrenergic tone, and treatment with diuretics, analgesics, sedatives, or beta blockade is appropriate. PAD may trigger sustained supraventricular or ventricular tachyarrhythmias that require treatment with β-blocking agents, verapamil, or class IA antiarrhythmic drugs.[4]

Premature Ventricular Depolarizations

The relatively common complaint of "palpitations" or "awareness of skipped beats" is frequently the reason for cardiac consultation during pregnancy, with PVD the most commonly identified cause. Skipped beats caused by PVD tend to be noticed more than those caused by PAD. Clinically, they are accompanied by a giant "a" (cannon) wave, visible in the neck as the PVD occurs against a closed tricuspid valve. Sudden distension of the pulmonary veins may elicit an associated spontaneous cough.

Premature ventricular depolarizations occur frequently in the general population. In a Holter monitor study of 50 healthy women, 54% had PVD (6% had >50 beats in 24 hours). The majority of pregnant women with PVD have no evidence of underlying heart disease. As with PAD, PVD may be associated with anxiety, intake of stimulants (caffeine, tobacco, alcohol), systemic infection, electrolyte abnormalities, hypoxia, and a variety of medications. Correction of underlying causes and avoidance of stimulants may reduce or eliminate PVD.

As a general rule, pharmacologic therapy should be avoided and treatment with lidocaine for multifocal PVD occurring at a rate more than 5 per minute is not recommended unless there is hemodynamic compromise. Occasionally, in severely symptomatic women, antiarrhythmic drugs are indicated. Quinidine (class IA) has a good safety record in pregnancy. Low-level beta blockade is as effective as quinidine in suppressing symptoms. Among class IB antiarrhythmic drugs, the safest appears to be lidocaine, as long as serum levels are monitored and maternal and fetal effects followed closely. Current indications for treatment are included in Table 2–6. A small subset of patients with mitral valve prolapse (MVP) and long QT interval syndrome have a predisposition to ventricular tachycardia, which, if sustained, may be associated with embolic events and sudden death. Given a history of PVD, MVP, and long QT interval, prophylactic antiarrhythmic treatment may be warranted.

Supraventricular Dysrhythmias

Supraventricular tachycardia (SVT) is characterized by a narrow QRS complex (except for cases of pre-existing bundle branch block or aberrant conduction) with a regular R-R interval and a rate between 150 and 250 bpm (Table 2–7). SVT encompasses a variety of tachyarrhythmias originating in the SA node, atria, and AV junction. Atrial depolarization is retrograde, resulting in inverted P waves in ECG leads II, III, and aVF. The P wave may occur just before, during, or after the QRS complex, and it is not seen if it arises during the QRS complex. Reciprocating tachycardias involving anomalous (accessory) AV or nodal-ventricular pathways are included even though both atrium and ventricle are part of the re-entrant circuit. The premature beat starting the tachycardia may originate in the ventricle, not necessarily above the ventricle.

Paroxysmal SVT (PSVT)

Paroxysmal SVT (PSVT) is a distinct clinical syndrome characterized by repeated episodes (paroxysms) of tachycardia with an abrupt onset, lasting from a few seconds to several hours. PSVT may stop spontane-

TABLE 2–6. INDICATIONS FOR TREATMENT OF PVD IN PREGNANCY

PVD in presence of significant hemodynamic compromise

Symptomatic PVD sustained over a long period of time

PVD with underlying structural abnormality of the heart predisposing to life-threatening ventricular dysrhythmia (controversial)

PVD = premature ventricular depolarizations

ously, as suddenly as it started, or it may stop as a consequence of another ectopic supraventricular beat interrupting the circus movement.[7]

Electrophysiologically, SVT is the result of (1) re-entry, which may occur at the level of the sinus node, atria, or AV junction; (2) abnormal automaticity; and (3) triggered activity.

Abnormal automaticity and triggered activity are the mechanisms responsible for 10% or less of supraventricular tachycardias. More than 90% of PSVT is due to re-entry, and the initial event is frequently a premature atrial complex. Approximately 60% of PSVT cases are due to re-entry in the AV node, involving the AV node alone or AV node plus an extra-AV nodal bypass tract. In the majority of patients with AV nodal re-entrant tachycardia, anterograde conduction occurs over a slow alpha pathway and retrograde conduction over a fast beta pathway (typical AV nodal re-entrant tachycardia; P wave buried within QRS complex). In 5 to 10% of patients with AV nodal re-entry, anterograde conduction occurs over the fast pathway and retrograde conduction over the slow pathway (atypical AV nodal re-entrant tachycardia; P wave appears long after QRS; RP greater than PR interval). Fifteen to twenty percent of re-entrant SVT occurs over a "concealed" bypass tract. These tachycardias use a macro re-entrant circuit, which involves both atria and ventricles. In the orthodromic AV reciprocating tachycardia, anterograde conduction occurs over the AV node and His-Purkinje system and retrograde conduction occurs over the accessory pathway. On a surface ECG, the P wave is buried within, or it closely follows, a narrow QRS.[4]

Symptoms such as palpitations, lightheadedness, dyspnea, anxiety, angina, and syncope depend on the HR, duration of dysrhythmia, and presence of underlying heart disease. Angina, pulmonary edema, and syncope may occur in women with heart disease; the symptoms are due to myocardial ischemia, heart failure, and decreased cerebral circulation, respectively. These hemodynamic events result from a decrease in left ventricular filling and cardiac output.[7] Pulmonary edema is most likely to occur if SVT lasts longer than 6 hours or in the presence of underlying heart disease, such as mitral stenosis.

In Pregnancy. PSVT is a relatively common dysrhythmia that may occur in the absence of underlying structural heart disease. The estimated incidence during pregnancy is as high as 2.6% but, in those with a prior history, there may be more frequent and severe exacerbations.[4, 8, 9] Not infrequently, a diagnosis of PSVT is made for the first time during pregnancy. PSVT occurs more often during pregnancy in women with a prior history of PSVT, in those with Wolff-Parkinson-White syndrome associated dysrhythmias,[4, 8] and in those treated with beta-agonists for premature labor.[10] The most common cause of a sustained dysrhythmia in pregnancy is re-entrant supra-

TABLE 2–7. SUPRAVENTRICULAR DYSRHYTHMIAS IN PREGNANCY

Dysrhythmias	Rate/Rhythm	P wave/PR	QRS	Clinical Importance	Treatment
PADs	Regular with "skipped" beats	P wave contour abnormal; PR > 120 msec	Normal	Common (64%) Occasionally may trigger sustained SVT or VT Underlying heart disease uncommon Precipitating factors: stress, infection, alcohol, caffeine (tea, coffee, colas), nicotine (cigarettes), stimulant drugs (sympathomimetic asthma meds, decongestants); occult heart failure	Reassurance Avoid stimulants Usually no drug treatment required
PSVT	AR 140–220 bpm 2:1 AV block (usual) Rhythm regular	? P waves (inv P in II, III, avF); PR normal or ↑	Normal or ↑	2.6% pregnancies Usually well tolerated Serious sequelae can occur Can mimic VT if aberrant QRS Abrupt onset and offset	Goal: Slow AV conduction: Vagal Drugs Cardioversion
Atrial tachycardia: Nonparoxysmal Multifocal	AV block	P wave in or follows QRS RP > PR	—	Multifocal AT frequently associated with respiratory failure	
Atrial flutter	Type I (classic): AR 300, VR 150; 2:1 AV conduction; Type II: AR > 350	Sawtooth flutter waves	Normal	Less common than atrial fibrillation Underlying heart disease usual	Rapid atrial pacing (Type I) Drugs (Type II) Cardioversion
Atrial fibrillation	AR 350–600 VR 100–200 Irregular	No P waves	Narrow complexes	Uncommon in pregnancy Can occur in structurally normal hearts (paroxysmal form) Chronic form associated with myocardial and systemic disease	Convert to SR Drugs Cardioversion Pacemaker Slow VR Drugs Prevent recurrence Drugs

PSVT = paroxysmal supraventricular tachycardia; AR = atrial rate; AV = atrioventricular; SR = sinus rhythm; VR = ventricular rhythm; AT = atrial tachycardia

ventricular tachycardia. In the obstetric literature PSVT is often called paroxysmal auricular, atrial, or supraventricular tachycardia, with the underlying electrophysiologic mechanism rarely defined.[4]

Treatment

In the absence of coexisting heart disease, the majority of supraventricular tachycardias, of the atrioventricular nodal re-entrant type, are well tolerated in young people.[11] When treatment is required, as a result of hemodynamic compromise or underlying structural heart disease, it is directed at slowing AV nodal conduction and using vagal maneuvers and/or drug regimens. Vagal stimulation maneuvers (carotid sinus massage [Table 2–8], Valsalva maneuver, or gagging) may abort PSVT or significantly slow the ventricular rate in up to 75% of cases.[7, 12] Eyeball massage should *never* be performed because it may result in retinal detachment.[11]

Various drugs, including adenosine, verapamil, β-blockers, and class IA antiarrhythmic drugs, successfully terminate SVT.[13–15] Adenosine is currently the drug of choice and 6 mg given intravenously is often immediately effective.[13] Propranolol is only half as effective as adenosine and verapamil in terminating acute tachyarrhythmias,[14] and propranolol must be used with caution in women with heart disease or asthma. Cholinergic agents, such as edrophonium, and pressor agents, such as phenylephrine, are other classes of drugs that have been used to stop PSVT in the presence of normal and low blood pressures, respectively.[7] In severe hemodynamic compromise or resistance to drug therapy, synchronized direct-current cardioversion (10–50 joules) is the treatment of choice. Rapid atrial pacing is also effective in stopping PSVT and may be useful for those cases refractory to drug therapy.[16]

It can be difficult to differentiate supraventricular ectopic beats, or SVT with aberrant conduction, from ventricular ectopic beats or VT. The typical narrow QRS complex of PSVT is not seen if a pre-existent or rate-dependent bundle branch block (BBB) is present, or if an anterograde conduction to the ventricles occurs over an accessory AV nodal pathway, such as a Kent bundle. The clinical importance of differentiating PSVT

and VT is considerable. Supraventricular dysrhythmias are generally less dangerous than the more ominous, potentially life-threatening, ventricular tachycardia, which requires immediate treatment.

Wide-QRS tachycardias, especially those of uncertain origin, should be considered VT until proven otherwise. They should be treated accordingly (with IV lidocaine, procainamide, electrocardioversion). Treatment of rapid, wide, regular QRS tachycardia with agents such as verapamil, in the belief that they represent supraventricular tachycardia with aberrant conduction, can have disastrous consequences (e.g., precipitation of ventricular fibrillation) if the tachycardia is ventricular.

Prevention of PSVT depends on the frequency and severity of acute attacks. Verapamil, quinidine, or propranolol may be given. In some, pacemaker implantation may be necessary; implantation avoids medical therapy. When appropriate, ablation procedures that destroy part of an accessory re-entrant pathway are done. Such procedures can result in a long-term cure.[11]

Atrial Tachycardia and Atrial Flutter

Atrial tachycardia may be classified as nonparoxysmal atrial tachycardia or multifocal atrial tachycardia, with the latter commonly seen in patients with severe pulmonary disease.

Atrial flutter is less common than atrial fibrillation. Paroxysmal forms of atrial flutter may occur in the absence of structural heart disease, but in its chronic form, atrial flutter is almost always associated with underlying heart disease.[4, 7] Atrial flutter is frequently unstable, reverting to sinus rhythm or degenerating into atrial fibrillation.[7]

Electrocardiography reveals a sawtooth morphology in the inferior leads. Atrial flutter is classified into two types: type I (classic), which is an atrial rate of 300 bpm, ventricular rate of 150 bpm (2:1 AV conduction); and type II, which is a flat baseline with a positive flutter wave in the inferior leads and a rate usually greater than 350 bpm. Type I disease originates close to the sinus node and activates the right atrium in a counter-clockwise direction. Type II disease appears to originate in the lateral wall, and the depolarization wave occurs usually in a clockwise direction.

In Pregnancy

Relatively few cases of atrial flutter have been reported in pregnancy. Atrial flutter has been reported in association with a wide variety of conditions such as Graves disease,[6] rheumatic heart disease,[4] and postsurgical correction of congenital heart disease.[4, 17]

Treatment

The treatment is dictated by hemodynamic status. In hemodynamically stable patients, verapamil, digoxin,

---

TABLE 2–8. CORRECT APPLICATION OF CAROTID SINUS MASSAGE

With fingertips of left hand, palpate the carotid sinus region of the right neck—opposite the level of the thyroid cartilage, medial to the sternocleidomastoid muscle (carotid pulse palpable)

Get patient to *take a maximal inspiration (hold)* and apply firm pressure in a posterior direction over the carotid sinus

While continuing to press firmly for 30–60 sec, get patient to exhale

and beta-blocking agents may control the ventricular rate and occasionally terminate the dysrhythmia. To avoid 1:1 conduction, class IA antiarrhythmic drugs (e.g., procainamide), should be administered only after control of the ventricular rate. Rapid atrial pacing is effective in converting type I atrial flutter, provided that the atria are paced at a rate approximately 20% faster than the flutter rate, with a maximal current (usually 20 amps) from a site high in the right atrium. This pacing should continue for approximately 30 seconds following the interruption of atrial flutter. A change in morphology of the flutter pattern is a sign of overdrive suppression. If suppression does not occur, it is usually because of inadequate rate, pacing time, or current.[18]

Frequently, type II flutter cannot be converted by rapid atrial pacing. In hemodynamically unstable patients, electrical cardioversion beginning with low energy levels is indicated. Prevention of atrial flutter is similar to that for PSVT. Digoxin alone, or in combination with quinidine, is effective. If quinidine is used, it is important that the diagnosis of flutter be correct and that the patient be digitalized first, *because quinidine alone accelerates AV node conduction.* Monotherapy with verapamil, digoxin, β-blocking agents, or class IA antiarrhythmic drugs may be equally effective.[4]

Atrial Fibrillation

Atrial fibrillation is characterized by totally disorganized atrial depolarization at a rate of 350 to 600 bpm. Most atrial impulses are blocked because of concealed conduction within the AV node, and the ventricular rate is irregular at 100 to 200 bpm. As with atrial flutter, paroxysmal atrial fibrillation can occur in normal hearts, whereas the chronic form is associated with myocardial and systemic disease (Table 2–9). In patients with cardiovascular disease, atrial fibrillation is associated with doubling of morbidity and mortality.[19]

The hemodynamic consequences of atrial fibrillation depend on the severity of underlying disease and the ventricular rate. Atrial fibrillation develops more often in patients with enlarged left atria (>40 mm). In patients with mitral stenosis, a higher HR shortens the diastolic filling time and increases the transvalvular pressure gradient. Sudden onset of atrial fibrillation with rapid ventricular rates raises left atrial pressure, leading to symptoms of dyspnea and possibly pulmonary edema. Because normal left atrial contraction con-

TABLE 2–9. PREDISPOSING CAUSES OF ATRIAL FIBRILLATION IN PREGNANCY

Congenital heart disease (corrected, uncorrected)

Acquired heart disease: Rheumatic, hypertensive, ischemic, cardiomyopathy, pericarditis, post-cardiac surgery

Thyrotoxicosis

tributes up to 30% of the presystolic transvalvular pressure gradient, abrupt loss of atrial contraction can decrease cardiac output by 20%. Ventricular filling is restricted more by the rapid HR than by the loss of atrial contraction. When left ventricular dysfunction with reduced ventricular compliance is present, cardiac output may drop more dramatically.

A significant increase occurs in the frequency of embolic stroke and peripheral embolization in patients with chronic atrial fibrillation and underlying heart disease (especially mitral stenosis). Clinically symptomatic emboli develop in approximately 35% of patients with mitral valve disease, 18% with ischemia and hypertension, and 10% with hyperthyroidism. Postmortem examination of patients with chronic atrial fibrillation demonstrates emboli in 45% of those with valvular disease and in 35% of those with ischemia and hypertension. The risk of embolization is much less in the absence of heart disease.[4]

In Pregnancy

Atrial fibrillation and atrial flutter are rare in women of reproductive age and therefore warrant investigation when they are diagnosed during pregnancy. Atrial fibrillation in pregnancy has been reported most often in women with rheumatic heart disease, especially mitral valve disease. Mendelson[6] reviewed 92,315 pregnancies and identified 3252 (3.5%) women with organic heart disease. Atrial fibrillation was identified in 31 (1%) women with organic heart disease, with 29 having rheumatic heart disease. Nineteen women were classified as having New York Heart Association (NYHA) class III and IV disease, and the associated maternal and fetal mortality was 19% and 58%, respectively. Five patients had embolic complications.

In a review of 8843 pregnancies, 99 of 112 women with organic heart disease had rheumatic heart disease.[20] Atrial fibrillation occurred in two patients with severe rheumatic heart disease, and both patients died. *Both of the aforementioned references were written 40–50 years ago, when the prevalence of rheumatic heart disease was higher than it is today. Atrial fibrillation secondary to rheumatic heart disease is a possibility, however, in areas of the world where women are deprived of health care and sanitary living conditions.*

Widerhorn and coworkers[4] reported on 118 women with rheumatic heart disease and revealed 15 cases of cardiac dysrhythmia, nine of which were atrial fibrillation. Six of the nine patients had atrial fibrillation before pregnancy. In the same series, atrial fibrillation was observed in three of 24 women with congenital heart disease.

Treatment

Correction is made of any contributing or underlying cause, when applicable, and either conversion of the dysrhythmia to sinus rhythm or slowing of the ventricular response in those in whom conversion does not occur is performed. Intravenous drugs used to convert acute atrial fibrillation include esmolol, procainamide, and amiodarone (popular in Europe). The use of esmolol and amiodarone in pregnancy is controversial.[44] Digitalis, calcium channel blockers and/or β-blockers are given to control the HR in chronic atrial fibrillation, which cannot be converted to sinus rhythm. In the operating room and intensive care unit, intravenous calcium channel blockers and β-blocking drugs are particularly useful because they quickly slow ventricular response, although they do not restore normal sinus rhythm. Digoxin is not as effective in the acute setting, because it usually requires more than 1 hour to slow ventricular response significantly. Adenosine slows ventricular response briefly, aiding in the diagnosis, but not the treatment, of atrial fibrillation.

When atrial fibrillation is part of a tachycardia-bradycardia syndrome, pacing may be required in addition to drug therapy. Electrical cardioversion is reserved for patients who are not responsive to drug therapy. The decision to proceed to electrical cardioversion should be made after careful evaluation of underlying heart disease, duration of the atrial fibrillation, left atrial size, and condition of the patient and fetus. Successful conversion and sustained sinus rhythm are most likely in patients with small left atria and atrial fibrillation of less than several months' duration. Administration of quinidine (after digitalization) for a few days before electrical cardioversion is recommended, because 10 to 15% of cases convert to sinus rhythm during this time. Despite successful conversion, hemodynamic improvement may not be seen immediately, because left atrial contraction may remain depressed up to several weeks.[18] Long-term therapy with digoxin and quinidine may be indicated to prevent recurrence of atrial fibrillation.

The incidence of embolization during cardioversion is 1 to 3%. If elective cardioversion is planned, special consideration should be given to thromboembolic prophylaxis. Anticoagulation is recommended in the presence of mitral stenosis; in recent-onset atrial fibrillation of more than 4 days' duration; and in association with a history of recurrent and recent emboli, prosthetic mitral valve, and dilated cardiomyopathy. If not contraindicated, anticoagulation with heparin for 2 weeks before, and several weeks following, cardioversion may help to decrease embolic complications.

Ventricular Dysrhythmias

Ventricular Tachycardia

On routine ECG, ventricular tachycardia (VT) is suggested by bizarre QRS complexes of a duration longer than 120 msec, fusion beats, capture beats, and AV dissociation. Fifty percent have retrograde conduction to the atria. Occasionally, differentiation from wide-QRS tachycardia of supraventricular origin may be difficult. For example, rapid atrial fibrillation with conduction over a bypass tract appears as a grossly irregular, rapid (200–300 bpm), wide-QRS tachycardia on ECG. Vagal maneuvers or drug therapies that slow conduction over the AV node may help in the differential diagnosis. Occasionally, electrophysiologic testing may be required. Wide-QRS tachycardia of uncertain origin should be considered as VT until proved otherwise, and it should be treated accordingly (IV lidocaine, procainamide, electrocardioversion).

VT develops by one of three mechanisms: (1) re-entry (majority); (2) abnormal automaticity; and (3) triggered activity. Most cases of VT are due to re-entry. Triggered activity occurs when the impulse is a result of early or delayed after-depolarizations. Calcium ions and slow, inward calcium channels are involved in the latter, and calcium channel blocking drugs (e.g., verapamil) may be helpful. Triggered activity may also be involved in arrhythmias associated with congenital or acquired long-QT syndrome or excess catecholamines.[4]

Some VTs occur in the absence of obvious structural cardiac abnormalities (primary electrical disease). VT in pregnancy usually falls into this category, and it may arise for the first time during pregnancy.[21–25]

Generally, the patient's prognosis is good if there is no structural heart disease, although sudden death can occur.[26, 27] Factors noted to precipitate paroxysmal VT include emotional upset, fear, exercise, caffeine, smoking, alcohol, trauma, changes in posture, hypokalemia, hypomagnesemia,[28] and imbalance of the autonomic system. Some catecholamine-sensitive, nonsustained VTs can be prevented by treatment with beta-blocking drugs and avoidance of exercise and other triggers.

VT in the presence of underlying structural heart disease has a less favorable prognosis. In descending order of frequency, VT is seen with ischemic heart disease, cardiomyopathy (dilated and hypertrophic), mitral valve prolapse, other valvular lesions, and congenital disease.

In Pregnancy

VT is rare in pregnancy. About 30 case reports have appeared in the literature over the past 50 years.[4] Overall, maternal outcome was good except for two cases of cardiac death. One maternal death involved a 19-year-old woman who died during her sixth month of pregnancy, 3 weeks after initiation of procainamide.[29] The second involved a woman with hypertrophic cardiomyopathy who died from VT at 39 weeks' gestation.[30] Paroxysmal ventricular tachycardia in women without demonstrable heart disease is reported to be more frequent in pregnancy. From the information available, it is unclear as to whether this statement is true. It is also not clear if there is a pattern of variability during various trimesters of pregnancy.[4]

Treatment

If VT is well tolerated hemodynamically, drug treatment with IV lidocaine or procainamide is initiated. If VT is unresponsive to drug therapy, direct-current cardioversion is indicated, and low energy synchronized shock (20–50 joules) is often successful in restoring normal sinus rhythm. If the patient's condition is clinically unstable, immediate treatment with cardioversion is required. VT associated with digitalis toxicity should be treated with potassium, lidocaine, propranolol, and/or phenytoin, as indicated. In those patients with a prior history of VT, continued antiarrhythmic medication throughout pregnancy is necessary.[4] Some antiarrhythmic medications increase the propensity to other arrhythmias (proarrhythmia), and these may increase the risk of sudden death. Drugs currently considered to have less proarrhythmic potential include β-blockers, mexiletine, and amiodarone. Safety of these drugs in pregnancy needs to be considered. The risks and benefits of each medication must be assessed on an individual basis.

Ventricular Fibrillation (VF)

Ventricular fibrillation should be treated according to the current ACLS protocol,[11] always with care to maintain left uterine displacement to ensure adequate venous return (see Chapter 3).

AV Blocks

First Degree AV Block

A prolonged PR interval is found in approximately 0.5% of the normal population and may be a manifestation of increased vagal tone, drug effect, and ischemic or rheumatic heart disease.[4] During pregnancy, it is associated mainly with rheumatic heart disease; but if no underlying pathology can be identified, first degree AV block has no clinical significance.

Second Degree AV Block

Mobitz type I (Wenckebach) second degree AV block is characterized by a progressive lengthening of the PR interval until an impulse is blocked (i.e., no QRS follows the blocked P wave). The condition is relatively benign and may occur during sleep or whenever vagal tone is increased. The block, which usually occurs in the AV node, is often transient and reversible. It is commonly associated with rheumatic fever, ischemia, and inferior wall myocardial infarction, or it may be a manifestation of drug effects. The block seldom progresses to complete AV block.[4] Treatment with pacing

in patients with Mobitz type I block is indicated only in seriously symptomatic patients.

Mobitz type II second degree AV block is characterized by the sudden stoppage of an impulse without previous prolongation of PR interval. Mobitz type II block *may progress to symptomatic complete heart block.* When it occurs in the presence of an acute myocardial infarction, it is usually associated with larger infarcts and higher morbidity. An accompanying BBB, frequently involving the His-Purkinje system, may be seen on ECG. Permanent pacing is recommended for pregnant women with symptomatic Mobitz type II AV block.

In Pregnancy

The incidence of second degree AV block during pregnancy is very low. The majority of cases reviewed by Mendelson[6] were acquired, occurring in association with rheumatic heart disease and infection. Among 26 cases of acquired heart block, six had second degree AV block. Only one of 21 women with congenital heart block had a second degree block.[6]

Third Degree AV Block

Third degree AV block (complete heart block—CHB) occurs when no supraventricular impulses are conducted to the ventricles. Complete AV dissociation is present, with the atrial and ventricular rates determined by their own independent pacemakers. The ventricular rate is usually low (junctional=45–50 bpm; idioventricular rate=35–45 bpm) with a faster atrial rate. Congenital third degree AV block is often nodal, resulting from immunologic offense by maternal antibodies against the fetal AV node.[31] Acquired third degree AV block is usually infranodal, involving the His-Purkinje system.

In Pregnancy

The first case of complete heart block in pregnancy was reported in 1914. Mendelson[6] reviewed the literature from 1937 to 1957 and found 47 reported cases of CHB in pregnancy, 40 of which he analyzed. Fifty percent of the patients had acquired AV block with the etiologies being rheumatic (11 cases), infection (6 cases), myocarditis (2 cases), and coronary artery disease (one case). The other 50% had congenital heart block, 10 of which were associated with ventricular septal defect. The maternal and fetal mortality rates were 13% and 15%, respectively.

Maternal and fetal prognosis for women with CHB is now much improved because of the development and success of artificial pacemakers.[32] Women with congenital CHB (Table 2–10) and normal QRS duration are usually asymptomatic and have uneventful pregnancies[33] in contrast to those with acquired heart

TABLE 2–10. CONGENITAL COMPLETE HEART BLOCK IN PREGNANCY

Incidence = 1:15,000–1:22,000 live births
ECG criteria for diagnosis (usually narrow QRS)
Slow pulse from an early age
No history of infection (diphtheria, rheumatic fever, others)
No evidence of ischemic heart disease or cardiomyopathy
No history of cardiac surgery
May present during pregnancy

block.[4] Heart block, by itself, rarely affects the course or outcome of pregnancy if the ventricular rate remains in the range of 50 to 60 bpm. If the rate slows suddenly, syncope may occur. Stokes-Adams attacks, and limited HR responses to stress, may occur. It may be necessary to insert a temporary pacemaker to manage the increased hemodynamic burden of labor and delivery. Permanent AV sequential pacing is a desirable option in symptomatic women.[4] After pacemaker placement for CHB, pregnancy is usually well tolerated (see Pacemaker section).

Dysrhythmias Associated With Heart Disease

Heart disease is congenital or acquired. Dysrhythmias associated with acquired organic heart disease are outlined in Table 2–11.

Advances in the medical and surgical management of children with congenital heart disease (CHD) over the past 25 years have resulted in an increasing number of affected females reaching childbearing age (see Chapter 1). From 1970 to 1983, CHD rose in frequency from 20 to 42% as a cause of heart disease complicating pregnancy (Table 2–12).

Specific Lesions

Patients with CHD often present with dysrhythmia in pregnancy, including (1) atrial septal defect (ASD) (women with uncorrected ASD may develop supraventricular dysrhythmias during pregnancy); (2) CHB (see earlier); (3) cyanotic CHD; and (4) mitral valve prolapse.

TABLE 2–11. DYSRHYTHMIAS ASSOCIATED WITH ORGANIC HEART DISEASE IN PREGNANCY

Aortic valve disease	Ventricular dysrhythmias PVD (84%) Multifocal PVD, couplets, runs of ventricular tachycardia (73%)
Aortic stenosis	↑ risk of severe hemodynamic problems with atrial fibrillation or junctional rhythm (loss of atrial contraction) Avoid volatile anesthetic-induced junctional rhythms
Congestive heart failure	Supraventricular dysrhythmias with atrial dilation CHF + dilated cardiomyopathy 　PVD (80%) 　Nonsustained ventricular tachycardia (50%) 　Decreasing heart chamber size may decrease atrial and ventricular dysrhythmias
IHSS	Sudden death Ventricular tachycardia
Ischemic heart disease	Ischemia/coronary vasospasm Atrial dysrhythmias Ventricular dysrhythmias Anti-ischemic therapy (nitroglycerin) may be therapeutic and more efficacious than antiarrhythmics
Mitral stenosis	Atrial fibrillation Decreased left ventricular filling/cardiac output Increased LAP and LA volume → CHF Thrombus formation atrial appendage
Mitral valve prolapse	Atrial dysrhythmias (PSVT) Ventricular dysrhythmias Prolonged Q-T Avoid hypovolemia and vasodilation (decrease LV size: ↑ prolapse)
Pericarditis	Atrial dysrhythmias ECG changes: 　Low voltage QRS complexes 　Electrical alternans 　ST segment elevation (diffuse) 　T wave inversion 　PR segment depression
Peripartum cardiomyopathy	Dysrhythmias common ECG: 　Nonspecific ST-T changes 　Infarct pattern Avoid hyperkalemia (can exacerbate dysrhythmias)

PVD = premature ventricular contraction; LAP = left atrial pressure; LA = left atrium; CHF = congestive heart failure; IHSS = idiopathic hypertrophic subaortic stenosis

TABLE 2–12. DYSRHYTHMIAS ASSOCIATED WITH CONGENITAL HEART DISEASE IN PREGNANCY

Atrial septal defect	Supraventricular dysrhythmias
Congenital heart block	Bradyarrhythmias
Ebstein anomaly	Supraventricular dysrhythmias
Eisenmenger complex	Sudden death
Mitral valve prolapse	Atrial and ventricular dysrhythmias
Tetralogy of Fallot	Conduction system disorders, heart block, bradycardia, and ventricular dysrhythmias
Transposition of the great arteries	Loss of sinus rhythm Supraventricular dysrhythmias Heart block
Tricuspid atresia, double-outlet right ventricle or single ventricle	Atrial fibrillation, sinus bradycardia, and complete AV block

Ebstein's Anomaly

Women with Ebstein's anomaly are at risk for re-entrant paroxysmal tachycardia, often via a bypass tract as seen in Wolff-Parkinson-White syndrome. The course of the pregnancy is determined by the severity of the tricuspid regurgitation, stenosis, and right-to-left shunting across the ASD. This anomaly is usually mild in the adult and some women remain asymptomatic, successfully completing pregnancy. During pregnancy, cyanosis may appear for the first time. Right ventricular failure can occur from an increase in tricuspid regurgitation. After surgical tricuspid valve reconstruction, pregnancy may result in worsening of residual tricuspid regurgitation, dysrhythmias, and endocarditis.

Eisenmenger's Complex and Pulmonary Hypertension

Death may occur suddenly, although symptomatic dysrhythmias are not often a problem until late in the natural history of the disease. Pregnancy is not tolerated well (50% maternal mortality; >40% fetal mortality), and consideration is usually given to termination of pregnancy in the first trimester.

Surgically Repaired Tetralogy of Fallot (TOF)

Important postoperative electrophysiologic sequelae, including bradycardia, conduction system disease, heart block, ventricular dysrhythmias, and sudden death, have been reported following repair of TOF.[34] Affected patients should be evaluated periodically for the presence of serious dysrhythmias.

Transposition of the Great Arteries

Most people with transposition of the great arteries undergo surgical repair before reaching childbearing age. The most common postoperative complications of the surgical procedures (atrial switch with a Senning or a Mustard procedure) are supraventricular tachycardias, loss of sinus rhythm, and heart block.[35]

Tricuspid Atresia, Double-Outlet Right Ventricle, and Single Ventricle

The electrophysiologic sequelae of the surgical repairs include atrial fibrillation, sinus bradycardia, and complete AV block.[34] In preconception counseling, these women should know that dysrhythmias may increase during pregnancy.

Mitral Valve Prolapse

Atrial and ventricular dysrhythmias occur with greater frequency, especially in those patients with resting ST segment and T wave abnormalities (Table 2–13). PSVT involving AV nodal re-entry or accessory AV connections (see later) is the most common tachyarrhythmia. A very small subset of patients with a diagnosis of mitral valve prolapse (MVP) and long QT interval syndrome may have a predisposition to ventricular tachycardia, which can result, rarely, in sudden death.

Dysrhythmias Associated With Cardiac Transplantation

The transplanted heart is denervated (Table 2–14) (see Chapter 11). The transplanted heart shows an increased sensitivity to catecholamines, but normal vagal

TABLE 2–13. MITRAL VALVE PROLAPSE IN PREGNANCY

Associated Conditions	Clinical Importance	Course
Accessory AV connections (WPW syndrome and variants) ASD Ebstein anomaly of tricuspid valve Hypertrophic cardiomyopathy Marfan syndrome Ostium secundum Long Q-T syndrome	Prolapse aggravated by hypovolemia and vasodilation Atrial dysrhythmias (PSVT) Ventricular dysrhythmias ↑ risk VT with MVP and long Q-T combined	Benign Progressive degeneration of mitral valve Mitral regurgitation Complex dysrhythmias

WPW = Wolff-Parkinson-White syndrome; VT = ventricular tachycardia; PSVT = paroxysmal supraventricular tachycardia

TABLE 2–14. CARDIAC RESPONSES AFTER HEART TRANSPLANTATION

Loss of normal vagal tone and reflex activity (denervated heart)
Delayed heart rate (HR) increase in response to stress and exercise
Attenuated HR decrease during recovery
Normal contractility
↑ sensitivity to catecholamines
Dysrhythmias (due to ↑ sensitivity to catecholamines or manifestation of rejection)

tone and reflex activity are lacking. Normal contractility is present, but chronotropic responses to stress and exercise are altered. HR increase with exercise may be delayed, and initial adaptation occurs as a result of the Frank-Starling mechanism. The usual decrease in HR during recovery is attenuated. Dysrhythmias that occur may result from the increased sensitivity to catecholamines. The dysrhythmias may be a manifestation of rejection. Only direct-acting cardiac drugs exert inotropic or chronotropic effects.

Dysrhythmias Associated With Electrolyte Abnormalities

Potassium. Ventricular dysrhythmias may occur with serum potassium (K^+) levels less than 3.0 mEq/L. Hypokalemia and hypomagnesemia may attenuate the effects of antiarrhythmic drugs. The serum K^+ level should be kept above 4.0 mEq/L.

Magnesium. Low serum magnesium (Mg) levels reduce sodium-potassium (Na^+-K^+) pump activity, which increases Na^+/Ca^{++} exchange, raises intracellular Ca^{++} levels, and reduces intracellular K^+ concentrations. It is difficult to restore intracellular K^+ in the presence of a low Mg level. Chronic Mg depletion may occur with diuretic and aminoglycoside therapy, alcohol abuse, secondary aldosteronism, and malabsorption syndromes. Serum Mg levels may not accurately reflect intracellular Mg levels, especially in chronic depletion. Reduced intracellular Mg decreases extrusion of Ca^{++} (via the Ca-adenosine triphosphatase [ATPase] pump), resulting in increased Ca^{++} currents, which are arrhythmogenic in triggered automaticity models. Mg reduces the incidence of ventricular and supraventricular dysrhythmias following myocardial infarction and after cardiac bypass operations. Mg is also beneficial in digitalis toxic dysrhythmias, torsades de pointes, and refractory ventricular dysrhythmias, even when the serum Mg level is within normal limits. Two grams of $MgSO_4$ IV, given over 2 to 3 minutes, can be used to treat ventricular dysrhythmias refractory to lidocaine or procainamide.[36]

Pre-excitation Syndromes

Definition

Pre-excitation results when an impulse originating in the atrium activates (depolarizes) the whole, or part, of the ventricular myocardium earlier than expected. The clinical syndromes that accompany short PR intervals and anomalous QRS complexes are shown in Table 2–15. Collectively they constitute the pre-excitation syndromes.[37] The incidence of pre-excitation in the normal population is 0.01 to 0.3%.[38] It occurs with increased frequency in certain conditions, such as mitral valve prolapse[39] and Ebstein's anomaly, but in the majority of cases there is no evidence of underlying heart disease.

Pathophysiology

Ventricular muscle is activated earlier than expected because an atrial impulse is conducted along anomalous myocardial muscular connections instead of along normal conduction pathways of the heart. These anomalous accessory pathways may be located anywhere around the atrioventricular rings (accessory atrioventricular bypass tracts), with left-sided pathways more common than right-sided. Nodoventricular and fasciculoventricular connections (Mahaim fibers) also exist. Ten percent of those patients with pre-excitation have multiple accessory pathways. In the best known pre-excitation syndrome, the Wolff-Parkinson-White (WPW) syndrome, conduction occurs over an accessory atrioventricular bypass tract (Kent bundle).

ECG

The ECG is characterized by a short PR interval and anomalous QRS complexes. In WPW syndrome, the typical ECG shows a PR interval of less than 120 msec with a slurred onset (δ wave) and ST-T waves directed in the opposite direction from the QRS vector (Figs. 2–2 and 2–3).

Dysrhythmias

Approximately 50% of individuals with pre-excitation develop supraventricular tachycardia at some time. Ten percent of individuals with recurrent SVT have WPW syndrome. Paroxysmal atrial tachycardia (PAT) and re-entrant AV tachycardia are the supraventricular dysrhythmias that occur most frequently in the pre-excitation syndromes. Atrial flutter or fibrillation and ventricular tachycardia, flutter, or fibrillation, however, may also occur and can be life-threatening.

Approximately 80% of the tachyarrhythmias are of the reciprocating antidromic or orthodromic type. In the antidromic variety, anterograde conduction is via the bypass tract and retrograde conduction through the AV node. In this subtype, atrial fibrillation occurs in 15 to 30%, and there is a high risk of developing very rapid ventricular rates, which may lead to ventricular fibrillation (possibly because of very rapid conduction over the accessory pathway). In the orthodromic variety, anterograde conduction occurs through the normal

TABLE 2-15. PRE-EXCITATION SYNDROMES

Type	ECG	Arrhythmias	Clinical Implications	Treatment
Wolff-Parkinson-White (WPW) syndrome Type A: premature excitation of LV via anomalous pathway Type B: premature excitation of RV	Short PR <120 ms; wide QRS >120 ms; delta wave; ST-T directed opposite delta wave + QRS vectors	Recurrent tachyarrhythmia 14–90% WPW AV re-entrant tachycardia, atrial fibrillation, atrial flutter Most often precipitated by premature beat arising in atrium, ventricle or AV junction	↑ Frequency arrhythmias in pregnancy Associated conditions: MVP Ebstein's anomaly Balloon mitral valve +/− MR ASD/forme fruste Cardiomyopathy Fetus with WPW predisposed to arrhythmias in utero	1. PSVT with wide* QRS: DC cardioversion (50–100 joules) Suspect atrial fib/flutter Procainamide IV [*adenosine contraindicated] 2. Surgical interruption of accessory pathway after epicardial mapping (when not pregnant)
Lown-Ganong-Levine syndrome variants	PR usually short; QRS normal; refractory period normal or reduced	Variety of tachyarrhythmia can be life-threatening; Tachycardia with regular narrow QRS Atrial fib with rapid ventricular response VT/VF		1. AV re-entrant tachycardia (PSVT) with narrow QRS: IV adenosine or verapamil (Alternative: digoxin or propranolol) 2. Cryoablation of AV node-His bundle
Nodoventricular + Fasciculoventricular		Re-entrant tachycardias	Associated conditions: Ebstein anomaly	

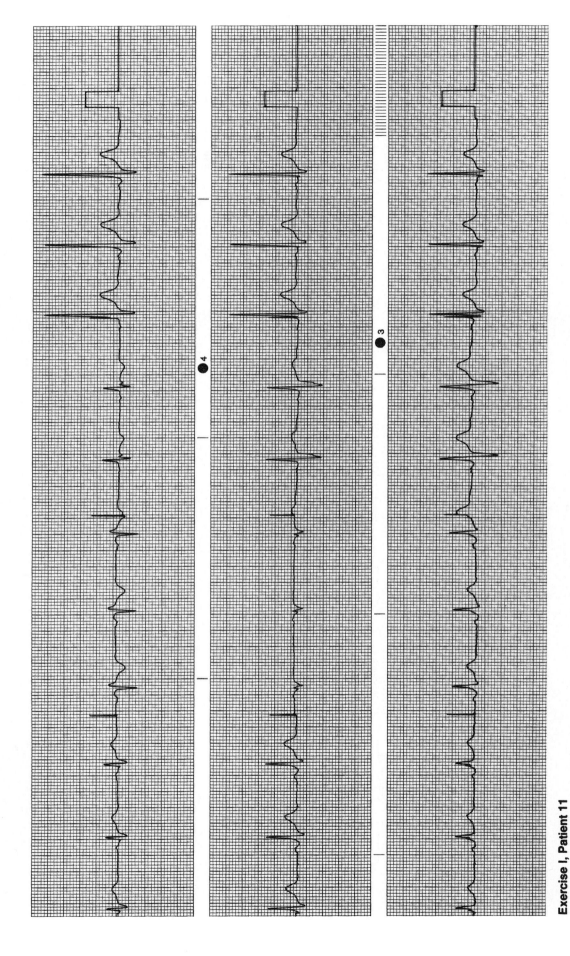

Exercise I, Patient 11

Figure 2–2. ECG tracing showing characteristics of Wolff-Parkinson-White syndrome. The R wave in V_1 is prominent, and there is T wave inversion. A short PR interval and delta waves in leads II, III, aVF, V_3 and V_4 are other features. (From Underwood DA. Clinical Electrocardiography: Self Assessment and Review. Philadelphia, WB Saunders, 1993.)

Exercise III, Patient 14

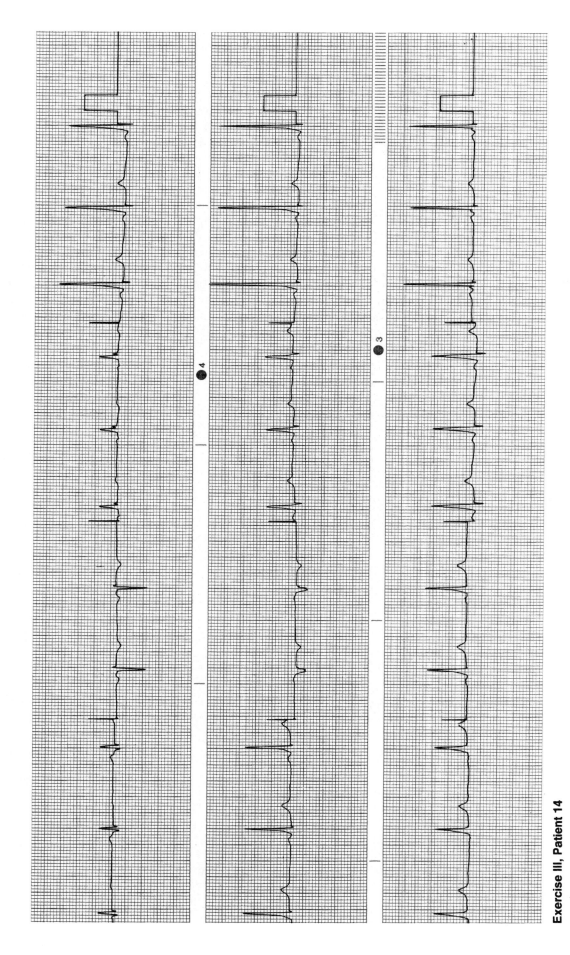

Figure 2–3. Delta waves. This ECG tracing shows sinus rhythm with delta waves throughout. The tracing is typical for WPW syndrome. (From Underwood DA. Clinical Electrocardiography: Self Assessment and Review. Philadelphia, WB Saunders, 1993.)

conduction system and retrograde conduction via the bypass tract.

In Pregnancy

As noted earlier, pregnancy may predispose women to the development of tachyarrhythmias. Women with known WPW syndrome whose condition has been stable in the nonpregnant state have developed arrhythmias during pregnancy (Table 2–16). Monitoring a parturient at risk sufficiently to identify a tachydysrhythmia, plus monitoring of the fetus to detect adverse fetal effects of a dysrhythmia is important.

Treatment

Asymptomatic women with ECG evidence of pre-excitation usually do not require treatment. Vagal stimulation (carotid sinus massage; Valsalva maneuver) is chosen frequently as the initial treatment for supraventricular tachycardia (see Table 2–8). More definitive therapy for AV tachycardia is frequently required, however. DC cardioversion is the treatment of choice when there is hemodynamic instability or when drug therapy has failed. Cardioversion has been used successfully, with no adverse effects on pregnancy, mother, or fetus, with the exception of transient fetal dysrhythmias.[41] For those who are symptomatic and hemodynamically stable, intravenous procainamide (a class IA drug) is the drug of choice to treat AV tachycardia. Various other drugs, including quinidine, disopyramide, amiodarone, and ajmaline, have been given to successfully block or decrease accessory pathway conduction in nonpregnant patients. Procainamide and quinidine may not be tolerated because of side effects, particularly nausea and vomiting. Amiodarone has been used successfully in some drug-refractory cases,[43] but its safety during pregnancy requires further evaluation.[44] Beta-adrenergic blocking drugs may also be used to slow AV node conduction. For long-term prophylaxis, oral class IA antiarrhythmic drugs alone or in combination with beta-adrenergic blocking drugs or verapamil are recommended.

Verapamil, lidocaine, and digitalis are contraindicated as single drug therapy in patients with pre-exci-

TABLE 2–16. REPORTS OF WPW IN PREGNANCY SINCE 1981

Reference	Clinical Presentation	ECG	Treatment	Outcome
Gleicher[40]	Known WPW type A Forceps delivery, oxytocin 10 u (pt 1) Chest pain, palpitations	Atrial fibrillation VR 190	Lidocaine—no response Procainamide: conversion NSR	Good
	22 wks: Palpitations and chest discomfort Chest radiograph: Bilateral interstitial infiltrates (pt 2)	HR: 240 WPW	Edrophonium, metaraminol—no response Propranolol: conversion NSR	Intermittent recurrences One prolonged episode cardioversion Good outcome
	18 wk. palpitations when walking (pt 3)	WPW Type A	Discontinue caffeine, CSM prn	Good
Klepper[41]	Three episodes tachyarrhythmias: WPW			Elective labor induction, failure to progress Cesarean section
	1. Palpitations × 12 hrs	PSVT: 180–210	CSM, Valsalva, practolol, disopyramide: no effect DC cardioversion 400 j to nodal then NSR	Good outcome
	2. 1 month later	SVT 160–170	Practolol followed by DC cardioversion	
	3. Postpartum SVT	SVT	Verapamil, DC cardioversion	
Afridi et al[42]	7 mo: Dizziness, palpitations During labor Prior to CS	SVT 230, narrow complex	Vagal maneuvers: no effect Adenosine: conversion NSR	During SVT, FHR deep variables, resolved with conversion NSR
		SVT 230	Adenosine: no effect 6 mg; 12 mg conversion NSR	
		SVT 230	Adenosine 12 mg: conversion NSR	
Widerhorn[38]	26-wk sudden-onset palpitations, lasting few min to 30 min, dizziness, SOB Symptomatic WPW	Runs of atrial tachycardia to 182	Procainamide 3 g/day	Good

WPW = Wolff-Parkinson-White syndrome; VR = ventricular rate; PSVT = paroxysmal supraventricular tachycardia; NSR = normal sinus rhythm; SVT = supraventricular tachycardia; SOB = shortness of breath; FHR = fetal heart rate; CS = cesarean section; DC = direct current; CSM = carotid sinus massage

tation syndromes. Verapamil and lidocaine may increase the ventricular rate and precipitate ventricular fibrillation. Digitalis can shorten the refractory period of the accessory pathway and, in the presence of atrial fibrillation, cause an accelerated ventricular rate. Adenosine has no effect on ventricular tachycardia or pre-excitation tachycardia[71] and can be given in the management of wide complex tachycardia of uncertain etiology. After pregnancy, women with pre-excitation and symptomatic, hemodynamically significant tachyarrhythmias should undergo electrophysiologic evaluation. Surgical or radiofrequency catheter ablation of the bypass tracts represents a definitive treatment option.[4]

Anesthesia

Tachydysrhythmias may develop during anesthesia in individuals with known WPW and other pre-excitation syndromes. Women presenting for anesthesia with an established tachycardia are, of course, best treated by first correcting the dysrhythmia (Table 2–17). In general, agents and techniques likely to cause undue tachycardia and circulatory disturbance should be avoided.

Avoiding aortocaval compression is important. The effects of such an obvious insult to cardiac output, especially if a woman is already compromised by a tachydysrhythmia, can be disastrous.

Long QT Syndrome (LQTS)

The association of a prolonged QT interval with recurrent attacks of syncope, sudden death, and malignant ventricular arrhythmias is known as the long QT syndrome (LQTS). The ventricular tachyarrhythmias are often of the distinct torsades de pointes type (twisting of the points), characterized by phasic changes in amplitude and polarity of the QRS complexes so that the peaks appear to be twisting around an imaginary isoelectric baseline. Cardiac output and blood pressure tend to fall dramatically with resultant syncope. Most

TABLE 2–17. TREATMENT: SUPRAVENTRICULAR TACHYCARDIA IN WPW

Acute Tachyarrhythmia	Rationale
Vagal maneuver	To slow conduction AV node
Drug of choice =	↓ accessory pathway
IV procainamide	conduction;
Avoid	
Lidocaine	May ↓ refractory period in
Verapamil	accessory pathway, ↑
? Adenosine	ventricular rate and precipitate VF
Cardioversion (with sedation or GA)	If symptomatic, hemodynamically unstable
Prevention	
Procainamide ± β-blocker or verapamil	↓ accessory pathway conduction; β-blockers slow AV conduction

TABLE 2–18. LQTS: CLASSIFICATION AND ETIOLOGY

Classification	Etiology
Congenital LQTS	
Inherited	Jervell, Lange-Nielsen syndrome (autosomal recessive)
	Romano-Ward syndrome (autosomal dominant)
Sporadic	
Acquired LQTS	
Drug-induced Cardiac	Antiarrhythmics*: Class Ia agents: quinidine, procainamide, disopyramide Class Ic agents: flecainamide, encainide, indecainide, lidocaine Class III agents: amiodarone, sotalol Coronary vasodilator: prenylamine
Anesthetic	Thiopentone, succinylcholine, epinephrine, norepinephrine
Psychotropic	Phenothiazines, tricyclics, tetracyclic drugs
Miscellaneous	Organophosphorus insecticides, other
Central nervous system diseases	Intracranial hemorrhage Acute cerebral thrombosis
Cardiac diseases	Bradyarrhythmias: Sick sinus syndrome, high-grade AV block Structural heart disease Ischemic heart disease, mitral valve prolapse
Electrolyte and temperature imbalance	Hypokalemia, hypomagnesemia, hypocalcemia
Metabolic abnormalities	Hypothyroidism, hypothermia

*Vaughan Williams classification of antiarrhythmic drugs

tachyarrhythmic episodes stop spontaneously with return of consciousness, but some may degenerate into ventricular fibrillation with resultant death. The long QT syndrome is classified into congenital and acquired forms (Table 2–18). Acquired LQTS is seen more commonly.

QT interval

Prolongation of the QT interval is defined as a QT interval *corrected for HR* (QTc) of more than 440 msec (Fig. 2–4). Optimal measurement of the QT interval, which varies with HR and autonomic tone, is obtained during a resting state with simultaneous recording of several limb leads and measurement of the QT interval in lead II (if T wave amplitude is reasonable). Using Bazett's formula, the QTc is obtained by dividing the measured QT interval by the square root of the preceding R-R interval, in seconds. The measured QT interval may also by compared against Simonson's age- and rate-adjusted normal range of values of the QT interval.[45] At the cellular level, the QT interval parallels the duration of the ventricular action potential. Hence, the QT interval reflects the phase of ventricular depolarization (QRS duration) as well as ventricular repolariza-

Exercise IV, Patient 4

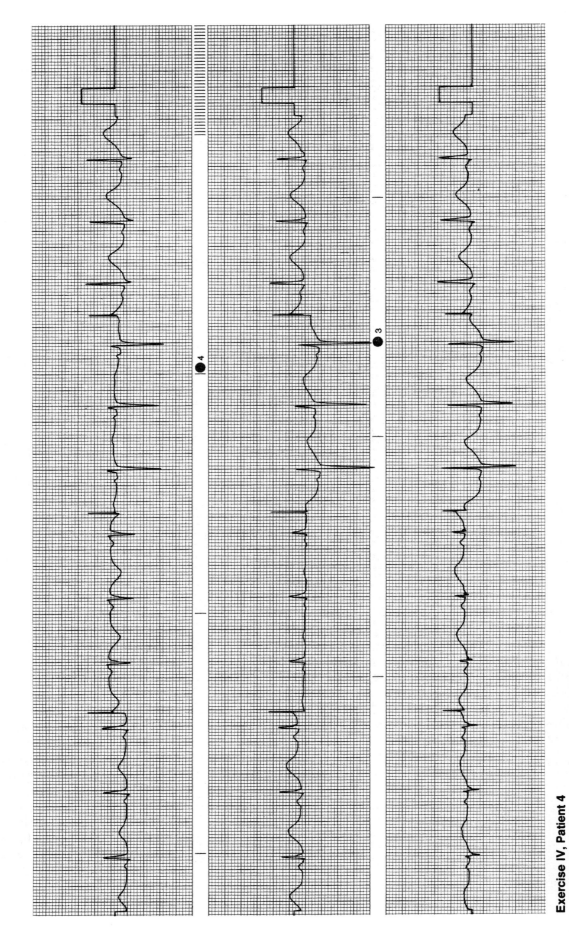

Figure 2–4. ECG tracing demonstrating a prolonged QT interval. (From Underwood DA. Clinical Electrocardiography: Self Assessment and Review. Philadelphia, WB Saunders, 1993.)

tion. A prolonged QT interval is generally taken to represent abnormal repolarization of cardiac muscle, and it is during the vulnerable relative refractory period of ventricular repolarization that ventricular dysrhythmias are most easily triggered.

Congenital LQTS

The congenital form of LQTS may be genetically determined (heritable features) or may occur sporadically (no heritable features).

Jervell, Lange-Nielsen Syndrome (Cardioauditory or Surdocardiac Syndrome):

This syndrome, first described in 1957,[46] is characterized by autosomal recessive inheritance, prolonged QT interval, and congenital bilateral sensorineural deafness. It accounts for about 30% of LQTS[47] and is estimated to occur in approximately 1% of children born with a perceptive hearing loss.[48]

Romano-Ward Syndrome

This syndrome, described in 1963 by Romano and in 1964 by Ward, is characterized by a prolonged QT interval, normal hearing, and autosomal dominance with varying expression pattern of inheritance. The fetus, due to genetic dominance, has up to a 50% probability of inheriting the disorder.[49]

Sporadic

This subgroup is characterized by prolonged QT, normal hearing, and no heritable features.

Clinical Features

The natural history and clinical presentation of the congenital syndromes vary considerably. Typically, recurrent attacks of presyncope or syncope due to torsades de pointes occur in early childhood or adulthood. Syncope tends to develop later in the sporadic LQTS subgroup. Ventricular dysrhythmias and symptoms are frequently triggered by increased sympathetic activity associated with acute emotional or physical stress. Multiple syncopal attacks and sudden death are common. The degree of QT prolongation itself does not seem to have any prognostic value.

The diagnosis of congenital LQTS combined with a family history of sudden death and a history of syncope and documented ventricular dysrhythmias, however, correlate with an increased risk for sudden death. Mortality is as high as 78% in untreated symptomatic patients with congenital LQTS. In addition to ventricular tachydysrhythmias, other dysrhythmias seen include low resting HR, sinus pauses, impaired HR increases to exercise, atrioventricular (AV) dissociation, and high-grade AV block.

The duration of the QT interval may vary from day to day, and in about one third of patients, significant prolongation of the QT interval is not seen until just before a syncopal attack or during emotional stress.

Pathophysiology

The fundamental pathogenic mechanism of congenital LQTS remains undefined.[46] Neuropathologic lesions (focal neuritis and neural degeneration within the sinus node, A-V node, His bundle, and ventricular myocardium; round cell ganglionitis of the stellate ganglia) have been identified consistently, but their exact prevalence and significance is unknown. Schwartz and coworkers[50] hypothesized that the basic defect in the syndrome involved sympathetic imbalance with relative dominance of left-sided adrenergic activity. In animals, anesthetized or unanesthetized, left stellate ganglion stimulation and/or right stellate ganglion ablation produce QT interval prolongation; episodes of T wave alternans; increased ventricular dysrhythmias during myocardial ischemia or intense psychological stress; and decreased threshold for ventricular fibrillation.[50] Similar effects have been documented in humans. Left cervicosympathectomy has been employed to suppress symptoms in patients with this syndrome.[50]

A direct cause-and-effect relationship between sympathetic imbalance and congenital LQTS has not been proven. Indirect evidence suggests that activation of the adrenergic system by fright, intense emotion, or arousal by auditory stimuli can precipitate ventricular tachyarrhythmias in vulnerable patients with LQTS. It is possible that the basic defect may be at the myocardial level involving some complex electrophysiologic mechanism as yet undefined. The sudden surges in left-sided adrenergic activity merely provide the trigger for malignant ventricular arrhythmias.[45]

Treatment

Treatment of congenital LQTS is directed toward blunting sympathetic activity, suppressing maternal ventricular tachydysrhythmias, and maintaining uteroplacental perfusion (Table 2–19).

Beta-adrenergic antagonists play a significant role in suppressing ventricular dysrhythmias in these patients. In someone with LQTS, suppression of PVD may be beneficial, because PVD can be a precursor of torsades de pointes or ventricular tachycardia. Therapy that reduces the number of syncopal episodes probably reduces the likelihood of sudden death. In full doses, β-adrenergic antagonists completely suppress, or significantly reduce, the frequency of symptoms, although the QT interval remains unaffected. An appropriate dose of propranolol is that which is maximally tolerated or produces symptomatic bradycardia. No inherent advantages exist to atenolol use, except that it is a longer acting cardioselective agent with fewer periph-

TABLE 2–19. **LQTS: TREATMENT IN PREGNANCY**

Clinical State	Treatment	Goal of Treatment
Congenital LQTS		
Benign LQTS—without syncope, family history of sudden death or complex ventricular dysrhythmias	No prophylactic treatment	1. ↓ excess sympathetic activity 2. Prevent and suppress ventricular tachydysrhythmia 3. Maintain uteroplacental perfusion
Asymptomatic LQTS—with family history of premature sudden death or with history of complex ventricular dysrhythmias	Full-dose* β-blocker	
Symptomatic LQTS		
a. ≥1 episode of syncope without prior treatment	a. Full-dose β-blocker ± phenytoin† ± phenobarb	
b. Recurrent syncope despite β-blocker ± left cervicothoracic ganglionectomy	b. Add phenytoin ± phenobarb Consider pacemaker	
c. Sustained life-threatening dysrhythmia (acute situation)	c. Temporary overdrive pacing	
Drug-refractory LQTS syncope despite intensive drug therapy or disabling drug side effects	Left cervicothoracic sympathetic ganglionectomy Chronic overdrive cardiac pacing	
Recurrent cardiac arrest	AICD‡	
Acquired LQTS		
Induced change in ECG pattern: Prolonged QTc interval (≥440 msec), ↑ PVDs ± bigeminy, VT, torsades de pointes	Discontinue causative drug Correct underlying electrolyte and metabolic abnormalities (hypokalemia, hypomagnesemia, hypocalcemia)	Early recognition Treat cause Avoid drugs and conditions that cause QT prolongation +/or potentiate ventricular dysrhythmias
Sustained torsades de pointes Prevention of recurrent malignant ventricular dysrhythmias	Electrical defibrillation Isoproterenol infusion Cardiac pacing	

*Full-dose β-blockers: β-blockers should be administered to the maximum tolerated dose/symptomatic bradycardia
†Not recommended for use in pregnancy
‡Automatic implantable cardiovertor defibrillator

eral side effects. For patients who report only partial relief of symptoms on full-dose β-blockers, the addition of phenytoin and/or phenobarbital is thought to decrease the frequency of symptoms.

Beta-adrenergic antagonists are classified as relatively safe during pregnancy and are considered acceptable treatment for important indications (e.g., significant hypertension). Phenytoin, however, has been placed in the not-recommended category, and its use in pregnancy is discouraged because of fetal hydantoin syndrome. Left cervicothoracic sympathectomy has been recommended for patients who have symptoms refractory to maximal drug therapy or those who develop intolerable drug side effects.[45] Left cervicothoracic sympathectomy meets with varied success, and recurrent symptoms that do not always respond to drug therapy can be a problem. Chronic overdrive pacing with or without β-blockers may be an effective option for these patients, as well as for those who develop significant bradyarrhythmias from β-blockers. Temporary overdrive pacing as a therapy for a life-threatening dysrhythmia is an effective treatment option.

With patients having recurrent cardiac arrest or symptoms refractory to all of the aforementioned modalities, implantation of an automatic implantable cardioverter/defibrillator (AICD) should be considered. It is recommended that patients with congenital LQTS avoid loud noises and vigorous physical exertion with sudden demands for maximal performance.

Acquired LQTS

Acquired LQTS, which is more common than congenital LQTS, is a heterogeneous syndrome with many possible causes, including drugs, central nervous system diseases, ischemic heart diseases, bradyarrhythmias, and metabolic and electrolyte abnormalities (see Table 2–18). A minority of patients with QT prolongation, from any cause, are at risk for developing torsades de pointes (ventricular tachydysrhythmia). The mechanism involved is unclear, and it is not known how to predict who is at risk for developing this serious dysrhythmia.[45]

Etiology

Effects of antiarrhythmic drugs are the most common cause of torsades de pointes. All drugs that cause QT interval prolongation (see Table 2–18) have been associated with torsades de pointes. Antiarrhythmic drug-induced torsades de pointes appears to be an idiosyncratic reaction with an estimated incidence of 1 to 2%.[45] Quinidine, procainamide, and disopyramide (class Ia drugs) cause torsades de pointes with about equal frequency. Flecainide, encainide, indecainide, lidocaine (class Ic drugs); amiodarone, sotalol (class III drugs); and prenylamine (coronary vasodilator) produce this dysrhythmia less commonly.[45] Torsades de pointes has not been reported with class Ib drugs, which shorten the QT interval, nor with pure β-adrenergic blockers or calcium antagonists. In about half of patients, drug-induced torsades de pointes occurs within the first 3 to 4 days of initiation of therapy, but late-onset occurrence (months to years later), usually in association with a change in drug dose, electrolyte imbalance, or bradyarrhythmia, is also seen.[45] Warning signs of an impending drug-induced torsades de pointes may be the new appearance of a peculiar ventricular bigeminy, with late cycle PVD and bizarre postpause T wave changes in association with a moderate QT prolongation.[45]

Phenothiazines and tricyclic antidepressant drugs, which are similar to quinidine electrophysiologically, increase the duration of the QRS complex, prolong the QT interval, and cause T wave flattening with U wave prominence. These ECG changes occur in about 50% of patients treated with phenothiazines (thioridazine >chlorpromazine or trifluoperazine) and in about 20% of patients treated with tricyclic antidepressants. Increased ventricular irritability is a potential complication with therapeutic, as well as toxic, doses of these psychotropic drugs. Although the risk of torsades de pointes dysrhythmia is relatively low, the condition has been documented to occur with the majority of psychotropic drugs, thioridazine being implicated most often.

LQTS is sometimes associated with central nervous system diseases such as intracranial aneurysm, acute cerebral thrombosis, and brain metastases. Torsades de pointes has been well documented in some cases of subarachnoid hemorrhage. Torsades de pointes can also be precipitated by severe hypokalemia and severe hypomagnesemia, alone or in combination, and by hypokalemia in combination with antiarrhythmic or psychotropic drug therapy. Although hypocalcemia may prolong the QT interval, it is seldom associated with the development of torsades de pointes. Torsades de pointes is a rare complication of liquid-protein modified-fast dieting in individuals who have had significant rapid weight loss over a short period of time and exhibit QT prolongation on ECG. Bradyarrhythmias can also cause torsades de pointes. Ventricular arrhythmias (some torsades de pointes in morphology) are implicated as a cause of syncope in 10 to 60% of patients with high-grade AV block and syncope, and in 4 to 7% with SSS and syncope.[45] Some patients with mitral valve prolapse, who also have QTc prolongation, have a higher prevalence of ventricular arrhythmias.

Treatment

Treatment of acquired LQTS is directed toward early diagnosis of torsades de pointes and correction, or elimination, of its etiologic factors. Failure to diagnose LQTS may lead to continued use of the offending agent as well as of antiarrhythmic drugs capable of further prolonging the QT interval, thus increasing the risk of developing a fatal dysrhythmia.

Immediate therapy should include withdrawal of the offending agents and correction of any underlying electrolyte abnormality. Sustained torsades de pointes can be terminated with electrical defibrillation. Subsequent recurrences are prevented by increasing the HR (shortens the QT interval) with an isoproterenol infusion or temporary cardiac pacing. Isoproterenol has the advantage of acting rapidly (within minutes), but it is not always effective and it carries some risks in patients with uncontrolled systemic hypertension, angina, or acute myocardial infarction. Temporary pacing abolishes torsades de pointes rapidly and is useful when isoproterenol is contraindicated. Atrial pacing, which maintains AV synchrony, as well as normal depolarization of the ventricles, may be superior to ventricular pacing. Other drugs that have been administered to treat torsades de pointes include lidocaine, atropine, phenytoin, magnesium sulfate, bretylium tosylate, and amiodarone. *Magnesium sulfate is currently the drug of choice.*[43]

LQTS in Pregnancy

Over 900 cases of LQTS have been described, but there are relatively few reports of LQTS in pregnancy. Table 2–20 summarizes the initial presentation, clinical course, and outcome for eight pregnant women with congenital LQTS reported in the literature from 1984 to 1995. Interpretation of fetal cardiotocographic monitoring may be difficult when full doses of β-adrenergic blocking drugs are administered to the mother, or when there is a possibility that the fetus may have inherited the cardiac conduction defect. Monitoring for fetal acidosis with periodic fetal scalp sampling may be the only way to adequately diagnose fetal distress. Neonatal bradycardia and hypoglycemia consequent to beta-blockade should be anticipated and managed as necessary.

Anesthetic Management

Several case reports can be found for the anesthetic management of the patient with LQTS (Table 2–21).[57–62] Because high levels of circulating catecholamines are postulated to precipitate dysrhythmias in patients with LQTS, it is important to allay emotional stress and anxiety. Drugs and techniques that minimize catecholamine release and cardiac sensitization to catecholamines should be selected. For those individuals who are profoundly deaf (those with Jervell or Lange-Nielsen syndrome), effective communication and reduction of stress and anxiety, may be enhanced by an interpreter skilled in deaf signage. Treatment of conditions

TABLE 2–20. **CONGENITAL LQTS IN PREGNANCY: CASE REPORTS**

Reference	Clinical Course	ECG	Treatment	Outcome
Freshwater[51]	JLN syndrome; deafness +, Hx syncope + + + Two uneventful pregnancies; both deliveries by elective CS with GA	QTc 530 msec No documented dysrhythmias	Propranolol	Good
Bruner[52]	LQTS, unspecified Uneventful pregnancy Forceps delivery with LEA	No information	Left stellate ganglion block	Good
Ryan[53]	JLN, deafness + +, syncope + + + Hx VF + cardiac arrest age 12 yr Uneventful pregnancy Fetal distress during labor → emergency CS with LEA 5 mo postpartum: cardiac arrest × 2	QTc 540 msec	Procainamide	Good
Gutgesell[54]	Romano-Ward, no syncope; history of multiple ventricular arrhythmias requiring cardioversion Uneventful pregnancy Spontaneous vaginal delivery with LEA	No information	Bretylium Propranolol Atenolol K+, Mg +, Spironolactone	Good
Wilkinson[47]	LQTS, syncope +, history of cardiac arrest Uneventful pregnancy Forceps delivery with LEA	QTc 520 msec	Propranolol	Twins with: congenital LQTS; treated with propranolol
Heidegger[49]	Romano-Ward, no syncope Uneventful pregnancy Immediately postpartum: isolated supraventricular extrasystoles (QT 510 msec)	QTc 470 msec ↑ QT prolongation (630 msec) during CS with GA	None	Good
McCurdy[55]	Romano-Ward, syncope at 29 wks with documented VT/VF, fetal distress with recovery CS with LEA	QTc 650 msec	Cardioversion Propranolol Esmolol	Maternal outcome good; Neonate: congenital LQTS treated with propranolol
Ganta[56]	Romano-Ward, no syncope, bradycardia, occasional PVD Emergency CS with LEA	QTc 420 msec	Atenolol Diltiazem	Good

CS = caesarean section; GA = general anesthesia; JLN = Jervell, Lange-Nielsen syndrome; LEA = lumbar epidural anesthesia; LQTS = long Q-T syndrome; VF = ventricular fibrillation; VT = ventricular tachycardia; PVD = premature ventricular depolarization

TABLE 2–21. **LQTS IN PREGNANCY: ANESTHETIC CONSIDERATIONS**

Assessment

1. Establish whether congenital or acquired LQTS
2. Assess status:
   a. Electrolytes
   b. Temperature
   c. Blood pressure

   d. Pain
   e. Physical/emotional stress and anxiety

3. History drugs known to cause QT interval prolongation
   a. Antidysrhythmics
   b. Psychotropic drugs
   c. Anesthetic drugs

4. History ventricular dysrhythmias + / − bradyarrhythmias

1. Continue (or establish) appropriate treatment
2. Avoid triggering cardiac dysrhythmias and increasing catecholamine (CA) levels:
   a. Correct hypokalemia, hypomagnesemia, hypocalcemia
   b. Correct hypothermia
   c. Avoid/correct hypotension (left uterine displacement, hydration, vasopressors)
   d. Adequate pain relief
   e. Avoid sudden loud noises. vigorous physical exertion (sudden demands for maximal performance) in congenital LQTS
   f. Provide information, reassurance, emotional support
   g. Deaf signage if needed (Jervell, Lange-Nielsen syndrome [JLN])
   h. Judicious use of anxiolytics
3. Avoid or use cautiously
   a. Quinidine, procainamide, disopyramide, flecainamide, encainamide, indocainamide, lidocaine, sotalol, prenylamine
   b. Phenothiazines, tricyclic antidepressants, lithium
   c. Thiopentone (minimal QT prolongation), succinylcholine, norepinephrine, ephedrine
4. Anticipate and be prepared to treat with drugs, defibrillation, overdrive pacing

Labor and Delivery

1. Monitors and special preparation

2. Interpretation of fetal cardiographic monitoring

3. Avoid aortocaval compression
4. Evaluate effects of therapy on fetus and neonate

1. Monitor mother and fetus, continuous monitoring if symptoms or dysrhythmia; defibrillator on standby: immediately available
2. Fetal heart rate (FHR) and pattern may reflect β-blocker therapy (or other antiarrhythmic drug) or possible inherited LQTS abnormality
   Fetal scalp sampling may be required to establish fetal acidosis and diagnose fetal distress
3. Ensure left uterine displacement
4. Diagnosis of fetal distress from FHR may be difficult, may need fetal scalp sampling. Treat neonatal bradycardia, hypoglycemia if indicated

Regional Anesthesia (RA)

1. Sympathetic nervous system blockade

2. Hemodynamic stability

3. Lumbar epidural anesthesia (LEA)

4. Subarachnoid block

1. Advantageous (decreases CA levels); avoid relative parasympathetic overdrive, sudden bradycardia (PR prolongation)
2. Avoid precipitous drop in BP, use direct and indirect vasopressors judiciously to avoid triggering dysrhythmias and consequences of hypotension and
3. Titrate local anesthetic cautiously. Allows more hemodynamic stability. Avoid epinephrine with LA or take precautions to avoid IV injection
4. Quality/density of block usually better (less pain)
   Block level less predictable and less controllable
   May be more hypotension—treat judiciously
   Treat significant bradycardia immediately with atropine/ephedrine

General Anesthesia

1. Rapid sequence induction and intubation

2. Catecholamine increases

3. Myocardial sensitization to CA
4. Drugs with sympathomimetic properties
5. Drugs with documented safety in LQTS

1. Minimize CA response; β-blocker useful (topical/IV lidocaine may prolong QT interval)
2. Maintain adequate depth of anesthesia; avoid hypoxia, hypercarbia, hypotension
3. Avoid halothane
4. Avoid or use cautiously (ketamine, pancuronium, atropine)
5. Thiopentone (minimal QT prolongation; clinically insignificant), vecuronium, fentanyl, isoflurane

LQTS = long QT syndrome; CA = catecholamine; LA = local anesthetic

known to aggravate QT prolongation, such as hypokalemia, hypomagnesemia, and hypocalcemia, should be undertaken and drugs like procainamide, quinidine, lidocaine, and phenothiazines avoided.

PACEMAKERS AND RELATED DEVICES IN PREGNANCY

Women with pacemakers have conceived and carried pregnancies to completion successfully. Pacemakers have also been implanted during pregnancy with good maternal and fetal outcomes. Current pacemakers and related devices provide more sophisticated support of the cardiovascular adaptations imposed by pregnancy than in the past. For example, rate-responsive pacemakers, which can be programmed to sense a variety of stimuli (e.g., muscle activity, minute ventilation) in addition to atrial and ventricular activity, respond by increasing the HR when there is a need for greater cardiac output.[63]

Pacemakers in Pregnancy

A parturient is most likely to present with or require a pacemaker or pacemaker-related device[64-67] (e.g., implantable cardioverter-defibrillator/ICD) for definitive or prophylactic treatment of an intrinsic or surgically-induced second degree (type II) or third degree heart block; a symptomatic, hemodynamically significant bradydysrhythmia or tachydysrhythmia (recurrent or unresponsive to drugs); or a potential life-threatening dysrhythmia. In a pregnant woman, such dysrhythmias or conduction problems are seen mostly in conjunction with an intrinsic cardiac condition (congenital, rheumatic, or ischemic heart disease; a pre-excitation syndrome; long QT syndrome) or in association with a cardiac surgical procedure. Pacemaker therapy is occasionally chosen because of drug refractoriness or intolerance to side effects.

Pacemaker/ICD-Associated Complications in Pregnancy

The probability of successful completion of pregnancy with a pacemaker is favorable (Table 2–22). Although uncommon in pregnancy (approximately 25 reports in the literature since 1962), there have been documented problems associated with pacemakers.[68] Appropriate recognition and treatment of these complications are essential to ensure optimal maternal and fetal outcomes.[69]

TABLE 2–22. PACEMAKER-ASSOCIATED COMPLICATIONS IN PREGNANCY

Discomfort at implantation site
Ulceration at implantation site
Pacemaker failure
New signs and symptoms
  Dizziness (exertion/rest)
  Dyspnea (exertion/rest)
  Pulmonary edema
  Dysrhythmia
  Extrasystoles
  Tachycardia
Intrauterine growth retardation
Fetal dysrhythmia

Anesthetic Management of the Parturient with a Pacemaker/ICD

Patients require careful evaluation of their functional status and a specific review of their underlying heart disease, seeking new or recurrent cardiac signs and symptoms (chest pain, confusion, dizziness, shortness of breath, syncope). A thorough assessment of pacemaker type and function should be performed (Tables 2–23 and 2–24). Depending on the pacemaker type and programming (e.g., antitachycardia pacemaker), there may be special adjustments required. Interference from electrical sources (cautery, transcutaneous electrical nerve stimulation) or from other stimuli (shivering, excess catecholamines, fever) may have important consequences (Table 2–25). Consultation with a cardiologist regarding appropriate programming is beneficial. Generally speaking, these patients benefit from good analgesia during labor. Epidural analgesia decreases catecholamine release and allows flexibility if operative intervention is required.

DRUG THERAPY DURING PREGNANCY

The reader is referred to a good general summary on drugs of choice (doses and effects) for common

TABLE 2–23. ANESTHETIC REVIEW: PAST HISTORY OF PACEMAKER

Assessment	Goal
Indications	Optimize pacemaker
Signs/symptoms at time of insertion	functioning to meet ↑ demands antepartum, labor/ delivery, postpartum
Course to date	
Type, model, response mode(s) of pacemaker See patient ID card if available	
Pulse generator: replacement due date (5–10 year lifespan device and operation mode(s))	
Date pacemaker most recently evaluated	

TABLE 2–24. ANESTHETIC ASSESSMENT: PACEMAKER FUNCTION

Component	Potential Problems	Action
Pulse generator pocket	Discomfort at implantation site Ulceration at implantation site May become mobile/loose with external manipulation	Identify problems with generator pocket (implantation site)
Location Pectoralis muscle (sc pocket) L or R subclavian area Abdomen LUQ	Usual location unless myopotential inhibition has been a problem Not an appropriate location during pregnancy	Note location of pulse generator Re-locate appropriately if necessary
Pulse generator (PG) Size/shape (usual = 2"×5") Components Microchip (contains program)	Malfunction Capture problems Sensing problems	Review ECG for appropriate sensing, pacing, capture† Confirm capture by demonstration of a pulse simultaneously with ECG Avoid absorption of toxic amounts of LA which can lead to loss of capture
Battery (= most of unit); runs the microchip	Battery failure Competitive inhibition (Electromagnetic interference) Transcutaneous electrical nerve stimulators (TENS) Electrocautery Peripheral nerve stimulators	Replace battery if battery is known to be at end-of-life or soon due for elective replacement Avoid or use very cautiously: Magnet in presence of electromagnetic interference TENS Electrocautery Peripheral nerve stimulator
Epicardial leads	Lead displacement/fracture: ↑ likelihood with newly placed or temporary leads/trauma Common sites: Lead/PG connection Insertion into subclavian vein Clavicle/1st rib	If necessary, chest radiograph can identify: Number, position, integrity of pacing leads Pacemaker ID code Caution regarding PAC monitoring with recently inserted pacemaker leads Ensure external pacemaker leads well-insulated from contact with any source of potential current leakage
Rate-responsive pacemakers (PM) Stimuli sensing options: Muscle activity—responsive MV(TV + RR)—responsive Evoke QT—responsive Temperature-responsive RV dP/dT (preload/afterload)	Competitive sensing/capture Fasciculations, shivering, seizures Positive pressure ventilation CA‡ triggered 'R on T' Body temperature changes Hemodynamic changes	Know how PM is programmed regarding response modes Beware potential problems, make appropriate adjustments and verify PM function afterward Avoid shivering/fasciculations; avoid Sux except RSI; nondepolarizing MRs preferable; RA not contraindicated Control TV RR Minimize CA discharge Keep temperature normal Consult cardiologist regarding appropriate programming

*Use in pregnant women only when definitely indicated
†Capture may be confirmed by demonstration of a pulse simultaneously with ECG monitoring
‡Catecholamine
MV = minute ventilation; PAC = pulmonary artery catheter; Sux = succinylcholine; RSI = rapid sequence induction; MR = muscle relaxant; TV = tidal volume; RR = respiratory rate

dysrhythmias.[43] When considering the appropriate therapeutic intervention in the pregnant woman, it is important to be aware of the effects on the fetus as well as on the mother. Concerns include their teratogenetic potential, possible adverse effects on the fetus and newborn, and drug transmission into breast milk. An excellent reference for up-to-date information on the safety and efficacy of drugs in pregnancy and lactation is available.[44] Each drug is assigned a fetal risk category and a recommendation is made. It is important to differentiate between the use of a drug in an emergency situation, such as treatment of a dysrhythmia in a hemodynamically unstable patient, and long-term ther-

apy, and the use during the period of organogenesis. The risks and benefits must be assessed for each individual situation. Drugs commonly chosen to treat dysrhythmias during pregnancy are summarized in Table 2–26.

Adenosine

Adenosine, now used commonly as the initial drug treatment for acute narrow complex tachycardia (PSVT), successfully terminates more than 90% of PSVT.[70, 71] Adenosine depresses SA node automaticity

37. Gallagher JJ, Pritchett ELD, Sealy WC, et al. The pre-excitation syndromes. Prog Cardiovasc Dis 1978;20:285.

38. Widerhorn J, Widerhorn ALM, Rahimtoola SH, et al. WPW syndrome during pregnancy: Increased incidence of supraventricular arrhythmias. Am Heart J 1992;123:796.

39. Fuenzalida CE. A selective advantage with mitral valve prolapse (letter). Ann Intern Med 1983;98:670.

40. Gleicher N, Meller J, Sandler JZ, et al. Wolff-Parkinson-White syndrome in pregnancy. Obstet Gynecol 1981;58:748.

41. Klepper I. Cardioversion in late pregnancy. The anaesthetic management of a case of Wolff-Parkinson-White syndrome. Anaesthesia 1981;36:611.

42. Afridi I, Moise KJ, Rokey R. Termination of supraventricular tachycardia with intravenous adenosine in a pregnant woman with Wolff-Parkinson-White syndrome. Obstet Gynecol 1991;80:481.

43. Drugs for cardiac arrhythmias. Med Lett 1996;38:75.

44. Briggs GG, Freeman RK, Yaffe SJ. Drugs in Pregnancy and Lactation, 4th ed. Baltimore, Williams & Wilkins, 1994.

45. Bhandari AK, Nguyen PT, Scheinman MM. Congenital and acquired long QT syndromes. In Chatterjee K, Chemlin MD, Karliner J, et al. (eds): Cardiology: An Illustrated Text/Reference, vol I. Philadelphia, J.B. Lippincott, 1991, p 6.258.

46. Jervell A, Lange-Nielsen F: Congenital deaf-mutism, functional heart disease with prolongation of the QT interval and sudden death. Am Heart J 1957;54:59.

47. Wilkinson C, Gyaneshwar R, McCusker C. Twin pregnancy in a patient with idiopathic QT syndrome. Case report. Br J Obstet Gynaecol 1991;98:1300.

48. Ratshin RA, Hunt D, Russell RO, et al. QT-interval prolongation, paroxysmal ventricular arrhythmias, and convulsive syncope. Ann Intern Med 1971;75:919.

49. Heidegger H, v. Hugo R, Plötz J. Hereditär verlängertes Qtintervall (Romano Ward Syndrom) im geburtshilflichen management. Geburtshilfe Frauenheilkunde 1993;53:201.

50. Schwartz PJ, Periti M, Malliani A. The long Q-T syndrome. Am Heart J 1975;89:378.

51. Freshwater JV. Anaesthesia for Caesarean section and the Jervell, Lange-Nielsen syndrome (prolonged Q-T interval syndrome). Br J Anaesth 1984;56:655.

52. Bruner JP, Barry MJ, Elliott JP. Pregnancy in a patient with idiopathic long QT syndrome. Am J Obstet Gynecol 1984;149:690.

53. Ryan H. Anaesthesia for Caesarean section in a patient with Jervell, Lange-Nielsen syndrome. Can J Anaesth 1988;35:422.

54. Gutgesell M, Overholt E, Boyle R. Oral bretylium tosylate use during pregnancy and subsequent breastfeeding: A case report. Am J Perinatol 1990;7:144.

55. McCurdy CM, Rutherford SE, Coddington CC. Syncope and sudden arrhythmic death complicating pregnancy. A case of Romano-Ward syndrome. J Reprod Med 1993;38:233.

56. Ganta R, Roberts C, Elwood RJ, et al. Epidural anesthesia for cesarean section in a patient with Romano-Ward syndrome (letter). Anesth Analg 1995;81:424.

57. Wilton NCT, Hantler CB. Congenital long QT syndrome: Changes in QT interval during anesthesia with thiopental, vecuronium, fentanyl, and isoflurane. Anesth Analg 1987;66:357.

58. Brown M, Liberthson RR, Ali HH, et al. Perioperative anesthetic management of a patient with long Q-T syndrome (LQTS). Anesthesiology 1981;55:586.

59. Medak R, Benumof JL. Perioperative management of the prolonged Q-T interval syndrome. Br J Anaesth 1983;55:361.

60. Galloway PA, Glass PSA. Anesthetic implications of prolonged QT interval syndromes. Anesth Analg 1985;64:612.

61. Ponte J, Lund J. Prolongation of the Q-T interval (Romano-Ward syndrome): Anaesthetic management. Br J Anaesth 1981;53:1347.

62. Owitz S, Pratilas V, Pratila MG, et al. Anaesthetic considerations in the prolonged Q-T interval (LQTS): A case report. Can Anaesth Soc J 1979;26:50.

63. Bourke ME. The patient with a pacemaker or related device. Can J Anaesth 1996;43:R24.

64. Gudal M, Kervancioglu C, Oral D, et al. Permanent pacemaker implantation in a pregnant woman with the guidance of ECG and two-dimensional echocardiography. PACE 1987;10:543.

65. Holdright DR, Sutton GC. Restoration of sinus rhythm during two consecutive pregnancies in a woman with congenital complete heart block. Br Heart J 1990; 64: 338.

66. Lau CP, Lee CP, Wong CK, et al. Rate responsive pacing with a minute ventilation sensing pacemaker during pregnancy and delivery. Pace 1990;13:158.

67. Matorras R, Diez J, Saez M, et al. Repeat pregnancy associated with cardiac pacemaker. Int J Gynecol Obstet 1991;36:323.

68. Jaffe R, Gruber A, Fejgin M, et al. Pregnancy with an artificial pacemaker. Obstet Gynecol Surv 1987;42:137.

69. Terhaar M, Schakenbach L. Care of the pregnant patient with a pacemaker. J Perinat Neonatal Nurs 1991;5:1.

70. Lerman BB, Belardinelli L. Cardiac electrophysiology of adenosine. Basic and clinical concepts. Circulation 1991;83:1499.

71. Camm AJ, Garratt CJ. Adenosine and supraventricular tachycardia. N Engl J Med 1991;325:1621.

72. Podolsky SM, Varon J. Adenosine use during pregnancy. Ann Emerg Med 1991;20:1027.

73. Harrison JK, Greenfield RA, Wharton JM. Acute termination of supraventricular tachycardia by adenosine during pregnancy. Am Heart J 1992;123:1386.

74. Leffler S, Johnson DR. Adenosine use in pregnancy: Lack of effect on fetal heart rate. Am J Emerg Med 1992;19:548.

75. Matfin G, Baylis P, Adams P. Maternal paroxysmal supraventricular tachycardia treated with adenosine (letter). Postgrad Med J 1993;69:661.

76. Mason BA, Ogunyemi D, Punla O, Koos BJ. Maternal and fetal cardiorespiratory responses to adenosine in sheep. Am J Obstet Gynecol 1993;168:1558.

77. Wheeler CPD, Yudilevish DL. Transport and metabolism of adenosine in the perfused guinea pig placenta. J Physiol 1988;405:511.

CARDIOPULMONARY RESUSCITATION
. . . .

Mark D. Johnson, M.D., Carol J. Luppi, R.N., and Dawn C. Over, M.B., F.R.C.A.

Cardiac arrest in the pregnant patient is a rare and unexpected event, which is currently estimated to occur about once in 30,000 pregnancies.[1] As a result, the obstetric team has limited experience with this problem and little opportunity to develop the reflex responses required for efficient management of such an emergency.

The incidence, however, may be increasing. In the past, most pregnant women were young and healthy. Advances in medical technology and changing social trends are increasing the size of the high-risk obstetric population. The new obstetric population includes older women who have postponed childbearing and are at greater risk for medical and obstetric complications. Drug-related complications, especially those related to abuse of powdered or "crack" cocaine, are seen with increasing frequency in pregnant patients. In addition, women afflicted with medical conditions that previously jeopardized their own lives are now surviving to childbearing ages. Intricate medical and surgical interventions are sometimes performed during pregnancy to optimize maternal and fetal well-being. These advanced care techniques often require sophisticated technology and inherently place the parturient at greater risk. Even the low-risk parturient is vulnerable to iatrogenic, traumatic, and pregnancy-induced complications that may lead to cardiac arrest.[2-5]

The application of the American Heart Association (AHA) Cardiopulmonary Resuscitation (CPR) protocol in response to a cardiac arrest in the general population has improved survival rates.[2, 6] The anatomic and physiologic changes of pregnancy and labor result in a significantly decreased cardiovascular and pulmonary reserve,[7-13] which complicates resuscitation. In addition, the fetus is both a complicating factor and a patient in its own right. Specific obstetric resuscitation protocols published by Lee and colleagues[14] and discussed in various lecture series by Harvey and colleagues[15] have addressed these issues. A review of the available clinical and experimental evidence suggests that further modification of these protocols may improve the chance of a successful outcome for mother and fetus.[14-16] An alternative protocol intended to increase the efficiency of resuscitation is discussed.

CAUSES OF CARDIOPULMONARY ARREST IN PREGNANCY

Cardiac arrest in pregnancy may arise as a result of pathologic processes within the patient; cardiac arrest may also result from iatrogenic factors or trauma.[3-5, 17-21] The causes are diverse and can affect even healthy parturients (Table 3–1).

Hemorrhage

Two of the most common causes of cardiopulmonary arrest in pregnancy are airway misadventure and hemorrhage. The clinical signs of hypovolemia and major hemorrhage may be subtle. The pregnant patient can lose up to 35% of her circulating blood volume before displaying the classic signs of hypovolemia.[22] A substantial part of the patient's circulating volume can be lost without external evidence (for example, placental abruption or post-laparotomy bleeding). Recognition of the severity of blood loss may be critically delayed. Obstetric hemorrhage may also be complicated by coagulopathy occurring as a result of amniotic fluid embolism or severe pregnancy-induced hypertension (PIH). The more subtle signs of early hypovolemia must be appreciated and sought (Table 3–2).

Local Anesthetic Toxicity

Another important cause of cardiopulmonary arrest in pregnancy is local anesthetic toxicity. Regional analgesia and anesthesia are widely used in obstetric practice. Cardiac arrest can arise from (1) direct cardiotoxicity from intravascular overdose; (2) hypotension caused by an excessively high regional block; and (3) rare severe allergic reaction. High regional blocks are, relatively easily, managed by prompt control of the airway and cardiorespiratory support. Intravascular toxicity is a more sinister problem. The definitive management may be different in each case. The local anesthetic agent is also relevant. A brief review of the

TABLE 3–1. **CAUSES OF CARDIOPULMONARY ARREST IN PREGNANCY**

Inadequate ventilation (see Chapter 5)	Failed intubation Esophageal intubation Pulmonary aspiration Airway obstruction
Hemorrhage	Uterine atony Placental abruption Placenta previa/accreta/increta/percreta DIC* Rare—ruptured splenic artery aneurysm
Ventilation/perfusion mismatch	Hypovolemia Bronchospasm (see Chapter 8) Pneumothorax (see Chapter 9) Pulmonary embolism (see Chapter 10)—thrombus, amniotic fluid, air, fat Pulmonary pathology Pulmonary aspiration
Iatrogenic anesthetic–related	Intravascular local anesthetic overdose Total spinal anesthesia Drug allergy (rare) Regional anesthetic induced sympathectomy
Severe pregnancy-induced hypertension	
Drug-related	Illicit drug abuse Drug error Anaphylaxis Drug overdose Hypermagnesemia (see Table 3–3)
Septic shock	
Trauma	
Cerebral pathology (see Chapter 16)	Subarachnoid hemorrhage Brainstem herniation (cerebral edema)
Pre-existing heart disease (see Chapter 1)	Congenital heart disease Acquired valvular disease Dysrhythmia Myocardial infarction
Recent-onset heart disease	Idiopathic peripartum cardiomyopathy Dysrhythmia (possible electrolyte imbalance) Traumatic myocardial contusion Myocardial infarction
Malignant hyperthermia (see Chapter 21)	

*DIC = disseminated intravascular coagulation.

problems associated with local anesthetic-induced cardiopulmonary arrest is therefore appropriate.

The mechanisms of local anesthetic cardiotoxicity have been extensively investigated in animal models. In high dosages, local anesthetics cause generalized depression of myocardial contractility[23]; progressively decrease the rate of phase-4 depolarization[24]; inhibit conduction of impulses from the SA node to atrial muscle[25]; prolong the effective refractory period[26, 27]; decrease the maximal rate of depolarization (V_{max}) of isolated ventricular muscle fibers[25, 28]; and decrease heart rate, stroke volume, cardiac output, and systemic vascular resistance.[26] These toxic effects are enhanced in the pregnant patient because physiologic alterations in blood volume, cardiac output, functional residual capacity, oxygen consumption, and plasma protein concentrations result in an increased volume of distribution of local anesthetics and a decreased cardiopulmonary reserve. Increased plasma progesterone concentrations in pregnancy render the heart more sensitive to membrane-depressant effects of local anesthetics.[29]

The more potent, lipid-soluble, longer acting local anesthetics (bupivacaine and etidocaine) have a narrower safety margin between the serum concentrations producing neurotoxicity (i.e., seizures) and cardiovascular collapse.[30] They also exhibit the most cardiotoxicity.[31] Bupivacaine appears to enter myocardial cells more easily than lidocaine[32] and inhibits atrial activity more severely than lidocaine. Bupivacaine cardiotoxicity is enhanced by concurrent hypoxia, acidosis,[31, 33, 34] and increased serum progesterone concentration.[29] In addition, the duration of bupivacaine cardiotoxic effects is prolonged when compared with that of lidocaine. Clarkson and Hondeghem[35] have postulated that, although lidocaine can readily dissociate from sodium channel binding sites (fast in–fast out theory) bupivacaine is more tightly bound (fast in–slow out theory).

Because bupivacaine is commonly given for obstetric

TABLE 3–2. CLASSIC CLINICAL SIGNS OF CONDITIONS THAT CAUSE CIRCULATORY FAILURE

Cause	Change
1. Hypovolemia	
Heart rate	↑
Blood pressure	↓
Capillary return time	>2 seconds
CVP/JVP	↓
Urine output	↓
Arterial trace swings with respiration	
ABG	Base deficit
2. Heart Failure	
Heart rate	↑ or ↓
Blood pressure	↑ or ↓
Capillary return time	↑
CVP/JVP	↓ or ↑
+/− pulmonary edema	
3. Pulmonary Embolus	
If mild, may be no signs	
If severe—Blood pressure	↓
Heart rate	↑
CVP/JVP	↑
Oxygenation of blood	↓
Right heart strain on ECG	(possible S_1, Q_3, T_3 pattern)
4. Cardiac Tamponade	
If mild, may be no signs	↓
If severe—Blood pressure	
Heart rate	↑ initially
CVP/JVP	↑
Oxygenation of blood	↓

*Classic signs of 2–4 may be absent/altered if hypovolemia is also present
CVP = central venous pressure; JVP = jugular venous pressure; ABG = arterial blood gas

regional anesthesia, the potential for prolonged myocardial dysfunction (and/or a form of ventricular fibrillation resistant to standard treatment regimens) must be anticipated.[36] Experimental evidence also shows that concurrent occlusion of the inferior vena cava, as in the pregnant patient, prolongs the time to successful resuscitation.[37] In clinical practice it is necessary to differentiate between partial intravascular cardiotoxicity leading to dysrhythmias, total intravascular cardiotoxicity resulting in prolonged cardiac standstill (totally anesthetized heart), allergic reactions to local anesthetics, and high spinals. Local anesthetic–related cardiotoxicity may be of sufficient severity and duration to require cardiac pacing (although cardiac pacing is ineffective in a fully anesthetized heart) or cardiopulmonary bypass. Cardiac arrest caused by high spinal anesthesia, in contrast, is managed usually by standard resuscitation techniques, volume resuscitation, and vasopressors.

Experimentally, lidocaine has been administered successfully in treatment of the ventricular dysrhythmias.[38] Kasten and Martin,[39] however, found that lidocaine enhanced the cardiotoxic effects of bupivacaine, whereas de Coussaye and coworkers pointed out that it was not logical to use one local anesthetic to treat the toxic effects of another.[40] Evidence exists for the efficacy of bretylium alone or in combination with epinephrine.[41] A case report and study have, however, cast doubt upon this suggestion.[42, 43] Other possibilities include the administration of amiodarone[43] or clonidine and dobutamine in combination.[44] The administration of hypertonic saline before a toxic dose of bupivacaine has been shown to protect against dysrhythmias.[45] No clinical evidence exists of its efficacy, however, if it is administered after the toxic dose of local anesthetic.

In light of the conflicting evidence, which is obtained mainly from animal studies, we suggest that in cases of bupivacaine-induced bradycardia, the drug of choice is atropine (to a maximum dose of 2 mg) with isoproterenol as the second-line agent. Cardiac pacing may assist in the management of moderate cardiotoxicity. Pacing is not, however, effective in severe cardiotoxicity when the myocardium is fully anesthetized. Bretylium, with or without epinephrine, is the drug of first choice in cases of ventricular tachydysrhythmias; however, it may take as long as 20 minutes from the time of bretylium administration until ventricular stabilizing activity is seen. In addition, bretylium may be associated with an initial increase in blood pressure, followed by a later decrease in blood pressure. This latter effect may further complicate resuscitation of the patient. The administration of hypertonic saline may also be considered.

In severe bupivacaine or etidocaine cardiotoxicity, a prolonged resuscitation period should be anticipated. Early employment of open-chest cardiac massage is appropriate if external CPR is ineffective after the first 5 to 15 minutes. In centers where cardiopulmonary bypass is available, its use is indicated when it is clear that the cardiotoxicity is unresponsive to closed-chest massage and usual drug therapy. Massive cardiac poisoning with bupivacaine results in long-term (10–20 hour) myocardial and Purkinje fiber dysfunction. In this setting, closed-chest cardiac massage is not adequate. Open-chest cardiac massage for extended periods may be traumatic and is not practical. Cardiopulmonary bypass can maintain effective organ perfusion for extended periods and may actually serve to lower blood concentrations of local anesthetic through binding effects to bypass equipment components. Open-heart massage may be utilized to transport a patient to a facility where cardiopulmonary bypass capability is available.

To summarize, direct local anesthetic cardiotoxicity may be partial or total. Partial anesthesia of the myocardium and conduction system can cause dysrhythmias, especially ventricular fibrillation. In more severe cases, total anesthesia of the myocardium leads to cardiac standstill. The resulting dysrhythmias and/or asystole may be resistant to standard resuscitation techniques. Open-chest cardiac massage and cardiopulmonary bypass are indicated in such cases.

Magnesium Toxicity

Magnesium toxicity can also lead to cardiac arrest. The uses of magnesium sulfate in pregnancy include preterm labor tocolysis and eclamptic seizure prophylaxis and treatment. An awareness of the early signs of magnesium overdose limits the occurrence of this complication (Table 3–3).

Cardiac Disease

Patients with pre-existing or pregnancy-related cardiac disease are more susceptible to hypoxemia, hypovolemia, and hypervolemia (see Chapter 1). Dysrhythmias, especially supraventricular tachycardias, are relatively common in the pregnant patient. Although most dysrhythmias are relatively benign, some progress to more sinister rhythms and cardiac arrest (see Chapter 2). Treatment of dysrhythmias in pregnancy is complicated by altered responses to some medications.[46]

PHYSIOLOGIC CHANGES OF PREGNANCY

Pregnancy is associated with significant changes in maternal anatomy and physiology (Table 3–4). Many of these changes increase the probability of maternal and fetal death or permanent injury following cardiopulmonary arrest. In addition, the same factors limit the effectiveness of standard cardiopulmonary resuscitation regimens.

The most significant physiologic changes relative to cardiopulmonary resuscitation are outlined in the following sections.

Altered Airway Anatomy

The larynx is more anterior and cephalad. The associated edema and friability of the laryngeal and pharyngeal mucosa contribute to the increased incidence of failed intubation (up to 1 in 300) in the pregnant female.[47]

Increased Oxygen Consumption

Basal metabolic rate, oxygen consumption, and carbon dioxide production are all increased by about 20% in late pregnancy from the metabolic demands of the fetus, uteroplacental unit, and hypertrophied breasts.[48]

Altered Respiratory Mechanics

The gravid uterus displaces the diaphragm 4 to 7 cm cephalad, causing a decreased functional residual capacity.[13, 49] Uterine size, in combination with the increased oxygen consumption, predisposes the pregnant patient to precipitous drops in arterial and venous oxygen tension during periods of reduced ventilation.[14, 50] Oxygenation and ventilation of the pregnant patient during cardiopulmonary resuscitation (CPR) are further complicated by the decrease in chest compliance resulting from diaphragmatic displacement, breast hypertrophy, and physiologic anemia.

Decreased Buffering Capacity

Hyperventilation occurs in response to the changes in basal metabolic rate, oxygen demand, and carbon dioxide production.[12] Increased progesterone production further stimulates respiration. Compensation for the resulting chronic respiratory alkalosis is provided by increased renal excretion of bicarbonate, which, in turn, produces a low serum bicarbonate level, mild metabolic acidosis, and diminished buffering capability. Arterial blood gas samples from healthy pregnant women reflect these changes (see Table 3–4).

Circulatory Changes

Pregnancy produces dramatic changes in cardiovascular physiology that significantly affect the circulatory aspects of CPR.[6, 10] Maternal blood volume increases by an average of 45%.[10] The final plasma volume increase totals about 1200 ml by 30 to 40 weeks' gestation. The final increase in red blood cell volume is usually proportionately smaller than that of the plasma volume increase and contributes to the physiologic anemia of pregnancy. Maternal heart rate, in the supine patient, increases by an average of 30% by gestational week 36. Heart rate changes are, however, positional.[10] Systemic vascular resistance (SVR) is decreased owing to the effects of progesterone and the enlarged uteroplacental bed, which receives a large portion of the cardiac out-

TABLE 3–3. **CLINICAL PRESENTATION OF SERUM MAGNESIUM LEVELS**

Plasma level (mEq/l)	Clinical Presentation
1.5 to 2.0	Normal plasma levels
4.0 to 8.0	Therapeutic range
5.0 to 10	ECG changes
	Prolonged P-R interval
	Widened QRS complex
10 to 12	Loss of deep tendon reflexes
15	Respiratory paralysis
	Sinoatrial and atrioventricular block
25	Cardiac arrest (secondary to respiratory arrest)

TABLE 3–4. **PHYSIOLOGIC CHANGES OF PREGNANCY RELEVANT TO CARDIOPULMONARY RESUSCITATION**

Parameter	Change	
Cardiovascular System		
Total blood volume	Increased 45%	
Plasma volume	Increased 55%	
Red cell volume	Increased 30%	
Cardiac output	Increased 50%	
Heart rate	Increased 25%	
Systolic blood pressure	Unchanged	
Systemic vascular resistance	Decreased 20%	
Central venous pressure	Unchanged	
Pulmonary capillary wedge pressure	Unchanged	
Ejection fraction	Increased	
Femoral venous pressure	Increased 15%	
Uterine blood flow	Increased tenfold	
Asymptomatic pericardial effusion is common		
Respiratory System		
Minute ventilation	Increased 45%	
Alveolar ventilation	Increased 45%	
Tidal volume	Increased 45%	
Respiratory rate	Unchanged	
Functional residual capacity	Decreased 20%	
Residual volume	Decreased 15%	
Oxygen consumption	Increased 20%	
Arterial pH	Slightly increased	Average 7.40–7.45
Pa_{O_2} (mm Hg)	Increased	104–108 mm Hg
Pa_{CO_2} (mm Hg)	Decreased	30–34 mm Hg
Renal System		
Renal blood flow	Increased 75%	
Glomerular filtration rate	Increased 50%	
Upper limit of blood urea nitrogen	Decreased 50%	
Upper limit of serum creatinine	Decreased 50%	
Hepatic System		
Total plasma protein concentration	Decreased 20%	
Pseudocholinesterase concentration	Decreased 25%	
Coagulation factors	Mainly increased	
Gastrointestinal System		
Gastric emptying	Delayed ⎫ in labor/after opioids	
Gastric fluid volume/acidity	Increased ⎭	
Gastroesophageal sphincter tone	Decreased	

put. The resulting decrease in SVR contributes to a 35 to 50% increase in resting cardiac output and a decrease in arterial blood pressure. Uterine contractions in labor can further raise cardiac output by up to 20%.

Aortocaval Compression

The presence of the gravid uterus has significant effects on both cardiovascular and respiratory mechanics.[9, 51] Cardiovascular changes include displacement of the heart, diaphragm, and abdominal contents by the expanding uterus.[11] Compression of the abdominal aorta by the gravid uterus causes significant aortic outflow obstruction with secondary decreases in renal and uterine blood flow.[9] Compression of the inferior vena cava by the gravid uterus decreases venous return to the heart. This phenomenon is seen as early as gestational week 20; it worsens as the pregnancy pro-

gresses.[9, 11] Compression of the inferior vena cava and major pelvic veins may sequester as much as 30% of the circulating blood volume.[14] In consequence, up to 10% of normal patients, in late pregnancy, develop hypotension, bradycardia, and dramatic decrease in cardiac output in the supine position. Hypovolemic patients or patients in cardiac arrest are especially vulnerable to these adverse effects. Because perfusion during CPR is dependent on both venous return and forward flow, the effects of uterine compression on the vena cava and aorta significantly impede successful cardiopulmonary resuscitation.

MAJOR ISSUES IN CARDIOPULMONARY RESUSCITATION

Differential Diagnosis

Cardiopulmonary arrest in the pregnant woman is the final common pathway of many pathologic processes. Although initial resuscitation is identical regardless of etiology, definitive management varies depending on the primary cause. For example, although prompt transfusion is indicated in management of hypovolemic cardiopulmonary arrest, transfusion does little to help the patient with intractable dysrhythmias due to severe local anesthetic toxicity. Optimal management, therefore, demands early, correct diagnosis. No time for delay is allowed, however, and it is rarely practical to obtain a complete history, detailed physical examination, or complex laboratory investigation. A simplified approach to rapidly diagnosing the cause of the arrest is suggested in Table 3–5.

Airway problems are a prominent cause of cardiopulmonary arrest during pregnancy.[52-69] Failed intubation is the most common precipitant (see Chapter 5). In the intubated patient who suffers an arrest, misplacement of the tube in the esophagus, pharynx, or main bronchus must be considered. Purely respiratory causes of cardiopulmonary arrest are more rare. Possibilities include severe asthma provoked by histamine-releasing drugs or prostaglandins, pneumothorax, or traumatic chest injuries (see Chapter 8).

Circulatory failure is the second etiology to be ruled out. The classic patterns associated with hypovolemia, heart failure, pulmonary embolism, or cardiac tamponade may be detected (see Table 3–2). The history may also provide useful evidence of pre-existing cardiac disease, dysrhythmias, or trauma.

Drug-related causes must always be excluded. These include (1) accidental administration of the wrong drug; (2) intravascular overdose of opioids, local anesthetics, antihypertensive agents, or general anesthetic agents; (3) severe anaphylactic or anaphylactoid drug reactions; and (4) deliberate drug abuse. Abuse of cocaine, in powdered and crack form, in particular is associated with premature coronary artery disease and myocardial dysfunction. Increased progesterone production in pregnancy potentiates these cardiotoxic effects.

Ventilation/perfusion mismatch is indicated by poor oxygenation of the blood with associated evidence of (a) adequate circulation but poor ventilation; or (b) adequate ventilation but poor circulation. Pulse oximetry, except in the hypovolemic or hypothermic patient, assists in diagnosis of ventilation/perfusion ($\dot{V}/\dot{Q}$)

TABLE 3–5. CARDIOPULMONARY ARREST—RAPID DIAGNOSIS

Mnemonic : AHEAD – C/S
Airway
Hemorrhage
Embolism
Anesthesia
Drugs

Cerebral
Septic shock

mismatch. Severe $\dot{V}/\dot{Q}$ mismatch associated with overwhelming local anesthetic cardiotoxicity or massive pulmonary embolism is a scenario in which cardiopulmonary bypass may be the only therapy. In these situations, the decision to proceed to cardiopulmonary bypass must be timely to avoid irreversible ischemic damage.

Cardiac arrest preceded by convulsions requires a neurologic assessment. A history of cerebral disease, pregnancy-induced hypertension, or drug ingestion should be sought. Evidence for acute intracranial pathology includes sluggish pupillary reflexes, increased or unequal pupillary size, and signs of motor dysfunction. The most likely acute cerebral problems in pregnancy are subarachnoid hemorrhage and cerebral herniation caused by cerebral hemorrhage and edema.

Trauma-induced cardiac arrest is possible. An estimated 6 to 7% of pregnant patients suffer traumatic injuries. Trauma is the leading cause of nonobstetric death.[5] External evidence of injury is usually obvious. Diagnosis, however, may be hampered by the physiologic and anatomic changes of pregnancy. Abdominal viscera are displaced by the gravid uterus and are more vulnerable to damage during upper abdominal and lower thoracic trauma. In addition, visceral and peritoneal pain responses are diminished.[5]

A high index of suspicion for concealed visceral injury or hemorrhage is advised. Peritoneal lavage, via an open, supraumbilical approach, may assist in the diagnosis with an accuracy rate of 98% following blunt abdominal trauma in pregnancy.[5] Myocardial contusion, which may behave like a recent myocardial infarction, should be considered in the patient who has suffered blunt trauma to the chest. Patients may require inotropic, chronotropic, pressor, or vasodilator therapy in addition to standard resuscitation drugs. The presence of penetrating chest wounds should alert the resuscitation team to the possibility of cardiac tamponade or tension pneumothorax.

Septic shock can be associated with chorioamnionitis, prolonged retained products of conception, intrauterine fetal death, and pyelonephritis. Septicemia can progress extremely rapidly in pregnancy, perhaps resulting from an altered immune status. Septicemic patients are likely to require continued inotropic support following successful resuscitation. The definitive treatment is to remove or treat the precipitating cause. Extreme cases of synergistic infection rapidly attacking the myometrium have been observed. The lifesaving treatment is immediate hysterectomy. Invasive hemodynamic monitoring, including a pulmonary artery catheter, is required in many cases.

Airway Management

During CPR *prompt intubation of the trachea to protect the airway is imperative.* Airway management in preg-

TABLE 3–6. ENDOTRACHEAL DRUG ADMINISTRATION

Epinephrine 2.0 mg
Lidocaine 200 mg
Atropine 2.0 mg
Narcan 0.8 mg

1. Dilute with normal saline to a total volume of 5–10 ml
2. Instill via medication atomizer or catheter
3. Hyperinflate lungs for 5–10 breaths for dispersal

*Pulmonary pathology may affect dispersal and absorption

nancy is detailed in Chapter 5 and thus is not repeated here. Once an endotracheal tube is in place it can provide a rapid route for drug administration when central venous access is not available (Table 3–6).[70, 71]

Closed-chest CPR With Manual Left Uterine Displacement

Closed-chest Massage

In the past it was believed that artificial circulation during closed-chest massage was achieved by compression of the heart between the spine and sternum.[72–74] Experimental observations now suggest that closed-chest massage produces an artificial circulation by phasic fluctuations of intrathoracic pressure.[75–82] These changes in intrathoracic pressure are transmitted equally to the vessels and the cardiac chambers, with the heart acting as a passive conduit rather than as a pump. For forward flow to occur, a pressure gradient from the arterial to the venous circulation must be generated. Artificial circulation can be generated only in vasculature protected by competent venous valves able to inhibit retrograde flow from the great intrathoracic veins.[75, 83–85] Efficient external cardiac massage requires 60 pounds of force to depress the sternum by 1 ½ to 2 inches.

The options for maintenance of artificial circulation include closed-chest massage, open-chest massage, and cardiopulmonary bypass. Attempted resuscitation involving external cardiac massage has a long history.[86, 87] External cardiac massage is intended only to preserve circulation to vital organs for a few minutes during the treatment of dysrhythmias. Prolonged external cardiac massage is not effective and can at best generate 30% of a nonpregnant patient's cardiac output.[87–96] The associated myocardial perfusion may be less than 5% of the pre-arrest value.[91, 97, 98] The resulting progressive increase in myocardial $PaCO_2$ correlates with a decreased probability of successful resuscitation as time passes.[99] It is also well documented that the benefits achieved with closed-chest cardiac massage decline when external massage is prolonged over 15 minutes.[98, 100]

Closed-chest CPR is incapable of maintaining adequate organ perfusion for more than a few minutes without administration of exogenous adrenergic agonists.[101] These agonists increase aortic diastolic pressure, venous return to the heart, and resistance of the carotid arteries to collapse.[102, 103]

Investigational Variations of CPR Techniques

Several variations of conventional CPR have also been investigated. "New CPR" involves the use of simultaneous positive-pressure ventilation and chest compression. Employing the new CPR is controversial. Studies have shown that this method can produce higher carotid artery blood flow and radial artery pressures than the standard CPR techniques.[104–106] Clear evidence exists that the resulting high intrathoracic pressures cause obstruction of venous outflow from the major cerebral veins and can raise intracerebral pressure (by elevating cerebrospinal fluid pressure) and reduce cerebral perfusion.[107] In the form of "cough CPR" in the conscious patient, there is evidence for the efficacy of this method.[108–110]

Other variants include the simultaneous implementation of abdominal compression[111–115] and military antishock trousers (MAST) to enhance venous return during closed-chest CPR.[116] Adverse effects associated with these techniques include impaired coronary artery blood flow and rupture of the liver and spleen. A technique not studied in pregnancy employs a hand-held suction device to perform active compression and decompression CPR. The cardiovascular physiologic adaptations to pregnancy (see Table 3–4) may limit the utilization of these promising techniques.[117] Regardless of which method of closed-chest CPR is chosen, it is unlikely that external cardiac massage can provide sufficient flow for the higher cardiac output and oxygen demands of pregnancy.

Complications of CPR in pregnancy affect both the mother and fetus. The mother may sustain lacerations to the liver, uterine rupture, hemothorax, or hemoperitoneum. Fetal central nervous system toxicity may also occur as a result of maternal antiarrhythmic drug therapy. The most significant fetal effect from maternal cardiopulmonary arrest is deficient uteroplacental blood flow.

The cardiovascular consequences of aortocaval compression by the gravid uterus have been described. The effects of aortocaval compression on CPR are also significant. These effects can be caused by the gravid or the postpartum uterus. Perfusion during CPR is dependent on both venous return and forward flow. Clinical reports of resuscitation of pregnant patients confirm that aortocaval compression significantly impedes successful CPR.[118–121]

Some relief from aortocaval compression can be achieved by routinely placing pregnant patients in lateral positions that rotate the pelvis at least 30° from the horizontal. This position may be achieved by placing a wedge beneath the patient's right hip or laterally tilting the working surface. Tilting the patient only partially relieves the aortocaval compression, however. In addition, the efficiency of CPR is decreased when the patient is wedged or tilted. A study by Rees and Willis in 1988 investigated the efficacy of resuscitation at various angles of inclination employing a patient model and a special Cardiff wedge.[1] Effective CPR is impossible with the patient in a full lateral position; these investigators recommend that the best compromise is achieved by wedging the patient at an angle of 27°. At this angle, only about 80% of the maximal resuscitative force for external cardiac massage can be provided by the rescuer. Chest compression is more effective and less tiring to perform with the patient supine and on a hard surface. If the supine position is utilized, aortocaval compression must be relieved with manual uterine displacement for successful resuscitation to be achieved. Whatever method is chosen, there is no technique that fully relieves aortocaval compression by the gravid uterus.

If resuscitation is not achieved within the first few minutes after onset of maternal cardiopulmonary arrest, an emergency cesarean delivery should be performed to maximize the chances of maternal and fetal survival.

Defibrillation

Standard Advanced Cardiac Life Support (ACLS) defibrillation guidelines are applicable in the pregnant patient. In pregnancy, pressure from the gravid uterus results in dextroversion of the maternal heart. Anteroposterior electrode positioning may maximize the defibrillation charge.

Cardiac monitoring is not routinely performed in the obstetric setting, and staff members may be unfamiliar with the equipment. Unfortunately, many dysrhythmias require rapid direct-current therapy. A simple, user-friendly monitoring and defibrillation system is recommended. Various disposable, combined monitoring and defibrillation self-adherent pads are on the market. The pads provide a one-step approach to monitoring the cardiac rhythm and consistently delivering the defibrillation charge. Variations exist among products, but many of the electrodes remain effective for up to 50 direct-current shocks and can be left in place for up to 24 hours.[122] Sterile internal defibrillation paddles and instructions regarding appropriate defibrillator energy settings should also be immediately available during open-chest cardiac massage.

As with other recommended resuscitation techniques and equipment, personnel should become competent with all of the functions of the defibrillator before an emergent event occurs. Training may be conducted through regular inservice and mock code sessions coordinated by the departments of anesthesia, nursing, and obstetrics.

Application of Resuscitation Drugs in Pregnancy

The standard ACLS/American Heart Association (AHA) resuscitation algorithms are applicable to the management of cardiac arrest in the pregnant patient. The most common concern regarding resuscitation drugs and the pregnant patient is whether these drugs have negative effects on the fetus. The paramount concern, however, should be resuscitation of the parturient. Any drug required to maintain maternal hemodynamic function is necessary and appropriate. Most resuscitation drugs cross the placenta and have some fetal effects. These effects should be treated once the baby is delivered.

Lidocaine. Lidocaine crosses the placenta and at therapeutic levels is not associated with adverse fetal effects.[14]

Atropine. High-dose atropine may cause fetal tachycardia (a relatively benign complication). Alternatively, glycopyrrolate may be used. Glycopyrrolate does not cross the placenta to any significant degree, but its slow onset, relative to atropine, may be disadvantageous to the mother.

Epinephrine. Epinephrine and other alpha-adrenergic agonists can cause uteroplacental vasoconstriction. As a result, it has been suggested that vasopressors be used with caution during resuscitation from cardiac arrest in pregnancy. In established cardiac arrest, however, it is probable that uteroplacental vasoconstriction is already severe. In addition, it is well recognized that exogenous administration of epinephrine is essential to maintain peripheral vascular constriction and adequate coronary and cerebral filling pressure during CPR.[101-103] It is reasonable to assume that the same applies to the uteroplacental bed. It is necessary and appropriate that epinephrine be administered according to the ACLS algorithms. Concerns about the ill effects of repeated dosing become less relevant if the new protocol, described later, is employed.

Sodium Bicarbonate. During cardiopulmonary arrest, metabolic acidosis develops rapidly. The pregnant patient is prone to rapid, severe metabolic acidosis from an increased metabolic rate and a decreased buffering capacity. Uteroplacental vasoconstriction is also provoked by acidosis and, for this reason, a more liberal approach to the use of bicarbonate has been suggested in cases of cardiopulmonary arrest during pregnancy.[14]

Administration of sodium bicarbonate is not without complications, however. Clinically, a large, abrupt bo-

TABLE 3–7. **PERIMORTEM CESAREAN DELIVERIES WITH SURVIVING INFANTS WITH REPORTS OF TIME OF DEATH OF THE MOTHER UNTIL DELIVERY (FROM 1900–1986)**

Time (mins)	Number of Patients	Outcome	Percentage
0–5	42	Normal infants	70
6–10	7	Normal infants	13
	1	Mild neurological sequelae	
11–15	6	Normal infants	12
	1	Severe neurological sqeuelae	
16–20	1	Severe neurological sequelae	1.7
21+	2	Severe neurological sequelae	
	1	Normal infant	3.3
Total	61		100

From Katz VL, Dotters DJ, Droegemueller W. Perimortem cesarean delivery. Obstet Gynecol 1986; 68:571. (Reprinted by permission from the American College of Obstetricians and Gynecologists.)

lus of sodium bicarbonate may precipitate fetal intracerebral bleeding. The recipient must be adequately ventilated to prevent adverse rises in carbon dioxide concentration, although excessive ventilation may be counterproductive because it may reduce coronary, cerebral, and placental perfusion. Sodium bicarbonate can form precipitates when administered concomitantly with other standard resuscitation drugs and is irritant to tissues if administered outside the vein. Concerns about the potential adverse effects of excessive amounts of bicarbonate upon cerebral resuscitation have caused the ACLS/AHA to recommend that sodium bicarbonate be administered only in response to absolute evidence of metabolic acidosis. When possible, sodium bicarbonate should be administered via a separately running high-flow intravenous line.

Other Drugs. Many other antiarrhythmic, inotropic, and chronotropic drugs cross the placenta and have an effect on the fetus. This caution should not, however, prevent appropriate medication of the mother when indicated. Large volumes of glucose-containing intravenous solutions should be avoided because of the risks of worsening maternal cerebral edema and causing severe hypoglycemia in the neonate.

Perimortem Cesarean Section

Perimortem cesarean section has a long and successful history.[118–121, 123–128] A review of perimortem cesarean section by Katz and coworkers in 1986 (Table 3–7)[128] concluded that "Unequivocally, if a pregnant woman suffers a cardiopulmonary arrest from any cause during the third trimester, a perimortem section should be performed. The benefits are the high probability of a healthy normal infant and the possibility that the operation will aid in cardiopulmonary resuscitation" and that "perimortem cesarean delivery initiated within four minutes of maternal cardiac arrest will yield the highest rates of maternal survival."

In the past, many such operations have been performed with the primary aim of salvaging the infant. Reports are available of sudden and dramatic maternal revival, after apparently unsuccessful standard CPR, following perimortem cesarean delivery undertaken for the sole intention of fetal rescue.[118–121] Delivery of the baby and placenta (of greater than 20 weeks' gestational size) decreases maternal oxygen requirements and aortic outflow obstruction, and allows return of normal vena cava flow. Production of carbon dioxide and hydrogen ions by the uteroplacental unit is also decreased. Although the fetus may not be independently viable at this age, perimortem cesarean section can be justified in terms of the significant cardiorespiratory benefits to the mother. If the mother does not survive, the fetus will not survive. Additional concerns regarding perimortem cesarean delivery include legal liability. Interestingly, *no physician has been found liable for performing a perimortem cesarean section.*[129]

Hemorrhage

Hemorrhage is the primary cause of cardiac arrest in pregnancy.[130] The average nonpregnant patient, without complicating disease or medications, can lose up to 30% blood volume before demonstrating the classic signs of hypovolemia (see Tables 3–2 and 3–8).[131] The loss of a further 10% more blood results in signs of severe hypovolemia with critically diminished major organ perfusion.

TABLE 3–8. **SIGNS OF BLOOD VOLUME LOSS**

0–15% Blood loss*
  Minimal tachycardia
  No measurable changes in
    Blood pressure
    Pulse pressure
    Respiratory rate
    Capillary refill test
15–30% Blood loss*
  Tachycardia
  Decreased pulse pressure
  Anxiety
  Positive capillary return test
  Urine output decreased—about 20–30 ml/hour
30–40% Blood loss*
  Tachycardia + +
  Tachypnea +
  Altered mental status
  Decreased systolic blood pressure
  Urine output decreased − +
40% + Blood loss (imminently life-threatening)*
  Tachycardia + + +
  Decreased systolic blood pressure + + +
  Pulse pressure decreased + + + (or diastolic pressure unobtainable)
  Severely depressed mental status (loss of consciousness at 50% or more)
  Urine output negligible

*% of total blood volume.
Total blood volume at term is 80–85 ml/kg (singleton pregnancy) or 95–100 ml/kg (twin pregnancy).

In the pregnant patient, compensation for blood loss is even more efficient. Up to 35 to 40% of circulating blood volume may be lost before overt signs of hemorrhage are revealed.[22] The ability to compensate for such large blood loss is provided by the physiologic expansion in blood volume, together with compensatory mechanisms that maintain maternal perfusion at the expense of the uteroplacental unit. Once these mechanisms are exhausted, however, cardiovascular collapse is dramatically abrupt.

It is vital, therefore, that the more subtle signs of blood volume loss (see Table 3–8) be appreciated. It is also prudent to suspect hemorrhage when the etiology of hemodynamic instability is unclear. Whereas obstetric hemorrhage is often overt and dramatic, internal hemorrhage may remain undetected for some time. The clinician must maintain a high index of suspicion to prevent critical hypoperfusion and ensure adequate volume resuscitation.[130]

Vascular Access

The three significant vascular access issues related to CPR are rapid drug administration, volume resuscitation, and hemodynamic monitoring.

Central venous access is recommended during CPR. Central venous access allows a more accurate assessment of volume status and provides an efficient route for drug administration. The subclavian approach may be preferable because of the chest compression and ventilation activities during CPR. Any route is acceptable, and practitioners should choose the method with which they are most familiar. Whichever route of central access is utilized, the largest cannula available should be introduced. Initial placement of a Cordis-type cannula is advantageous. Various monitoring catheters can be introduced through this wide-bore cannula, and the side port provides a 14-gauge, high-flow, low-resistance route for rapid volume resuscitation.

Drug Administration

Resuscitation drugs may be administered into the circulation via intravenous, endotracheal, intraosseous, and intracardiac routes during cardiopulmonary arrest.[71, 132]

Obstetric patients routinely have peripheral venous access in place. Kuhn and coworkers[133] have shown that dye injected into such a peripheral vein may take over 300 seconds to reach a central artery during cardiac arrest, despite the performance of chest compressions. For this reason, central venous drug delivery is the preferred technique and should be established early in the resuscitation process. Until central access can be secured, peripheral venous access can be utilized. Drug delivery by the peripheral route can be improved by

following each drug injection by 20 to 30 ml of crystalloid solution. The extremity may also be elevated above the level of the heart to further speed access into the central circulation.

As stated earlier, the endotracheal tube can be used as an alternative route for initial CPR drug administration until adequate vascular access can be established (see Table 3–6); however, pulmonary pathology may affect drug absorption.

The insertion of cannulae into the marrow cavities of long bones provides an intraosseous approach to the circulation and may be an effective means of delivering all resuscitation drugs, with the exception of bretylium. The intraosseous route has been most commonly used for resuscitation of children, but there are reports of its success in adults. Aspirated bone marrow can be utilized for crossmatching of blood, and administered drugs can rapidly reach the central circulation. The intraosseous route is not recommended, however, as a first-line technique in the adult because the post-childhood obliteration of the bone marrow cavities and the hardness of the adult bone may make it difficult to gain access to a vascular area.

The utilization of the intracardiac route *is not encouraged*. A postmortem study of the accuracy of intracardiac injection revealed that only 72% were made directly into the heart. Moreover, the study identified hemothorax, pneumothorax, hemopericardium, and direct damage to the myocardium and coronary arteries as complications.[134] The altered heart position in pregnancy also increases the likelihood of misplacement of the needle.

Volume Resuscitation

Pregnant patients have the potential for massive hemorrhage. It is essential that specific equipment be readily available for rapid replacement of blood volume. This equipment should include some form of a wide-bore, Cordis-type cannula and a pressurized system for infusion of temperature-regulated fluid. In the presence of hemorrhage, a minimum of two wide-bore intravenous cannulae should be placed.

A cell-saver system may also be helpful. Such systems have not yet found favor in the obstetric area because of concerns that contamination of the retransfused fluid may cause amniotic fluid embolism. Preliminary evidence suggests that cell savers can effectively separate amniotic fluid from blood and can be used in cases of massive obstetric hemorrhage.[135] For added safety, it is advised that the majority of the amniotic fluid released during uterine incision be suctioned away before cell saver collection is started.

Monitoring

Monitoring of cardiac and respiratory parameters should be instituted as rapidly as possible to guide resuscitation therapy.

Electrocardiogram

Any resuscitation algorithm requires continuous accurate analysis of the cardiac rhythm by electrocardiogram (ECG).

Pulse Oximetry

Pulse oximetry may provide information regarding adequacy of resuscitative efforts when the patient's volume status is adequate. Persistent low oxygen saturation readings with adequate pulses and adequate ventilation (with 100% oxygen) suggest $\dot{V}/\dot{Q}$ mismatch (e.g., massive pulmonary embolism, amniotic fluid embolism).

Capnography

Capnography is a valuable indicator of correct placement of the endotracheal tube. A persistently low end-tidal carbon dioxide concentration alerts the resuscitation team to the inadequacy of circulatory resuscitation and the possibility of pulmonary embolism. Inexpensive, disposable (phenolphthalein-chemical indicator) end-tidal carbon dioxide devices are available commercially to qualitatively indicate tracheal intubation.

Noninvasive Blood Pressure

Noninvasive blood pressure monitoring may be less reliable during active resuscitation. Early use of an intra-arterial pressure monitoring system is advised. The pressure monitoring system permits accurate assessment of the progress of resuscitation[136] and access for arterial blood gas sampling. Massive peripheral vasoconstriction associated with volume resuscitation and pressors can render the peripheral arterial line useless. When this occurs during cesarean section, sterile (saline-filled) arterial tubing attached to a needle can be provided to the surgeon so that pressures can be transduced from the abdominal aorta.

Temperature

Volume resuscitation with cool or partially warmed fluids may cause critical hypothermia. Hypothermia below 30°C can result in malignant dysrhythmias that are refractory to antiarrhythmic drugs. Cardiopulmonary bypass has been utilized to rewarm patients with hypothermia resulting from massive volume replacement in the treatment of obstetric hemorrhage.

Fetal Heart Rate

It has been suggested that fetal heart rate monitoring be continued during resuscitation to determine the need for urgent cesarean section. Accurate monitoring of the fetus cannot be achieved easily during CPR. During CPR, it can be assumed that uteroplacental perfusion is decreased and is suboptimal. Attempts to acquire this data may detract from the primary task of resuscitation. Maintaining electronic fetal monitoring during resuscitation and defibrillation may also become a safety hazard. External or internal fetal monitoring attachments can act as an alternative route to ground during defibrillation. Severe maternal or fetal burns and damage to the monitor may result. For these reasons, it is suggested that fetal monitoring be discontinued during initial maternal CPR. All fetal monitoring cables should be unplugged and placed on the bed with the patient during defibrillation attempts. Fetal monitoring can be re-established at a later stage, if appropriate.

Open-chest Massage

Numerous reports document successful resuscitation with open-chest massage following failure of external cardiac massage.[137-144] Closed-chest CPR generates increased intrathoracic pressure, which in turn generates increased intracerebral pressure. Increased intrathoracic pressure beyond physiologic normal values reduces net coronary perfusion. Raised intracerebral pressure beyond physiologic normal values reduces net cerebral perfusion. Open-chest CPR does not increase intrathoracic pressures. In addition, with intrathoracic pressure at atmospheric level, cerebral venous outflow obstruction is minimized, intracranial pressure falls, and cerebral perfusion pressure is maximized. Open-chest CPR generates greater cardiac output and does not impede cerebral or coronary perfusion pressures.

The findings regarding open-chest massage are confirmed by clinical and research reports. In 1965, Del Guercio and coworkers showed that open-chest cardiac massage can double the cardiac output.[90] Human and animal studies have shown clearly that open-chest massage can produce superior hemodynamic effects[117, 144-153] and cerebral perfusion.[149, 150, 152]

Other studies have shown that open-chest massage is often the only effective measure for patients with chest trauma, tension pneumothorax, massive pulmonary embolism, cardiac tamponade, profound hypovolemia, and hypothermia.[137-139, 143] The pregnant patient, whose resuscitation is hindered by the previously described anatomic and physiologic changes, also belongs on this list. Perimortem cesarean delivery also decreases intra-abdominal pressures. Lower intra-abdominal pressure reduces intrathoracic pressure and may make closed-chest CPR, theoretically, less effective. Tapping or squeezing the heart through the diaphragm to augment cardiac massage during perimortem cesarean delivery has been reported.[154] Formal open-chest CPR may be more effective.

Many physicians are alarmed at the prospect of performing open-chest cardiac massage. If this option is to be considered, qualified and experienced surgeons should be included in developing the arrest code response plan for the unit. Open-chest cardiac massage may offer the only chance of survival for patients in the high-risk groups described, and it should be considered early in the management of a cardiac arrest. Open-chest massage can be performed via a traditional thoracotomy incision or a formal sternotomy. Internal thoracic massage is performed by holding the posterior part of the heart in the palm of the hand while the fingers compress the anterior heart. Alternatively, the heart can be compressed against an intact sternum. The internal mammary artery is at risk for laceration during the initial thoracotomy incision, and the potential for substantial blood loss must be anticipated. If substantial blood loss occurs, it must be effectively treated.

Cardiopulmonary Bypass

Cardiopulmonary bypass may be the only means of effective resuscitation in limited clinical situations. Bypass must be rapidly initiated to prevent irreversible anoxic damage when there is evidence of oxygen desaturation despite maximal resuscitative efforts. This situation indicates a $\dot{V}/\dot{Q}$ mismatch. Indications for cardiopulmonary bypass also exist in situations in which an adequate oxygen saturation can be maintained but prolonged resuscitation effort is required. These indications include any situation in which adequate cardiac rhythm cannot be restored, as with hypothermia and local anesthetic toxicity.

Cardiopulmonary bypass is not a panacea for every arrest, but it has been shown to be a lifesaving maneuver in limited situations. In any hospital with both obstetric and cardiac facilities, a well-organized plan should be established to ensure that the appropriate personnel and equipment are made available to manage these rare, but potentially treatable, emergencies. Most maternity units are, by design, relatively "low-tech" environments. Many clinicians may not have immediate access to on-site cardiopulmonary bypass equipment. Immediate access may also be lacking in some units with large delivery rates and high-risk patient populations. In fact, many maternity centers are freestanding and geographically remote. Cardiopulmonary bypass is a final clinical option when available and is not a standard of care.

Route of Access

Vascular access for cardiopulmonary bypass can be obtained utilizing the femoral-femoral or median sternotomy route. Each approach has its own limitations and advantages. The femoral route effects rapid access with limited equipment. Aortocaval compression before delivery of the baby limits the effectiveness of the femoral route, as does any abdominal vascular catastrophe. A median sternotomy permits adequate access for both the cardiac surgeon and the resuscitator performing open-chest cardiac massage. The sternal route requires specialized equipment (sternal saw, power source, rib spreader) and may be more time-consuming. Establishing cardiopulmonary bypass requires extensive coordination of the cardiac operating room team, perfusionist team, obstetric team, and anesthesiology team. Any condition that warrants cardiopulmonary bypass is an indication for early open-chest cardiac massage. Closed-chest cardiac massage is minimally effective after about 15 minutes of continued resuscitation, and it will be some time before the patient's condition is completely stable on bypass.

Clinical Indications

1. $\dot{V}/\dot{Q}$ mismatch resulting in inadequate oxygenation of the blood. Possible causes include thrombotic or amniotic fluid pulmonary embolism and severe recalcitrant hemorrhage/hypovolemia.
2. Severe local anesthetic toxicity, especially when it is related to bupivacaine or etidocaine because the duration of cardiac dysrhythmias or cardiac standstill is likely to be prolonged.
3. Hypothermia-related dysrhythmias, especially if they are associated with bupivacaine toxicity
4. Penetrating chest trauma

MANAGEMENT OF CARDIOPULMONARY ARREST

Historical Development of Parturient CPR Protocol

Three major protocols have been used in the past to guide CPR of the pregnant patient.

Lee, Rodgers, White, and Harvey Protocol

These investigators[14] recognized the potential benefits offered by early perimortem delivery and open-chest cardiac massage. In 1986, they published a protocol more likely to result in successful outcome for the mother and fetus. Considerations of fetal gestational age and viability were used to define the appropriate management plan. This work resulted in the three-stage management approach in Tables 3–9 and 3–10.

At the time of publication the authors believed that "before the onset of fetal viability (about the 24th gestational week), the objectives of cardiopulmonary resuscitation can be directed almost exclusively to maternal considerations," but that "when fetal viability has been reached, the decision to expedite delivery in the face of maternal cardiac arrest is dependent on fetal status

TABLE 3–9. LEE AND COWORKERS' PROTOCOL: RECOMMENDED APPROACH TO CARDIOPULMONARY RESUSCITATION (CPR) DURING PREGNANCY ACCORDING TO GESTATIONAL AGE

Less Than 25 Weeks	25 to 32 Weeks	32 Weeks or More
Continue CPR until appropriate end point Consider open-chest cardiac massage after 15 minutes of continuous CPR; sooner if maternal hypoxia or inadequate circulation uncorrected by closed-chest CPR	Position patient to decrease aortocaval compression by uterus Special attention to fetal status, especially with: Defibrillation Lidocaine, verapamil Epinephrine Consider open-chest massage when decision to perform emergency cesarean section is made Emergency cesarean section after 15 minutes continuous CPR; sooner if maternal hypoxia or inadequate circulation uncorrected by CPR Continue CPR during and after delivery	Position patient to decrease aortocaval compression by uterus Special attention to fetal status, especially with: Defibrillation Lidocaine, verapamil, beta-blockers Epinephrine Emergency cesarean section after 15 minutes continuous CPR; sooner if maternal hypoxia or inadequate circulation uncorrected by CPR or fetal distress Continue CPR during and after delivery Consider open-chest massage if maternal condition after delivery warrants

From Lee RV, Rodgers BD, White LM, Harvey RC: Cardiopulmonary resuscitation of pregnant women. Am J Med 1986; 81:311.

as well as on maternal status." External fetal monitoring and ultrasound examination were suggested as means of assessing fetal status.

In patients between weeks 24 and 32 of gestation, these workers advised that "thoracotomy and open-chest cardiac massage should be considered if standard cardiopulmonary resuscitation is ineffective for more than 15 minutes." In addition, they stated that "If they are not successful for five minutes, emergency cesarean section is mandatory." For patients at more than 32 weeks' gestation, it was advised that "proceeding directly to emergency cesarean section seems appropriate if standard cardiopulmonary resuscitation is ineffective for more than 15 minutes."

Close reading of the text and protocol reveals that the researchers clearly recognized that when closed-chest CPR is ineffective, open-chest CPR or emergency cesarean section should be performed sooner than the ACLS/AHA time scales stipulated, which are discussed later. The Lee and coworkers' protocol was a dramatic improvement over the previously available guidelines.

TABLE 3–10. LEE AND COWORKERS' PROTOCOL: APPROACH TO CARDIOPULMONARY RESUSCITATION DURING PREGNANCY

Time	Resuscitative Action	Diagnostic Action	Pharmacologic Action
0	Chest thump Ventilation (mouth-to-mouth) External cardiac massage Defibrillate Intravenous access: central line	Electrocardiography for rhythm Check for pulses and perfusion Determine gestational age	Intravenous fluids Ventricular fibrillation—lidocaine Supraventricular tachyarrhythmia—digitalis/beta-blocker as appropriate
1 to 2 minutes	Endotracheal intubation plus ventilation with oxygen	Measure arterial blood gases Check for pulses and perfusion Check fetal heart, sonography	pH less than 7.3—sodium bicarbonate Asystole/bradyarrhythmia—atropine Pulmonary edema—furosemide
2 to 5 minutes	Defibrillate as needed Position to move uterus to left	Electrocardiography for rhythm Electrocardiography for rhythm Quick measure of blood pressure, pulses, perfusion Portable chest radiography	Ventricular fibrillation—lidocaine Ventricular fibrillation—bretylium Electromechanical dissociation—calcium chloride, epinephrine (one time only), isoproterenol
5 to 10 minutes	Continue ventilation plus external massage Begin preparation for operative procedure as appropriate Arterial line Defibrillate as needed	Measure arterial blood gases Check fetal heart, sonography Check for tension pneumothorax, cardiac tamponade, hypovolemia Measure arterial blood gases	pH less than 7.3—sodium bicarbonate pH less than 7.3—sodium bicarbonate
15 minutes	Open-chest cardiac massage and/or emergency cesarean section as appropriate	Continue as above	Continue as above

From Lee RV, Rodgers BD, White LM, Harvey RC: Cardiopulmonary resuscitation of pregnant women. Am J Med 1986; 81:311. (Reprinted with permission from Excerpta Medica Inc.)

The ACLS/AHA Protocols

The ACLS/AHA protocols are an excellent guide to resuscitation (Figures 3–1 through 3–4). To apply these algorithms to the pregnant patient, some modifications should be considered. The 1987 edition of the ACLS manual, for example, states that "If 5–10 minutes of standard CPR, leftward displacement of the gravid uterus, airway management, fluid volume restoration, and defibrillation (if indicated) fail to restore effective circulatory function, an attempt to evaluate fetal viability via external monitoring or real-time ultrasound, though difficult, may be useful in deciding if and when open-chest heart massage and/or cesarean section is required," and that "If standard measures are not successful within 15 minutes of the onset of arrest, thoracotomy and open-chest massage should be performed

if the fetus is still viable. If there is no return of spontaneous effective maternal circulation or there is evidence of fetal distress after 5 minutes of CPR with open-chest cardiac massage, some have recommended that cesarean section be performed immediately."[155]

A few issues need to be considered in light of the current literature. These issues are as follows:

1. The emphasis on the use of open-chest cardiac massage and/or emergency cesarean delivery only as a means of salvaging the infant when maternal resuscitation has failed
2. Fetal monitoring during initial resuscitation
3. The delay of perimortem cesarean section beyond 5 minutes.

A more aggressive approach to early (within 4–5 minutes of cardiac arrest) cesarean delivery is advocated in the report of the 1992 National Conference on Cardiopulmonary Resuscitation and Emergency Cardiac Care.[6] Once again, the major emphasis appears to be directed toward the salvage of the fetus. The decision to perform a perimortem cesarean section is described as "complex," and no clear guidelines are given regarding its timing.[156]

In general, these recommendations may place excessive emphasis on the fetus, and the time scales suggested may be too long. Further literature suggests that the guidelines may require modification.

Troiano, Harvey, and Associates

In 1989, a further development occurred when the Troiano group[15] published the protocol shown in Table 3–11. As can be seen, the same three management categories are defined according to fetal gestational age. As with the earlier protocol of Lee and coworkers, the presence or absence of fetal distress is employed to define the need for open-chest CPR or emergency cesarean section. This protocol also includes recommendations for earlier performance of open-chest cardiac massage and emergency cesarean section.

A Modified Protocol for Cardiopulmonary Resuscitation

The new protocol, described later, was developed based on the existing protocols combined with the available clinical and current literature. The modifications were based on (1) the special needs of the pregnant patient and fetus; (2) the outcomes following cardiopulmonary arrest; and (3) the infrequent occurrence rate of cardiopulmonary arrest in pregnancy. The protocol was intended as a user-friendly guideline for obstetric staff who are rarely confronted with this

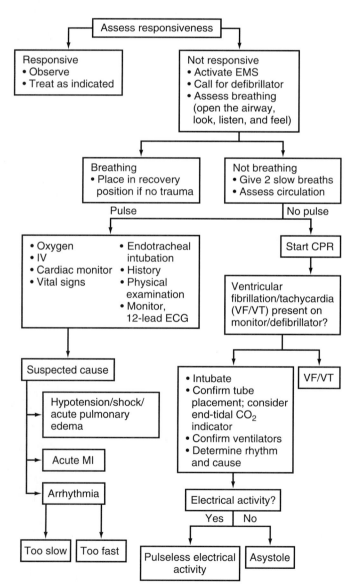

Figure 3–1. ACLS universal algorithm. (Reproduced with permission. © Textbook of Advanced Cardiac Life Support, 1994. Copyright American Heart Association.)

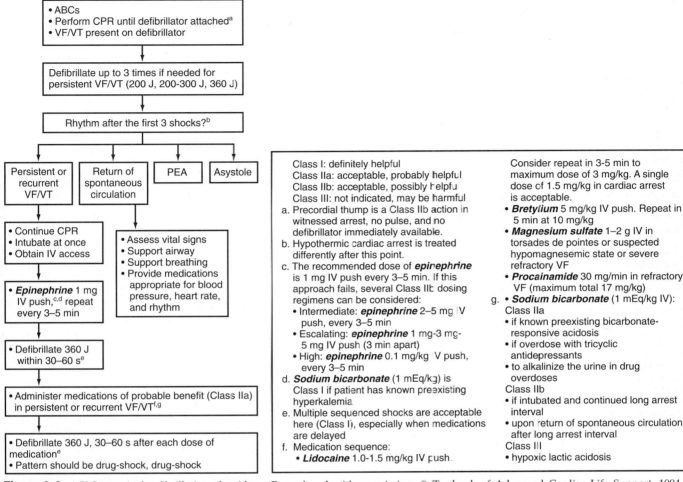

Figure 3-2. ACLS ventricular fibrillation algorithm. (Reproduced with permission. © Textbook of Advanced Cardiac Life Support, 1994. Copyright American Heart Association.)

TABLE 3-11. **TROIANO PROTOCOL**

Time min	≤24 weeks		24–32 weeks		>32 weeks
0	Initiate CPR ↓		Initiate CPR ↓		Initiate CPR ↓
	If NO favorable maternal response		Evaluate fetus ↓		If NO favorable maternal response
	↓	Fetal distress ↓	Fetus satisfactory	Fetus satisfactory	↓
5		Emergent C/S	Mother poor ↓	Mother favorable ↓	Emergent C/S ↓
	Open chest cardiac massage		Other chest cardiac massage	Cont. CPR Deliver if any fetal distress	
			No response ↓	↓	If NO favorable maternal response ↓
			Emergent C/S		Open chest cardiac massage
				If CPR is still necessary, open chest CPR and emergent C/S	

From Troiano N. J Perinat Neonat Nurs 1989;3:1.

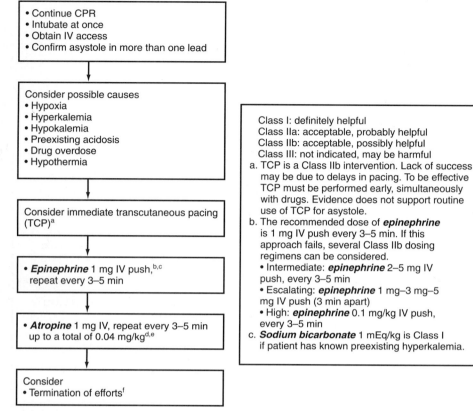

Figure 3–3. ACLS asystole algorithm. (Reproduced with permission. © Textbook of Advanced Cardiac Life Support, 1994. Copyright American Heart Association.)

emergency. Two of us (MDJ and CJL) developed an earlier version of this new protocol for obstetric resuscitation at The Brigham and Womens Hospital in Boston, Massachusetts. The version shown subsequently reflects the experience gained during real and mock code exercises at that hospital.

The protocol focuses on an aggressive and organized approach to CPR of the parturient, emphasizing the hemodynamic effects of the physiologic adaptations to pregnancy. The most important features of the new protocols are shown in Tables 3–12 through 3–15. The personnel allocations were designed for one particular hospital. Variations in facilities, staffing levels, and physical design of individual hospitals mean that local modifications are required for the protocol's employment in other hospitals.

Issues considered in the modifications of existing protocols included the following:

1. *The decreased cardiopulmonary reserves of the pregnant patient* place both mother and fetus at increased risk. The apneic pregnant patient becomes hypoxic much faster than the nonpregnant patient.
2. *The maternal oxygen reserve* is limited. Maternal brain damage is likely after 4–6 minutes of sustained cardiac arrest.[2, 50] A delay of even 6–9 minutes may lead to irreversible brain damage in the mother.[123]

3. *The fetal oxygen reserve* is approximately 2 minutes.[49] Clinically, the fetus may survive undamaged for slightly longer. Katz and coworkers[128] report that most intact fetal survivors are delivered within 5 minutes of maternal arrest.
4. *The fetoplacental unit* mechanically inhibits effective resuscitation, consumes maternal oxygen reserves, and generates carbon dioxide and hydrogen ion.

TABLE 3–12. **IMPORTANT FEATURES OF NEW RESUSCITATION PROTOCOL**

Airway	Intubate trachea as soon as possbile
Breathing	Control ventilation
Circulation	Central venous access ASAP
	Closed-chest massage
Displacement	Manual left uterine displacement ASAP
Defibrillate	As per ACLS protocol
Drugs	As per ACLS protocol
Delivery	Deliver fetus and placenta within 5 minutes if standard resuscitation techniques are not successful
Document	
Consider	
Open-chest cardiac massage	Within *15 minutes* if standard resuscitation techniques are not successful
Cardiopulmonary bypass	When indicated

ASAP = as soon as possible; ACLS = advanced cardiac life support

5. *Maternal hypoxia, hypotension, and lactic acidosis* can result in uteroplacental vasoconstriction and acidosis in the fetus.

6. *Aortocaval compression* occurs, and experimental and clinical evidence have shown that successful re-

Includes	• Electromechanical dissociation (EMD)
	• Pseudo-EMD
	• Idioventricular rhythms
	• Ventricular escape rhythms
	• Bradyasystolic rhythms
	• Postdefibrillation idioventricular rhythms

• Continue CPR • Intubate at once	• Assess blood flow using Doppler ultrasound, end-tidal CO_2, echocardiography, or arterial line

Consider possible causes
(Parentheses=possible therapies and treatments)
• Hypovolemia (volume infusion)
• Hypoxia (ventilation)
• Cardiac tamponade (pericardiocentesis)
• Tension pneumothorax (needle decompression)
• Hypothermia
• Massive pulmonary embolism (surgery, **thrombolytics**)
• Drug overdose such as tricyclics, digitalis, β-blockers, calcium channel blockers
• Hyperkalemia[a]
• Acidosis[b]
• Massive acute myocardial infarction

• Epinephrine 1 mg IV push,[a,c] repeat every 3–5 min

• If absolute bradycardia (<60 beats/min) or relative bradycardia, give **atropine** 1 mg IV
• Repeat every 3–5 min up to a total of 0.04 mg/kg[d]

Class I: definitely helpful
Class IIa: acceptable, probably helpful
Class IIb: acceptable, possibly helpful
Class III: not indicated, may be harmful

a. **Sodium bicarbonate** 1 mEq/kg is Class I if patient has known preexisting hyperkalemia.
b. **Sodium bicarbonate** 1 mEq/kg:
   Class IIa
   • if known preexisting bicarbonate-responsive acidosis
   • if overdose with tricyclic antidepressants
   • to alkalinize the urine in drug overdoses
   Class IIb
   • if intubated and continued long arrest interval
   • upon return of spontaneous circulation after long arrest interval
   Class III
   • hypoxic lactic acidosis
c. The recommended dose of **epinephrine** is 1 mg IV push every 3–5 min.
   If this approach fails, several Class IIb dosing regimens can be considered.
   • Intermediate: **epinephrine** 2–5 mg IV push, every 3–5 min
   • Escalating: **epinephrine** 1mg–3 mg–5 mg IV push (3 min apart)
   • High: **epinephrine** 0.1 mg/kg IV push, every 3–5 min
d. Shorter **atropine** dosing interval (3 min) is possibly helpful in cardiac arrest (Class IIb).

Figure 3–4. ACLS electromechanical dissociation algorithm. (Reproduced with permission. © Textbook of Advanced Cardiac Life Support, 1994. Copyright American Heart Association.)

TABLE 3–13. ANTEPARTUM CPR GUIDELINES

1. Call Code Blue, CB code team, code location
2. Closed-chest CPR with *manual left uterine displacement*
3. *Endotracheal intubation* as soon as possible
   Consider use of transtracheal medications
4. *Rapid central access* for large-volume replacement
   Consider subclavian approach
   Send blood for:
   Venous or arterial blood gases
   Electrolytes
   Hemoglobin and hematocrit
   Coagulation studies
   Avoid hypothermia
5. Monitoring
   Pulse oximeter
   ECG
   Early use of arterial monitoring
   Consider aortic arterial line
6. Assess for hemorrhage
   Control site of bleeding
   Consider manual aortic tamponade
   Consider ligation of hypogastric arteries
7. *By 4 minutes*
   Consider *perimortem cesarean section* if maternal resuscitation is failing and uterine size is *20 weeks* or more (fundus at level of umbilicus or above)
8. *By 5 minutes*
   Ensure delivery of baby
   Delay abdominal closure until hemodynamic stability ensured
9. *By 15 minutes*
   If maternal resuscitation remains inadequate consider *direct cardiac massage* via: Transabdominal left thoracotomy or median sternotomy
10. Evaluate need for *cardiopulmonary bypass*:
    Poor $\dot{V}/\dot{Q}$ matching
    Pulmonary embolism
    Massive hemorrhage
    Electromechanical dissociation
    Disseminated intravascular coagulation
    Drug/anesthesia overdose
    Bupivacaine toxicity
    Hypothermia-related dysrhythmia
Also:
    Remove existing IV and epidural infusion fluids
    Keep for analysis
    Diagnose the cause of the arrest

suscitation is unlikely when the vena cava is occluded.[37, 118] Following delivery of the fetus, venous return via the inferior vena cava is restored, aortic outflow obstruction is reduced, and cardiac output can increase to as much as 80% above predelivery values.[157]

7. *Closed-chest cardiac massage* becomes less effective with time and is virtually ineffective in the pregnant patient after 15 minutes.

8. *Perimortem cesarean section* is a consideration. Delivery of the fetus and placenta after 20 weeks' gestation decreases maternal oxygen requirements, decreases aortic outflow obstruction, allows return of normal vena cava blood flow, and allows independent resuscitation of the mother and fetus. Both mother and fetus stand to gain significant benefit from this procedure. Clear evidence exists that emergency cesarean delivery should be completed within

TABLE 3–14. **POSTPARTUM CPR GUIDELINES**

1. Call Code Blue, OB code team, code location
2. Closed chest CPR with *manual left uterine displacement*
   Uterus may be filled with blood
3. *Endotracheal intubation* as soon as possible
   Consider use of transtracheal medications
4. *Rapid central access* for large-volume replacement
   Consider subclavian approach
   Send blood for:
      Venous or arterial ABGs
      Electrolytes
      Hgb and Hct
      Coagulation Studies
   Avoid hypothermia
5. Monitoring
   Pulse oximeter
   ECG
   Early use of arterial monitoring
   Consider aortic arterial line
6. Assess for hemorrhage
   Control site of bleeding
   Consider opening/re-opening the abdomen
   Delay abdominal closure until hemodynamic stability ensured
   Consider manual aortic tamponade
   Consider ligation of hypogastric arteries
7. *By 15 minutes*
   If maternal resuscitation remains inadequate consider *direct cardiac massage* via transabdominal left thoracotomy, or median sternotomy
8. Evaluate need for *cardiopulmonary bypass*
   Poor $\dot{V}/\dot{Q}$ matching
   Pulmonary embolism
   Massive hemorrhage
   Electromechanical dissociation/disseminated intravascular coagulation
   Drug/anesthesia overdose
   Bupivacaine toxicity
   Hypothermia-related dysrhythmia
Also
   Remove existing IV and epidural infusion fluids
   Keep for analysis
   Diagnose the cause of the arrest

ABGs = arterial blood gases; Hgb = hemoglobin; Hct = hematocrit

the first 5 minutes of maternal arrest. There is no time to waste.

9. *Fetal viability* must be considered. Effective maternal resuscitation offers the best chance for both mother and baby. In general terms, if the mother's condition is bad, the baby's is worse, and what is good for the mother is good for the baby.

Modification to Existing Protocols

The modified protocol is simplified by identifying only two treatment groups that are defined by relative uterine size of 20 weeks' gestation or less. Aortocaval compression becomes hemodynamically significant at 20 weeks' gestational size. Definition of actual gestational *age* may be difficult. A uterus of 20 gestational weeks' *size* can, however, be identified by palpation of the fundus at, or above, the level of the umbilicus. When standard resuscitation techniques have not been successful and the uterus is at 20-week size or greater, emergency cesarean delivery should be underway by

4 minutes from the maternal arrest (*the 4-minute rule*). It is the intention that the baby be delivered by 5 minutes from the start of the arrest (*the 5-minute rule*).

Further modifications to existing protocols include the following:

1. Early intubation of the trachea is emphasized to safeguard the high-risk airway of the pregnant patient.
2. The use of manual left uterine displacement, rather than the use of tilt or wedging, is performed to limit aortocaval compression.
3. Early access to the central circulation is encouraged.
4. Early use of open-chest cardiac massage is encouraged in light of experimental data regarding the low cardiac outputs produced initially and their rapid decline when external cardiac massage is performed during CPR.
5. Early consideration of differential diagnosis of the precipitating cause is emphasized.
6. Indications for cardiopulmonary bypass are outlined.
7. Early discontinuation of existing intravenous and epidural infusions is suggested due to the possibility of an iatrogenic cause for the cardiopulmonary arrest.
8. Because of the controversy surrounding its efficacy and the technical difficulties during resuscitation, assurance of fetal well-being may be best achieved through maternal condition stabilization.

Practical Issues Associated With Perimortem Cesarean Section

The potentially lifesaving effects of perimortem cesarean section are well documented and should not be delayed in the hope of achieving preoperative cardiovascular stability. Protocols describing this procedure should be developed in consultation with involved disciplines. Lines of communication need to be established before the resuscitation emergency. Logistics vary from institution to institution, based on available resources.

Perimortem cesarean section is most effectively and rapidly performed with a vertical abdominal incision. Following delivery of the baby, hemostasis must be promptly achieved. In the absence of pathologic uterine bleeding, a rapid running wound closure assists. Wound closure should not occur, however, until adequate maternal resuscitation has been achieved and all major bleeding points have been identified. Blood loss before wound closure can be limited by packing the abdomen with warm, wet laparotomy packs or, if necessary, surgical drapes.

Uterine atony may respond to administration of oxytocin (Pitocin) (10 units in 10 ml of normal saline) by direct intramyometrial injection at divided sites. In cases of persistent pathologic bleeding, a temporary

TABLE 3–15. EXAMPLE OF INDIVIDUAL RESPONSIBILITIES DURING CARDIOPULMONARY RESUSCITATION IN LABOR AND DELIVERY

Primary Nurse

Ascertains cardiopulmonary arrest and *notes time*
  Unresponsive
    Calls for help
      AMBU bag
      Back board
      Code team
      Defibrillator
      Positions patient:
        Head of bed flat
        Left uterine displacement
  Airway
    Opens airway with jaw-thrust/head-tilt maneuver
    Assesses for airway obstruction
  Breathing
    Looks, listens, feels for breathing
    Obtains mask-valve device (in bedside table)
    Provides two rescue breaths
  Circulation
    Assesses carotid pulse
    Begins chest compression
  Initiates one-person CPR (if alone) *or* two-person CPR if other
    person in room
  1 (One) person CPR—15:2 ratio*
  2 (Two) person CPR—5:1 ratio
  Provides report to code team personnel
  Disconnects electronic fetal monitor prior to defibrillation

---

(*Chest compression to lung ventilation ratio)

Secretary

Calls hospital code operator
  States "Code Blue, OB code team, labor and delivery"
  Operator activates alpha-numeric OB code team beepers and
    hospital-wide intercom system
  When a private physician's patient—also calls "Code Blue, Dr.
    _____, Labor and Delivery"
Calls blood bank to report code status
Code secretary identified by nurse-in-charge (NIC)
  Second secretary called to Nursing Station to help
Identifies code phone—not main extension
Prepares extra patient labels and lab forms
  Code status written on lab forms
Communicates all lab results and phone messages to NIC
Notifies Cardiac Surgery service per surgical service senior resident
  Calls main Operating Room for support personnel/equipment

Second Nurse

Brings code cart *outside* of room
  Obtains oral airway and Ambu bag from code cart
  Connects Ambu bag to wall oxygen outlet at full flow
  Obtains backboard from code cart and assists primary nurse in
    placing it under patient, maintaining left uterine
    displacement
Calls for Defibrillator
Assists with two-person CPR
  Provides lung ventilation
  Compression to ventilation ratio = 5:1
Becomes recorder when anesthesiologist arrives to perform lung
  ventilation

Third Nurse

Manual Left Uterine Displacement

Fourth Nurse

Prepares drugs/ABG syringes/IVs at the code cart
  Lidocaine
  Epinephrine
  Atropine
  Dopamine—never IV push, always as an infusion
  Naloxone (Narcan)
Recorder until anesthesiologist arrives
Encourages universal precautions—face shields/goggles/gloves

Obstetric Anesthesia Fellow

Calls for anesthesia code cart to be brought *outside* of room
Brings transport monitoring device to room
  Portable pulse oximeter/NIBP monitor
Performs endotracheal intubation ASAP
  Intubation kit on nursing code cart
  OB code intubation kit (see Table 3–16) on the defibrillator cart
    Cricothyroidotomy kit
    Combitube
Provides large-volume central access
  Central Access Tray. Cordis, single- and triple-lumen catheters on
    nursing Code Cart

Obstetric Anesthesia Attending—Code Team Leader

Defibrillator Nurse

Applies defibrillator pads and connects cable
  To the right of the sternum below the clavicle and at the 4th
    intercostal space on the mid-axillary line
  Never over bone
  The heart is shifted anteriorly and to the left during pregnancy
Defibrillator to be maintained with defibrillator pads and cable
  assembled
Provides rhythm strip and defibrillation capability in one step
Turns defibrillator ON
Ascertains that the machine is in the correct mode
Charges the defibrillator according to team leader order
Assists in clearing all personnel from the bed *before* defibrillation

Obstetric Attending/Physician of Record

Upon entry to room, ascertains time of maternal arrest. Dons
  gloves, surgical gowns, opens perimortem cesarean section kit
  and loads blade onto handle.
Calls for perimortem cesarean section at 4 minutes from maternal
  arrest to effect delivery within 5 minutes from maternal arrest
  (when uterine size ≥20 weeks' gestation size = at umbilicus)
Perimortem cesarean section kit on defibrillator cart
Delay closure of abdomen until maternal pulse/BP is restored to
  ensure hemostasis
Saline packs and Vy drape
Continue to monitor postpartum uterus to avoid aortocaval
  compression and excessive blood loss

Obstetric Chief Resident

Same as Obstetric attending/physician of record

Neonatal ICU Attending Physician/NICU Triage Nurse

Provides NICU code cart, neonatal resuscitation personnel and
  transport Isolette

Labor and Delivery Nurse-in-charge

Delegates nursing responsibilities
  Assigns nursing roles—considering critical care obstetric (CCOB)
    team resources
  Assigns a "code" unit secretary
Facilitates code logistics
Removes support person(s) (if present) and obtains personnel to
  assist them
Designates neonatal resuscitation location
Provides crowd control
Provides "volume" control
Encourages personnel to respond only to code team leader

**Surgical Service Senior Resident On-call and Cardiac Surgery
Service**

Consider thoracotomy for direct cardiac massage per protocol
Thoracotomy kit and bypass kit on defibrillator cart
Surgical service resident to carry code beeper for immediate
  availability to perform thoracotomy
Notify cardiac surgery service ASAP
Call main operating room for support personnel/equipment
Consider *cardiopulmonary bypass* if indicated per cardiac surgery/
  protocol
    Sternotomy saw—on defibrillator cart
    Nitrogen tank—next to defibrillator cart

but effective measure is compression of the abdominal aorta by the surgeon's hand or a vascular clamp.

Postoperatively, continuing hemorrhage can refill the uterus. In severe cases this can cause significant hypovolemia and aortocaval compression. Persistent shock or recurrent need for resuscitation at this stage mandates examination of the uterus and, if necessary, reopening of the operative wound.

Logistics and Planning

Following cardiopulmonary arrest in the pregnant patient, permanent damage to the mother and/or fetus may occur within 4 to 6 minutes of sustained arrest.[2, 50] If resuscitation is to be successful it must be handled promptly and efficiently. Prior planning and practice are essential in achieving success. Advance preparation helps to identify the unexpected, but often significant, local problems that impair the smooth running of the resuscitation process. Advance planning and practice also promote development of an efficient team. It is well recognized that individual resuscitation skills diminish when not used regularly.[158–160] Time spent practicing "mock codes" is valuable in terms of education of the involved personnel.

A suitable resuscitation protocol designed and agreed upon by the involved members of the various disciplines is essential. Regardless of how good the resuscitation protocol looks on paper, it is useless unless all individuals have practiced their roles and have established lines of communication. An efficient communication system should be available to promptly summon the required personnel. Once a plan has been agreed upon it must be well publicized. All involved personnel must be identified in advance and made fully aware of their specific roles and responsibilities.

A wide variety of equipment may be required, and it must be immediately available. Because of the varied locations in which cardiopulmonary arrest can occur, this equipment should be readily portable. Table 3–16 shows equipment that should be available during resuscitation of a pregnant patient.

Three team leaders should be preassigned. These leaders should be immediately identifiable. All communication and instruction within the resuscitation area should originate with the team leaders to minimize noise and confusion. The three team leaders are the senior anesthesiologist present, who coordinates CPR; the senior obstetrician present, who coordinates surgical management and delivery of the baby; and the senior nurse present, who manages the resuscitation cart, data recording, and supervision of nursing personnel. The responsibilities of these individuals must be clearly designated and practiced in advance.

Medical and nursing staff are extremely busy at this time. An appropriately trained medical secretary can play an invaluable role by ensuring that all necessary

TABLE 3–16. ESSENTIAL EQUIPMENT FOR MANAGEMENT OF CARDIOPULMONARY ARREST IN PREGNANCY

1. Standard code cart equipment
2. Defibrillator
    Defibrillator pads and cables with concomitant ECG monitoring capability
    Sterile internal paddles and matching energy data
3. Monitoring equipment
    Pulse oximeter
    Noninvasive blood pressure machine
    Invasive arterial blood pressure cannulae/transducers/lines
4. Intravenous equipment
    Large-bore IV cannulae
    Pressure infusion bags
    Colloid for use until blood available
        25% albumin/hetastarch
    High-volume pressure infuser/warmer
5. Portable airway kit
    Datta handle laryngoscope (1)
        Mac 3 blade (1)
        Miller 2 blade (1)
    #7 Endotracheal tube with stylette and syringe in place (1)
    6.5 Endotracheal tube with stylette and syringe in place (1)
    Laryngeal mask airway size 3 (1)
    Laryngeal mask airway size 4 (1)
    Sheridan Combitube (1)
    Knife handle (1) with #10 blade
    Skin hook (1)
    10 ml/100 mg lidocaine prefilled syringe (1)
    10 ml vial of 10 mg/ml succinylcholine (1)
    500 mg sodium pentothal (1)
    Betadine packet
6. Portable perimortem cesarean section kit
    Knife handle with #10 blade (1)
    Kelly clamps (4)
    Mayo scissors (1)
    Bandage scissors (1)
    Tooth forceps (2)
    Needle holders (2)
    864 sutures (4)
    Lap packs (2)
    Vy drape (1)
    1-ml oxytocin vials (2)
    10-ml normal saline vials (2)
    10-ml syringe with 21 g 1½" needle (1)
    Betadine packet
7. Portable kit for open-chest cardiac massage/cardiopulmonary bypass
    Streamlined thoracotomy kit—per surgical service preference
8. Other useful equipment
    Level-1 pressure infuser
    Cell saver
    Cardiopulmonary bypass machine
    Nitrogen tank
    Sternotomy saw

personnel are present, communicating with staff outside the room, dealing with laboratory samples, and ensuring that results reach the team leaders.

A designated recorder of events should be identified. An accurate record of events assists in making a diagnosis of the cause of the arrest and assesses the progress of resuscitation. The record is also important for medicolegal purposes.

CONCLUSIONS

The efficiency of CPR is significantly impaired by the anatomic and physiologic changes of pregnancy.

We have presented modifications of standard resuscitation algorithms for cardiopulmonary arrest in the pregnant patient. These include the following:

1. Early endotracheal intubation
2. Closed chest massage on a firm, flat surface with manual uterine displacement
3. Perimortem cesarean delivery within 5 minutes of maternal arrest when resuscitation attempts are unsuccessful and uterine size is greater than 20 weeks' gestation.
4. Open-chest cardiac massage within 15 minutes, if delivery does not improve maternal condition.
5. Cardiopulmonary bypass for

   - Persistent and severe $\dot{V}/\dot{Q}$ mismatch
   - Massive hemorrhage
   - Drug/anesthesia overdose
   - Hypothermia-related dysrhythmia.

Fortunately, cardiopulmonary arrest during pregnancy is an extremely uncommon event. Successful outcomes depend upon a simplified protocol, teamwork, communication, and advanced preparation and practice.

Acknowledgments

We wish to acknowledge Jackie Wiley (Department of Anesthesiology, University of Texas Southwestern Medical Center, Dallas, Texas), research nurse, for her assistance in obtaining and reviewing research references.

References

1. Rees GAD, Willis BA. Resuscitation in late pregnancy. Anaesthesia 1988;43:347.
2. American Heart Association. Textbook of Advanced Cardiac Life Support. Dallas, AHA, 1987.
3. Songster GS, Clark SL. Cardiac arrest in pregnancy—what to do. Contemp Obstet Gynecol 1985;26:141.
4. Newkirk EJ, Fry ME. Trauma during pregnancy: Nursing assessment in the emergency department. Focus Crit Care 1985;12:30.
5. Rozycki GS, Champion HR, Drass MJ. Traumatic injuries in the pregnant patient. Hosp Physician 1989;25:20.
6. American Heart Association Subcommittee on Emergency Cardiac Care: Guidelines for Cardiopulmonary Resuscitation and Emergency Cardiac Care. JAMA 1992;268:2172.
7. Sullivan JM, Ramanathan KB. Management of Medical Problems in Pregnancy—Severe Cardiac Disease. N Engl J Med 1985;313:304.
8. Brinkman CR III, Woods JR. Effects of hypovolemia and hypoxia upon the conceptus. In Buchsbaum HJ (ed): Trauma in Pregnancy. Philadelphia, WB Saunders, 1979, p 52.
9. Bieniarz J, Branda LA, Maqueda E, et al. Unreliability of the sphygmomanometric method in estimating uterine artery pressure. Am J Obstet Gynecol 1968;102:1106.
10. Ueland K, Novy JM, Peterson EN, Metcalfe J. Maternal cardiovascular dynamics: IV. The influence of gestational age on the maternal cardiovascular response to posture and exercise. Am J Obstet Gynecol 1969;104:856.
11. Kerr MG. The mechanical effects of the gravid uterus in late pregnancy. J Obstet Gynecol Br Commonw 1965;72:513.
12. Weinberger SE, Weiss ST, Cohen WR, et al. Pregnancy and the lung. Am Rev Respir Dis 1980;121:559.
13. Gee JBL, Packer BS, Millen JE, Robin ED. Pulmonary mechanics during pregnancy. J Clin Invest 1967;46:945.
14. Lee RV, Rodgers BD, White LM, Harvey RC. Cardiopulmonary resuscitation of pregnant women. Am J Med 1986;81:311.
15. Troiano N. Cardiopulmonary resuscitation of the pregnant woman. J Perinat Neonat Nurs 1989;3:1.
16. Mauer D, Dick W, Leyser K, et al. Characteristics of cardiopulmonary resuscitation in pregnant women. Anaesthetist 1990;39:393.
17. DeSwiet M. Thromboembolism. In DeSwiet M (ed): Medical Disorders in Obstetric Practice. London, Blackwell Scientific Publications, 1984.
18. Clark SL, Montz FJ, Phelan JP. Hemodynamic alterations associated with amniotic fluid embolism: A reappraisal. Am J Obstet Gynecol 1985;151:617.
19. Hanson GC. Cardiac arrest. In Baldwin RWM, Gillian CR, Hanson GC (eds): The Critically Ill Obstetric Patient. London, Farrand Press, 1984.
20. Hands ME, Johnson MD, Saltzman DH, et al. The cardiac, obstetric and anesthetic management of pregnancy complicated by acute myocardial infarction. J Clin Anesth 1990;2:258.
21. Caplan RA, Ward RJ, Posner K, et al. Unexpected cardiac arrest during spinal anesthesia. A closed claims analysis of predisposing factors. Anesthesiology 1988;68:5.
22. Crosby WM. Traumatic injuries during pregnancy. Clin Obstet Gynecol 1983;26:902.
23. Lynch C III. Depression of myocardial contractility in vitro by bupivacaine, etidocaine and lidocaine. Anesth Analg 1986; 65:551.
24. Wojtczak JA, Griffin RM, Pratilas V, et al. Mechanisms of arrhythmias during bupivacaine intoxication in rabbits—in vitro and in vivo study (abstract). Anesth Analg 1985;64:A302.
25. Wheeler DM, Bradley EL, Woods WT. The electrophysiologic actions of lidocaine and bupivacaine in the isolated perfused canine heart. Anesthesiology 1988; 68: 201.
26. Kasten GW. Amide local anesthetic alterations of the effective refractory period temporal dispersion: Relationship to ventricular arrhythmias. Anesthesiology 1986; 65: 61.
27. de La Coussaye JE, Brugada J, Allessie MA. Electrophysiologic and arrhythmogenic effects of bupivacaine. A study with high-resolution ventricular epicardial mapping in rabbit hearts. Anesthesiology 1992; 77:132.
28. Moller RA, Covino BG. Cardiac electrophysiologic effects of lidocaine and bupivacaine. Anesth Analg 1988; 67: 107.
29. Moller RA, Datta S, Fox J, Johnson M, Covino BG. Effects of progesterone on the cardiac electrophysiologic action of bupivacaine and lidocaine. Anesthesiology 1992;76:604.
30. Vogulgaropoulos DS, Johnson MD, Covino BG. Local anesthetic toxicity. Semin Anesth 1990;9:8.
31. Albright GA. Cardiac arrest following regional anesthesia with etidocaine and bupivacaine. Anesthesiology 1979;51:285.
32. de La Coussaye JE, Bassoul B, Albat B, et al. Experimental evidence in favor of intracellular actions of bupivacaine in myocardial depression. Anesth Analg 1992;74:698.
33. Sage DJ, Feldman HS, Arthur GR, et al. Influence of lidocaine and bupivacaine on isolated guinea pig atria in the presence of acidosis and hypoxia. Anesth Analg 1984;63:1.
34. Heavner JE, Dryden CF, Sanghani V, et al. Severe hypoxia enhances central nervous system and cardiovascular toxicity of bupivacaine in lightly anesthetized pigs. Anesthesiology 1992;77:142.
35. Clarkson CW, Hondeghem LM. Mechanism for bupivacaine depression of cardiac conduction. Fast block of sodium channels during the action potential with slow recovery from block during diastole. Anesthesiology 1985;62:396.
36. Reiz S, Nath S. Cardiotoxicity of local anaesthetic agents. Br J Anaesth 1986;58:736.
37. Kasten GW, Martin ST. Resuscitation from bupivacaine-induced cardiovascular toxicity during partial inferior vena cava occlusion. Anesth Analg 1986;65:341.
38. de Jong RH, Davis NL. Treating bupivacaine arrhythmias: Preliminary report. Reg Anesth 1985;6:99.

39. Kasten GW, Martin ST. Bupivacaine cardiovascular toxicity: Comparison of treatment with bretylium and lidocaine. Anesth Analg 1985;64:911.

40. de La Coussaye JE, Bassoul BP, Gagnol JP, et al. Experimental treatment of bupivacaine induced cardiotoxicity. What is the best choice? Reg Anesth 1991;16:120.

41. Kasten GW, Martin ST. Succesful cardiovascular resuscitation after massive intravenous overdose in anesthetized dogs. Anesth Analg 1985;64:491.

42. Long WB, Rosenblum S, Grady IP. Successful resuscitation of bupivacaine-induced cardiac arrest using cardiopulmonary bypass. Anesth Analg 1989;69:403.

43. Haasio J, Pitkanen MT, Kytta J, Rosenberg PH. Treatment of bupivacaine-induced cardiac arrhythmias in hypoxic and hypercarbic pigs with amiodarone or bretylium. Reg Anesth 1990;15:174.

44. de La Coussaye JE, Bassoul B, Brugada J, et al. Reversal of electrophysiologic and hemodynamic effects induced by high dose of bupivacaine by the combination of clonidine and dobutamine in anesthetized dogs. Anesth Analg 1992;74:703.

45. Scalabrini A, Simonetti M dos P, Velasco IT, et al. Hypertonic NaC1 solution prevents bupivacaine-induced cardiovascular toxicity. Circ Shock 1992;36:231.

46. Dimich I, Pal Singh P, Herschman Z, et al. Role of adenosine in the diagnosis and treatment of postoperative supraventricular tachyarrhythmias. J Clin Anesth 1993;5:325.

47. Rosen M. Difficult and failed intubation in obstetrics. In Latto IP, Rosen M (eds): Difficulties in Tracheal Intubation. London, Bailliere, 1985, p 152.

48. Prowse CM, Gaensler EA. Respiratory and acid base changes during pregnancy. Anesthesiology 1965;26:381.

49. Greenberger PA, Patterson R. Management of asthma during pregnancy. N Engl J Med 1985;313:517.

50. Archer GW, Marx GF. Arterial oxygen tension during apnoea in parturient women. Br J Anaesth 1974;46:358.

51. Kerr MG, Scott DB, Samuel E. Studies of the inferior vena cava in late pregnancy. Br Med J 1964;1:532.

52. Sachs PB, Oriol NE, Ostheimer GW, et al. Anesthetic related maternal mortality, 1954–1985. J Clin Anesth 1989;1:333.

53. Glassenberg R. General anesthesia and maternal mortality. Semin Perinatol 1991;15:386.

54. Heyman HJ. Risk management and malpractice issues in obstetric anesthesia. Semin Anesth 1991;1:82.

55. Arthure H, Tomkinson J, Organe G, et al. Report on Confidential Enquiries into Maternal Deaths in England and Wales (1967–1969). London, Her Majesty's Stationery Office 1972.

56. Arthure H, Tomkinson J, Organe G, et al. Report on Confidential Enquiries into Maternal Deaths in England and Wales (1970–1972). London, Her Majesty's Stationery Office 1975.

57. Tomkinson J, Turnbull A, Robson G, et al. Report on Confidential Enquiries into Maternal Deaths in England and Wales (1973–1975). London, Her Majesty's Stationery Office 1979.

58. Tomkinson J. Turnbull A, Robson G, et al. Report on Confidential Enquiries into Maternal Deaths in England and Wales (1976–1978). London, Her Majesty's Stationery Office 1982.

59. Turnbull A, Tindall V, Robson G, et al. Report on Confidential Enquiries into Maternal Deaths in England and Wales (1979–1981). London, Her Majesty's Stationery Office 1986.

60. Turnbull A, Tindall V, Robson G, et al. Report on Confidential Enquiries into Maternal Deaths in England and Wales (1982–1984). London, Her Majesty's Stationery Office 1989.

61. Kaunitz AM, Hughes JM, Grimes DA, et al. Causes of maternal mortality in the United States. Obstet Gynecol 1985;65:605.

62. Rochat RW, Koonin LM, Atrash HK, et al. Maternal mortality in the United States: Report from the Maternal Mortality Collaborative. Obstet Gynecol 1988;72:91.

63. Atrash HK, Koonin LM, Lawson HW, et al. Maternal mortality in the United States, 1979–1986. Obstet Gynecol 1990;76:1055.

64. Endler GC, Mariona FG, Sokol RJ, et al. Anesthesia related maternal mortality in Michigan, 1972–1984. Am J Obstet Gynecol 1988;159:187.

65. May WJ, Greiss FC Jr. Maternal mortality in North Carolina: A forty year experience. Am J Obstet Gynecol 1989;161:555.

66. Taylor G, Larson CP Jr, Prestwich R. Unexpected cardiac arrest during anesthesia and surgery. An environmental study. JAMA 1976;236:2758.

67. Keenan RL, Boyan CP. Cardiac arrest due to anesthesia: A study of incidence and causes. JAMA 1985;253:2373.

68. Lunn JN, Mushin WW. Mortality associated with anaesthesia. London, The Nuffield Provincial Hospitals Trust, 1987.

69. Buck N, Devlin HB, Lunn JN. The Report of a Confidential Enquiry into Perioperative Deaths. London, The Nuffield Provincial Hospitals Trust, 1982.

70. Greenberg MI, Roberts JR, Baskin SI. The use of endotracheal medications in cardiac emergencies. In Rund DA, Wolcott BW (eds): Emergency Medicine Manual 1983. Norwalk, CT, Appleton-Century-Crofts, 1983, p 91.

71. Lindsay SL, Hanson GC. Cardiac arrest in near-term pregnancy. Anaesthesia 1987;42:1074.

72. Kouwenhoven WB, Ing Dr, Jude JR, Knickerbocker, GG, Baltimore MSE. Closed-chest cardiac massage. JAMA 1960;173:1064.

73. Deshmukh HG, Weil MH, Rackow EC, Trevino R, Bisera J. Echocardiographic observations during cardiopulmonary resuscitation: A preliminary report. Crit Care Med 1985;13:904.

74. Maier GW, Tyson GS, Olsen CO, et al. The physiology of external cardiac massage: High-impulse cardiopulmonary resuscitation. Circulation 1984;70:86.

75. Weisfeldt ML, Chandra N. Physiology of cardiopulmonary resuscitation. Annu Rev Med 1981;32:435.

76. Sanders AB, Meislin HW, Ewy GA. The physiology of cardiopulmonary resuscitation. An update. JAMA 1984;252:3283.

77. Niemann JT, Garner D, Rosborough J, Criley JM. The mechanism of blood flow in closed chest cardiopulmonary resuscitation. Circulation 1979;59 and 60(Suppl II):74.

78. Niemann JT. Cardiopulmonary resuscitation. N Engl J Med 1992;327:1075.

79. Rudikoff MT, Maughan WL, Effron M, et al. Mechanisms of blood flow during cardiopulmonary resuscitation. Circulation 1980;61:345.

80. Werner JA, Greene HL, Janko CL, Cobb LA. Visualization of cardiac valve motion in man during external chest compression using two-dimensional echocardiography. Implications regarding the mechanism of blood flow. Circulation 1981;63:1417.

81. Peters J, Ihle J. Mechanics of the circulation during cardiopulmonary resuscitation: Pathophysiology and techniques (Part II). Intens Care Med 1990;16:20. (Part I) Intens Care Med 1990;16:11.

82. Guerci AD, Weisfeldt ML. Mechanical-ventilatory cardiac support. Crit Care Clin 1986; 2: 209.

83. Fisher JF, Vaghaiwalla F, Tsitlik J, et al. Determinants and clinical significance of jugular venous valve competence. Circulation 1982; 65: 188.

84. Niemann JT, Rosborough JP, Hausknecht M, et al. Pressure synchronised cineangiography during experimental cardiopulmonary resuscitation. Circulation 1981;64:985.

85. Paradis NA, Martin GB, Goetting MG, et al. Simultaneous aortic, jugular bulb and right atrial pressures during cardiopulmonary resuscitation in humans: insights into mechanisms. Circulation 1989;80:361.

86. Sladen A, Kouwenhoven WB, Jude JR, Knickerbocker GG. Landmark perspective: Closed chest massage. JAMA 1984; 251:3137.

87. Del Guercio LRM, Coomaraswamy RP, State D. Cardiac output and hypoxic acidosis during external cardiac massage in man. Surg Forum 1963;14:286.

88. Standards for cardiopulmonary resuscitation (CPR) and emergency cardiac care (ECC). JAMA 1980;244:453.

89. Montgomery WH, Herrin TJ, Lewis AJ. Basic Life Support for Physicians. Dallas, American Heart Association, 1983, p 8.

90. Del Guercio LRM, Feins NR, Cohn JD, et al. Comparison of blood flow during external and internal cardiac massage in man. Circulation 1965;32[Suppl]:171.

91. Del Guercio LRM, Coomaraswamy RP, State D. Cardiac output and other hemodynamic variables during external cardiac massage in man. N Engl J Med 1963;269:1398.

92. Mackenzie GJ, Taylor SH, McDonald AH, Donald KW. Haemodynamic effects of external cardiac compression. Lancet 1964; 1:1342.

93. American Heart Association. Standards and guidelines for cardiopulmonary resuscitation and emergency cardiac care. JAMA 1980;244:453.

94. Safar P, Bircher NG. Cardiopulmonary Cerebral Resuscitation.

A Manual for Physicians and Paramedical Instructors. Philadelphia, WB Saunders, 1981.

95. Niemann JT. Differences in cerebral and myocardial perfusion during closed chest resuscitation. Ann Emerg Med 1984;13:849.

96. Robertson C, Holmberg S. Compression techniques and blood flow during cardiopulmonary resuscitation. A statement for the Advanced Life Support Working Party of the European Resuscitation Council 1992;24:123.

97. Ditchley RV, Winkler J, Rhodes CA. Relative lack of coronary blood flow during closed chest resuscitation in dogs. Circulation 1982;66:297.

98. Krause GS, Kumar K, White BC. Ischemia, resuscitation and reperfusion. Am Heart J 1986;11:768.

99. Kette F, Weil MH, Gazmuri RJ, et al. Intramyocardial hypercarbic acidosis during cardiac arrest and resuscitation. Crit Care Med 1993;21:901.

100. Jackson RE. Haemodynamics of cardiac massage. Emerg Med Clin North Am 1983;1:501.

101. Brown CG, Werman HA. Adrenergic agonists during cardiopulmonary resuscitation. Resuscitation 1990;19:1.

102. Paradis NA, Koscove EM. Epinephrine in cardiac arrest. A critical review. Ann Emerg Med 1990;19:1288.

103. Michael JR, Guerci AD, Koehler RC, et al. Mechanisms by which epinephrine augments cerebral and myocardial perfusion during cardiopulmonary resuscitation in dogs. Circulation 1984;69:822.

104. Chandra N, Rudikoff M, Weisfeldt ML. Simultaneous chest compression and ventilation at high airway pressure during cardiopulmonary resuscitation. Lancet 1980;1:175.

105. Wilder RJ, Weir D, Rush BF, et al. Methods of coordinating ventilation and closed chest massage in the dog. Surgery 1963;53:186.

106. Babbs CF. New versus old theories of blood flow during CPR. Crit Care Med 1980;8:191.

107. Swenson RD, Weaver WD, Niskanen RA, et al. Hemodynamics in humans during conventional and experimental methods of cardiopulmonary resuscitation. Circulation 1988;78:630.

108. Criley JM, Blaufuss AH, Kissel GL. Cough-induced cardiac compression. Self-administered form of cardiopulmonary resuscitation. JAMA 1976;236:1246.

109. Niemann JT, Rosborough JP, Brown D, et al. Cough-CPR: Documentation of systemic perfusion in man and in an experimental model—a window to the mechanism of blood flow in external CPR. Crit Care Med 1980;8:141.

110. Robertson C. The precordial thump and cough techniques in advanced life support. A Statement for the Advanced Life Support Working Party of the European Resuscitation Council. Resuscitation 1992;24:133.

111. Harris LC, Kirimli B, Safar P. Augmentation of artificial circulation during cardiopulmonary resuscitation. Anesthesiology 1967;28:730.

112. Chandra, N, Snyder LD, Weisfeldt ML, et al. Abdominal binding during cardiopulmonary resuscitation in man. JAMA 1981;246:351.

113. Niemann JT, Rosborough JP, Ung S, Criley JM. Hemodynamic effects of continuous abdominal binding during cardiac arrest and resuscitation. Am J Cardiol 1984;53:269.

114. Ralston SH, Babbs CF, Niebauer MJ. Cardiopulmonary resuscitation with interposed abdominal compression in dogs. Anaesth Analg 1982;61:645.

115. Redding JS. Abdominal compression in cardiopulmonary resuscitation. Anesth Analg 1971;50:688.

116. Bircher N, Safar P, Stewart R. A comparison of standard, MAST-augmented, and open-chest CPR in dogs. Crit Care Med 1980;8:147.

117. Cohen TJ, Goldner BG, Maccaro PC, et al. A comparison of active compression-decompression cardiopulmonary resuscitation with standard cardiopulmonary resuscitation for cardiac arrests occurring in the hospital. N Engl J Med 1993;329:1918.

118. DePace NL, Betesh JS, Kotler MN. Postmortem cesarean section with recovery of both mother and offspring. JAMA 1982;248:971.

119. Oates S, Williams GL, Rees GAD. Cardiopulmonary resuscitation in late pregnancy. Br Med J 1988;297:404.

120. O'Connor RL, Sevarino FB. Cardiopulmonary arrest in the pregnant patient: A report of a successful resuscitation. J Clin Anesth 1994;6:60.

121. Marx GF. Cardiopulmonary resuscitation of late-pregnant women. Anesthesiology 1982;56:156.

122. Crockett PJ, Droppert BM, Higgins SE. Defibrillation—What You Should Know, 3rd ed. Physio Control Corporation, 1991, p 1.

123. Weber CE. Postmortem cesarean section: Review of the literature and case reports. Am J Obstet Gynecol 1971;110:158.

124. Arthur RK. Postmortem cesarean section. Am J Obstet Gynecol 1978;132:175.

125. Buchsbaum HJ, Cruikshank DP. Postmortem cesarean section. In Buchsbaum HJ (ed): Trauma in Pregnancy. Philadelphia, WB Saunders, 1979, p 236.

126. Ritter OW. Postmortem cesarean section. JAMA 1961;175:715.

127. Kelly JV, Winston HG. Successful postmortem cesarean section. Am J Obstet Gynecol 1956;72:203.

128. Katz VL, Dotters DJ, Droegemueller W. Perimortem cesarean delivery. Obstet Gynecol 1986;68:571.

129. Manner RI. Family Law-Court ordered surgery for the protection of a viable fetus. West N Engl Law Rev 1982, p 125.

130. Pritchard JA, MacDonald PC, Gant NF. Obstetrics in broad perspective. In Pritchard JA, MacDonald PC, Gant NF, et al (eds). Williams' Obstetrics, 17th ed. New York, Appleton-Century-Crofts 1985, p 3.

131. Advanced Trauma Life Support Manual. American College of Surgeons, Chicago, 1988, p 61.

132. Hapnes SA, Robertson C. CPR-drug delivery routes and systems. A statement for the Advanced Life Support Working Party of the European Resuscitation Council. Resuscitation 1992;24:137.

133. Kuhn GJ, White BC, Swetnam RE, et al. Peripheral vs central circulation times during CPR: A pilot study. Ann Emerg Med 1981;10:417.

134. Sabin HI, Coghill SB, Khunti K, et al. Accuracy of intracardiac injection determined by post-mortem study. Lancet 1993; 2:1054.

135. Thornhill ML, O'Leary AJ, Lussos S, et al. An *in vitro* assessment of amniotic fluid removal through cell saver processing (abstract). Anesthesiology 1991;75:A830

136. Rivers EP, Lozon J, Enriquez E, et al. Simultaneous radial, femoral and aortic arterial pressures during human cardiopulmonary resuscitation. Crit Care Med 1993;21:878.

137. Russell ES. Cardiac arrest: (A) Survival after two and one-half hours of open chest cardiac massage and (B) survival after closed chest cardiac massage. Can Med Assoc J 1962;87:512.

138. Stewart JSS, Stewart WK, Gillies HG. Cardiac arrest and acidosis. Lancet 1962;2 964.

139. Cooper DR. Cardiac arrest on the myelographic tilt table. JAMA 1964;187:674.

140. Sykes MK, Ahmed N. Emergency treatment for cardiac arrest. Lancet 1963;2:347.

141. Shocket E, Rosenblum R. Successful open cardiac massage after 75 minutes of closed massage. JAMA 1967;200:333.

142. Linton AL, Ledingham IM. Severe hypothermia with barbiturate intoxication. Lancet 1966;1:24.

143. Bayne CG, Josing W. Reversal of inadequate cardiac output and perfusion during CPR by open-chest cardiac massage. Am J Emerg Med 1984;2:138.

144. Brunette DD, Biros M, Mlinek EJ, et al. Internal cardiac massage and mediastinal irrigation in hypothermic cardiac arrest. Am J Emerg Med 1992;10:32.

145. Cohn JD, Del Guercio LRM, Feins NR, et al. Cardiorespiratory determinants of cardiopulmonary arrest. Surg Forum 1983; 1:182.

146. Weiser FM, Adler LN, Kuhn LA. Hemodynamic effects of closed and open chest cardiac resuscitation in normal dogs and those with acute myocardial infarction. Am J Cardiol 1962;10:555.

147. Weale FE, Rothwell-Jackson RL. Efficiency of cardiac massage. Lancet 1962;1:990.

148. Byrne D, Pass HI, Neely WA, et al. External versus internal cardiac massage in normal and chronically ischemic dogs. Am Surg 1980;46:657.

149. Bircher N, Safar P. Comparison of standard and new closed-chest CPR and open-chest CPR in dogs. Crit Care Med 1981;9:384.

150. Alifimoff JK, Safar P, Bircher N. Cardiac resuscitability and cerebral recovery after closed-chest, MAST augmented and open chest CPR (abstract). Anesthesiology 1980;3:S151.
151. Robertson C. The value of open chest CPR for non-traumatic cardiac arrest. Resuscitation 1991;22:203.
152. Bartnett WM, Alifimoff JK, Paris PM, et al. Comparison of open-chest cardiac massage techniques in dogs. Ann Emerg Med 1986;15:408.
153. Babbs CF. Hemodynamic mechanisms in CPR: A theoretical rationale for resuscitative thoracotomy in non-traumatic cardiac arrest. Resuscitation 1987;15:37.
154. White CS. The role of heart massage in surgery. Surg Gynecol Obstet 1909;4:388.
155. American Heart Assocation: Textbook of Advanced Cardiac Life Support. Dallas, AHA, 1987, p 233.
156. American Heart Association Subcommittee on Emergency Cardiac Care: Guidelines for Cardiopulmonary Resuscitation and Emergency Cardiac Care. JAMA 1992;268:2249.
157. Ueland K, Hansen JM. Maternal cardiovascular hemodynamics. III: Labor and delivery under local and caudal analgesia. Am J Obstet Gynecol 1969;103:8.
158. Kaye W, Mancini MF, Rallis S, Handel LP. Education aspects: Resuscitation training and evaluation. In Kaye W, Bircher NG (eds): Cardiopulmonary Resuscitation. Scientific Basis, Current Standards and Future Trends. Clin Crit Care Med 1989;16:124.
159. Lowenstein SR, Hansborough JF, Libby LS, et al. Cardiopulmonary resuscitation by medical and surgical house-officers. Lancet 1981;2:679.
160. Stross JK, Bole GG. Maintaining competency in advanced cardiac life support skills. JAMA 1983;249:3339.

VASCULAR DISEASES

. . . .

Jack A. Stecher, M.D., and David R. Gambling, M.B.

OCCLUSIVE THROMBOARTEROPATHY

Occlusive thromboarteropathy (OTAP) or Takayasu's arteritis is an idiopathic condition characterized by obliterative arteritis. Symptoms are related to the organ systems involved by stenosis and obliteration of large and intermediate arteries.[1] This chronic disease can affect any artery, but significant signs and symptoms arise as a result of involvement of the aorta, its major branches, and the pulmonary arteries.[2] Upper extremity involvement has led to the name *pulseless disease*. Inflammation and subsequent fibrosis affect the arterial media, intima, and adventitia, with intimal involvement being the direct cause of arterial stenosis and obliteration.[2, 3] The characteristic pathologic change observed in affected vessels is fibrosis. Signs and symptoms of OTAP reflect the vascular beds and organs to which blood flow has been diminished.

Occlusive thromboarteropathy affects women almost six times as often as men,[1, 4] and it affects Asian and Latino women predominantly.[5] Although the onset of the disease occurs between the ages of 11 and 48 years,[6] it arises predominantly during the second and third decades of life[5]; therefore, pregnancy can be a coexisting condition.

Classification and Prognosis

Several classifications of OTAP have been proposed with most based on the site of the anatomic lesions.[2, 6, 7] As an example, Ueno and coworkers have suggested a comprehensive anatomic description,[7] which has been further modified by Lupi and coworkers[2] (Table 4–1).

Ishikawa presented a clinical classification of OTAP "with special reference to the natural history and prognosis" of the disease (Table 4–2).[8]

Takayasu's retinopathy is considered mild or moderate if there is dilatation or microaneurysm formation of the small retinal vessels. Severe disease reflects formation of arteriovenous anastomoses or visual changes.[8]

Hypertension is classified as mild if the brachial systolic pressure is 140 to 159 and/or the diastolic pressure is 90 to 94 mm Hg, or the popliteal systolic pressure is 160 to 179 mm Hg and/or the diastolic pressure is 90 to 94 mm Hg. Hypertension is severe if the systolic brachial artery pressure is 200 mm Hg or higher and/or the diastolic pressure is 110 mm Hg or higher or the popliteal systolic pressure is 230 mm Hg or higher and/or the diastolic pressure is 110 mm Hg or higher. Pressures between the limits of mild and severe hypertension are considered moderate.

The severity of aneurysms of the aorta and its main branches are determined angiographically. An aneurysm is classified as severe if its diameter is more than twice that of the normal vessel. The severity of aortic regurgitation is estimated either angiographically or clinically; however, criteria for its severity are not described.[8]

Although OTAP is a chronic disease with survival of up to 14 years, periods of remission are common.[9] Ishikawa stresses the importance of starting treatment (steroids and anticoagulants) early to slow progression of the disease and its consequences. Despite ongoing treatment, the 5-year mortality rate for patients with group IIb or group III disease in Ishikawa's study was 30%. Survival for groups I and IIa was significantly better, with only one death among the 31 patients in those categories. Death resulted from congestive heart failure or cerebrovascular accident.[8]

OTAP and Pregnancy

Pregnancy in patients with early OTAP is not associated with an increased risk for obstetric complications.[10] If OTAP is symptomatic, 50% of pregnant patients require management of hypertension. OTAP is not associated with an increased rate of premature labor, but intrauterine growth retardation is seen often in the fetus. Neonatal outcome is worse with advanced maternal vascular involvement, with severe hypertension during pregnancy (especially in the presence of pre-eclampsia), and with delayed management of

TABLE 4–1. **UENO AND LUPI's CLASSIFICATION OF OTAP**

Type I	Lesions restricted to the aortic arch and major branches (Shimizu and Sano Type)
Type II	"Atypical coarctation of the aorta" with involvement of the thoracic descending aorta and the abdominal aorta without aortic arch involvement (Kimoto type)
Type III	Features of both type I and type II (Inada type)
Type IV	Any involvement of the pulmonary arteries

Data from Ueno A, Awane Y, Wakabayashi A, et al. Successfully operated obliterative brachiocephalic arteritis (Takayasu) associated with the elongated coarctation. Jpn Heart J 1967;8:538; and Lupi E, Sanchez G, Horwitz S, et al. Pulmonary artery involvement in Takayasu's arteritis. Chest 1975;67:69.

OTAP. Induction of labor and cesarean section are performed for the usual obstetric indications.[10]

Some patients with OTAP have resolution or improvement of their symptoms during pregnancy,[11] whereas others have either no change in, or worsening of, their condition.[12] Pregnancy is said to have an unfavorable effect on the patient when the OTAP classification of Ishikawa changes from I to II, or II to III (see Table 4–2).

The risk of cerebral ischemia is increased during pregnancy, especially during the first trimester and the early postpartum period. A small reduction in mean arterial blood pressure in patients with severe occlusive disease has the potential for syncope or severe cerebral ischemia.[12]

Cerebrovascular accidents (CVA) are likely when patients have

■ Severe narrowing of the branches of the aortic arch
■ Elevated systolic blood pressure during the first stage of labor
■ Complications in groups IIb or III

Avoiding pregnancy, or elective termination of pregnancy, is recommended for patients whose disease is characteristic of group IIb or III disease.[12] For women who decline termination of pregnancy, hospitalization and symptomatic management, as required, are recommended. Elective cesarean section often is used for women whose disease is in groups IIb or III who

TABLE 4–2. **ISHIKAWA'S AND MATSUURA'S CLASSIFICATION OF OTAP**

Group I	Narrowing or occlusion in any part of the aorta and/or its main branches with or without pulmonary artery involvement
Group II*	OTAP with one of the following complications: Takayasu's retinopathy secondary hypertension aortic regurgitation aortic or arterial aneurysm
Group III	OTAP with two or more of the complications listed in Group II

Data from Ishikawa K, Matsuura S. Occlusive Thromboaortopathy (Takayasu's Disease) and pregnancy. Am J Cardiol 1982;50:1293.
*Group II is subdivided into mild and moderate (Group IIa) and severe (Group IIb) disease. See text for description.

reach near term, especially those with retinopathy and severely elevated systolic blood pressure (BP) in early labor. Ishikawa and Matsuura recommend elective cesarean section for women with groups IIb and III disease if BPs are not obtainable in either arm, because monitoring BPs in the lower extremities in women in labor is difficult. They also recommend elective cesarean section for women with groups I and IIa disease if elevation of systolic BP is severe despite aggressive medical management.[12]

Anesthetic Management

The anesthetic management of OTAP must take into account the susceptibility of the patient to severe hypertension with its concomitant risk of CVA and cardiac failure. Hypotension is poorly tolerated and may result in cerebral ischemia. Other considerations include the risk of pulmonary hypertension and the difficulty of hemodynamic monitoring, due to the nature of the disease.

Hemodynamic Monitoring

The need for invasive hemodynamic monitoring must be assessed for each patient. Early consultation is desirable to define the arterial involvement, review the aortography, assess the cardiovascular status, and control the BP.[13, 14]

Patients with group I or IIa disease have a mild form with little hemodynamic compromise. Electrocardiogram, pulse oximetry, and noninvasive blood pressure monitoring are adequate. When OTAP affects peripheral arteries, however, noninvasive pressures may be inaccurate or unobtainable. In such cases a peripheral arterial catheter should be inserted,[5] but occasionally a central arterial catheter introduced via the femoral artery may be required.[14] The use of such catheters carries a risk of arterial occlusion at the site of insertion.[15–17]

When OTAP is associated with heart failure it is necessary to monitor central venous, right heart, and pulmonary capillary wedge pressures. Calculation of cardiac output and systemic vascular and pulmonary vascular resistance aids in the prevention of heart failure and in the maintenance of adequate cerebral and renal perfusion.[1, 13, 14, 18]

Choice of Anesthetic

For labor and delivery, epidural analgesia has the advantage of providing effective pain relief, preventing acute catecholamine release associated with labor pain. The anesthesiologist should carefully titrate the dose of local anesthetic to produce a level satisfactory for delivery without causing severe hypotension, which could lead to cerebral ischemia.[19] Giving patients oxygen by mask and encouraging them to experience labor in the lateral position help ensure adequate oxygen delivery to the fetus.

Bupivacaine 0.25% in 2- to 3-ml increments can be given to produce an initial T10 sensory block. Bupivacaine (0.1%–0.0625%) with fentanyl (2–3 µg/ml), infused at a rate of 12 to 14 ml/hr, maintains analgesia throughout labor and delivery. A central infusion of vasopressors (phenylephrine 0.05–0.25 $\mu g \cdot kg^{-1} \cdot min^{-1}$) or vasodilators (nitroprusside 1–8 $\mu g \cdot kg^{-1} \cdot min^{-1}$) should be available to prevent dangerous swings in arterial pressure.

For cesarean section, epidural anesthesia must be induced slowly and incrementally using 2% lidocaine or 0.5% bupivacaine and fentanyl 1 to 1.5 µg/kg. Three percent 2-chloroprocaine may be administered to produce a surgical level of anesthesia rapidly in cases of fetal distress when an epidural catheter is already in place.[4, 5, 14, 17] It is our opinion that epidural epinephrine should be avoided in parturients with OTAP.

One advantage of epidural anesthesia for cesarean section is that the patient remains awake. This gives the anesthesiologist a clinical assessment of cerebral perfusion, which central or peripheral arterial pressures may not accurately reflect.

General anesthesia can be given for cesarean section, although evaluation of cerebral perfusion becomes more difficult or impossible even with an electroencephalogram (EEG). Patients with severe carotid disease, however, should have EEG monitoring to help prevent cerebral ischemia during general anesthesia. Pretreatment with beta adrenergic blockers (labetalol in 5- to 10-mg increments titrated to the desired response), nitroglycerin 50 to 100 µg, or lidocaine 1 to 1.5 mg/kg intravenously can attenuate the rise in systolic blood pressure that accompanies intubation. Rapid-sequence induction with thiopental and succinylcholine is then performed and the airway secured. During tracheal intubation, extreme extension of the patient's neck must be avoided because stenosis of the carotid arteries predisposes to occlusion and hence the risk of cerebral ischemia. Nitrous oxide must be avoided if pulmonary vasoconstriction and hypertension are present. Nitrous oxide has been used without adverse reaction in a parturient with Takayasu's arteritis, but pulmonary hypertension was ruled out before its administration.[20]

Following delivery of the neonate, general anesthesia is maintained with a volatile agent and opioids. Oxytocin has been given to provide uterine contraction safely following delivery, but prostaglandin $F_{2\alpha}$ and ergot alkaloids should be given cautiously as they can cause systemic and pulmonary hypertension.

Spinal anesthesia in OTAP is controversial because of an increased risk of hypotension. Preoperative volume expansion with 15 to 20 ml/kg of a glucose-free crystalloid solution and judicious use of ephedrine or other pressors are especially important in maintaining BP

and vital organ perfusion during spinal anesthesia.[15] Left uterine displacement is even more critical in these patients when regional anesthesia is administered.

Patients with OTAP frequently receive anticoagulant and corticosteroid therapy. Coagulation abnormalities must be corrected before instituting regional anesthesia to avoid epidural hematoma. Adrenal supression may be assumed and supplemental steroids considered.

PRIMARY PULMONARY HYPERTENSION

Primary pulmonary hypertension (PPH) is a disease of unknown origin that produces a sustained rise of at least 25 mm Hg in mean pulmonary artery pressure.[21] This elevated pressure inevitably leads to right ventricular dilatation and right ventricular hypertrophy progressing to right ventricular failure and death.[21, 22] The course of PPH usually is slow, but unrelenting, with death 4 to 6 years after the initial diagnosis. Its course may be as short as 6 months from first symptoms to death, however.

Primary pulmonary hypertension affects women four to five times more often than men. It may arise at any age, but is most prevalent in the third and fourth decades,[23] with a mean age at diagnosis of 27 years.[24] Among the prognostic indicators of survival the most powerful and easily obtainable is the systemic arterial oxygen saturation (SpO_2). When SpO_2 is greater than 63%, the rate of 3-year survival is 55%. When SpO_2 is less than 63%, the rate of 3-year survival is only 17%.[23]

Sudden death is caused by tachycardia and loss of effective atrial systole, acute pulmonary embolism from deep venous thromboses, or right ventricular ischemia or infarction.[22] A rapid increase in venous return to the right heart, and subsequently to the lungs, may produce a vagally mediated bradycardia and a fall in cardiac output, which can be lethal.[25]

In most cases, postmortem microscopic examination of the lungs reveals that both lungs are affected by diffuse pulmonary vascular changes characterized by intimal proliferation, medial hypertrophy, and perivascular lymphocytic cuffing—described as plexogenic arteriopathy.[26] Thrombotic pulmonary arteriopathy has been reported as a more likely cause of pulmonary hypertension.[23] PPH caused by pulmonary veno-occlusive disease with intimal proliferation and fibrosis of intrapulmonary veins and venules occurs less frequently.[22]

Signs and Symptoms

The signs and symptoms of PPH are related to right ventricular compromise and failure. Dyspnea is caused by decreased cardiac output and ventilation/perfusion ($\dot{V}/\dot{Q}$) mismatch. Syncope is due to a fixed cardiac output and an inability of the heart to respond to a demand for increased output. Angina is common and is probably related to right ventricular ischemia and increased right ventricular afterload. Other signs and symptoms include fatigue, edema, and peripheral cyanosis. Occasionally, hoarseness develops owing to the pressure of an enlarging pulmonary artery on the recurrent laryngeal nerve, which is known as Ortner's syndrome.[22]

A right ventricular heave may be present, and an ejection click may be heard over the pulmonic area. The second heart sound usually is split, with accentuation of the pulmonic component. There may be an ejection murmur and a regurgitant murmur over the pulmonary valve. Jugular venous distension and prominent A wave usually are evident. Chest radiography demonstrates right ventricular enlargement, hilar enlargement, and peripheral vasculature pruning (Fig. 4–1). The electrocardiogram shows right ventricular hypertrophy and right axis deviation (Fig. 4–2). Pulmonary function tests may indicate restrictive disease due to decreased lung compliance as a result of elevated pulmonary vascular pressure.[22]

Association With Pregnancy

Among women of reproductive age, approximately 8% of PPH is associated with pregnancy.[26] It is possible

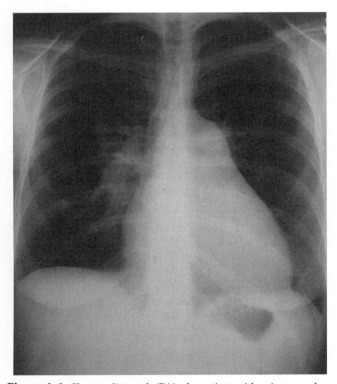

Figure 4–1. Chest radiograph (PA) of a patient with primary pulmonary hypertension. Note the large hilum bilaterally, representing large right and left pulmonary arteries and the ischemic peripheral vessels, indicative of pruning of the peripheral vasculature. Right ventricular enlargement would be seen on the lateral view.

that pregnancy initiates PPH in some women, but it is more likely that symptoms of pre-existing disease are unmasked by the increased hemodynamic stress of pregnancy.[26] When symptoms arise during pregnancy, the diagnosis of PPH is made only after excluding other causes of pulmonary hypertension. These include amniotic fluid embolism, trophoblastic embolism, thromboembolism, obliterative hypertension, and Eisenmenger syndrome.[26]

Primary pulmonary hypertension and pregnancy is an ominous combination. Maternal mortality ranges from 36 to 56%,[21, 24, 27] with death often during delivery, or 4 days to 6 weeks after delivery—despite intensive postoperative management.[21] Death usually is sudden, precipitated by acute right heart failure. Absolute pulmonary artery pressure is a poor indicator of the extent of the disease. A poor prognosis in pregnancy, however, is associated with right ventricular hypertrophy, low cardiac index ($2–2.5 \, l \cdot min^{-1} \cdot m^{-2}$), increased right atrial pressure (10 mm Hg) and high pulmonary vascular resistance ($>1000–1500$ dynes-sec $\cdot \, cm^{-5}$).[21]

Anesthetic Management

The principal goals of management of PPH include avoiding increases in pulmonary vascular resistance and pulmonary artery pressure, preventing changes in right ventricular preload, and maintaining left ventricular afterload and right ventricular contractility.[28, 29] Potent titratable drugs should be readily available in the event of hemodynamic instability. The need for inotropes (dopamine or dobutamine), vasopressors (phenylephrine or ephedrine), or afterload reducers (nitroprusside or phentolamine) during labor and delivery or cesarean section should be anticipated.

Before the onset of labor, the severity of pulmonary hypertension by pulmonary artery catheterization can be assessed in addition to the response of the pulmonary vasculature to vasoactive drugs.[28, 30] Preoperative adenosine and nifedipine have been shown to reduce pulmonary vascular pressure.[31] These may be useful adjuncts to oxygen therapy at the time of parturition. It is important to measure right- and left-sided pressures continuously during labor and delivery. Multiple pulmonary capillary wedge pressure (PCWP) measurements should be discouraged because of the risk of pulmonary artery rupture.

During delivery, an increase in pulmonary vascular resistance can occur as a result of hypercarbia, acidosis, hypoxia, stress, and pain.[30] Epidural analgesia provides excellent pain control and attenuates many of these adverse effects. Investigators have reported successful management of labor using various doses of epidural local anesthetics, with and without fentanyl.[21, 25, 30, 32–36] Ackerman and Juneja have questioned the addition of fentanyl to labor epidural infusions out of concern of its causing myocardial depression in patients with compromised hearts.[37] It seems unlikely that 2 μg/ml fentanyl at 10 to 15 ml/hr would produce serum levels that would be clinically important in this regard. Care should be taken to titrate the level of analgesia to avoid hypotension and reduction in right ventricular preload. Excellent pain relief also has been obtained in patients with pulmonary hypertension using 1 mg intrathecal morphine.[38, 39] Forceps or vacuum extraction is often used to help prevent the untoward hemodynamic effects caused by maternal pushing.

Cesarean section can be performed after careful extension of an epidural block to T4-5 without significant risk of severe hypotension when provision to support blood pressure has been taken. Both epidural anesthesia[40, 41] and general anesthesia have been administered successfully for cesarean section[33, 42] and tubal ligation[43] in patients with PPH. Invasive monitoring was also used during these procedures.

Proponents of general anesthesia usually cite the risk of decreased afterload, decreased preload, and acute right heart failure that may be precipitated by sympathetic blockade induced by epidural or spinal analgesia.[42] Supporters of regional anesthesia suggest that careful titration of the level of the block and judicious use of vasoactive drugs allow for satisfactory management in these parturients. In addition, pulmonary hemodynamic changes associated with laryngoscopy,[44] which increase the risk for precipitating right heart failure, are avoided with regional anesthesia.

If general anesthesia is selected, it is recommended that nitrous oxide be avoided owing to its tendency to promote increased pulmonary vascular resistance. Isoflurane is the volatile anesthetic agent of choice for general anesthesia because it has the least depressant effect on the myocardium. It should be given with an air and oxygen mixture.[43] In patients with labile disease, and/or in those with severe disease, we recommend invasive monitoring. Spinal anesthesia is contraindicated due to the risk of rapid-onset, deleterious hemodynamic changes.

PULMONARY ARTERIOVENOUS MALFORMATIONS

Pulmonary arteriovenous malformations (PAVM) are rare, thin-walled vascular lesions that may complicate pregnancy because of rapid enlargement or rupture. They occur as discrete or multiple lesions, in one or more lobes, and in one or both lungs.[45, 46] Many small AVM may be scattered throughout the lungs.[46, 47] There is an 11% mortality in patients with untreated PAVM.[45, 48]

About 60% of patients with PAVM suffer from Osler-Weber-Rendu disease (OWR), a disease with autosomal dominant transmission, also called *hereditary hemorrhagic telangiectasia*.[49, 50] About 15% of patients with OWR have PAVM,[45, 49, 51] and patients frequently exhibit multiple cutaneous and mucous membrane AVM, which are visible on the lips, labia, and oral mucosa. Epistaxis arising from lesions of the nasal mucosa is highly characteristic.[50] Pregnant women who have a family history of OWR or have mucocutaneous signs of the disease should be evaluated for occult pulmonary lesions.[50, 52]

Most PAVM are congenital, but patients are not diagnosed until the second decade.[45] Most PAVM occur singly and grow slowly.[50] Patients with OWR, however, tend to have a high incidence of multiple PAVM that seem to grow more rapidly and produce more complications than in patients without OWR.[47]

Complications associated with the pulmonary lesions include vascular shunts, mitral valve disease, congestive heart failure (CHF), bacterial endocarditis, hemoptysis and hemothorax due to rupture, and cerebral embolism, thrombosis, and abscess.[46, 53] Most shunts are right-to-left, but left-to-right shunts of the bronchial, internal mammary, and intercostal arteries have been described.[46] Paradoxical emboli may arise in the systemic circulation and pass through the enlarged and engorged PAVM to affect the cerebral circulation.[46] Likewise, thrombi may originate on diseased valves or within PAVM, due to the sluggish flow characteristic of AVM, and may shower the cerebral circulation. Paradoxical air emboli can occur when air enters the pulmonary circulation following rupture of a PAVM.[50] Such a rupture is rare, but when it occurs it is frequently massive and fatal. Rapid recognition, response, and repair or resection are necessary if the patient is to survive.[50]

Pregnancy and Pulmonary Arteriovenous Malformations

Pregnancy increases the risk of PAVM enlargement and rupture.[48, 50, 51, 54, 55] The increase in size is a result of the increase in blood volume and cardiac output.[52] In addition, the hormonal changes of pregnancy directly affect the compliance of the blood vessel, with an elevation in the level of progesterone causing relaxation of arteriolar smooth muscle and further dilatation of the PAVM.[51, 52, 56, 57] Estrogens are associated with the formation of spider telangiectasia and may contribute to an increase in PAVM size during pregnancy.[47] During pregnancy there is a gradual increase in venous distensibility, which is greatest (150% of normal) just before delivery, similar to the 20 to 30% increase in venous distensibility observed during the menstrual cycle.[57–59]

The structure of the AVM contributes to its fragility. The vascular spaces are lined by a single layer of endothelial cells on a continuous basement membrane.[60] Smooth muscle cells within the walls of the

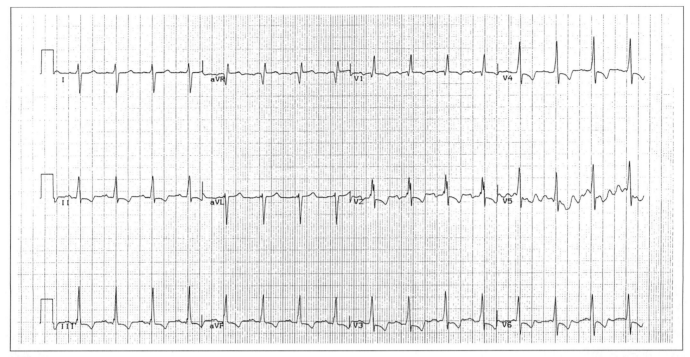

Figure 4–2. Electrocardiogram of a patient with primary pulmonary hypertension. Note large-voltage QRS complexes in the right precordial leads, which represent right ventricular hypertrophy. (Other changes on this ECG are not necessarily related to primary pulmonary hypertension.)

AVM are irregularly shaped and do not form a continuous structure around the blood vessels. Both endothelial cells and smooth muscle cells are vacuolated, which suggests degeneration. There is no elastic tissue within the walls. Thus, the walls of the AVM appear to be insufficient as a contractile element and are unable to respond to the increased stress associated with the increased blood volume and cardiac output of pregnancy.[60] The walls of the AVM, therefore, are unable to contract and control hemorrhage when they rupture.[50, 60] In addition, Waring and coworkers suggest that there may be an elevation in tissue plasminogen activator (TPA) in the endothelium of AVM, which impairs clot formation when bleeding occurs.[52]

Signs and Symptoms of Pulmonary Arteriovenous Malformations

The usual symptoms of PAVM—dyspnea, cyanosis, and clubbing—are caused by hypoxemia due to right-to-left shunt. Hypoxemia induces bone marrow to increase its production of hemoglobin and red blood cells, and it may cause polycythemia. A shunt of at least 25% is required to produce clubbing and polycythemia.[45, 46] Although plasma volume remains normal, the red blood cell mass and volume increase.[45] Frequent minor hemorrhages may prevent polycythemia.[46]

Hemoptysis and hemothorax occur when a lesion ruptures into the airway and pleural cavity, respectively. A cerebrovascular accident may occur following thromboembolic events.[50]

Bruits often are audible on the chest wall over the AVM.[45, 46, 50] A continuous hum is accentuated by systole and deep inspiration. The characteristic features on chest radiograph are those of a peripheral, circumscribed, lobulated, noncalcified structure connected to the hilum by tortuous vessels (Fig. 4–3). Fluoroscopy of the lesion shows pulsations with each heart beat, and increase and decrease in size with Müller and Valsalva maneuvers (inspiration and expiration against a closed glottis), respectively.[45, 46]

According to Peery, cardiomegaly is "conspicuously absent" in patients with right-to-left shunt.[61] If cardiomegaly is present on the radiograph, the clinician should suspect concomitant right heart disease or left-to-right shunt.[61] Rib notching occurs when left-to-right shunt via an enlarged and tortuous intercostal AVM exists. The definitive diagnosis of a PAVM is made by angiography.

Management of the Pregnant Patient with PAVM

When PAVM become symptomatic during pregnancy, they can be managed successfully utilizing spring coil[50–52, 62] or balloon[48, 50, 62] embolization. These procedures are done using local anesthesia, and successful occlusion usually resolves the hypoxemia and high-output CHF.

When multiple lesions exist, they may not be amenable to embolization, and pulmonary lobule or lobe resection is necessary to eliminate them. This surgery

A significant fall in SVR and an increase in right-to-left shunt must be avoided by carefully raising the level of the epidural to T10. SVR is supported with an ephedrine or a phenylephrine drip if required, while the fetal heart rate is monitored. Arterial and pulmonary artery pressure monitoring is necessary when heart failure is suspected, but PCWP measurement may be hazardous because of the risk of PAVM rupture. An arterial line also is necessary when titrating drugs to increase SVR.

Cesarean section may be performed for obstetric reasons employing regional or general anesthesia. General anesthesia has the potential disadvantage of intubation hypertension and the possibility of high pulmonary inflation pressures adversely affecting the integrity of the AVM.

Dyspnea improves when the patient reclines. In the supine position there is decreased venous return due to the pressure of the gravid uterus on the vena cava, decreased distension of the PAVM, and decreased shunt. Hemoglobin saturation improves. Thus, it may be beneficial for the patient with symptomatic PAVM to experience labor without uterine displacement. We recommend that if this approach is attempted, the well-being of the fetus be carefully monitored. Postpartum, the effect of the gravid uterus on venous return is abolished, and autotransfusion of blood from within the gravid uterus increases venous return and shunt. It is imperative that the patient be monitored carefully after delivery for any deterioration from an increased shunt—because resection or embolization of the PAVM may be necessary.

Arteriovenous malformations of the oral, pharyngeal, or tracheal mucosa may exist. Therefore, the upper airway must be thoroughly examined when considering general anesthesia and intubation in these patients so as to avoid inadvertent trauma to the mucosal lesions.

MARFAN SYNDROME

Marfan syndrome is a disorder of connective tissue that is transmitted as an autosomal dominant characteristic without gender or racial preference. There is nearly 100% penetrance, but pleiotropy and variability affect its expression.[68] Marfan syndrome occurs in 4 to 6 of 100,000 births.[69] Although there is often a family history, 15% of cases are thought to arise as new mutations.[69] The syndrome's manifestations affect the ocular, skeletal, pulmonary, and cardiovascular systems.[70, 71]

The life span is shortened with a mean expectancy of only 32 years.[69] Ninety percent of the mortality is due to cardiovascular disease, which thus presents the greatest challenge in providing analgesia and anesthesia for pregnant patients with this condition.[71]

Common ocular disorders that have been described

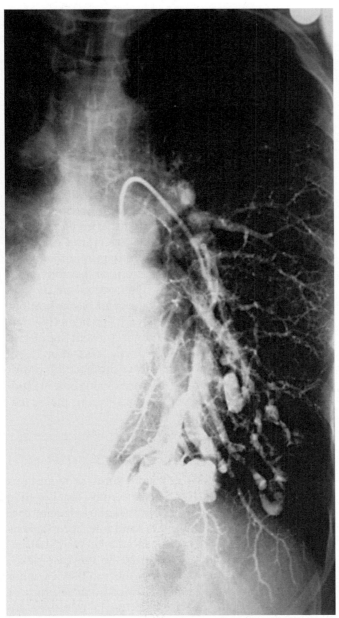

Figure 4–3. Pulmonary arteriogram (AP) of a young woman with pulmonary arterovenous malformation of the left lung. Note the large densely opacified feeding pulmonary artery and the less densely opacified pulmonary vein, which define this diagnosis.

is most safely performed during the second trimester to avoid the period of fetal organogenesis and reduce the risk of preterm labor.

Epidural analgesia is acceptable for the laboring patient. Placement of the epidural catheter is performed using loss of resistance to saline to avoid the risk of introducing air into the vascular system and the risk of paradoxical air emboli. Because there may be coexisting epidural AVM, care must be taken to seek signs of epidural hematoma following epidural insertion (i.e., persistent paresthesia, pain, or paralysis after expected resolution of analgesia).[63–67] Hence, short-acting local anesthetics are more suitable.

include ectopia lentis and myopia. Common skeletal abnormalities include arachnodactyly, pectus deformity, kyphoscoliosis, high narrow palate, and increased length of the long bones. As a consequence of connective tissue weakness and kyphoscoliosis, the patients have a propensity to develop pneumothorax, bullous emphysema, and restrictive lung disease. Therefore, it is prudent to maintain a high index of suspicion for pneumothorax when using positive-pressure ventilation.[68, 72]

Cystic medial necrosis (collagenous metachromatically staining mucoid material) is the characteristic histologic change. The weakness imparted by the defect is believed to be the cause of progressive dilatation, dissection, and aorta rupture. The ascending aorta is the most frequent site of dissection because it sustains the greatest stress during systole.[72]

Mitral valve prolapse (most frequently of the posterior leaflet) and myxomatous degeneration of the mitral valve occur frequently. Mitral valve pathology is detectable by echocardiography in at least 80% of these patients.[72] Mitral valve prolapse is suggested by the presence of a systolic click, which is best heard just medial to the cardiac apex.[69, 72] Early onset of coronary artery disease may occur, producing a high rate of arrhythmias and conduction disturbances.[72]

For patients with Marfan syndrome, aortic dilatation begins early in childhood. Progressive dilatation occurs slowly but at varying rates between individuals.[71] Life-threatening complications of aortic disease are more common after the aortic root dilates to more than 60 mm. The normal aortic root diameter is about 22 mm.[69, 72] The aortic root lies in the cardiac shadow on chest radiographs, and thus aortic dilatation often is unappreciated unless echocardiography, computed tomography, or magnetic resonance imaging is performed.[72] Patients should have a cardiac echocardiogram performed annually to look for changes in the aortic root diameter.

Pregnancy and Marfan Syndrome

During pregnancy there is a 30 to 40% increase in cardiac output by the second trimester, being made up by an equal increase in heart rate and stroke volume.[68, 73] During labor this level is more profound (100% greater than prepregnancy levels), and immediately following delivery the stroke volume may rise a further 40 to 50% above prepregnancy levels.[74–77]

The high serum estrogen concentration of pregnancy causes connective tissue changes at the subcellular level that produce collagen "softening."[73] The increased stress placed on the aortic root by the increased cardiac output, pre-existing cystic medial necrosis, and estrogen effects all contribute to an increased risk for aortic dissection during pregnancy. Half of all dissections

that occur in women of childbearing age are during pregnancy.[73] The actual risk is difficult to determine because of the variability of its expression.[71]

Patients with known Marfan syndrome who are pregnant or wish to become pregnant should first be counselled that one half of their children will be affected by the disease. If pregnancy is desired, the parturient should have a thorough cardiovascular assessment including an echocardiogram. Patients with mild cardiovascular symptoms before conception and aortic roots smaller than 40 mm in diameter seldom have serious cardiovascular complications during pregnancy, and thus they tolerate pregnancy well.[71]

Those patients whose aortic root diameters exceed 40 mm should be counselled against becoming pregnant. Pyeritz states, "patients with more than minimal aortic root dilatation, aortic regurgitation, or hemodynamically significant mitral valve dysfunction are at high risk of life-threatening cardiovascular complications during or shortly after pregnancy."[71] The hemodynamic changes associated with pregnancy present significant predisposing risk factors for aortic dissection.[78] All pregnant women with Marfan syndrome are considered high-risk patients and require evaluation, including echocardiograms, every 6 weeks during their pregnancies.[71]

Anesthetic Management

If the parturient does not have signs or symptoms of cardiac failure, and if the aortic root is smaller than 40 mm in diameter, she does not require special care during labor and delivery.[71] Antibiotic prophylaxis against bacterial endocarditis should be provided because of the occult collagen changes in this disorder.[69]

The principles for managing the woman in labor with aortic root enlargement of more than 40 mm or significant valvular disease are to (1) minimize increases in cardiac contractility and (2) minimize abrupt swings in blood pressure.[72] Invasive arterial pressure monitoring is therefore recommended.

Most patients at risk for aortic dissection are usually followed by a cardiologist and are treated with beta-blockers to prevent a rise in cardiac contractility and blood pressure. The medications include atenolol or metoprolol, but an intravenous labetalol infusion can provide rapid BP control.[79, 80] Calcium channel blockers also are helpful in controlling blood pressure in these patients.[70] Beta-agonists, vagolytics, and ergot derivatives should be avoided because these agents may cause a rapid rise in cardiac output and may increase the risk of dissection. Atropine must be administered carefully to treat bradycardia-induced hypotension.[68]

Significant hypotension is treated with phenylephrine to avoid the beta-agonist effect of ephedrine. Judicious phenylephrine therapy is unlikely to cause untoward effects in the uncompromised fetus.[68] Vasodilators, such as nitroglycerin and nitroprusside, when used as a sole agent, cause an increase in left ventricular ejection velocity by reducing systemic vascular resistance (SVR) and afterload, which in turn leads to stress on the aortic root. If hypertension occurs, therefore, it is best managed by adding labetalol.[72]

Vaginal delivery is permissible for the asymptomatic patient. Epidural analgesia for labor should be initiated early to prevent pain-induced catecholamine release, elevated blood pressure, and increased cardiac output. A saline intravenous fluid load is required and can be administered slowly in 250-ml aliquots up to 750 ml, as required. The epidural level must be titrated carefully to T10 to prevent a sudden fall in SVR and blood pressure. Epinephrine-containing solutions should be avoided.

Cesarean section usually is indicated for obstetric reasons. It may be performed using regional or general anesthesia. The same caveats apply to epidural anesthesia for cesarean section as for labor and vaginal delivery.

For general anesthesia, combined beta-blockade and vasodilator therapy should be employed to prevent a sudden rise in blood pressure and cardiac output during intubation. Halothane may be the ideal volatile agent for these parturients because it decreases cardiac contractility.[72] Positive-pressure ventilation must be utilized carefully to avoid inducing pneumothorax.

Aortic dissection in the near-term parturient with Marfan syndrome has been reported by several investigators.[70, 73, 79, 81] Immediately post partum, the patient experiences the greatest stress on the aortic root because of the autotransfusion of blood from the uterus to the systemic circulation. Vigilance for cardiovascular catastrophes should be maintained for several days after delivery. In three reported cases maternal systolic BP was stabilized (<100 mm Hg), cesarean section performed, and aortic repair undertaken 48 hours to 72 hours post partum.[73, 79, 81] One patient, whose condition was stabilized after delivery, was discharged without aortic repair.[70] Delaying the aortic repair gives the uterus time for involution, and the placental implantation site becomes fully hemostatic before anticoagulation is instituted for vascular surgery.

PERIPHERAL PULMONARY ARTERY STENOSIS

Peripheral pulmonary artery stenosis (PPAS) is a congenital condition of unknown etiology that accounts for 2 to 4% percent of congenital heart disease in women. It is characterized by multiple coarctations of the distal pulmonary arteries.[82] PPAS may occur together with pulmonary stenosis, atrial septal defect, ventricular septal defect, or tetralogy of Fallot. This condition occurs alone in approximately 40% of cases.[83]

There may be an association of PPAS in offspring of women who contracted rubella during pregnancy.[84]

Peripheral pulmonary artery stenosis usually is not considered a serious condition. Often it is diagnosed in early childhood when a loud, asymptomatic, continuous systolic murmur is investigated. Only when involvement of the peripheral pulmonary arteries is so extensive that it produces pulmonary hypertension is there a risk to the patient. Such a condition is uncommon.[82]

Four cases of PPAS and pregnancy have been reported.[82-84] In none of the cases did PPAS present a management problem for the anesthesiologist. During pregnancy cardiac catheterization should be performed to detect elevated right heart pressures and assess the relative risk for heart failure during or after pregnancy. If the patient has pulmonary hypertension, she should be managed as described for the patient who has PPH. If right heart pressures are normal or only mildly elevated, the patient requires no special management.

PULMONARY ARTERY ANEURYSM

Pulmonary artery aneurysms occur rarely and affect the main pulmonary artery or a major branch of the pulmonary vascular tree. Their incidence is approximately 1:10,000 to 1:20,000 of the general population.[85] Associated conditions include the following:

- Patent ductus arteriosus
- Marfan syndrome (cystic medial necrosis of the pulmonary artery)
- Persistent pulmonary artery hypertension (primary or associated with congenital cardiac defects that produce left-to-right shunting)
- Infundibular stenosis
- Infective endocarditis.

The following contribute to the development of pulmonary artery aneurysm and rupture:[85, 86]

- Atherosclerosis
- Trauma
- Syphilis.

Rupture of aneurysms of the pulmonary arteries may produce massive and fatal hemoptysis. Death may also be caused by cardiac tamponade if a pulmonary artery ruptures into the pericardial sac.[85, 86] An increased risk of aneurysm formation and rupture during pregnancy[87] exists as a result of

- An increase in intravascular volume
- The pain and expulsive efforts of labor
- Involution of the uterus post partum which produces increased flow through the pulmonary arteries and raises vessel wall stress
- Increased deposition of mucopolysaccharides in the

media of major blood vessels which occurs during pregnancy and may contribute to weakening of the artery.

Signs and Symptoms

Pulmonary artery aneurysm may cause shunting and cardiac failure, and patients present with exertional dyspnea, cough, hemoptysis, and chest tightness.[85] The following heart sounds and mumurs may be heard on clinical examination:

- Those consistent with patent ductus arteriosus (e.g., a to-and-fro murmur heard best at the left second intercostal space, a midsystolic hyperdynamic flow murmur of the mitral valve, and a paradoxical splitting of S2)
- Intracardiac shunts (i.e., usually fixed, wide split S_2) and murmur of increased pulmonic flow
- Pulmonary hypertension (i.e., tricuspid regurgitation characterized by a holosystolic murmur that increases with respiration or pulmonic and aortic regurgitation characterized by decrescendo diastolic murmurs).

Chest radiographs may show pulmonary artery enlargement, cardiac hypertrophy, and decreased peripheral vascular markings characteristic of pulmonary edema (Figs. 4–4 and 4–5). The definitive diagnosis of a pulmonary artery aneurysm and its dissection, however, is based on results of angiography, computed tomography, or magnetic resonance imaging. The ECG usually shows right axis deviation due to right ventricular hypertrophy.[85, 86]

Anesthetic Management

Pulmonary artery aneurysm and dissection almost invariably are associated with pulmonary hypertension.[87] Thus, the anesthetic management is similar to that for primary pulmonary hypertension. The presence of a pulmonary artery aneurysm is life-threatening. Because it occurs rarely, however, there is no consensus as to the best management. The options are predelivery repair and expectant management of pregnancy, labor, and delivery without repair.

During labor, the goal should be to minimize hemodynamic stresses such as systemic hypertension and profound swings in preload and afterload. This goal is best achieved with a labor epidural, using an infusion of dilute bupivacaine and/or intrathecal opioids. Epidural analgesia is induced gradually to a level of T10 to abolish the pain of labor and delivery and to prevent a catecholamine-induced rise in cardiac output and pulmonary artery pressure. Forceps or vacuum delivery helps to shorten the second stage of labor and avoids the need for expulsive effort by the parturient. As in patients with primary pulmonary hypertension, peripheral arterial, central venous, and pulmonary artery catheters can provide good information and are mandatory if rapidly titratable vasoactive medications are given to optimize cardiovascular function.

The principles for managing cesarean delivery in these patients are the same as those for patients with pulmonary hypertension and Marfan syndrome. Carefully titrated epidural anesthesia is preferable to subarachnoid block because the degree and acuity of hemodynamic changes are less extreme. Intrathecal anesthesia for cesarean delivery, however, is not absolutely contraindicated.

MOYAMOYA DISEASE

Moyamoya disease is a rare, progressive, vaso-occlusive disorder of unknown origin that affects the internal carotid arteries and their distal branches.[88] This disease may be associated with intracranial aneurysms in about 15% of cases.[89] Moyamoya disease is most frequently found in young females; the disease may show a familial disposition.[90]

Signs and Symptoms

Patients with moyamoya disease may present with signs of cerebral ischemia, including dysarthria, head-

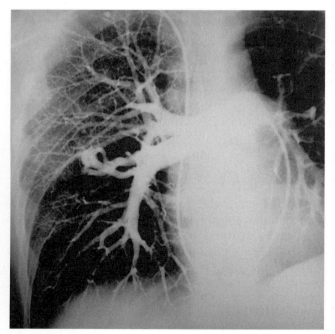

Figure 4–4. Pulmonary angiogram (AP) of a young woman with a small peripheral branch pulmonary artery aneurysm. Note the larger branch pulmonary artery feeding the small aneurysm in the right mid-lung field. Note that there is no draining vein to suggest an arteriovenous malformation.

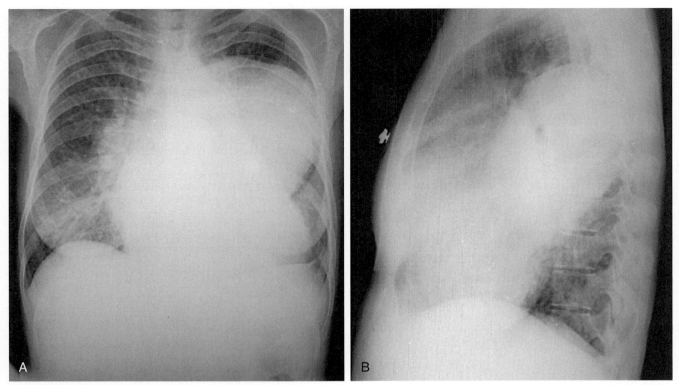

Figure 4–5. (*A* and *B*) PA and lateral chest radiographs of a young woman with a very large pulmonary aneurysm of the left main pulmonary artery. The mass is not diagnostic on the plain radiograph alone, and would require confirmation by other imaging modalities such as CT scan, MRI, or angiography.

ache, hemiplegia, and seizure.[91] Children with this condition usually experience transient ischemic attacks with paroxysmal hemiplegia,[92] whereas adults often present with subarachnoid hemorrhage.[93] Symptoms may be precipitated by hypocarbia due to hyperventilation, or by hyperthermia causing an increase in the cerebral metabolic rate for oxygen ($CMRO_2$).[94–97] The increase in cardiac output, which occurs during pregnancy and parturition, may precipitate intracranial hemorrhage.[98]

Angiograms characteristically show narrowing of the carotid arteries and/or their distal branches, particularly at the origin of the anterior cerebral and middle cerebral arteries.[99] Compensatory enlargement of the perforator arteries around the basal ganglia accompanies the changes in the carotid vessels.[100, 101] In Japanese, moyamoya means "something hazy" (like a puff of smoke), and haziness is the characteristic appearance of the vasculature around the basal ganglia seen on angiography.[102] Periventricular pseudoaneurysms and saccular aneurysms of the circle of Willis can also be seen angiographically in some patients.[103] Confirmatory diagnosis is based on the angiographic findings. Typically the patients receive anticoagulants (warfarin), aspirin for platelet inactivation, and nimodipine for cerebral vasodilation to help prevent cerebral ischemia. Patients with seizure disorders are maintained on anticonvulsant therapy.[88]

Anesthetic Management

The goal of anesthetic management is to provide a pain-free vaginal delivery or cesarean section while maintaining cerebral blood flow. Hypotension and hyperventilation must be avoided because they decrease cerebral perfusion. At the same time, increased cardiac output and hypertension, which may accompany endotracheal intubation, should be anticipated and managed with intravenous lidocaine and antihypertensive drugs, such as labetalol. This regimen minimizes the risk of cerebral hemorrhage, particularly in those who have intracranial aneurysms. Ideally, operative vaginal or abdominal delivery should be performed to prevent the hemodynamic consequences of maternal effort.

An arterial catheter is recommended for continuous arterial pressure monitoring during labor and delivery.[88] After 500 to 750 ml of intravenous crystalloid is given, epidural analgesia is induced using bupivacaine 0.25%, followed by bupivacaine 0.0625% with fentanyl 2 µg/ml at 12 to 14 ml/hr to maintain a T8–T10 level of analgesia. Care should be taken, as always, to avoid aortocaval compression associated with the supine position.

If cesarean section is required, the block may be raised to T4–T6 with lidocaine 2% or bupivacaine 0.5% in incremental doses. Left uterine displacement is mandatory until delivery of the neonate.

If general anesthesia is unavoidable, titratable vasodilators can be administered to prevent significant hypertension during intubation of the trachea. Conversely, vasopressors such as ephedrine and phenylephrine should be available to treat sustained hypotension, which may cause cerebral ischemia. Normocapnea should be maintained at all times.

References

1. Ramanthan S, Gupta U, Chalon J, et al. Anesthetic considerations in Takayasu's Arteritis. Anesth Analg 1979;58:247.
2. Lupi E, Sanchez G, Horwitz S, et al. Pulmonary artery involvement in Takayasu's Arteritis. Chest 1975;67:69.
3. Nasu T. Pathology of pulseless disease: Systematic study and critical review of twenty-one autopsy cases reported in Japan. Angiology 1962;14:225.
4. Crofts SL, Wilson E. Epidural analgesia for labour in Takayasu's arteritis: Case report. Br J Obstet Gynecol 1991;98:408.
5. McKay RSF, Dillard SR. Management of epidural anesthesia in a patient with Takayasu's Disease. Anesth Analg 1992;74:297.
6. Nakao K, Ikeda M, Kimata S, et al. Takayasu's arteritis: Clinical report of eighty-four cases and immunological studies of seven cases. Circulation 1976;35:1141.
7. Ueno A, Awane Y, Wakabayashi A, et al. Successfully operated Obliterative Brachiocephalic Arteritis (Takayasu) associated with the elongated coarctation. Jpn Heart J 1967;8:538.
8. Ishikawa K. Natural history and classification of Occlusive Thromboaortopathy (Takayasu's Disease). Circulation 1978; 57:27.
9. Hauth JC, Cunningham FG, Young BK. Takayasu's Syndrome in pregnancy. Obstet Gynecol 1977;50:373.
10. Wong VCW, Wang RYC, Tse TF. Pregnancy and Takayasu's Arteritis. Am J Med 1983;75:597.
11. Ishikawa K, Matsuura S. Occlusive Thromboaortopathy (Takayasu's Disease) and pregnancy: Clinical course and management of 33 pregnancies and deliveries. Am J Cardiol 1982;50:1293.
12. Thorburn JR, James MFM. Anaesthetic management of Takayasu's arteritis. Anaesthesia 1986;41:734.
13. Winn HN, Setaro JF, Mazor M, et al. Severe Takayasu's arteritis in pregnancy: The role of central hemodynamic monitoring. Am J Obstet Gynecol 1988;159:1135.
14. Matsumura A, Moriwaki R, Numano F. Pregnancy in Takayasu's arteritis from the view of internal medicine. Heart Vessels 1992;7:S120.
15. Hampl KF, Schneider MC, Skarvan K, et al. Spinal anaesthesia in a patient with Takayasu's disease. Br J Anaesth 1994;72:129.
16. Gaida BJ, Gervais HW, Mauer D, et al. Anesthesiology problems in Takayasu's Syndrome. Anaesthetist 1991;40:1.
17. Beilin Y, Bernstein H. Successful epidural anaesthesia for a patient with Takayasu's arteritis presenting for Caesarean section. Can J Anaesth 1993;40:64.
18. Warner MA, Hughes DR, Messick JM. Anesthetic management of a patient with Pulseless Disease. Anesth Analg 1983;62:532.
19. Wiebers DO. Ischemic cerebrovascular complications of pregnancy. Arch Neurol 1985;42:1106.
20. Herrema I. Takayasu's disease and Caesarean section. Int J Obstet Anesth 1992;1:117.
21. Roberts NV, Keast PJ. Pulmonary hypertension and pregnancy: A lethal combination. Anaesth Intensive Care 1990;18:366.
22. Rich S. Primary pulmonary hypertension. Prog Cardiovasc Dis 1988;31:205.
23. Fuster V, Steele PM, Edwards WD, et al. Primary pulmonary hypertension: Natural history and the importance of thrombosis. Circulation 1984;70:580.
24. Takeuchi T, Nishii O, Okamura T, et al. Primary pulmonary hypertension in pregnancy. Int J Gynecol Obstet 1988;26:145.
25. Nelson DM, Main E, Crafford W, et al. Peripartum heart failure due to primary pulmonary hypertension. Obstet Gynecol 1983;62:58S.
26. Dawkins KD, Burke CM, Billingham ME, et al. Primary pulmonary hypertension and pregnancy. Chest 1986;89:383.
27. Feijen HWH, Hein PR, van Lakwijk-Vondrovicova EL, et al. Primary pulmonary hypertension and pregnancy. Eur J Obstet Gynec Reprod Biol 1983;15:159.
28. Breen TW, Janzen JA. Pulmonary hypertension and cardiomyopathy: Anaesthetic management for Caesarean section. Can J Anaesth 1991;38:895.
29. Sullivan JM, Ramanathan KB. Management of medical problems in pregnancy: Severe cardiac disease. N Engl J Med 1985;313:304.
30. Slomka F, Salmeron S, Zetlaoui P, et al. Primary pulmonary hypertension and pregnancy: Anesthetic management for delivery. Anesthesiology 1988;69:959.
31. Nootens M, Rich S. Successful management of labor and delivery in primary pulmonary hypertension. Am J Cardiol 1993;71:1124.
32. Robinson DE, Leicht CH. Epidural analgesia with low-dose bupivacaine and fentanyl for labor and delivery in a parturient with severe pulmonary hypertension. Anesthesiology 1988; 68:285.
33. Smedstad KG, Cramb R, Morison DH. Pulmonary hypertension and pregnancy: A series of eight cases. Can J Anaesth 1994;41:502.
34. Power KJ, Avery AF. Extradural analgesia in the intrapartum management of a patient with pulmonary hypertension. Br J Anaesth 1989;63:116.
35. Bredgaard Sorensen M, Korshin JD, Fernandes A, et al. The use of epidural analgesia for delivery in a patient with pulmonary hypertension. Acta Anaesth Scand 1982;26:180.
36. Roessler P, Lambert TF. Anaesthesia for Caesarean section in the presence of primary pulmonary hypertension. Anaesth Intensive Care 1986;14:317.
37. Ackerman WE, Juneja MM. Should epidural fentanyl be given for labor and delivery in a patient with severe pulmonary hypertension? Anesthesiology 1988;69:284.
38. Abboud TK, Raya J, Noueihed R, et al. Intrathecal morphine for relief of labor pain in a parturient with severe pulmonary hypertension. Anesthesiology 1983;59:477.
39. Leduc L, Kirshon B, Diaz SF, et al. Intrathecal morphine analgesia and low-dose dopamine for oliguria in severe maternal pulmonary hypertension: A case report. J Reprod Med 1990;35:727.
40. Weeks SK, Smith JB. Obstetric anesthesia in patients with primary pulmonary hypertension (editorial). Can J Anaesth 1991;38:814.
41. Atanassoff P, Alon E, Schmid ER, et al. Epidural anesthesia for Caesarean section in a patient with severe pulmonary hypertension. Acta Anaesth Scand 1989;33:75.
42. Batson MA, Longmire S, Csontos E. Alfentanil for urgent Caesarean section in a patient with severe mitral stenosis and pulmonary hypertension. Can J Anaesth 1990;37:685.
43. Myles PS. Anaesthetic management for laparoscopic sterilisation and termination of pregnancy in a patient with severe primary pulmonary hypertension. Anaesth Intensive Care 1994;22:465.
44. Hjort Sorensen C, Bredgaard Sorensen M, Jacobsen E. Pulmonary hemodynamics during direct diagnostic laryngoscopy. Acta Anaesth Scand 1981;25:51.
45. Hodgson CH, Burchell HB, Good CA, et al. Hereditary hemorrhagic telangiectasia and pulmonary arteriovenous fistula. N Engl J Med 1959;261:625.
46. Hodgson CH, Kaye RL. Pulmonary arteriovenous fistula and hereditary hemorrhagic telangiectasia: A review and report of 35 cases of fistula. Dis Chest 1963;43:449.
47. Chanatry BJ. Acute hemothorax owing to pulmonary arteriovenous malformation in pregnancy. Anesth Analg 1992;74:613.
48. LaRoche CM, Wells F, Shneerson J. Massive hemothorax due to enlarging arteriovenous fistula in pregnancy. Chest 1992;101:1452.
49. Swinburne AJ. Pregnancy and pulmonary arteriovenous fistula (editorial). N Y State J Med 1992;92:515.
50. Bevelaque FA, Ordorica SA, Lefleur R, et al. Osler-Weber-Rendu disease: Diagnosis and management of spontaneous hemothorax during pregnancy. N Y State J Med 1992;92:551.

51. Gammon RB, Miksa AK, Keller FS. Osler-Weber-Rendu disease and pulmonary arteriovenous fistulas. Chest 1990;98:1522.

52. Waring PH, Shaw B, Brumfield CG. Anesthetic management of a patient with Osler-Weber-Rendu syndrome and rheumatic heart disease. Anesth Analg 1990;71:96.

53. Baumgardner DJ, Kroll MR. Pulmonary arteriovenous malformations in pregnancy. Am Fam Physician 1993;48:1032.

54. Swinburne AJ, Fedullo AJ, Gangemi R, et al. Hereditary telangiectasia and multiple pulmonary arteriovenous fistulas: Clinical deterioration during pregnancy. Chest 1986;89:459.

55. Robinson JL, Hass CS, Sedzimir CB. Arteriovenous malformations, aneurysms, and pregnancy. J Neurosurg 1974;41:63.

56. Livneh A, Langevitz P, Morag B, et al. Functionally reversible hepatic arteriovenous fistulas during pregnancy in patients with hereditary hemorrhagic telangiectasia. South Med J 1988;81:1047.

57. McCausland AM, Hyman C, Winsor T, et al. Venous distensibility during pregnancy. Am J Obstet Gynecol 1961;81:472.

58. McCausland AM, Holmes F, Trotter AD. Venous distensibility during the menstrual cycle. Am J Obstet Gynecol 1963;86:640.

59. Pritchard JA. Changes in the blood volume during pregnancy and delivery. Anesthesiology 1965;26:393.

60. Jahnke V. Ultrastructure of hereditary telangiectasia. Arch Otolaryngol 1970;91:262.

61. Peery WH. Clinical spectrum of hereditary hemorrhagic telangiectasia (Osler-Weber-Rendu disease). Am J Med 1987;82:989.

62. Burke CM, Safai C, Nelson DP, et al. Pulmonary arteriovenous malformations: A critical update. Am Rev Respir Dis 1986;134:334.

63. Newquist RE, Mayfield FH. Spinal angioma presenting during pregnancy. J Neurosurg 1960;17:541.

64. Fields WS, Jones JR. Spinal epidural hemangioma in pregnancy. Neurol 1957;7:825.

65. Nelson DA. Spinal cord compression due to vertebral angiomas during pregnancy. Arch Neurol 1964;11:408.

66. Martin RA, Howard FM, Salamone CR, et al. Spinal cord vascular malformations with symptoms during menstruation. J Neurosurg 1977;47:626.

67. Lam RL, Roulhac GE, Erwin HJ. Hemangioma of the spinal canal and pregnancy. J Neurosurg 1951;8:668.

68. Gordon CF, Johnson MD. Anesthetic management of the pregnant patient with Marfan syndrome. J Clin Anesth 1993;5:248.

69. Pyeritz RE, McKusick VA. The Marfan syndrome: Diagnosis and management. N Engl J Med 1979;300:772.

70. Chow SL. Acute aortic dissection in a patient with Marfan's syndrome complicated by gestational hypertension. Med J Aust 1993;159:760.

71. Pyeritz RE. Maternal and fetal complications of pregnancy in the Marfan Syndrome. Am J Med 1981;71:784.

72. Wells DG, Podolakin W. Anaesthesia and Marfan's syndrome: Case report. Can J Anaesth 1987;34:311.

73. Pumphrey CW, Fay T, Weir I. Aortic dissection during pregnancy. Br Heart J 1986;55:106.

74. Robson SC, Hunter S, Boys RJ, et al. Serial study of factors influencing changes in cardiac output during human pregnancy. Am J Physiol 1989;256:H1060.

75. Robson SC, Hunter S, Moore M, et al. Haemodynamic changes during the puerperium: a Doppler and M-mode echocardiographic study. Br J Obstet Gynaecol 1987;94:1028.

76. Capeless EL, Clapp JF. Cardiovascular changes in early phase of pregnancy. Am J Obstet Gynecol 1989;161:1449.

77. Katz R, Karliner JS, Resnik R. Effects of a natural volume overload state (pregnancy) on left ventricular performance in normal human subjects. Circulation 1978;58:434.

78. Elias S, Berkowitz RL. The Marfan Syndrome and pregnancy. Obstet Gynecol 1976;47:358.

79. Ferguson JE, Ueland K, Stinson EB, et al. Marfan's syndrome: Acute aortic dissection during labor, resulting in fetal distress and cesarean section, followed by successful surgical repair. Am J Obstet Gynecol 1983;147:759.

80. Murdoch JL, Walker BA, Halpern BL, et al. Life expectancy and causes of death in the Marfan Syndrome. N Engl J Med 1972;286:804.

81. Rosenblum NG, Grossman AR, Gabbe SG, et al. Failure of serial echocardiographic studies to predict aortic dissection in a pregnant patient with Marfan's syndrome. Am J Obstet Gynecol 1983;14:470.

82. Marks F, Santos A, Leppert P, et al. Peripheral pulmonary artery stenosis in pregnancy. A report of two cases. J Reprod Med 1992;37:381.

83. Landsberger EJ, Grossman JH. Multiple peripheral pulmonic stenosis in pregnancy. Am J Obstet Gynecol 1986;154:152.

84. Togo T, Sugishita Y, Tamura T, et al. Uneventful pregnancy and delivery in a case of multiple peripheral pulmonary stenosis. Acta Cardiologica 1983;38:143.

85. Hankins GDV, Brekken AL, Davis LM. Maternal death secondary to a dissecting aneurysm of the pulmonary artery. Obstet Gynecol 1985;65:45S.

86. D'Arbela PG, Mugerwa JW, Patel AK, et al. Aneurysm of pulmonary artery with persistent ductus arteriosus and pulmonary infundibular stenosis: Fatal dissection and rupture in pregnancy. Br Heart J 1970;32:124.

87. Green NJ, Rollason TP. Pulmonary artery rupture in pregnancy complicating patent ductus arteriosus. Br Heart J 1992;68:616.

88. Sharma SK, Wallace DH, Gajraj NM, et al. Epidural anesthesia for a patient with moyamoya disease presenting for cesarean section. Anesth Analg 1994;79:183.

89. Konishi Y, Kadowaki C, Hara M, et al. Aneurysms associated with moyamoya disease. Neurosurgery 1985;16:484.

90. Kitahara T, Ariga N, Yamaura A, et al. Familial occurrence of moyamoya disease: Report of three Japanese families. J Neurol Neurosurg Psychiatr 1979;42:208.

91. Karasawa J, Kikuchi H, Furuse S, et al. Treatment of moyamoya disease with STA-MCA anastomosis. J Neurosurg 1978;49:679.

92. Golden GS. Stroke syndromes in childhood. Neurol Clin 1985;3:59.

93. Aoki N, Mizutari H. Does moyamoya disease cause subarachnoid hemorrhage? Review of 54 cases with intracranial hemorrhage confirmed by computerized tomography. J Neurosurg 1984;60:348.

94. Kurokawa T, Chen YJ, Tomita S, et al. Cerebrovascular occlusive disease with and without the moyamoya vascular network in children. Neuropediatrics 1985;16:29.

95. Fukuyama Y, Umezu R. Clinical and cerebral angiographic evolutions of idiopathic progressive occlusive disease of the Circle of Willis ("moyamoya" disease in children). Brain Develop 1985;7:21.

96. Tagawa T, Naritomi H, Mimaki T, et al. Regional cerebral blood flow, clinical manifestations, and age in children with moyamoya disease. Stroke 1987;18:906.

97. Sumikawa K, Nagai H. Moyamoya Disease and anesthesia. Anesthesiology 1983;58:204.

98. Miyakawa I, Huei CL, Haruyama Y, et al. Occlusive disease of the internal carotid arteries with vascular collaterals (moyamoya disease) in pregnancy. Arch Gynecol 1986;237:175.

99. Kurehara K, Ohnishi H, Touho H, et al. Cortical blood flow response to hypercapnia during anaesthesia in moyamoya disease. Can J Anaesth 1993;40:709.

100. Savit JM, Levy LA, Reiner MA, et al. Moyamoya Disease. N Y State J Med 1983;83:237.

101. Suzuki J, Takaku A. Cerebrovascular "Moyamoya" Disease. Arch Neurol 1969;20:288.

102. Bingham RM, Wilkinson DJ. Anaesthetic management in moyamoya disease. Anaesthesia 1985;40:1198.

103. Hashimoto K, Fujii K, Nishimura K, et al. Occlusive cerebrovascular disease with moyamoya vessels and intracranial hemorrhage during pregnancy. Neurol Med Chir (Tokyo) 1988;28:588.

AIRWAY OBSTRUCTION AND DIFFICULT TRACHEAL INTUBATION

■ ■ ■ ■ ■ ■ ■

Glenn K. Shopper, M.D., and Mark D. Johnson, M.D.

One fundamental obligation of the anesthesiologist to the patient is to preserve alveolar ventilation and tissue oxygenation; breach of this responsibility can result in disastrous consequences. Airway mishaps currently account for the majority of anesthesia-related maternal deaths, with inadequate ventilation, esophageal intubation, and aspiration as the three leading causes.[1-4] Although the maternal death rate has been decreasing by approximately 7% per year, the contribution attributable to anesthesia has, until lately, remained stable. Anesthetic misadventure accounted for approximately 10 to 13% of maternal deaths and has been the third most common cause of maternal deaths over the past 20 years, behind pre-eclampsia/eclampsia and pulmonary embolism. Further statistics, however, show anesthesia contributing to between 3.3 and 4.4% of maternal deaths.[5, 6] Whether this trend is a reflection of better anesthetic care and whether it will continue to improve remain to be seen.

For many reasons, management of the parturient's airway is more difficult than that of the nonpregnant patient. Changes in lung volumes, oxygen consumption, and respiratory mucosa characteristics[7] all contribute to make management of the pregnant patient's airway more difficult and prone to failure. Although total lung capacity is unchanged, the gravid uterus elevates the diaphragm and decreases functional residual capacity (FRC), a measure of oxygen stores during periods of apnea, by 20%. Oxygen consumption is increased 20 to 35% during pregnancy. Thus hypoxia can be expected to occur much sooner during induction of general anesthesia if alveolar ventilation is not restored promptly.

Gastric emptying may be delayed during labor especially if parenteral opioids have been administered.[7] Barrier pressure is decreased in pregnancy because the resting tone of the gastroesophageal sphincter is reduced and intragastric pressure is higher, particularly in the lithotomy position. As a result, parturients are at a higher risk for regurgitation of stomach contents into the esophagus than nonparturients. Few cesarean sections are performed after an 8-hour fast. The net result is an increased risk for pulmonary aspiration of gastric contents.[8, 9]

Airway edema[10-24] can occur during pregnancy, especially in the case of pre-eclampsia, requiring the availability of smaller endotracheal tubes. Furthermore, capillary engorgement of the nasal mucosa makes nasal intubation plus insertion of nasal airways a potential cause of severe epistaxis.

Airway management in the parturient is further complicated by a well-documented, increased incidence of difficult intubation. The rate of failed obstetric intubations is eight times the rate of all other failed intubations.[25-27] It is unclear why pregnancy results in increased difficulty in visualization of the vocal cords during direct laryngoscopy. Increased breast size, full dentition, and changes in body water content leading to laryngeal edema, tongue enlargement, and immobility have been implicated.[28] Other possibilities include physician fatigue or inexperience, inadequate preoperative evaluation, poor positioning of the patient, inappropriate application of cricoid pressure, and prompt use of a failed intubation drill in obstetrics.[26]

UNCOMMON CAUSES OF AIRWAY OBSTRUCTION

Although iatrogenic airway obstruction is not uncommon, cases of maternal airway obstruction from less common etiologies have been described (Table 5–1). As stated, the respiratory changes of pregnancy include increased minute ventilation, limited diaphragmatic excursion, and capillary engorgement of respiratory tract mucosa. A relatively small decrease in airway caliber can result in dramatic decompensation.

Tracheal stenosis in the parturient is fortunately very rare, although it can be misdiagnosed as asthma.[29] Spirometry with flow-volume loops and evidence of lack of improvement with bronchodilators can facilitate diagnosis. Four cases have been reported with diverse

TABLE 5–I. SOME REPORTED UNCOMMON CAUSES OF AIRWAY OBSTRUCTION

Tracheal stenosis
- Radiotherapy
- Trauma (external or post-intubation/tracheostomy)
- Congenital web

Laryngeal edema
- Infection
- Pre-eclampsia
- Fluid overload
- Allergy
- Prolonged pushing/straining
- Tracheal intubation

Thyroid pathology
Intratracheal tumors
Acute epiglottitis
Vocal cord paralysis
Laryngospasm
Foreign body
Sleep apnea syndrome*

*From Mercer M. Caesarean section and sleep apnoea syndrome (Letter). Anaesthesia 1996;51:992.

etiologies, each amenable to different management options.[29–32]

Balloon tracheal dilatation using local anesthesia[30] was well tolerated in a patient with a possible congenital tracheal web. Balloon dilatation resulted in a significant improvement in pulmonary function and complete relief of symptoms. Because the frictional resistance of turbulent gas flow varies with density, a helium and oxygen mixture results in greater gas flow through a partially obstructed trachea. This mixture has been used for symptomatic relief of dyspnea during delivery in a patient with tracheal stenosis following tracheostomy.[31]

Regional anesthesia was given for cesarean section in a patient with tracheal stenosis due to radiotherapy for adenocystic carcinoma of the larynx.[32] Intraoperative hemorrhage, however, required induction of general anesthesia and intubation with a 4.0-mm tracheal tube under direct laryngoscopy. Hypercapnia and marginal oxygenation required the utilization of the Hayek oscillator cuirass ventilator to achieve acceptable levels of blood gases.

A term parturient with a remote history of laryngeal trauma was found to have a cricotracheal separation and multiple fractures of the tracheal rings upon evaluation of progressive dyspnea.[29] It is notable that the diagnostic fiberoptic bronchoscopy resulted in dyspnea sufficient to warrant tracheal intubation, tracheostomy, and cesarean delivery.

To date, there have been 21 reported cases of laryngeal edema occurring in conjunction with pre-eclampsia,[10–24] prolonged labor and pushing,[18, 22, 23] fluid overload,[15, 22, 23] weight gain,[24] upper respiratory infection,[11] and recent intubation.[13–15, 19, 20] In all cases in which laryngeal edema was noted on laryngoscopy, a smaller tracheal tube (5.0–7.0) was necessary. In two cases intubation was unsuccessful, with surgery continuing by

mask[12] or epidural anesthesia.[10] All investigators attempted intubation after induction of general anesthesia except one[17] who performed successful awake intubation and one[11] who avoided intubation through the successful use of steroids and regional anesthesia. In all reports, except three,[11, 16, 17] no preoperative stridor or dyspnea was reported. In only seven cases was facial or neck edema noted.[15–18, 21]

Acute airway compromise resulting from thyroid pathology can occur during pregnancy. Hemorrhage into a thyroid cyst during pregnancy can compress the trachea. The patient presents as if having an asthma attack.[33] Negative-pressure pulmonary edema as a result of airway obstruction from a progressively enlarging euthyroid goiter has also been reported.[34] Both cases required tracheal intubation shortly after admission; intubation was performed without difficulty after the induction of general anesthesia. Subtotal thyroidectomy relieved the tracheal obstruction in both cases.

In a review of airway obstruction resulting from thyroid pathology,[35] of the 19 female patients admitted, two were in their third trimester of pregnancy. Thyroidectomy relieved their symptoms. A thyroid mass can cause posterior displacement of the epiglottis. This has been implicated in causing the Sellick maneuver to completely obstruct the airway during attempts to mask-ventilate a patient who could not be intubated.[36] Mask ventilation was performed when cricoid pressure was released, and surgery was subsequently performed using epidural anesthesia. Another case of airway obstruction from cricoid pressure following undiagnosed laryngeal trauma has been reported.[37]

Intratracheal tumors are rare but have been reported during pregnancy. Kaposi's sarcoma of the trachea was present, during the second trimester, in an HIV-positive patient who required rigid bronchoscopy to improve stridor.[38] A tracheal cylindroma has been reported in a woman pregnant with twins[39] whose dyspnea had been misdiagnosed as asthma. The tumor was removed by rigid bronchoscopy using general anesthesia and a spontaneously breathing barbiturate and halothane technique.

Two cases of ectopic intratracheal thyroid tissue occurring during pregnancy have been reported.[40] One patient, who was admitted in active labor, required endotracheal intubation for "asthma" and subsequently died of respiratory failure. Two intratracheal nodules revealing follicular thyroid carcinoma were found 2 cm inferior to the vocal cords. The other patient, a sister of the first patient, noted only increasing neck swelling and dyspnea during pregnancy. Years later a mass composed of normal thyroid tissue was excised from her trachea.

Acute epiglottitis during pregnancy has been reported[41]; the patient required intubation for 48 hours. Following antibiotic treatment and extubation, the remainder of her pregnancy was uneventful. Necrotizing epiglottitis secondary to infectious mononucleosis has been reported[42] during the first trimester. Dyspnea occurred after symptoms of sore throat, fever, neck swelling, and dysphagia developed over a period of 2 weeks. The patient required tracheal intubation, and she had a spontaneous abortion.

Paradoxical vocal cord movement causing stridor and necessitating tracheal intubation has been reported following general anesthesia for cesarean section.[43] Although the etiology in that case was unclear, the condition can mimic asthma, aspiration, laryngospasm, allergic reaction, and vocal cord paralysis. The diagnosis is made by laryngoscopy during an episode. Treatment is usually supportive, but occasionally the patient requires tracheal intubation. Psychogenic laryngospasm during epidural anesthesia for cesarean section has occurred,[44] which caused a decreased oxygen saturation but resolved spontaneously.

THE DIFFICULT AIRWAY

Definition

The incidence of difficult intubation varies according to its degree and its definition. There is a continuum from successful intubation after one or multiple attempts, blades, or laryngoscopists; to unsuccessful intubation but ventilation by mask possible; to complete inability to intubate the trachea or ventilate the lungs. The incidence of difficult but successful intubation is 1 to 18%. Airways that cannot be intubated but in which mask ventilation is possible occur in 0.05 to 0.35% of patients. The extreme in difficult airways, those that cannot be either intubated or mask-ventilated are rare, occurring in only 0.01 to 2 per 10,000 patients.[45] The fact that these extremely difficult airways are encountered so infrequently is a mixed blessing. Many anesthesiologists may have had little experience managing this type of airway. It is easy to forget, however, that airway-related mishaps are still a significant cause of anesthesia-related maternal mortality.

The need for an accurate predictor of difficult intubation has resulted in the development of many methods of preoperative airway evaluation. Although the apparent difficulty of an airway intubation can vary along the continuum from easy to impossible, its subsequent management centers on only two options: intubation after the induction of anesthesia and awake laryngoscopy and/or intubation. Therefore, the ideal airway evaluation would provide a yes/no answer, rather than a probability of difficult intubation. Such an evaluation would yield a reliable correlation between external airway anatomy and subsequent success or failure of intubation. Obviously, this perfect airway evaluation has not been found. Current methods suffer from both false-positive and false-negative evaluations. Because

the ultimate success of intubation is dependent upon the skills of the intubator, these tests, at best, yield information resulting in only the expected view or probability of difficult intubation.

The subject of false-positive and false-negative evaluations deserves additional comment. Although both of these errors ideally are avoided, a false-negative error carries greater risk to the patient. A false-positive error (in which an airway appears difficult to intubate but is subsequently found to be easy) exposes the patient to the discomfort and delay in inducing anesthesia while an awake laryngoscopy or intubation is performed. A false-negative error, however, can lead to induction of general anesthesia in a patient whose airway cannot be intubated. Even though one must weigh the risks to the fetus by delaying delivery with the risks of maternal airway compromise, most agree that maternal airway concerns take precedence over those of fetal well-being. Advanced planning and suitable preparation significantly reduce the risk to the fetus.

Numerous conditions associated with difficult intubations have been described (Table 5–2).[46] These have formed the basis for methods of preoperative airway evaluation that attempt to identify and characterize risk factors and correlate them to the incidence of difficult intubation. Most tests of airway evaluation become more sensitive if an objective measure of difficulty, such as exposure of laryngeal structures, is used. Such an objective measure allows for a graded assessment of successful intubation of the trachea. The goal of most current tests of airway evaluation is to find a correlation between preoperative predictors and subsequent degrees of laryngeal exposure. Originally described by Cormack and Lehane,[47] laryngeal exposure was graded on a four-point scale (Fig. 5–1):

- Grade I, full exposure of the vocal cords
- Grade II, partial exposure of the vocal cords with posterior corniculate cartilages seen
- Grade III, only epiglottis seen
- Grade IV, not even the epiglottis seen

Although most anesthesiologists have successfully

TABLE 5–2. **ANATOMIC FACTORS PROPOSED TO PREDICT DIFFICULT INTUBATION**

Short muscular neck with full dentition
Receding mandible
Protruding incisors
Poor mobility of mandible
Long, high-arched palate
Increased alveolar-mental distance
Decreased mentothyroid cartilage distance
Poor mobility of atlanto-occipital joint (stiff neck)
Inability to visualize soft palate, uvula, faucial pillars
Obesity

Modified from Malan TP, Johnson MD. The difficult airway in obstetric anesthesia: Techniques for airway management and the role of regional anesthesia. J Clin Anesth 1988;1:104.

Grade 1

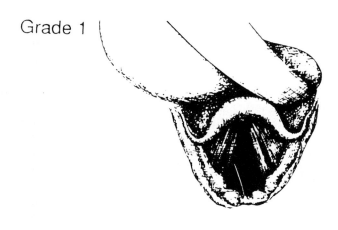

Grade 2

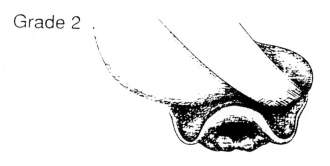

Grade 3

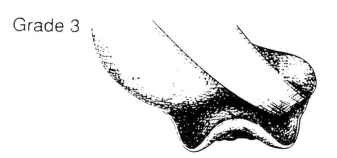

Grade 4

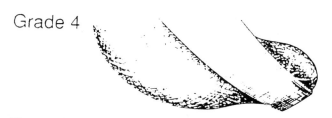

Figure 5–1. Graded laryngoscopic views of the glottis. (From Cormack RS, Lehane: Difficult tracheal intubation in obstetrics. Anaesthesia 1984;39:1105.)

intubated grade III and even grade IV airways, we arbitrarily designate the laryngeal exposure afforded by classes I and II as "adequate" and classes III and IV as "inadequate."

Specific Tests

One common airway test uses the ratio of the size of the tongue to the oropharynx. Described by Mallam-

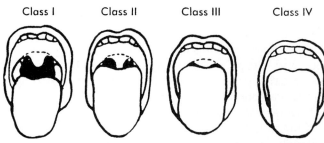

Figure 5–2. Pictoral classification of the pharyngeal structures, as seen when conducting the modified Mallampati test. (From Samsoon GLT, Young JRB: Difficult tracheal intubation: A retrospective study. Anaesthesia 1987;42:487.)

pati and coworkers,[48] this method requires that the patient sit up, open her mouth, and protrude her tongue maximally. Phonation was not elicited. A grading system was described:

- Class I, ability to visualize the faucial pillars and uvula completely
- Class II, ability to visualize the base of the uvula
- Class III, ability to visualize the soft palate only
- Class IV [a modification by Samsoon[25]], visualization of the hard palate only (Fig. 5–2).

From Mallampati's data, it is apparent that a correlation exists between the ability to visualize pharyngeal structures preoperatively and the degree of laryngeal exposure during direct laryngoscopy (Table 5–3). All of the 155 class I patients had an adequate exposure, and all but one of the 15 class III patients had an inadequate exposure.

Unfortunately, it is equally apparent that some significant shortcomings exist within this system. This

TABLE 5–3. **CORRELATION BETWEEN VISIBILITY OF FAUCIAL PILLARS, SOFT PALATE, AND UVULA, AND EXPOSURE OF GLOTTIS BY DIRECT LARYNGOSCOPY**

Visibility of Structures No. Pts (%)	Laryngoscopy Grade			
	Grade 1 No. Pts (%)	Grade 2 No. Pts (%)	Grade 3 No. Pts (%)	Grade 4 No. Pts (%)
Class I 155 (73.8%)	125 (59.5%)	30 (14.3%)	—	—
Class II 40 (19%)	12 (5.7%)	14 (6.7%)	10 (4.7%)	4 (1.9%)
Class III 15 (7.14%)	—	1 (0.5%)	9 (4.3%)	5 (2.4%)

From Mallampati SR, Gatt SP, Gugino LD, et al. A clinical sign to predict difficult tracheal intubation: A prospective study. Can Anaesth Soc J 1985; 32:429.

Class I: Faucial pillars, soft palate and uvula could be visualized. Class II: Faucial pillars and soft palate could be visualized, but uvula was masked by the base of the tongue. Class III: Only soft palate could be visualized. (See Figure 5–2.) Grade 1: Glottis (including anterior and posterior commissures) could be fully exposed. Grade 2: Glottis could be partly exposed (anterior commissure not visualized). Grade 3: Glottis could not be exposed (corniculate cartilages only could be visualized). Grade 4: Glottis including corniculate cartilages could not be exposed. (See Figure 5–1.)

method evaluates just one anatomic factor, tongue size, from a list of many factors that can predict difficult intubation. Additionally, this method did not evaluate the incidence of failed or difficult intubations; rather it evaluated only laryngeal exposure. This study was conducted on a nonpregnant population, and its applicability to the management of the airway of the obstetric patient is suspect. Furthermore, even stringent performance of this test in the context of an academic study has resulted in a wide distribution of preoperative scores.[49] Even among experienced anesthesiologists this evaluation is frequently performed incorrectly; common examples include performing the test on a supine patient, asking her to phonate,* and even reporting a general "gestalt" of the airway rather than a depiction of pharyngeal structures seen. ("I didn't see the uvula at all, but she opens wide and has a large thyromental distance, so I'd give her a grade II.") Another problem with this evaluation in pregnancy is the fact that the score can change in the same woman between the first and third trimesters[50] and during labor.[51]

Most disturbingly, this test lacks both sensitivity and specificity. Of the 28 inadequate exposures, only 14 occurred in class III patients. If a class III rating is considered predictive of difficult intubation, the sensitivity (the proportion of difficult intubations that were correctly predicted) is 50%, with a false-positive rate of 7%. Other investigators have found sensitivities of 42%[49] to 46%[52] with a 9 to 16% false-positive rate. Thus, approximately half of the difficult intubations occurred in patients with normal-appearing upper airway anatomy (class I and II). For patients with class II ratings, there is a further deterioration of the relationship between Mallampati class and degree of laryngeal exposure. Of the patients with class II ratings studied, only 65% were considered to have adequate exposure, 25% had a grade III view, and 10% had a grade IV view. Because almost one fifth of the patients studied were judged to fall within the class II category, this presents a dilemma: When managing such a patient, does one perform an awake fiberoptic intubation when there is a 65% chance of her having an adequate airway? Or does one induce general anesthesia on a patient who has a 35% chance of being a difficult intubation? Obviously, this method, by itself, is unsatisfactory and other methods to evaluate the airway further must be sought.

Rocke and coworkers[53] studied 1500 patients receiving general anesthesia for cesarean section. The Mallampati/Samsoon classification was evaluated preoperatively, along with other facial and physical characteristics that could affect intubation. In addition to recording laryngeal exposure, the ease and success of intubation were noted. From the portion of data that used the tongue and pharynx's relative size as a predictor, the results were similar to those of Mallampati. Inadequate exposure occurred more frequently in class IV and III airways (7 and 3.4%) than in class II and I airways (1.6 and 0.2%). A sensitivity of only 59% was seen, however. Only 16 of 27 inadequate exposures occurred in class III or IV airways, with the remainder in class I and II airways. There was only one grade IV exposure, occurring in a class II patient. Failed intubation happened twice (0.13%), once in a class II airway and once in a class III airway.

Wilson[54] identified five risk factors for difficult intubation. These were weight, head and neck movement, jaw movement, receding mandible, and "buck" teeth (Table 5–4). Note that buck teeth and receding mandible were judged on a subjective scale of severity. The tongue and pharynx size were not evaluated. A score of zero to two was given for the presence and severity of each risk factor for a total score of zero to ten. The risk factors were obtained and then tested prospectively. If a clinician considers that a Wilson score of two is diagnostic of a difficult intubation, 75% of all difficult airways can be correctly identified, although at a cost of a 12.1% false-positive rate. An additional study[49] of the Wilson test revealed a decreased sensitivity of 42%, with 8% false-positive results. Although this low rate of false-positives may appear reasonable, given an incidence of difficult intubation of 1.5%, for every difficult intubation correctly identified approximately 10 will be incorrectly identified as difficult.

Recommendations

It is clear that no individual test can identify every difficult intubation, especially without a prohibitive

TABLE 5–4. **RISK FACTORS COMPARED AMONG "NORMAL" AND "DIFFICULT" PATIENTS**

Risk Factor	Risk Level	Normal	Difficult	P
Weight	0	533 (95%)	45 (90%)	0.05
	1	27 (5%)	3 (6%)	
	2	1 (0.2%)	2 (4%)	
Head and neck movement	0	297 (91%)	27 (54%)	0.001
	1	21 (6%)	11 (22%)	
	2	8 (3%)	12 (24%)	
Jaw movement	0	457 (92%)	19 (38%)	0.001
	1	36 (7%)	17 (34%)	
	2	2 (0.4%)	14 (28%)	
Receding mandible	0	506 (97%)	29 (58%)	0.001
	1	16 (3%)	16 (32%)	
	2	1 (0.2%)	5 (10%)	
Buck teeth	0	504 (96%)	32 (64%)	0.001
	1	18 (3%)	12 (24%)	
	2	2 (0.4%)	6 (12%)	

P = probability that the difference between normal and difficult groups could arise by chance. For weight, the risk levels 0 and 1 were pooled and the difference calculated by Fischer's Exact test; all other differences were calculated by chi squared test.
Risk level 0 to 2: see text and Wilson, et al.[54]

---

*Editors' note: Phonation is permissible according to some experts—personal communication with Dr. John Benumof.

TABLE 5–5. **RELATIVE RISK OF FACTORS ASSOCIATED WITH DIFFICULTY AT TRACHEAL INTUBATION COMPARED WITH UNCOMPLICATED MALLAMPATI CLASS I SCORES**

Risk Factor	Regression Coefficient (SE)	Relative Risk (95% CI)
Mallampati class		
II	−0.233 (0.3266)	3.23 (1.70; 6.13)
III	0.620 (0.3173)	7.58 (4.07; 14.12)
IV	1.019 (0.4127)	11.30 (5.03; 25.38)
Short neck	1.612 (0.3746)	5.01 (2.40; 10.450)
Receding mandible	2.273 (0.8292)	9.71 (1.91; 49.32)
Protruding maxillary incisors	2.080 (0.8554)	8.0 (1.50; 42.50)

From Rocke DA, Murray WB, Rout CC, Gouws E. Relative risk analysis of factors associated with difficult intubation in obstetric anesthesia. Anesthesiology 1992;77:67.

number of false-positive results. How can the clinician screen effectively for difficult intubation? There are three points worth mentioning in answer to this question: First, the best test (or group of tests) can only offer an estimate of the probability of difficult intubation. In the Rocke study,[53] a group of four factors and their relative risk were described (Table 5–5); it included high Mallampati score, short neck, receding mandible, and protruding maxillary incisors. The contribution they made to difficult intubation is seen in Figure 5–3.

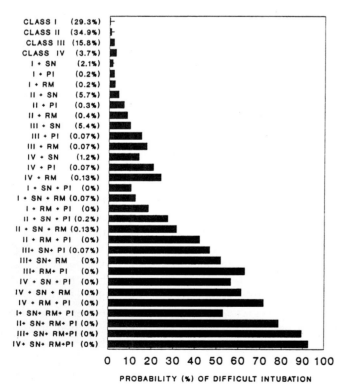

Figure 5–3. Probability of experiencing difficult intubation for varying combinations of risk factors ([%] = observed incidence of the combination of risk factors; SN = short neck; PI = protruding maxillary incisors; RM = receding mandible). (From Rocke DA, Murray WB, Rout CC, Gouws E: Difficult intubation in obstetric anesthesia. Anesthesiology 1992;77:67.)

Although this information is very useful, the result provides only a probability of difficult intubation. The anesthesiologist's dilemma is in utilizing these imperfect indicators to make a yes/no decision of whether to intubate before or after inducing anesthesia. The decision to perform an awake intubation is affected by experience of the laryngoscopist, concern for fetal welfare, and tolerance for false-negative and false-positive errors.

Because 50% of all difficult intubation incidents are unexpected, a difficult intubation drill must be developed in advance, with all emergency airway adjuncts (e.g., jet ventilators, cricothyrotomy kits, laryngeal mask airways, small endotracheal tubes) ready at all times. Communication with the obstetric team is essential. Obstetricians must be informed that a potential airway problem may take precedence over fetal indications for an expeditious delivery.

If parturients are denied a traditional rapid induction of general anesthesia, an alternate method of anesthesia must be offered if possible. The role of regional anesthesia in this situation is obvious. In addition to epidural anesthesia, continuous spinal anesthesia is particularly suited for this situation.[46] A catheter can be placed for immediate use, or one may be placed simply in anticipation of a possible cesarean section. Two drawbacks have tempered the use of spinal catheters: The potential for neurologic complications and occurrence of post-dural puncture headaches (PDPH). Although repeated administrations of inappropriately large doses of hyperbaric 5% lidocaine via microcatheters have been implicated in cauda equina syndrome,[55] the 20-gauge "epidural" catheter and hyperbaric bupivacaine should mitigate this risk. A more common problem, PDPH, may dissuade many practitioners from utilizing spinal catheters; however, in our opinion, this is a relatively minor nuisance compared with the possibility of losing an airway. Additionally, another study[56] indicated a surprisingly low incidence of PDPH after continuous spinal anesthesia in a population of morbidly obese parturients, a group in whom a spinal catheter may offer a particular advantage.

Although many practitioners consider regional anesthesia to be the method of choice in the parturient with a potentially difficult airway, one caveat must be considered—the risk of losing the natural airway. Because the possibilities of intravascular injection of local anesthetic, total spinal anesthesia, and intraoperative hemorrhage are real, the anesthesiologist must be prepared for sudden loss of consciousness and circulatory collapse in the patient who cannot be intubated. A reasonable alternative is to secure the airway by awake intubation electively, especially if help is not readily available and if the patient is at increased risk for bleeding.

In addition to regional anesthesia for the management of the "bad airway, bad baby" scenario, performing the cesarean section using local anesthesia should be considered.[57, 58] There are many shortcomings to this technique; near-toxic local anesthetic levels may result from the large volumes required, even with dilute, epinephrine-containing solutions. Maternal discomfort can be expected, and generous sedation is often necessary. Not surprisingly, local anesthetic infiltration for cesarean section is seldom performed electively, and most obstetricians are inexperienced in performing field blocks.

When uncertain whether a patient can be intubated easily, an "awake look" is a technique that can rapidly resolve this dilemma. With a gentle hand, good topical anesthesia or glossopharyngeal nerve block, and a frank discussion with the patient, an anesthesiologist can often perform direct laryngoscopy simply and atraumatically. This technique (especially in the context of fetal distress and questionable airway) can be performed while awaiting help or additional equipment. If adequate glottic exposure is obtained, anesthesia may be induced without further delay. [Many consider that if you take an "awake look" at the vocal cords and see them clearly, an endotracheal tube should be inserted immediately. General anesthesia is then induced shortly after. It is possible that relaxation of the patient, with anesthetic induction agents, may alter the position of the glottis.] If, however, the vocal cords cannot be visualized, the anesthesiologist can stand resolute, knowing that the patient is not a candidate for the usual "crash" anesthetic induction.

MANAGEMENT OF THE ANTICIPATED DIFFICULT AIRWAY

The management of a difficult airway depends on when it is discovered to be difficult. The American Society of Anesthesiologists' difficult airway algorithm[59] (Fig. 5–4) has two limbs, one for the spontaneously breathing patient with an anticipated bad airway, and one for the apneic patient with an airway found to be difficult after induction of anesthesia. It is imperative that the reader be familiar with this algorithm; it is likely to be invoked in emergency situations and at inconvenient times. The anesthesiologist must be both comfortable and confident when faced with an airway emergency.

If difficult intubation is anticipated, subsequent management centers on maintaining the patient's natural airway until tracheal intubation is accomplished. After discussion with the patient and administration of topical anesthesia of the airway, options include the following:

- Direct, awake laryngoscopy
- Awake fiberoptic bronchoscopy
- Retrograde wire intubation

- Use of a Bullard laryngoscope or light wand
- Intubation through a laryngeal mask airway (LMA, vide infra)
- Awake cricothyrotomy or tracheostomy using local anesthesia.

Although the administration of respiratory depressant drugs to the mother is usually discouraged, awake intubations are frequently facilitated by the judicious use of sedation (0.5 mg increments of intravenous [IV] midazolam and 25–50 μg IV fentanyl), which should not be withheld if it will result in a more expedient, atraumatic, and successful securing of the airway.

MANAGEMENT OF THE UNEXPECTEDLY DIFFICULT AIRWAY

If initial attempts at intubation are unsuccessful after inducing anesthesia, a few additional attempts at intubation are appropriate before considering the case a difficult airway. Replicating the same conditions for subsequent attempts, however, only wastes time and traumatizes the airway. The clinician must change laryngoscope blades, head position, or laryngoscopist with each attempt. Patients die from hypoxemia, not from failure to intubate. If the trachea cannot be intubated after these adjustments, management centers on introducing oxygen into the trachea with a face mask, if possible. If ventilation is difficult with a face mask and oral airway, options are limited to placing a laryngeal mask airway (LMA) or Combitube or performing a cricothyrotomy.

CANNOT INTUBATE, CANNOT VENTILATE

Transtracheal Jet Ventilation

This situation is obviously the most dire and the one in which the majority of anesthesia-related maternal deaths occur. If LMA or Combitube insertion fails (see later), the management preference of many is the performance of percutaneous needle cricothyrotomy and transtracheal jet ventilation (TTJV). A needle or intravenous cannula inserted through the cricothyroid membrane, directed caudad and attached to a high-pressure oxygen source, can instill oxygen into the trachea and maintain oxygenation and, frequently, normocarbia. A large-bore needle should be inserted into the trachea while aspirating with a syringe containing saline. When the needle has entered the trachea, bubbles are seen in the syringe. The cricothyroid ligament is easily located; it is avascular and below the vocal cords. We routinely locate and mark the cricothyroid ligament before induction on patients who may prove to have difficult airways.

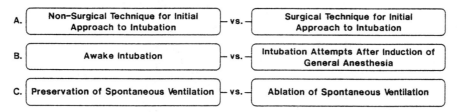

DIFFICULT AIRWAY ALGORITHM

1. Assess the likelihood and clinical impact of basic management problems:

    A. Difficult Intubation

    B. Difficult Ventilation

    C. Difficulty with Patient Cooperation or Consent

2. Consider the relative merits and feasibility of basic management choices:

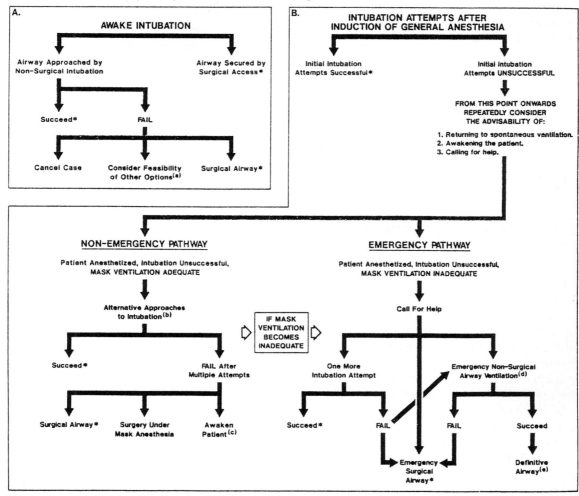

Figure 5–4. Difficult airway algorithm. (From American Society of Anesthesiologists: Practice guidelines for management of the difficult airway—a report by the American Society of Anesthesiologists Task Force on management of the difficult airway. Anesthesiology 1993;78:597.)

Most anesthesiologists are comfortable in performing cricothyroid puncture, and if a jet ventilator is not available, a high-pressure oxygen source can be fashioned from easily obtainable materials.[60-62] Although lifesaving, TTJV must be tempered with the following caveats: (1) a route for egress of exhaled gas must be present; and (2) in the case of laryngospasm or upper airway obstruction, the intrathoracic pressure rises rapidly and dramatically. TTJV cannot protect against aspiration, and cricoid pressure must be interrupted to perform TTJV. The possibility of barotrauma can further complicate airway management. We are aware of subcutaneous and mediastinal emphysema occurring rapidly after TTJV, impinging on the trachea and obscuring landmarks. Furthermore, in the case of a cesarean section for fetal asphyxia, TTJV can forestall profound hypoxia; however, it does not provide a means to continue the anesthetic. We consider TTJV to be of greatest utility for nonemergent situations in which it is acceptable to allow the patient to awaken after initiating TTJV.

Cricothyrotomy

Numerous percutaneous cricothyrotomy kits are available (e.g., Pertrach [Fig. 5–5], Melker), using a variant of the Seldinger technique, introducing a wire through the cricothyroid ligament and then a dilator and cuffed tracheostomy tube over the wire. Although more invasive than a needle TTJV, this technique allows for a cuffed tube to be placed into the trachea, protecting the lungs from gastric aspiration and allowing an emergent cesarean section to proceed.

In an emergency, many surgeons may offer to perform a tracheostomy. It should be stressed that an emergency tracheostomy is rarely appropriate; it takes longer to perform than a cricothyrotomy, and its prox-

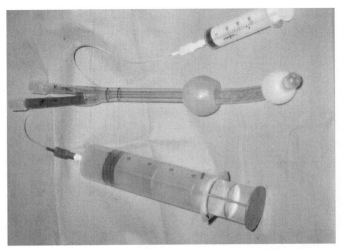

Figure 5–5. The esophageal-tracheal Combitube (ETC).

imity to the thyroid gland results in brisk bleeding if meticulous dissection is not performed. Because few surgeons (and fewer obstetricians) are familiar with performing a cricothyrotomy, anesthesiologists, by nature of their knowledge of airway anatomy, must be capable of performing this procedure, as described elsewhere.[63]

Esophageal-tracheal Combitube

Development of the esophageal-tracheal Combitube (ETC, Fig. 5–6) has stemmed from an attempt to improve upon the drawbacks of the esophageal obturator airway (EOA). It is composed of two lumens, one resembling an endotracheal tube, one similar to an EOA. Two balloons are placed on the ETC; the proximal one is filled with 100 cc of air and forms a seal in the oropharynx; the distal balloon forms a seal with 10 to 15 cc of air. The device is inserted blindly, usually into the esophagus, although tracheal placement is possible. When placed in the esophagus, the ETC functions similarly to an EOA, with the seal of the pharyngeal balloon obviating the need to achieve a good mask seal (Fig. 5–7A). In the event of tracheal placement of the ETC, ventilation can be performed through the cuffed distal lumen, which functions as an endotracheal tube (see Fig. 5–7B).

The ETC is efficacious when used by clinicians with a modicum of training. When done as an alternative to tracheal intubation, no failures of insertion were reported when the tube was placed by experienced physicians,[64-66] with two tracheal placements in 79 uses. Placement of the ETC was more rapid (27.3 sec) than regular tracheal intubation (39 sec). When the ETC was used by intensive care unit nurses[67] and paramedics[68] trained in its application, success rates decreased to 94% and 69%, respectively. A majority of the failed insertions were the result of improper insertion angle

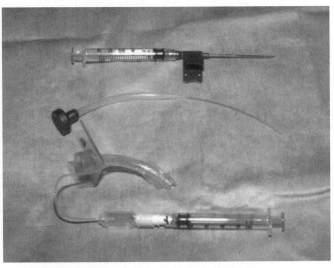

Figure 5–5. The Pertrach—a surgical airway.

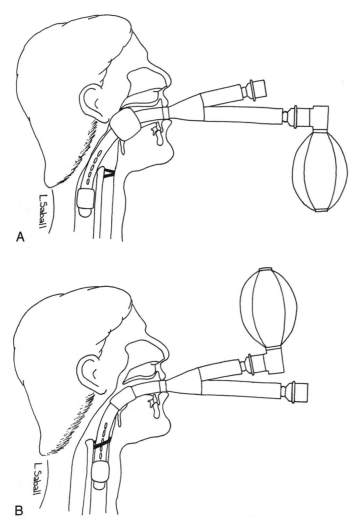

Figure 5–7. Two potential placements of the ETC. (A) ETC placed in the esophagus, proximal cuff inflated, tracheal cuff deflated, ventilation through the proximal lumen. (B) ETC placed in the trachea, proximal cuff deflated, tracheal cuff inflated, ventilation through the distal lumen.

and poor retention of training. The ETC is labeled for single use only, making training and retention of technique relatively expensive. When used in the parturient and inserted into the esophagus, any swelling around the tracheal orifice may limit air entry to the trachea. The ETC may also provide incomplete protection against pulmonary aspiration.

Laryngeal Mask Airway

The LMA (Fig. 5–8A) was developed in the early 1980s as an alternative to a face mask[69] and has enjoyed great popularity outside the US. It is inserted blindly into the pharynx until the tip sits upon the upper esophageal sphincter, and the elliptical cuff overlies the epiglottis and forms a seal around the perimeter of the laryngeal inlet (see Fig. 5–8B). Although contraindicated if a risk of aspiration exists, the LMA has found

a place in obstetric anesthesia, because it can be inserted easily and rapidly and may still allow ventilation even if grossly malpositioned.[70]

Although the low-pressure seal of the pharyngeal cuff can allow gas leakage if higher inspiratory pressures are applied, numerous case reports have demonstrated the usefulness of LMAs in the management of difficult airways.[71-77] In a survey of anesthesiologists in the UK, 72% supported the use of the LMA when intubation had failed and ventilation was inadequate.[78] Success rates for LMA insertion, ranging from 74 to 98% on first attempt, have been reported when three attempts are allowed.[79-82] Insertion times averaged 20 sec.[82] It is notable that the lower overall success rates were obtained with unskilled and inexperienced personnel. A learning curve was demonstrated, in that fewer than 15 LMA insertions are associated with 88 to 94% success. Success of 100% was seen in personnel with an experience of more than 15 insertions.

The *triple airway maneuver* (mouth opening, head extension, and jaw thrust) can facilitate insertion of the LMA.[83] Although ventilation following all insertions with and without this maneuver was successful, fiberoptic confirmation of LMA position showed improved epiglottic visibility and less epiglottic downfolding after insertion with the triple airway maneuver. Many alternative insertion techniques have been described, including inflating the cuff before insertion and backwards insertion of the LMA, then rotating it 180°. No alternative technique, however, has improved upon inserting the LMA fully deflated, with the deflated rim posterior, and using a midline approach, as originally described by Brain.[69] Full and partial inflation of the cuff resulted in more insertion failures, and rotation of the LMA was associated with a high success rate but significant residual rotation to the coronal plane.[86]

Although it was thought initially that the LMA, aimed toward the esophagus, might be easier to insert in patients who were difficult to intubate, this speculation has not been supported by the data. Studies have failed to show a correlation between Mallampati classification and ease or success of LMA insertion[83] or fiberoptic confirmation of LMA position.[86, 87] One additional study[88] concluded that a Mallampati class III airway was associated with a 20% failure rate; no failures occurred in the other groups. Further, the successful insertions in the Mallampati III group required an average of 2.4 attempts, versus one attempt for Mallampati class I airways.

The effect of cricoid pressure on the ease of LMA insertion has been the matter of much debate. Because the application of cricoid pressure can prevent the distal portion of the mask from projecting into the hypopharynx, it appears reasonable that the success rate is lessened with cricoid pressure. The data appear to support this contention. Although one study[89] reported

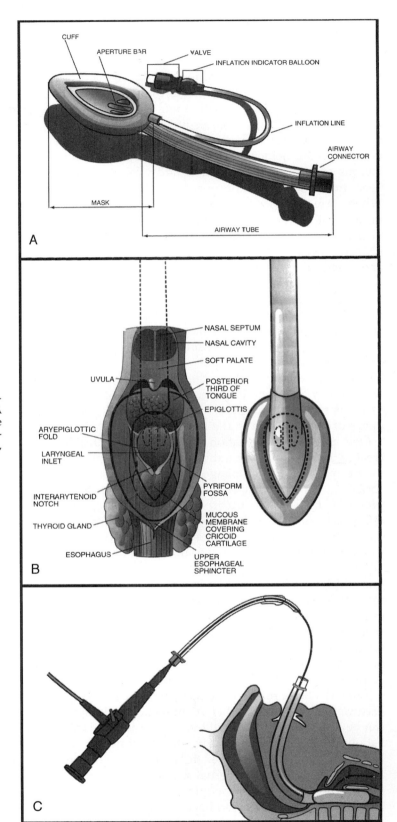

Figure 5–8. Laryngeal mask airway (LMA). *(A)* Three components of the LMA. *(B)* Anatomic relationships of the LMA when fully inserted. *(C)* Fiberoptic intubation through the LMA. (Reproduced from Brain AIJ, Denman WT, Goudsouzian NG: LMA Instruction Manual. San Diego, Gensia Inc., 1995.)

no effect of cricoid pressure upon successful LMA placement, numerous other studies[87, 90–92] have shown that LMA placement is impaired by cricoid pressure, resulting in failure rates greater than those without cricoid pressure and ranging from 4 to 86%. Although variable, cricoid pressure appears to have a detrimental effect on LMA placement. Variations in the degree of hindrance have been ascribed to variations in the techniques of cricoid pressure, neck support, head position, and cricoid pressure force.

The LMA was not developed as a replacement for tracheal intubation and is not indicated for patients at risk for aspiration. Its utility as a lifesaving maneuver when neither tracheal intubation nor mask ventilation was possible, however, has resulted in its success for patients with cesarean sections[72–75] and bowel obstructions[76] without evidence of pulmonary aspiration. Numerous reports of regurgitation and aspiration have been made with an appropriately placed LMA.[93–99] When correctly placed, the tip of the LMA usually lies in, and may even occlude, the esophagus. Fiberoptic visualization of the esophagus within the bowl of the LMA occurred in 6%,[100] 9%,[101] and 10%[87] of placements and occurred more frequently when cricoid pressure was applied during LMA insertion.[87] Dye studies in a nonpregnant population have been performed with a methylene blue capsule ingested just before anesthesia and ventilation via LMA or face mask. Although the incidence of pharyngeal staining of 0%[102] and 4%[103] have been reported with LMAs, one study[104] found a 25% incidence of dye within the LMA. The esophagus was seen by fiberoptic inspection in less than one third of patients who regurgitated dye. There was no evidence of regurgitation in the face mask group.

One possible explanation for the apparently increased incidence of aspiration in the LMA group is the decreased lower esophageal sphincter pressure associated with LMA placement.[105] If the reaction to the presence of the LMA tip in the esophagus causes a reflex relaxation of the lower esophageal sphincter similar to that produced by a bolus of food in the esophagus, the decrease in barrier pressure can allow regurgitation. The application of cricoid pressure may obviate this effect, however. An LMA in situ does not compromise the effectiveness of cricoid pressure in preventing reflux of gastric contents, even with intragastric pressures approximately twice those during twin gestations.[106] Nonetheless, cricoid pressure applied to a correctly placed LMA has been reported to force the vocal cords to close and obstruct ventilation.[87]

The LMA has a role in the management of the airway predicted to be difficult before induction, because it can be used as an aid to facilitate awake tracheal intubation. When placed properly, the apertures of the LMA are positioned just over the glottic opening, and a well-lubricated 6-mm internal diameter (ID) endotracheal tube, gum elastic bougie (GEB), or fiberoptic bronchoscope can be passed beyond the LMA, into the trachea. Heath and Allagain[89] reported a 90% success rate for blind intubation through an LMA, including a 6% failure of LMA insertion and only 2 of 50 attempts at intubation via the LMA abandoned. The application of cricoid pressure, however, resulted in only 56% of blind intubations through the LMA meeting with success; an additional 30% were intubated after release

of cricoid pressure. These investigators recommended rotating the endotracheal tube 90° to the left to bring the bevel of the tube anteriorly, facilitating passage through the aperture bars.

The LMA compares very favorably with the Williams Airway Intubator,[107] with median intubating times of 8.9 sec (LMA) versus 12.9 sec (Williams Airway Intubator). The LMA can also be employed when secretions, blood,[108] or anterior glottic positioning[109] have resulted in failure of fiberoptic intubation without the LMA. Using a fiberoptic bronchoscope through an LMA has been described for awake intubation in the patient at risk for aspiration[110] and for the patient having cesarean section (see Fig. 5–8C).[111] The LMA has been utilized as a guide to pass a GEB blindly into the trachea and then intubate over it.[112] Of note is that the LMA was used with a fiberoptic bronchoscope and GEB on awake patients who were under topical anesthesia and was well tolerated. Thus, two potential ways of employing the LMA as a bridge to tracheal intubation can be done: when the LMA is placed emergently in the asleep patient unable to be intubated or ventilated, and in the awake patient, to facilitate the intubation.

CANNOT INTUBATE, CAN VENTILATE

The case of "cannot intubate, can ventilate" offers the anesthesiologist numerous options and, as such, has generated significant controversy. One reasonable and justifiable course is to allow the patient to wake up and to have the anesthesiologist perform an awake intubation, as outlined in the algorithm for the airway known to be difficult. Although discounting fetal well-being as a secondary consideration, this avenue allows the anesthesiologist to secure the airway before surgery. In cases of fetal asphyxia, and when mask ventilation is not difficult, most clinicians consider continuing to mask-ventilate (with constant application of cricoid pressure) and allowing surgery to begin.

Although the role of the LMA in the context of a failed intubation is still not defined, we advocate the following guidelines. If intubation is unsuccessful but ventilation with a face mask is easily accomplished, we do not place an LMA; we waken the patient or proceed with cesarean section using mask ventilation. If mask ventilation is difficult or impossible, we place an LMA initially, with cricoid pressure maintained; if this technique is unsuccessful, a second attempt is made after cricoid pressure is briefly released. If LMA placement is successful, we awaken the patient or proceed with cesarean section while attempting to intubate through the LMA with a fiberoptic bronchoscope. If intubation, mask ventilation, and LMA placement are impossible, we perform a cricothyroidotomy. Those with significant experience with ETC may prefer it as an alternative to cricothyroidotomy. The decision to perform a needle cricothyroidotomy and TTJV versus placing a percutaneous cuffed cricothyroidotomy tube may be determined by the fetal condition and the need to proceed with emergent operative delivery.

References

1. Tomkinson J, Turnbull A, Robson G, et al. Report on confidential enquiries into maternal deaths in England and Wales 1973–1975. London, Her Majesty's Stationery Office, 1979.
2. Tompkinson J, Turnbull A, Robson G, et al. Report on confidential enquiries into maternal deaths in England and Wales 1976–1978. London, Her Majesty's Stationery Office, 1982.
3. Turnbull AC, Tindall VR, Robson G, et al. Report on confidential enquiries into maternal deaths in England and Wales 1979–1981. London, Her Majesty's Stationery Office, 1986.
4. Turnbull AC, Tindall VR, Beard RW, et al. Report on confidential enquiries into maternal deaths in England and Wales 1982–1984. London, Her Majesty's Stationery Office, 1989.
5. Tindall VR, Beard RW, Sykes MK, et al. Report on confidential enquiries into maternal deaths in England and Wales 1985–1987. London, Her Majesty's Stationery Office, 1991.
6. Atrash HK, Koonin LM, Lawson HW, et al. Maternal Mortality in the United States, 1979–1986. Obstet Gynecol 1990;76:1055.
7. Conklin KA. Physiological changes of pregnancy. In Chestnut DH (ed): Obstetric Anesthesia, Principles and Practice. St. Louis, CV Mosby, 1994, p 17.
8. Awe WC, Fletcher WS, Jacob SW. The pathophysiology of aspiration pneumonitis. Surgery 1960;60:232.
9. Roberts RB, Shirley MA. Reducing the risk of acid aspiration during cesarean section. Anesth Analg 1974;53:859.
10. Brock-Utne JG, Downing JW, Seedat F. Laryngeal oedema associated with pre-eclamptic toxaemia. Anaesthesia 1977;32:556.
11. Seager SJ, Macdonald R. Laryngeal oedema and pre-eclampsia. Anaesthesia 1980;35:360.
12. Jouppila R, Jouppila P, Hollmen A. Laryngeal oedema as an obstetric anaesthesia complication. Acta Anaesth Scand 1980;24:97.
13. Rocke DA, Scoones GP. Rapidly progressive laryngeal oedema associated with pregnancy-aggravated hypertension. Anaesthesia 1992;47:141.
14. Hein HAT. Cardiorespiratory arrest with laryngeal oedema in pregnancy-induced hypertension. Can Anaesth Soc J 1984;31:210.
15. Salt PJ, Nutbourne PA, Park GR, Glazebrook CW. Laryngeal oedema after caesarean section. Anaesthesia 1983;38:693.
16. Brimacombe J. Acute pharyngolaryngeal oedema and pre-eclamptic toxaemia. Anaesth Intensive Care 1992;20:97.
17. Heller PJ, Scheider EP, Marx GF. Pharyngolaryngeal edema as a presenting symptom in preeclampsia. Obstet Gynecol 1983;62:523.
18. Mackenzie AI. Laryngeal oedema complicating obstetric anaesthesia. Anaesthesia 1978;33:271.
19. Keeri-Szanto M. Laryngeal oedema complicating obstetric anaesthesia. Anaesthesia 1978;33:272.
20. Stevens ID. ICU admissions from an obstetric hospital. Can J Anaesth 1991;38:677.
21. Ebert RJ. Post-partum airway obstruction after vaginal delivery. Anaesth Intensive Care 1992;20:365.
22. Procter AJM, White JB. Laryngeal oedema in pregnancy. Anaesthesia 1983;38:167.
23. Dobb G. Laryngeal oedema complicating obstetric anaesthesia. Anaesthesia 1978;33:839.
24. Spotoft H, Christensen P. Laryngeal oedema accompanying weight gain in pregnancy. Anaesthesia 1981;36:71.
25. Samsoon GLT, Young JRB. Difficult tracheal intubation: A retrospective study. Anaesthesia 1987;42:487.
26. Lyons G. Failed intubation: Six years' experience in a teaching maternity unit. Anaesthesia 1985;40:759.
27. Glassenberg R. General anesthesia and maternal mortality. Semin Perinatol 1991;15:386.
28. Boliston TA. Difficult tracheal intubation in obstetrics. Anaesthesia 1985;40:389.
29. Pare PD, Donevan RE, Nelems JM. Clues to unrecognized upper airway obstruction. Can Med Assoc J 1982;127:39.
30. Salama DJ, Body SC. Management of a term parturient with tracheal stenosis. Br J Anaesth 1994;72:354.
31. Mallett VT, Bhatia RK, Kissner DG, Sokol RJ. Use of a HeO₂ mixture in the management of upper airway obstruction during labor and delivery. J Reprod Med 1989;34:429.
32. Sutcliffe N, Remington SAM, Ramsay TM, Mason C. Severe tracheal stenosis and operative delivery. Anaesthesia 1995;50:26.
33. Mettam IM, Reddy TR, Evans FE. Life-threatening acute respiratory distress in late pregnancy. Br J Anaesth 1992;69:420.
34. Lagler U, Russi E. Upper airway obstruction as a cause of pulmonary edema during late pregnancy. Am J Obstet Gynecol 1987;156:643.
35. Shaha A, Alfonso A, Jaffe BM. Acute airway distress due to thyroid pathology. Surgery 1987;102:1068.
36. Georgescu A, Miller JN, Lecklitner ML. The Sellick maneuver causing complete airway obstruction. Anesth Analg 1992;74:457.
37. Shorten GD. Airway obstruction from cricoid pressure. Anesth Analg 1993;76:665.
38. Rajaratnam K, Desai S. Kaposi's sarcoma of the trachea. J Laryngol Otol 1988;102:951.
39. Ellis DJ, Millar WL, Karagianes TG. Anesthesia for laser resection of a tracheal tumor in a woman pregnant with twins. Anesthesiology 1988;68:629.
40. Donegan JO, Wood MD. Intratracheal thyroid—familial occurrence. Laryngoscope 1985;95:6.
41. Glock JL, Morales WJ. Acute epiglottitis during pregnancy. South Med J 1993;86:836.
42. Biem J, Roy J, Halik J, Hoffstein V. Infectious mononucleosis complicated by necrotizing epiglottitis, dysphagia, and pneumonia. Chest 1989;96:204.
43. Michelsen LG, Vanderspek AFL. An unexpected functional cause of upper airway obstruction. Anaesthesia 1988;43:1028.
44. Reuveni MA, Suresh A, Marx GF. Acute respiratory distress in a parturient under effective epidural analgesia. Can J Anaesth 1995;42:1063.
45. Benumof JL. Management of the difficult airway with special emphasis on awake tracheal intubation. Anesthesiology 1991;75:1087.
46. Malan TP, Johnson MD. The difficult airway in obstetric anesthesia: Techniques for airway management and the role of regional anesthesia. J Clin Anesth 1988;1:104.
47. Cormack RS, Lehane J. Difficult tracheal intubation in obstetrics. Anaesth 1984;39:1105.
48. Mallampati SR, Gatt SP, Gugino LD, et al. A clinical sign to predict difficult tracheal intubation: A prospective study. Can Anaesth Soc J 1985;32:429.
49. Oates JDL, Macleod AD, Oates PD, et al. Comparison of two methods for predicting difficult intubation. Br J Anaesth 1991;66:305.
50. Pilkington S, Carli F, Dakin MJ, et al. Increase in Mallampati score during pregnancy. Br J Anaesth 1995;74:638.
51. Farcon EL, Kim MH, Marx GF. Changing Mallampati score during labour. Can J Anaesth 1994;41:50.
52. Cohen SM, Laurito CE, Segil LJ. Oral exam to predict difficult intubations: A large prospective study (abstract). Anesthesiology 1989;71:A936.
53. Rocke DA, Murray WB, Rout CC, Gouws E. Relative risk analysis of factors associated with difficult intubation in obstetric anesthesia. Anesthesiology 1992;77:67.
54. Wilson ME, Spiegelhalter D, Robertson JA, Lesser P. Predicting difficult intubation. Br J Anaesth 1988;61:211.
55. Rigler Ml, Drasner K, Krejcie TC, et al. Cauda equina syndrome after continuous spinal anesthesia. Anesth Analg 1991;72:275.
56. Brown RS, Johnson MD, Zavisca F, et al. Morbid obesity in the parturient reduces the risk of post dural puncture headache after large bore continuous spinal anesthesia (abstract). Anesthesiology 1993;79:A1004.
57. Ranney B, Stanage WF. Advantages of local anesthesia for cesarean section. Obstet Gynecol 1975;45:163.
58. Busby T. Local anesthesia for cesarean section. Am J Obstet Gynecol 1963;87:399.
59. Practice guidelines for management of the difficult airway—a report by the American Society of Anesthesiologists Task Force

on management of the difficult airway. Anesthesiology 1993;78:597.

60. Meyer PD. Emergency transtracheal jet ventilation system. Anesthesiology 1990;73:787.

61. Sprague DH. Transtracheal jet oxygenation from capnographic monitoring components. Anesthesiology 1990;73:788.

62. Levinson MM, Scuderi PE, Gibson RL, Comer PB. Emergency percutaneous transtracheal ventilation (PTV). J Am Coll Emerg Physicians 1979;8:10.

63. Johnson MD, Ostheimer GW. Airway management in obstetric patients. Semin Anesth 1992;11:1.

64. Frass M, Frenzer R, Zdrahal F, et al. The esophageal tracheal combitube: Preliminary results with a new airway for CPR. Ann Emerg Med 1987;16:768.

65. Frass M, Frenzer R, Rauscha F, et al. Evaluation of esophageal tracheal combitube in cardiopulmonary resuscitation. Crit Care Med 1987;15:609.

66. Frass M, Franzer R, Rauscha F, et al. Ventilation with the esophageal tracheal combitube in cardiopulmonary resuscitation. Chest 1988;93:781.

67. Staudinger T, Brugger S, Watschinger B, et al. Emergency intubation with the combitube: Comparison with the endotracheal airway. Ann Emerg Med 1993;22:1573.

68. Atherton GL, Johnson JC. Ability of paramedics to use the combitube in prehospital cardiac arrest. Ann Emerg Med 1993;22:1263.

69. Brain AIJ. The Laryngeal Mask—a new concept in airway management. Br J Anaesth 1983;55:801.

70. Molloy AR. Unexpected position of the laryngeal mask airway. Anaesthesia 1991;46:592.

71. Baraka A. Laryngeal mask airway in the cannot-intubate, cannot-ventilate situation. Anesthesiology 1993;79:1151.

72. Storey J. The laryngeal mask for failed intubation at Caesarean section (letter). Anaesth Intensive Care 1992;20:118.

73. McClune S, Regan M, Moore J. Laryngeal mask airway for Caesarean section. Anaesthesia 1990;45:227.

74. Priscu V, Priscu L, Soroker D. Laryngeal mask for failed intubation in emergency Caesarean section. Can J Anaesth 1992;39:893.

75. Chadwick IS, Vorha A. Anaesthesia for emergency Caesarean section using the Brain laryngeal airway (letter). Anaesthesia 1989;44:261.

76. Brain AIJ. Three cases of difficult intubation overcome by the laryngeal mask airway. Anaesthesia 1985;40:353.

77. DeMello WF, Kocan M. The laryngeal mask in failed intubation. Anaesthesia 1990;45:689.

78. Gataure PS, Hughes JA. The laryngeal mask airway in obstetrical anaesthesia. Can J Anaesth 1995;42:130.

79. Smith I, White PF. Use of the laryngeal mask airway as an alternative to a face mask during outpatient arthroscopy. Anesthesiology 1992;77:850.

80. McCrirrick A, Ramage DTO, Pracilio JA, Hickman JA: Experience with the laryngeal mask airway in two hundred patients. Anaesth Intensive Care 1991;19:256.

81. Broderick PM, Webster NR, Nunn JF. The laryngeal mask airway. Anaesthesia 1989;44:238.

82. Davies PRF, Tighe SQM, Greenslade GL, Evans GH. Laryngeal mask airway and tracheal tube insertion by unskilled personnel. Lancet 1990;336:977.

83. Aoyama K, Takenaka I, Sata T, Shigematsu A. The triple airway manoeuvre for insertion of the laryngeal mask airway in paralyzed patients. Can J Anaesth 1995;42:1010.

84. Brimacombe J, Berry A. Insertion of the laryngeal mask airway—a prospective study of four techniques. Anaesth Intensive Care 1993;21:89.

85. Mahiou P, Narchi P, Veyrac P, et al. Is laryngeal mask easy to use in case of difficult intubation? (abstract) Anesthesiology 1992;77:A1228.

86. Brimacombe J, Berry A. Mallampati classification and laryngeal mask airway insertion. Anaesthesia 1993;48:347.

87. Brimacombe J, White A, Berry A. Effect of cricoid pressure on ease of insertion of the laryngeal mask airway. Br J Anaesth 1993;71:800.

88. McCrory CR, Moriarty DC. Laryngeal mask airway positioning is related to Mallampati grading in adults. Anesth Analg 1995;81:1001.

89. Heath ML, Allagain J. Intubation through the laryngeal mask. Anaesthesia 1991;46:545.

90. Brimacombe J. Cricoid pressure and the laryngeal mask airway. Anaesthesia 1991;46:986.

91. Ansermino JM, Blogg CE. Cricoid pressure may prevent insertion of the laryngeal mask airway. Br J Anaesth 1992;69:465.

92. Asai T, Barclay K, Power I, Vaughan RS. Cricoid pressure impedes placement of the laryngeal mask airway. Br J Anaesth 1995;74:521.

93. Nanji GM, Maltby JR. Vomiting and aspiration pneumonitis with the laryngeal mask airway. Can J Anaesth 1992;39:69.

94. Maroof M, Khan RM, Siddique MS. Intraoperative aspiration pneumonitis and the laryngeal mask airway. Anesth Analg 1993;77:409.

95. Griffin RM, Hatcher IS. Aspiration pneumonia and the laryngeal mask airway. Anaesthesia 1990;45:1039.

96. Koehli N. Aspiration and the laryngeal mask airway. Anaesthesia 1991;46:419.

97. Cyna AM, MacLoed DM. The laryngeal mask: Cautionary tales. (Letter) Anaesthesia 1990;45:167.

98. Campbell JR. The laryngeal mask: Cautionary tales. (Letter) Anaesthesia 1990;45:167.

99. Criswell J, John R. The laryngeal mask: Cautionary tales (letter). Anaesthesia 1990;45:168.

100. Payne J, Edwards J. The use of the fibreoptic laryngoscope to confirm the position of the laryngeal mask. Anaesthesia 1989;44:865.

101. John RE, Hill S, Hughes TJ. Airway protection by the laryngeal mask. Anaesthesia 1991;46:366.

102. El Mikatti N, Luthra AD, Healy TEJ, Mortimer AJ. Gastric regurgitation during general anaesthesia in the supine position with the laryngeal and face mask airways. Br J Anaesth 1992;69 529.

103. Akhtar TM, Street MK. Risk of aspiration with the laryngeal mask. Br J Anaesth 1994;72:447.

104. Barker P, Langton JA, Murphy PJ, Rowbotham DJ. Regurgitation of gastric contents during general anaesthesia using the laryngeal mask airway. Br J Anaesth 1992;69:314.

105. Rabey PG, Murphy PJ, Langton JA, et al. Effect of the laryngeal mask airway on lower oesophageal sphincter pressure in patients during general anaesthesia. Br J Anaesth 1992;69:346.

106. Strang TI. Does the laryngeal mask airway compromise cricoid pressure? Anaesthesia 1992;47:829.

107. Crichlow A, Locken R, Todesco J. The laryngeal mask airway and fibreoptic laryngoscopy. Can J Anaesth 1992;39:742.

108. Maroof M, Khan RM, Bonsu A, Raza HS. A new solution to fibreoptic intubation in the presence of blood and secretions. Can J Anaesth 1995;42:117.

109. Williams PJ, Bailey PM. Management of failed oral fibreoptic intubation with laryngeal mask airway insertion under topical anaesthesia. Can J Anaesth 1993;40:287.

110. Asai T. Use of the laryngeal mask for tracheal intubation in patients at increased risk of aspiration of gastric contents. Anesthesiology 1992;77:1029.

111. Godley M, Reddy ARR. Use of LMA for awake intubation for Caesarean section. Can J Anaesth 1996;43:299.

112. McCrirrick A, Pracilio JA. Awake intubation: A new technique. Anaesthesia 1991;46:661.

ADULT RESPIRATORY DISTRESS SYNDROME

Paul R. Howell, M.B.

Adult (or acute) respiratory distress syndrome (ARDS) is the severe form of acute respiratory failure that may develop as a consequence of acute lung injury. Although ARDS is uncommon in pregnancy (complicating almost 1 in 3000 deliveries[1]), it is clearly a highly significant condition that is associated with high mortality. In the latest maternal mortality report from the United Kingdom (UK), ARDS was the ultimate cause of death in 18.5% of maternal deaths.[2] In the US, the overall (nonobstetric) mortality rate from ARDS is reported to be between 10 and 90%,[3] although a figure around 60% is commonly accepted.[4] In two small obstetric series, 43 to 44% maternal mortality was reported,[1, 5] but the true overall mortality associated with pregnancy may be higher. It is disappointing that despite extensive research the prognosis appears to have changed little over the 30 years since Ashbaugh and coworkers' original description,[6] and there is still no drug therapy of proven value.[7]

ARDS is a lethal condition, and it must be taken seriously at the outset. Whenever the diagnosis is made it is vital to appreciate that ARDS represents the pulmonary component of that which is usually a serious and life-threatening multisystem disorder, and that early supportive therapy for other organs must be provided. Multiple organ failure is unfortunately common, and it develops in approximately 75% of patients.[1] All patients need expert management by senior staff in an intensive care environment, preferably by intensivists experienced in the particular problems presented by obstetric patients. The clinical complexity experienced in managing these patients is formidable.[8]

The diagnostic criteria for ARDS employed by different clinicians vary considerably, and there is obvious need for a universally respected definition.[9] The published report of the American-European consensus conference on ARDS clarifies the situation with a set of internationally agreed-upon diagnostic criteria (Table 6–1).[3] The diagnosis of ARDS requires information about left atrial pressure (or left ventricular function), which is usually inferred from the pulmonary artery occlusion pressure (PCWP) following balloon-tipped, flow-directed pulmonary artery catheterization. It is regrettable that in many of the cases reported in the obstetric literature the diagnosis is made without properly differentiating it from other causes of pulmonary edema (e.g., cardiogenic, fluid overload), and the value of these papers is hence undermined. Only when all clinicians are able to observe the same diagnostic rules will it be possible to effectively evaluate and compare the incidence, management, and prognosis of critically ill obstetric patients with ARDS.

PHYSIOLOGIC CHANGES OF PREGNANCY

Several of the normal, well-described, physiologic changes of pregnancy may predispose the parturient to the likelihood of pulmonary edema and ARDS, and their consequences.

Cardiac output increases steadily throughout pregnancy. Such increases are associated with increases in stroke volume, heart rate, plasma volume, and left ventricular dilation and hypertrophy. Mean arterial pressure falls owing to reduced systemic resistance, and mean pulmonary artery and occlusion pressures remain in the normal (nonpregnant) range. Pulmonary vascular resistance also falls, and pulmonary vasodilation leads to increased pulmonary blood volume. The capacity of the pulmonary circulation to compensate for further increases in circulating volume is impaired with a resultant higher risk of hydrostatic pulmonary

TABLE 6–1. DIAGNOSTIC CRITERIA FOR ARDS

Timing:	Acute onset
Oxygenation	$PaO_2/FiO_2 \leq 200$ mmHg (regardless of PEEP level)
Chest radiograph:	Bilateral infiltrates seen on frontal chest radiograph
PCWP:	≤ 18 mmHg when measured (or no clinical evidence of left atrial hypertension)

From Bernard GR, Artigas A, Brigham KL, et al. Report of the American-European consensus conference on ARDS: Definitions, mechanisms, relevant outcomes and clinical trial coordination. Intensive Care Med 1994;20:225. Copyright Springer-Verlag.

edema. Aortocaval compression may cause dramatic and destabilizing decreases in cardiac output.

Hyperventilation is normal during pregnancy, but the reduction in functional residual capacity compromises the oxygen storage capacity of the lungs, increasing the risk of hypoxemia. This problem is aggravated by increases in oxygen consumption and carbon dioxide production by up to 50% over the nonpregnant state. Reduction in the plasma protein concentration leads to a fall in the colloid oncotic pressure, which is another risk factor for the development of pulmonary edema.

CAUSES OF ARDS IN PREGNANCY

ARDS may be considered as the pulmonary component of a systemic inflammatory process frequently resulting from sepsis (Table 6–2).[10] In addition to all the usual causal events (not specifically related to pregnancy), ARDS may also develop from almost every reported major obstetric complication, but especially following infection, hemorrhage, pre-eclampsia/eclampsia, and pulmonary aspiration (see Table 6–2).[1,2] Several reports suggest pyelonephritis to be an important infective cause of ARDS in pregnancy, although not all cases fulfill true ARDS diagnostic criteria.[11–16] Common triggering events in pregnancy are shown in Figure 6–1. Although the inhalation of gastric contents (not necessarily anesthesia-related) has previously been shown to be a leading cause of ARDS in the UK,[2] it is anticipated that changing practice (increased use of regional anesthesia and H_2 antagonists) will reduce this occurrence.

The development of pulmonary edema following the prolonged use of β_2 adrenergic agonist agents for tocolysis in preterm labor is well known. In most reports there is little evidence that the specific diagnostic criteria of ARDS have been fulfilled, and direct fluid overload (aggravated by an antidiuretic effect) is probably the most likely cause.[17,18] Some patients, however, have

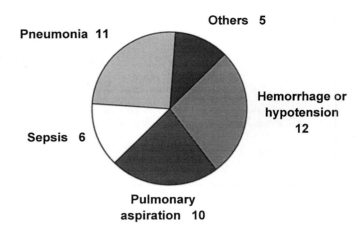

Figure 6–1. Maternal deaths from adult respiratory distress syndrome (ARDS) by triggering event in the United Kingdom from 1988 to 1990. (From Department of Health: Report on confidential enquiries into maternal deaths in the United Kingdom 1988–90. London, HMSO, 1994. Crown copyright is reproduced with the permission of the Controller of Her Majesty's Stationery Office.)

normal to low pulmonary artery occlusion pressures, suggestive of altered pulmonary vascular permeability.[19] The use of β_2 adrenergic agonists in the presence of maternal infection may predispose some to the development of pulmonary edema and ARDS.[20]

PATHOPHYSIOLOGY

The pathophysiologic processes behind ARDS have been extensively reviewed elsewhere,[4, 21–23] and the clinical effects are summarized in the following paragraphs.

Following the initial insult, a large number of interrelated inflammatory mediator systems are activated, producing widespread endothelial damage and increased vascular permeability. Pulmonary infiltrates and alveolar epithelial damage impair gas exchange, and increased permeability of pulmonary capillaries produces interstitial and alveolar edema and collapse. Surfactant production by type II pneumocytes is reduced, leading to falls in lung compliance and functional residual capacity. Hypoxemia results owing to increased ventilation-perfusion mismatch and right to left intrapulmonary shunting with increased clinical respiratory distress.

Pulmonary artery resistance and pressure frequently rise, and acute right ventricular dysfunction may develop. Right ventricular dysfunction, in turn, reduces left ventricular preload and cardiac output, decreasing oxygen delivery to other organs, where capillary membrane leakage is also a problem. In the absence of direct lung injury, ARDS may be considered as part of a systemic inflammatory response syndrome, with multiorgan failure a likely consequence.

TABLE 6–2. **PREGNANCY-RELATED CAUSES OF ARDS**

Infection	Rare
Generalized sepsis	Arsenic poisoning[48]
Pneumonia	Acetaminophen overdose[51]
Pyelonephritis	Tick-borne relapsing fever
Chorioamnionitis	(*Borrelia* spirochetemia)[52]
Inhalation of gastric contents	Orogenital sex (venous air
Hemorrhage and massive	embolism)[46]
transfusion	Pheochromocytoma[53]
Hypovolemic shock	Sickle cell disease[1]
Pre-eclampsia and eclampsia	Smoke inhalation[1]
Intrauterine fetal death	Thrombotic thrombocytopenic
Abruptio placentae	purpura[1]
Amniotic fluid embolism	
Thromboembolic disease	
Idiopathic	

CLINICAL MANIFESTATIONS

The precipitating event is usually obvious, and the clinical manifestations of ARDS develop insidiously over 12 to 72 hours. In 80% of patients acute lung injury is evident within 24 hours, and many of those with sepsis develop signs and symptoms within 6 hours.[21] Progressive tachypnea, dyspnea, cyanosis, and respiratory distress occur. Fine crepitations and rhonchi are heard on auscultation of the chest. Radiography shows bilateral, diffuse pulmonary infiltrates, and air bronchograms may be seen. Pulmonary function usually deteriorates rapidly, and local or systemic effects of the precipitating cause may escalate.

Worsening hypoxemia results in oxygen delivery to tissues that is inadequate to meet metabolic demands. Hemodynamic instability and multi-organ dysfunction become increasingly evident and are the main causes of death (i.e., not intractable respiratory failure). Acute renal failure is common, as is disseminated intravascular coagulopathy, and the development of hepatic failure is ominous. Nosocomial infection is a common late problem.

DIFFERENTIAL DIAGNOSIS

The diagnosis of ARDS is initially a clinical one and usually is confirmed by pulmonary artery catheterization. It is regrettable that precise diagnostic criteria vary between centers. An attempt to produce universally acceptable criteria is shown in Table 6–1.[3] It is important to exclude other causes of pulmonary edema (e.g., left ventricular failure, fluid overload) and chronic pulmonary disease, and echocardiography may be a good diagnostic tool.[24] In pregnancy, reduced colloid oncotic pressure may contribute to the development of pulmonary capillary leakage and alveolar edema.

MANAGEMENT OF ARDS

In view of the poor prognosis, whenever the diagnosis of ARDS is likely the patient should be transferred immediately to an appropriate intensive care unit for expert advice, invasive monitoring, and aggressive management. Deterioration of the condition of patients with established ARDS is associated with a high mortality rate, and transfer may be indicated to a center where particular expertise in the aggressive management of ARDS exists.

Treatment of ARDS is two-fold:

1. Treat the underlying cause
2. Provide supportive treatment
   a. Of the acute lung injury of ARDS
   b. To minimize secondary lung damage
   c. Of other organ dysfunction
   d. To minimize multisystem damage.

When the precipitating cause of ARDS is obvious there are clear goals to guide treatment of the underlying condition (e.g., antibiotics, resuscitation, blood transfusion). In the absence of obvious etiology, covert causes (e.g., intra-abdominal abscess, silent abruption) should be sought. When collapse is sudden and unexpected, however, supportive therapy under the guidance of invasive monitoring may be all that is possible in the initial phase. Cardiovascular monitoring should include pulmonary artery catheterization with facilities for cardiac output assessment and oxygen delivery and consumption studies as a minimum standard. All other treatment is aimed at minimizing secondary lung damage and other organ damage.

New management strategies for ARDS currently being evaluated are shown in Table 6–3.

Respiratory Support

Patients with true ARDS require intubation and positive-pressure ventilation to maintain adequate gas exchange. Particularly when the fetus is still in utero, the decision to intubate should be made early to optimize maternal condition and fetal oxygen delivery. Precautions against aspiration of gastric contents should be taken for endotracheal intubation (i.e., rapid sequence induction). Pharmacologic techniques for reducing the risks of aspiration and peptic ulceration (e.g., H_2 antagonist therapy, sucralfate) should be considered.

The hypoxemia of ARDS frequently requires high inspired oxygen concentrations to maintain adequate tissue oxygenation. Wherever possible, most clinicians attempt to limit the inspired oxygen concentration to 60% to minimize the risk of pulmonary damage due to oxygen toxicity.[25] The use of positive end-expiratory pressure (PEEP) to prevent alveolar collapse and increase functional residual capacity is almost universal, although excessive levels decrease cardiac output and oxygen delivery and increase the risk of barotrauma.

Reduced lung compliance results in high peak inflation pressures during positive-pressure ventilation

TABLE 6–3. NEW MANAGEMENT STRATEGIES FOR ARDS

Pulmonary	Systemic
High frequency (jet) ventilation	Parenteral nitric oxide synthase inhibitors
Inverse ratio ventilation	Selective decontamination of the digestive tract
Permissive hypercapnia	
Ventilation in prone position	Intravenous oxygenation (IVOX)
Inhaled nitric oxide	
Exogenous surfactant	Extracorporeal pulmonary support

with conventional ventilatory techniques (using relatively large tidal volumes), and barotrauma may exacerbate lung injury. Pressure-controlled ventilation seems preferable to volume control.[9] Unfortunately, ventilator-related complications are still common (occurring in 81% of patients in one study[1]) and include tension or recurrent pneumothorax, accidental extubation, and bronchopleural fistula formation.

New approaches to ventilation (e.g., inverse ratio ventilation, high-frequency jet ventilation, permissive hypercapnia, and prone positioning) may be helpful,[25-28] although there is little evidence that any of these techniques reduces mortality.[7] Two new nonpulmonary techniques, extracorporeal gas exchange (particularly the carbon dioxide removal component) and intravenous oxygenation (IVOX), are being pursued enthusiastically in a few centers, although their value in reducing mortality is still unproved.[27] Full recovery in a pregnant woman on maximal, traditional ventilatory support for ARDS and staphylococcal septicemia, however, has been reported following extracorporeal carbon dioxide removal.[29]

Much of the lung damage of ARDS is caused by a range of cascading mediator systems (including endotoxins, cytokinins, neutrophils, arachidonic acid metabolites, and complement activation), but pharmacologic attempts to combat the effects of these with inflammatory mediator antagonists have been singularly unsuccessful.[30] A deficiency in lung surfactant has been demonstrated in ARDS, but, unfortunately, contrary to the experience in neonates, there is little evidence that exogenous surfactant is useful in adults.[7]

At present the most promising therapeutic development is inhalation of vasodilator agents to reduce pulmonary vascular resistance in ventilated areas of the lung, thereby minimizing intrapulmonary shunt. Early experience with inhaled nitric oxide and aerosolized prostacyclin has been favorable.[31, 32] Initial studies also suggest that parenteral nitric oxide synthetase inhibitors (e.g., L-NMMA) may effectively increase peripheral vascular resistance in septic shock, although the overall effect on mortality is less clear.[33]

Multi-organ Failure

Most patients with ARDS die from multi-organ failure, and the main therapeutic goal in the protection of other organ systems is the maintenance of adequate oxygen delivery.[25] The value of goal-directed therapy as described by Shoemaker and coworkers[34] (aggressive use of inotropes to raise cardiac index and systemic oxygen delivery in nonsurgical patients) has been challenged,[35] however, and the debate continues. Initial enthusiasm for the use of monoclonal antibodies to endotoxin (HA-1A) in gram-negative septicemia has

not been sustained, and the product has now been withdrawn following reports of increased mortality.[35, 37]

Maintenance of normal gut function is considered important in preventing the release of gut-derived endotoxin, and early enteral feeding should be considered a high priority.[7] Selective decontamination of the digestive tract is still controversial,[38] although meta-analyses suggest it may be helpful in reducing the incidence of acquired pneumonia.[39-41] The impact on overall mortality, however, appears to be small. Gastric tonometry has been proposed as a useful and sensitive tool for assessing the effectiveness of oxygen delivery to the tissues.[42] Specific organ failure (e.g., acute renal failure) requires appropriate support with hemofiltration or hemodialysis.

Fluid Management

Several compounding factors make the management of fluids both critical and difficult in ARDS. Patients usually have a widespread capillary membrane leak, predisposing them to pulmonary edema and intravascular hypovolemia.[43] If the cardiac output falls as a result, oxygen delivery to tissues may be compromised. The danger of iatrogenic fluid overload in patients at risk of ARDS should also be appreciated because it may precipitate worsening pulmonary edema of multifactorial etiology.[14] Overaggressive fluid therapy in response to oliguria has probably been contributory to the dramatic increase in the number of pre-eclamptic deaths due to pulmonary complications (e.g., pulmonary edema and ARDS) in the UK in the late 1980s.[2] Despite current concerns about the overuse of pulmonary artery catheters, the development of pulmonary edema in pregnancy remains a clear indication for its early use.

Delivery

ARDS represents the nonspecific, common end-result of a wide range of physiologic insults that may occur during pregnancy and parturition. In many cases, delivery will already have been effected by the time of diagnosis. When the fetus is still in utero, however, careful consideration about the risks and benefits of delivery is required.

Perinatal mortality is markedly increased when the mother develops antenatal ARDS (23% in one series[1]). Fetal outcome depends greatly on the precipitating cause, and there are several reports of fetal survival. When the maternal condition is unstable or the precipitating cause is related to the fetoplacental unit (e.g., hemorrhage, amniotic fluid embolism), placental oxygen transfer may be compromised, and immediate delivery is usually indicated.

Several reports have appeared in the literature of vaginal delivery in ventilated patients with ARDS,[1, 44-47] but in some patients delivery has been successfully delayed until after recovery.[14, 16, 48] Fetal distress during attempted vaginal delivery may require conversion to cesarean section.[1] Termination of pregnancy (i.e., delivery) may be of benefit to the mother.[45] In the presence of disseminated intravascular coagulopathy (DIC) or other coagulopathies, however, blood loss at delivery may be difficult to control, and early clinical input from a hematologist is recommended. In addition, the problems associated with aortocaval compression must not be forgotten, and these patients must never lie supine without uterine displacement or tilt.

Reducing the Oxygen Demands of Delivery

The increased oxygen consumption during active labor is well known, as is the value of epidural analgesia in reducing it.[49] Epidural analgesia has been administered successfully in a hemodynamically stable, ventilated patient at 32 weeks' gestation with idiopathic ARDS.[47] Continuous mixed venous saturation ($S\bar{v}O_2$) monitoring with a pulmonary artery catheter demonstrated that the falls in $S\bar{v}O_2$ associated with uterine contractions were abolished after epidural analgesia was established. Further studies are needed, but continuous $S\bar{v}O_2$ monitoring appears to be useful. Opioid analgesia may have a similar effect in reducing oxygen demands in the intensive care situation,[50] although there is no information available specific to pregnant patients. Assisted vaginal delivery with forceps or vacuum extraction is recommended to minimize maternal effort and oxygen consumption.

OUTCOME

The mortality associated with ARDS in pregnancy is still disappointingly high despite many years of research, and the most optimistic series suggest a mortality rate over 40%.[1, 5] The lack of uniformity of diagnosis and reporting is a major limitation to our knowledge of the true outcome of ARDS in pregnancy, which may well be associated with a higher mortality rate than in the general population.

Mortality statistics from the UK suggest that ARDS is involved in almost one fifth of all maternal deaths and almost half the deaths due to pre-eclampsia.[2] In addition, a large proportion (41%) of maternal deaths due to ARDS were in women with pre-eclampsia or eclampsia. The inter-relationship of these conditions should not remain unnoticed. In the patients who die, multi-organ failure is an almost universal finding. Early deaths are mostly related to the precipitating event, whereas late deaths are usually due to sepsis.[21]

CONCLUSIONS

The significance of making the diagnosis of ARDS in a pregnant woman must not be underestimated, because it immediately marks her as a very high-risk patient. Expert care and early intervention with invasive monitoring and multisystem support are essential to reduce maternal and fetal morbidity and mortality. When antepartum patients are involved, the decision to deliver should normally be made on the basis of maternal condition. It is important that universally agreed upon diagnostic criteria for ARDS are established and observed.

References

1. Mabie WC, Barton JR, Sibai BM. Adult respiratory distress syndrome in pregnancy. Am J Obstet Gynecol 1992;167:950.
2. Department of Health. Report on confidential enquiries into maternal deaths in the United Kingdom 1988–90. London, Her Majesty's Stationery Office (HMSO), 1994.
3. Bernard GR, Artigas A, Brigham KL, et al. Report of the American-European consensus conference on ARDS: Definitions, mechanisms, relevant outcomes and clinical trial coordination. Intensive Care Med 1994;20:225.
4. Hankins GDV, Nolan TE. Adult respiratory distress syndrome in obstetrics. Obstet Gynecol Clin North Am 1991;18:273.
5. Smith JL, Thomas F, Orme JF, et al. Adult respiratory distress syndrome during pregnancy and immediately postpartum. West J Med 1990;153:508.
6. Ashbaugh DG, Bigelow DB, Petty TL, et al. Acute respiratory distress in adults. Lancet 1967;2:319.
7. Wenstone R, Wilkes RG. Clinical management of ARDS (editorial). Br J Anaesth 1994;72:617.
8. Turner JS, Evans TW, Hunter DN, et al. Royal Brompton grand rounds. Adult respiratory distress syndrome. Br Med J 1990;301:1087.
9. Beale R, Grover ER, Smithies M, Bihari D, et al. Acute respiratory distress syndrome ("ARDS"): No more than a severe acute lung injury? Br Med J 1993;307:1335.
10. Demling RH. Adult respiratory distress syndrome: Current concepts. New Horiz 1993;1:388.
11. Cunningham F, Lucas M, Hankins GD. Pulmonary injury complicating antepartum pyelonephritis. Am J Obstet Gynecol 1987;156:797.
12. Amstey MS. Frequency of adult respiratory distress syndrome in pregnant women who have pyelonephritis. Clin Infect Dis 1992;14:1260.
13. Towers CV, Kaminskas CM, Garite TJ, et al. Pulmonary injury associated with antepartum pyelonephritis: Can patients at risk be identified? Am J Obstet Gynecol 1991;164:974.
14. Elkington KW, Greb LC. Adult respiratory distress syndrome as a complication of acute pyelonephritis during pregnancy: Case report and discussion. Obstet Gynecol 1986;67:18S.
15. Seron C, Rubio S, Avallanas ML, et al. Acute respiratory failure complicating antepartum pyelonephritis. Intensive Care Med 1995;21:462.
16. Gurman G, Schlaeffer F, Kopernic G. Adult respiratory distress syndrome as a complication of acute pyelonephritis during pregnancy. Eur J Obstet Gynecol Reprod Biol 1990;36:75.
17. Clesham GJ, Scott J, Oakley CM, et al. β Adrenergic agonists and pulmonary oedema in preterm labour. Br Med J 1994;308:260.
18. Armson BA, Samuels P, Miller F, et al. Evaluation of maternal fluid dynamics during tocolytic therapy with ritodrine hydrochloride and magnesium sulfate. Am J Obstet Gynecol 1992;167:758.
19. Pisani RJ, Rosenow EC. Pulmonary edema associated with tocolytic therapy. Ann Intern Med 1989;110:714.
20. Hatjis CG, Swain M. Systemic tocolysis for premature labor is

associated with an increased incidence of pulmonary edema in the presence of maternal infection. Am J Obstet Gynecol 1988;159:723.

21. Hinds CJ, Watson D. Respiratory failure. In Hinds CJ and Watson D (eds): Intensive care—a concise textbook, 2nd edition. WB Saunders, London, 1995, p 125.

22. Eriksen NL, Parisi VM. Adult respiratory distress syndrome and pregnancy. Semin Perinatol 1990;14:68.

23. Neuhof H. Actions and interactions of mediator systems and mediators in the pathogenesis of ARDS and multi-organ failure. Acta Anaesthesiol Scand 1991;35[S95]:7.

24. Mabie WC, Hackman BB, Sibai BM. Pulmonary edema associated with pregnancy: Echocardiographic insights and implications for treatment. Obstet Gynecol 1993;81:227.

25. MacNaughton PD, Evans TW. Management of adult respiratory distress syndrome. Lancet 1992;339:469.

26. Marini JJ. Ventilation of the acute respiratory distress syndrome (editorial). Looking for Mr. Goodmode. Anesthesiology 1994;80:972.

27. Swami A, Keogh BF. The injured lung: Conventional and novel respiratory therapy. Thorax 1992;47:555.

28. Langer M, Mascheroni D, Marcolin R, et al. The prone position in ARDS patients. A clinical study. Chest 1988;94:103.

29. Greenberg LR, Moore TR. Staphylococcal septicemia and adult respiratory distress syndrome in pregnancy treated with extracorporeal carbon dioxide removal. Obstet Gynecol 1995;86:657.

30. Messent M, Griffiths MJD. Pharmacotherapy in lung injury. Thorax 1992;47:651.

31. Rossaint F, Falke KJ, Lopez F, et al. Inhaled nitric oxide for the adult respiratory distress syndrome. N Engl J Med 1993;328:399.

32. Walmrath D, Schneider T, Pilch J, et al. Aerosolised prostacyclin in adult respiratory distress syndrome. Lancet 1993;342:961.

33. Petros A, Lamb G, Leone A, et al. Effects of a nitric oxide synthase inhibitor in humans with septic shock. Cardiovasc Res 1994;28:34.

34. Shoemaker W, Appel P, Kram HB, et al. Prospective trial of supranormal values of survivors as therapeutic goals in high-risk surgical patients. Chest 1988;94:1176.

35. Hayes MA, Timmins AC, Yau EHS, et al. Elevation of systemic oxygen delivery in the treatment of critically ill patients. N Engl J Med 1994;330:1717.

36. Cross AS. Anti-endotoxin antibodies: A dead end? Ann Intern Med 1994;121:58.

37. McClosky RV, Straube RC, Sanders C, et al. Treatment of septic shock with human monoclonal antibody HA-1A. A randomized, double-blind, placebo-controlled trial. CHESS Trial Study Group. Ann Intern Med 1994;121:1.

38. Potgieter PD, Hammond JMJ. Selective decontamination of the digestive tract. Curr Opin Anesth 1995;8:114.

39. Selective Decontamination of the Digestive Tract Triallists' Collaborative Group. Meta-analysis of randomised controlled trials of selective decontamination of the digestive tract. Br Med J 1993;307:525.

40. Kolleff MH. The role of selective digestive tract decontamination on mortality and respiratory tract infections. A meta-analysis. Chest 1994;105:1101.

41. Heyland DK, Cook DJ, Jaeschke R, et al. Selective decontamination of the digestive tract. An overview. Chest 1994;105:1221.

42. Maynard N, Bihari D, Beale R, et al. Assessment of splanchnic oxygenation by gastric tonometry in patients with acute circulation failure. JAMA 1993;270:1203.

43. Eklund J. Management of the fluid balance in prevention and therapy of ARDS. Acta Anaesthesiol Scand 1991;35[S95]:102.

44. Sosin D, Krasnow J, Moawad A, et al. Successful spontaneous vaginal delivery during mechanical ventilatory support for the adult respiratory distress syndrome. Obstet Gynecol 1986;68:19S.

45. Daily WH, Katz AR, Tonnesen A, et al. Beneficial effect of delivery in a patient with adult respiratory distress syndrome. Anesthesiology 1990;72:383.

46. Kaufman BS, Kaminsky SJ, Rackow EC, et al. Adult respiratory distress syndrome following orogenital sex during pregnancy. Crit Care Med 1987;15:703.

47. Ackerman WE, Molnar JM, Juneja MM. Beneficial effect of epidural anesthesia on oxygen consumption in a parturient with adult respiratory distress syndrome. South Med J 1993;86:361.

48. Bolliger CT, van Zijl P, Louw JA. Multiple organ failure with the adult respiratory distress syndrome in homicidal arsenic poisoning. Respiration 1992;59:57.

49. Hagerdal M, Morgan CW, Sumner AE, et al. Minute ventilation and oxygen consumption during labor with epidural analgesia. Anesthesiology 1983;59:425.

50. Swinamer DL, Phang PT, Jones RL, et al. Effect of routine administration of analgesia on energy expenditures in critically ill patients. Chest 1988;93:4.

51. Ludmir J, Main DM, Landon MB. Maternal acetaminophen overdose at 15 weeks of gestation. Obstet Gynecol 1986;67:750.

52. Davis RD, Burke JP, Wright LJ. Relapsing fever associated with ARDS in a parturient woman. Chest 1992;102:630.

53. Feldman JM. Adult respiratory distress syndrome in a pregnant patient with a pheochromocytoma. J Surg Oncol 1985;29:5.

Cystic fibrosis (CF) is one of the most commonly occurring serious genetic disorders. It had been considered an illness of childhood. Cystic fibrosis was rarely seen in pregnancy. Dramatic advances in the management of CF have improved the life expectancy and quality of life, however, and more women with CF are now becoming pregnant. This change creates particular problems for the obstetrician and anesthesiologist. Few diseases demonstrate better the need for a multidisciplinary approach to management during pregnancy and the peripartum period.

CYSTIC FIBROSIS—THE DISEASE

Etiology

Cystic fibrosis is inherited in an autosomal recessive pattern with an incidence between 1:2000 and 1:5000 in Europeans. It occurs less commonly in the Afro-Caribbean and other racial groups. The gene responsible for CF is now known, and over 300 different mutations have been discovered.[1] The commonest mutation, deletion of phenylalanine at position 508 (ΔF_{508}), is responsible for approximately 70% of North European and North American cases. Cystic fibrosis is particularly prevalent among Ashkenazi Jews with three specific mutations being responsible for the majority of cases.[1]

The gene mutation causes a defect in the CF transmembrane conductance regulator which is a chloride channel protein that alters conductance of epithelial cells on mucosal surfaces. Epithelial cells of the respiratory tract, gastrointestinal tract, and exocrine glands produce protein-rich secretions that have important physiologic functions. The correct ionic, protein, and water composition of these secretions is vital. In CF, changes in the composition of these secretions result in a multisystem disorder with serious consequences, particularly in the cardiorespiratory and gastrointestinal systems.[2]

Although the phenotypic expression of CF is variable, there is evidence that certain genotype mutations are associated with specific clinical presentations. In particular, the patient with homozygous disease and ΔF_{508} mutation has a more severe disease and a poorer outcome than those with other genotypes.[1]

Where there is a family history of CF, deoxyribonucleic acid (DNA) screening allows detection of most CF gene mutations. Approximately 85% of carriers are now detected by testing for the four common mutations.[3] The relative value of selective prenatal, mass population, and neonatal screening is uncertain.[4]

Clinical Features

Cystic fibrosis commonly presents in childhood as respiratory disease, although occasionally malabsorption is the more debilitating condition (Table 7–1). Delayed puberty and growth retardation are common, and progressive cardiorespiratory decompensation is to be expected. Forty years ago, survival past infancy was unusual, but improved treatment has dramatically altered the prognosis, with a median survival of 29.4 years reported for the early 1990s.[5] Rarely, the diagnosis of CF in a woman is first made during pregnancy.[6]

Cardiorespiratory System

Patients are born with normal lungs, but pathologic changes rapidly result from abnormal mucous secretions. Hypersecretion; abnormal sodium, chloride, and water content; and phospholipid changes result in increased adhesiveness of and difficulty in clearing secretions. Airway colonization and chronic infection (from *Staphylococcus aureus*, *Haemophilus influenzae*, and *Pseudomonas* species) most commonly produce a chronic inflammatory response leading to airway scarring, bronchiectasis, distal hyperinflation, and areas of collapse. Pneumothorax and hemoptysis are potential serious complications. Increasing ventilation-perfusion ($\dot{V}/\dot{Q}$) imbalance results in chronic hypoxemia, but secondary polycythemia is rare.[7] Pulmonary hypertension and right ventricular dysfunction (cor pulmonale)

TABLE 7–1. SYSTEM INVOLVEMENT IN CYSTIC FIBROSIS

Organ System Involved	Percent of Patients Affected
Respiratory	
Upper: Nasal polyps	6–20
Pansinusitis	90–100
Lower: Bronchiolitis	Eventually 100
Bronchitis	Eventually 100
Bronchiectasis	Eventually 100
Aspergilloma	Rare
Hemoptysis	60
Pneumothorax	16
Respiratory failure	End stage
Gastrointestinal	
Pancreatic insufficiency	85
Meconium ileus	10
Meconium ileus equivalent	10–30
Rectal prolapse	20
Intussusception	1
Gastroesophageal reflux	?
Hepatobiliary	
Fatty liver	20
Focal biliary fibrosis	20
Cholelithiasis	12
Multilobar cirrhosis	5
Pancreatitis	5
Portal hypertension	Late finding
Cardiovascular	
Pulmonary hypertension	End stage
Cor pulmonale	End stage
Endocrine	
Diabetes mellitus	15
Delayed puberty	85
Reproductive	
Male: obstructive azoospermia	98
Sweat	
Chloride > 60 mEq/l	98

Adapted from Fiel SB. Clinical management of pulmonary disease in cystic fibrosis: Lancet 1993; 341:1070; and Di Sant'Agnese PA, Davis PB. Cystic fibrosis in adults. Am J Med 1979; 66:121.

appear as late sequelae, and end-stage disease is characterized by progressive respiratory failure (Fig. 7–1).

Gastrointestinal System

Cystic fibrosis may present in infancy as meconium ileus. A similar subacute obstruction occurs in adults.[8] Malabsorption is a common and important complication requiring aggressive management. Pancreatic insufficiency leads to maldigestion and malabsorption, with 15% of patients developing insulin-dependent diabetes mellitus. The absence of steatorrhea (i.e., in pancreatic-sufficient patients) is a good prognostic sign.[9, 10] Patients frequently suffer from a range of other gastrointestinal complaints, including intermittent abdominal pain, nausea, and gastroesophageal reflux. In late disease, biliary cirrhosis and portal hypertension may occur with abnormalities of hepatic function, hypoalbuminemia, and jaundice.

Reproductive System

Abnormal cervical mucous production may lead to female subfertility, although this probably also results from poor nutrition, chronic infection, and secondary amenorrhea.[11] In the male, obstructive azoospermia involving the vas deferens, epididymis, and seminiferous tubules is a frequent cause of infertility.

Diagnosis

The clinical diagnosis of CF is confirmed by a diagnostic sweat test (increased sodium chloride concentration of sweat following pilocarpine stimulation). This test is not reliable in neonates, and DNA testing to isolate the specific gene mutation now forms the definitive test. Chorionic villous sampling allows for antenatal testing of the fetus.

Current Treatment of Cystic Fibrosis

Although constantly evolving, the unchanging basis for treatment of CF involves effective bronchial toilet, aggressive treatment of acute respiratory infection (Table 7–2), and maintenance of adequate nutritional intake (Table 7–3). Many new drugs for combating respiratory problems are undergoing clinical evaluation and are reviewed elsewhere.[3, 5, 12, 13] Currently, there are no clear indications regarding the effectiveness of ion transport therapy, recombinant human DNAse (dornase alpha) or aerosolized antiproteases (Table 7–4). Heart-lung or bilateral single lung transplantation has been used successfully for patients with end-stage disease, although donor organ shortage is a constant limitation.[14]

Inadequate exocrine pancreatic function requires replacement therapy with lipase, protease, and amylase enzymes to prevent malabsorption. Treatment with the more effective pH-dependent, enteric-coated microspheres has replaced conventional pancreatic enzyme supplements.[15] Other therapies directed to improve gastrointestinal function are noted in Table 7–3.

Gene therapy offers the possibility of inserting genetic material to code for the production of normal CF transmembrane conductance regulator protein into the bronchial and bronchiolar respiratory epithelial cells of CF patients. Early trials of the use of recombinant adenovirus or liposomal vectors have produced encouraging results.[5, 16] The ultimate goal is to alter the genetic coding in stem cells for permanent correction of the CF defect. Unfortunately, this solution appears to be several years away.

CYSTIC FIBROSIS AND PREGNANCY

Effect of Pregnancy on CF

Early reports of pregnancy in CF patients paint a pessimistic picture. Just as the management and prog-

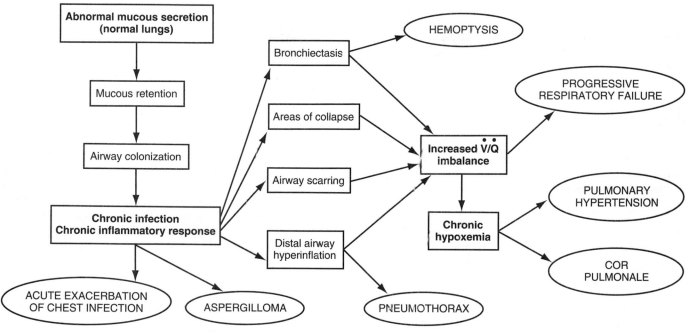

Figure 7–1. Cardiorespiratory effects of cystic fibrosis.

nosis of CF have changed dramatically over the past 30 years, so too has peripartum obstetric and anesthetic practice. Some reports suggest that pregnancy is usually well tolerated, and that deterioration in cardiorespiratory function is rare except in those women with severe pre-existing disease.[10, 17–19]

In a meta-analysis of the literature, the maternal death rate was 13.6% 2 years post partum, which is a figure similar to that in a group of nonpregnant women with CF.[20] The 1990 data from the Cystic Fibrosis Foundation National Patient Registry (CFFNPR) suggest that pregnancy does not result in a dramatic increase in short-term morbidity or mortality.[11] The largest published study of CF in pregnancy[21] found that poor maternal outcome correlated with breathlessness at rest, cyanosis, and moderately severe to severe lung disease (not defined). Current indicators of poor obstetric outcome are summarized in Table 7–5, although reports by Corkey[10] and Canny[17] and their coworkers suggest that a successful maternal outcome is possible even in severely compromised patients.

The obligatory increases in blood volume and cardiac output during pregnancy rarely present a prob-

TABLE 7–2. CURRENT PULMONARY TREATMENT FOR CYSTIC FIBROSIS

Bronchial Toilet	Postural drainage Chest percussion Exercise and mobility encouraged Positive expiratory pressure breathing Autogenic drainage
Antibiotics	Long-term treatment to minimize colonization Short-term treatment for acute exacerbations N.B. Drug resistance a major problem N.B. May need hospitalization for IV or aerosol therapy N.B. Fetal effects of newer antibiotics not known
Bronchodilators	Beta adrenergic agonists Ipratropium bromide 30% patients show some response N.B.: possible deterioration of lung function
Steroids	Prednisolone for short periods Long-term therapy marred by side effects
Oxygen	Routine for acute exacerbations Long-term/nocturnal oxygen controversial Mechanical ventilation only when awaiting transplant
Organ Transplantation	Heart-lung or bilateral single lung 3 year survival = 60% (1991)[13] Main 1st year problems = infection and rejection; obliterative bronchiolitis thereafter

TABLE 7–3. CURRENT GASTROINTESTINAL TREATMENT FOR CYSTIC FIBROSIS

Pancreatic enzymes:	Lipase, protease, and amylase supplementation See pH-dependent enteric-coated microspheres[15]
Nutrition	N.B. Nutritional state correlates with severity of pulmonary disease, prognosis and survival[43] High calorie diet Added fat-soluble vitamins Enteral feeding may be required (e.g., nasogastric, gastrostomy, jejunostomy) Parenteral feeding occasionally beneficial[27, 28]
Various	Opioid analgesics (for abdominal pain) Antiemetic agents Motility-stimulating drugs (e.g., Cisapride) Antacids and alginates

TABLE 7–4. NEW PULMONARY TREATMENT IN CF

Ion transport therapy	Aerosolized *amiloride* (sodium channel blocker) may reduce excessive sodium absorption from airway secretions[12] *Triphosphate nucleotides* (ATP, UTP) may stimulate alternative chloride channels[13]
Recombinant human DNAse (dornase alpha)	Promising early study results of *aerosolized rhDNAse* not sustained. Experience from US and Australia suggests it is not cost-effective. Not recommended in UK[44]
Aerosolized antiproteases	Excessive protease activity may cause airway destruction and bronchiectasis. *Aerosolized alpha-1 antitrypsin* currently being evaluated[12]
Gene therapy	? Insert genetic material for production of normal CFTR protein into bronchial and bronchiolar respiratory epithelial cells Early trials using recombinant adenovirus or liposomal vectors encouraging[5, 16] Routine use appears to be several years away Ultimate goal: alter genetic coding of stem cells to produce permanent correction of CF defect

lem, but they may precipitate cor pulmonale in the patient with severe CF. The increased ventilatory demands of pregnancy are usually well tolerated in patients with mild and moderate pulmonary disease. The normal physiologic hyperventilation of pregnancy, however, may not occur in patients with severe pulmonary disease.[22] Nonpregnant patients with chronic respiratory disease may depend on their hypoxic drive, and inappropriate oxygen therapy may produce hypoventilation. This does not, however, seem to be a significant problem in the pregnant patient with CF.

Women who do not require pancreatic enzyme supplements (i.e., pancreatic-sufficient patients) probably form a subgroup with better pulmonary function and prognosis and in whom pregnancy is better tolerated.[10] The increased nutritional demands of pregnancy are often difficult to maintain, particularly if hyperemesis occurs. Supplemental enteral or intravenous feeding may be necessary, therefore, for adequate weight gain.

TABLE 7–5. PREDICTORS OF POOR OBSTETRIC OUTCOME IN CF

FVC or FEV_1 <50–60% predicted	SaO_2 <90%
Weight <85% predicted	Cor pulmonale
Raised PCO_2	Schwachman score <80

(Data from Geddes DM. Cystic fibrosis and pregnancy. J Roy Soc Med 1992;85:536; and Kent NE, Farquharson DF. Cystic fibrosis in pregnancy. Can Med Assoc J 1993;149:809.)

Effect of CF on Pregnancy and the Neonate

Preterm labor is markedly increased (24%) in mothers with CF,[20] possibly due to poor nutritional status or hypoxemia. Preterm labor most commonly occurs in mothers with severe disease; poor maternal health, particularly poor weight gain, is an important predictive factor.[21] As a result of this increase in the rate of preterm delivery, the perinatal mortality rate is also high (7.9%),[20] although some reports indicate that better results are possible.[10, 17]

Data from the CFFNPR (1990) refute the belief that pregnancy occurs only in women with milder pulmonary involvement.[11] Although there appears to be a lower incidence of pancreatic insufficiency and diabetes mellitus, a significant proportion of CF pregnancies occur in patients with severe pulmonary disease.

Effect on Pregnancy of Drugs Used to Treat CF

In general, the risk to the fetus from poor maternal health is probably greater than the risk of drugs crossing the placenta.[23] The safety in pregnancy of many of the newer drugs is unknown, although, to date, no congenital anomalies have been reported with CF pregnancies.[23]

Cystic fibrosis patients frequently require multiple courses of antibiotics, often in combination. The older penicillins and cephalosporins appear safe. The effects of the quinolones are unknown, and fetal ototoxicity from the aminoglycosides does not appear to be a problem. The fetal side effects of tetracyclines (teeth and bone abnormalities), trimethoprim-sulfamethoxazole (teratogenicity), and sulfonamides (hyperbilirubinemia) suggest that these should be used only for specific indications. Early advice from a bacteriologist should always be sought.

Bronchodilators, the β_2 adrenergic agonists (e.g., salbutamol, terbutaline), are useful in a minority of patients and appear safe[24]; the benefit of maintaining maternal respiratory well-being outweighs potential harm to the fetus. These drugs are effective tocolytics, but the aerosol or nebulized route minimizes unwanted systemic effects. Oral therapy may cause hyperglycemia in patients with diabetes.[24]

Inhaled steroids are safe, but using systemic steroids during pregnancy is more controversial. Suppression of the fetal hypothalamopituitary-adrenal axis by maternal steroid therapy does not appear to occur with prednisone.[24]

ANTENATAL ASSESSMENT

The clinical status of the mother immediately prior to pregnancy is the most important determinant of outcome for both mother and baby. Pre-existing pulmonary status is the key prognostic factor,[21] although some suggest that a wider assessment is more useful.[18] Poor fetal and maternal outcome should be anticipated whenever maternal disease is severe. The patients should be reviewed throughout pregnancy by a multidisciplinary team that includes the chest physician, obstetrician, anesthesiologist, physiotherapist, and nutritionist. Involvement of an anesthesiologist should not be confined to the immediate peripartum period.

Various scoring systems are used to assess the severity of CF. Factors assessed are general activity, physical examination and pulmonary function test results, nutritional state, and chest radiographic appearance.[25, 26] Regular assessment of the cardiorespiratory system, particularly during the second and third trimesters, detects deterioration resulting from the changing demands of pregnancy. Simple pulmonary function tests (SaO_2, peak flow, spirometry) suffice for most patients, although patients with borderline respiratory failure may require sequential blood gas analysis. Good bronchial toilet, maintenance of normal medications, early involvement of physiotherapy, and vigorous treatment of respiratory infections are mandatory. Breathlessness at rest is an indicator of serious pulmonary compromise, and clinical evidence of right heart failure must be investigated.

It is important to assess and maintain optimal nutritional status during pregnancy, and this may necessitate enteral feeding. Long-term parenteral feeding has been advocated, although it is rarely required.[27, 28] Pancreatic sufficiency should be evaluated, pancreatic enzyme supplementation maintained, and diabetes mellitus closely controlled. Venous access may be difficult if there have been multiple admissions to the hospital for parenteral therapy, and a long-term subcutaneous intravenous access device (e.g., a Portacath and Hickman line) may be helpful.

In the first trimester, genetic counseling and screening should be offered to all women with CF to assess the risk of CF in the fetus. Women in whom there is a progressive deterioration in pulmonary function despite aggressive therapy should receive counseling about therapeutic abortion. Right heart failure, refractory hypoxemia unresponsive to low-flow oxygen, progressive hypercapnia, and respiratory acidosis are indications for pregnancy termination.[11]

LABOR AND DELIVERY

Principles of Obstetric Management

Discussion among the chest physician, obstetrician, and anesthesiologist allows early formulation of a labor and delivery plan that is based on the severity of the disease, the obstetric indications, and the patient's wishes. Because these patients have a wide range of respiratory and endocrine problems, they should be considered at high risk and managed in a high-dependency obstetric environment. The options for labor analgesia should be addressed early, as should the anticipated anesthetic management if cesarean section is required.

Spontaneous labor (preterm in 24% of pregnancies[20]) or planned induction of labor is appropriate unless there is a specific indication for cesarean section. Elective assisted delivery with ventouse extraction or forceps minimizes the cardiorespiratory demands of delivery and the consequent risk of maternal exhaustion or pneumothorax. Vigorous Valsalva maneuvers in the second stage can cause a pneumothorax, and this possibility must be excluded if the patient develops chest pain. Deterioration in maternal or fetal status may precipitate the need for rapid delivery and cesarean section. Overall, however, the incidence of cesarean section is the same as that in the general obstetric population.[17]

Other factors that need consideration during the peripartum period include maintenance of hydration (intravenous fluids) and normal CF medications, attention to rapidly changing insulin requirements in those with diabetes, and keeping the mother sitting upright for optimal pulmonary function. Regular H_2-receptor antagonist therapy during labor reduces the risk from accidental pulmonary aspiration. Additional antacids may be required.

Investigations and Monitoring

On admission to the delivery suite, the CF parturient should be carefully reassessed with particular reference to her previous pulmonary condition, nutritional status, and recent diagnostic investigations (Table 7–6).

TABLE 7–6. RECOMMENDED INVESTIGATIONS FOR WOMEN WITH CF IN LABOR

Investigation	Problem
Routine	
Full blood count	Anemia, polycythemia, infection
Urea and electrolytes	Renal function
Blood glucose	Diabetes
Liver function tests	Biliary cirrhosis, hypoalbuminemia
Coagulation screen	Coagulopathy
Peak expiratory flow	Pulmonary status
SaO_2	Pulmonary status, hypoxemia
FVC FEV$_1$	Pulmonary status
As indicated	
Arterial blood gases	Pulmonary status
Chest radiography	Infection, collapse, pneumothorax
ECG	Right heart strain, cor pulmonale
Echocardiography	Right heart failure
CVP	Right heart failure
PA catheter	Right heart failure, pulmonary hypertension

Pre-anesthetic assessment of the patient should be made at an early stage and venous access achieved.

Continuous SaO$_2$ monitoring should be established and humidified oxygen administered if the SaO$_2$ falls below 94% or if evidence exists of fetal compromise. Pulse and blood pressure are monitored on a regular basis to detect evidence of maternal exhaustion or incipient respiratory failure. Direct arterial pressure monitoring should be considered if cardiorespiratory function deteriorates. This monitoring also facilitates sequential blood gas analysis. Central venous pressure plus pulmonary artery monitoring is indicated when pulmonary hypertension or right heart failure is suspected. Chest radiography may be useful when pulmonary signs and symptoms are changing, although routine radiography is unnecessary. In severe disease, clinical, radiologic, and electrocardiographic evidence of cor pulmonale may be confirmed by echocardiography. Continuous electronic fetal heart rate monitoring is recommended because of the increased perinatal mortality rate.

Labor Analgesia

Despite the increasing reports of deliveries by CF women, few investigators have commented on the analgesic or anesthetic techniques used. The principal goals of the anesthesiologist are based on maintaining optimal cardiorespiratory function in the peripartum period. As the pain of uterine contractions increases both oxygen consumption and ventilatory requirements, effective pain relief should be provided early during the first stage of labor (Table 7–7).

Nitrous Oxide (Entonox)

Although widely administered in labor, nitrous oxide inhalation provides poor pain relief.[29, 30] In patients with obstructive airway disease it may be less effective because of the long time constants found in some areas of the lung. Although not described in CF pregnancies, there may be an increased risk of barotrauma due to air trapping. As a result, nitrous oxide for analgesia is not recommended.

Opioids

When epidural analgesia is contraindicated or unwanted, systemic or spinal opioids provide a less effective alternative. Although the respiratory depressant effect of opioids is well known, their effect on parturients with CF (who may or may not demonstrate pregnancy-induced hyperventilation) is uncertain. Intramuscular meperidine is poorly effective in labor.[29] It is associated with unpleasant side effects and is of little value to these high-risk patients. Intravenous patient-controlled analgesia (PCA) with opioids such as fentanyl is a more effective alternative.[31]

Intrathecal opioids produce little neonatal respiratory depression and have been used successfully for first-stage analgesia.[32] Pain in the second stage, however, is more difficult to control, and an additional local anesthetic block may be required for assisted delivery. Although not described in CF patients, the minimal degrees of motor and sympathetic block produced by a combined spinal-epidural technique with opioids and local anesthetics may be appropriate.[33] The risk of early or late respiratory depression with spinal opioids must not be forgotten, however.

Epidural Analgesia

Epidural analgesia provides the most effective analgesia and reduces the circulating catecholamines and the metabolic demands associated with labor and delivery.[34, 35] It has been administered successfully in women with CF[19, 22]; the epidural catheter should be placed as early as possible. Weak solutions of bupivacaine with opioid supplementation provide good-qual-

TABLE 7–7. **LABOR ANALGESIA**

Technique	Advantages	Disadvantages	Comments
Nitrous oxide (Entonox)	Easy to use Quick short-lived effect Obligatory oxygen	Poor analgesia Air-trapping—barotrauma	Not recommended
Opioids	Moderate 1st stage analgesia	Poor 2nd stage analgesia Side effects on mother Depressant effect on baby	? IV PCA more effective[31] ? Spinal opioids for 1st stage[32]
Epidural[32]	Supreme analgesia Allows assisted delivery ↓ metabolic "stress" of labor	Risk of respiratory embarrassment from high block Hypotension	Clear 1st choice for CF Establish early Use weak bupivacaine + opioid Aim for T8–T10 upper sensory level Maintain sitting position if possible Careful IV fluid management Consider infusion or PCEA ? Combined spinal-epidural[33]

ity analgesia with minimal hypotension, motor block, and respiratory compromise. By keeping the upper sensory level below T8 and avoiding excessive motor blockade, there is little deleterious effect on ventilatory performance. Slow incremental administration of the epidural drugs after a limited intravenous fluid preload avoids the rapid onset of destabilizing sympathetic blockade. Fluid overload must be avoided; when there is evidence of right heart failure, fluids should be administered in accordance with results of central venous pressure (CVP) monitoring. Some consider the risk of hypotension and the consequent need for corrective intravenous fluids and vasoconstrictors (e.g., ephedrine) a contraindication to epidural analgesia in CF.[32] If the epidural block is established slowly and with care, however, these complications are minimized.

Once established, the epidural analgesia may be maintained by intermittent "top-ups" or by infusion. Continuous infusion avoids the swings in analgesia and cardiovascular effects that may accompany intermittent "top-ups". Patient-controlled epidural analgesia (PCEA) has been described in a patient with CF.[19] As noted earlier, a combined spinal-epidural technique with low-dose bupivacaine and opioids is another option.[33] Epidural analgesia should be continued into the second stage of labor and may be "topped-up" for assisted delivery.[19]

Anesthesia for Cesarean Section

Cesarean section may become necessary for either maternal or fetal reasons. Whenever possible, the headlong rush to the operating room for a "crash" emergency cesarean section must be avoided. Close monitoring of the patient and pre-emptive action frequently allow time for a more controlled delivery and anesthetic. The choice between general or regional techniques should be made on the basis of individual circumstances, but scrupulous care must be taken to prevent aorto-caval compression.

From the literature it appears that almost all of the cesarean sections were performed using general anesthesia, but many of these cases occurred more than 20 years ago, before regional anesthesia was so common. It is likely that epidural anesthesia for cesarean section in CF patients is more prevalent in current practice than suggested by the paucity of published reports.

General Anesthesia

General anesthesia is well tolerated by most parturients with CF despite their impairment of pulmonary function. When cesarean section is performed for deteriorating maternal cardiac or respiratory function, general anesthesia with invasive monitoring is likely to be indicated. The advantages include improved ventilation and bronchial toilet via an endotracheal tube and the relative cardiovascular stability in comparison with regional techniques. In addition, many patients with severe pulmonary disease do not tolerate lying flat for procedures while they are under regional anesthesia.

The nature of the pulmonary disease in CF may lead to complications associated with general anesthesia. Bronchial hyper-reactivity may provoke bronchospasm, laryngospasm, and excessive coughing. Combined restrictive and obstructive lung disease may require high airway pressures, leading to barotrauma. Sputum retention, atelectasis, and fibrosis produce areas of low $\dot{V}/\dot{Q}$ ratio, and prolonged emergence from anesthesia is a potential problem. Hypoxemia is common, and high inspired oxygen concentrations may be required, as may a longer period of preoxygenation to produce effective denitrogenation.

Antisialogogue premedication should be avoided because of increased difficulty in clearing sticky secretions. The risk of aspiration from gastric acid secretions is reduced by administering an H_2 antagonist (e.g., ranitidine) and oral sodium citrate and by performing rapid-sequence induction and intubation with cricoid pressure. The patient is preoxygenated with 100% oxygen, ensuring a good seal with the face mask. In the absence of right heart failure and hepatic or renal dysfunction, standard doses of anesthetic drugs, including analgesics, are used. The anesthetic gases are humidified and good oxygenation maintained with an adequate inspired oxygen concentration. Positive-pressure ventilation with adequate tidal volumes and frequent suctioning reduces the risks of atelectasis and collapse. The inspiratory flow rates are adjusted to minimize the peak inspiratory pressure and the risk of barotrauma.

The majority of patients can be extubated at the end of surgery. Shorter-acting anesthetic agents (e.g., isoflurane) and muscle relaxants (e.g., vecuronium, atracurium) allow a more rapid return to normal consciousness. The nondepolarizing muscle relaxants are reversed with a mixture of an anticholinesterase (e.g., neostigmine) and an anticholinergic agent (e.g., atropine) to optimize ventilatory effort without excessive effect on bronchial secretions. Oxygen therapy is required for a variable amount of time postoperatively and should be guided by SaO_2 monitoring.

Regional Anesthesia

Epidural anesthesia for cesarean section is safe in women with CF.[10] If surgery is indicated and an epidural catheter is already sited and working, the patient should be encouraged to continue with epidural anesthesia. The clinician, however, must assess the patient's ability to lie flat (wedged) for surgery; her ability to cope with a higher, denser epidural block; and her level of cooperation. If the epidural is established de novo, an intravenous preload is administered and the local anesthetic solution injected slowly and incrementally. This technique minimizes the incidence of hypotension and the development of an unexpectedly high block. The addition of an opioid (fentanyl or sufentanil) to the local anesthetic improves the success of the block. It is prudent to aim for an upper sensory level of T6 to lessen the risk of respiratory embarrassment. Additional epidural medication or supplemental systemic drugs (e.g., intravenous opioids) may be given as necessary.

Spinal anesthesia produces a dense motor and sensory block that is difficult to control and is of very rapid onset. In the patient with more severe respiratory problems, the combination of this sudden high block and the need to lie flat (wedged) for surgery may precipitate a respiratory crisis. For these reasons, spinal anesthesia is a technique that is not recommended when epidural anesthesia is possible. A combined spinal-epidural technique is another option, although it too is not without problems.

Infiltration of local anesthesia for cesarean section has been reported in a woman with CF and idiopathic thrombocytopenic purpura.[36] The report did not expand on the reasons for this choice (it was used "since the risks of either inhalation or regional anesthesia were unacceptable"), but it is not a recommended technique!

Postoperative Management

Following cesarean section, these patients require attentive high-dependency care to ensure stability of hemodynamic and pulmonary function. The immediate postpartum period is a time of particular hazard when cor pulmonale exists. Patients with severe cardiopulmonary disease should be nursed in an intensive therapy unit (ITU). If general anesthesia was used, delayed extubation may then take place under controlled conditions. An early return to normal bronchial toilet and mobility should be encouraged, and adequate pain relief is important in achieving this.

Postoperative analgesia is usually provided by opioids in conjunction with nonsteroidal analgesic drugs (NSAIDs). Intravenous PCA opioids and spinal (epidural, intrathecal) opioids are replacing the traditional technique of intermittent, intramuscular opioids.[37] When epidural analgesia has been administered for delivery, however, it may be continued into the puerperium using weak opioid–local anesthetic solutions. Clinical respiratory status must be monitored regularly because the susceptibility of postpartum CF patients to opioid-induced respiratory depression is unknown. There is one report of the utilization of 3 mg of epidural morphine.[19] Supplementation with an NSAID (e.g., rectal diclofenac) reduces opioid consumption[38] and is beneficial for these patients.

In the past, breastfeeding by mothers with CF was discouraged because of the possibility of high sodium excretion into breast milk. Studies now suggest that the electrolyte composition of breast milk is normal, but the macronutrient content may be reduced, especially during exacerbations of pulmonary disease.[39] Hence, although breast-feeding is no longer discouraged, the usual benefits to the baby may be reduced. Additionally, the nursing mother may find it difficult to maintain adequate caloric intake.

Delivery Following Heart-Lung Transplantation

With the increasing success of heart-lung or bilateral single-lung transplantation, some women with severe CF may now have the opportunity to consider pregnancy. Current selection criteria for transplantation include patients with pre-existing diabetes but exclude patients who are malnourished and those who have had previous lung surgery for CF complications.

Following transplantation surgery, the patients are on long-term immunosuppressant therapy, including steroids. Pulmonary rejection and infection are the early causes of transplantation failure, whereas obliterative bronchiolitis is responsible for late failures.[40] Failed cases may require retransplantation.

Many consider that, in view of the increased risk of organ rejection during pregnancy and exposure of the fetus to potentially teratogenic drugs, pregnancy is unwise following transplantation.[41] When pregnancy does occur, however, the principles of early collaborative care by a multidisciplinary team apply.

Epidural anesthesia should be encouraged for labor and operative delivery, if required. In view of the increased risk of infection, the intrathecal route should be avoided. General anesthesia is the technique of choice if pulmonary function test results contraindicate an epidural. For a more detailed discussion of the potential problems, the reader is referred to a review article by Hou[42] and Chapter 11 in this book.

CONCLUSIONS

The world of CF is changing (Table 7–8), as new and improved treatments are studied in clinical trials. Gene therapy offers hope that in the near future many aspects of this multisystem disorder will be effectively eradicated. Evidence is growing that pregnancy can be safely managed in all but the most severely affected individuals. The important keys to success are the background health of the mother and the involvement of a multidisciplinary team. As the health of the CF population improves, there will be a corresponding decrease in maternal and neonatal morbidity and mortality.

TABLE 7–8. ANESTHESIA SUMMARY FOR DELIVERY OF WOMEN WITH CF

Problem	Action
Obstetric/delivery plan	Discuss with obstetric team
	Discuss with multidisciplinary team
	Nurse in obstetric high-dependency area
Dehydration	IV fluids
Diabetes mellitus	Check blood glucose regularly
	Dextrose + insulin infusion
Polypharmacy	Maintain all regular medications
Chest secretions	Active physiotherapy
	Usual chest drugs (+ nebulized)
	Sit up as much as possible
Hypoxia	Monitor SaO$_2$
	Humidified oxygen as indicated
Gastroesophageal reflux	Regular H$_2$ antagonist (e.g., ranitidine)
	Cisapride, antacids, alginates p.r.n.
Labor pains	Epidural analgesia:
	Establish early
	Use weak bupivacaine with opioid
	Consider infusion or PCEA
	Aim for T8–T10 upper sensory level
Maternal exhaustion	Epidural analgesia
	Elective assisted delivery
CS required	Use epidural if possible:
	"Top-up" epidural slowly
	Add opioid
	Aim for T6 upper sensory level
Puerperium	High-dependency care
	Analgesia
	Epidural opioid or IV PCA
	Oral or rectal NSAID
	Breast-feeding at will
	Attention to nutritional intake

References

1. Super M. Cystic fibrosis: Milestones in cystic fibrosis. Br Med Bull 1992;48:717.
2. McPherson MA, Dormer RL. Cystic fibrosis. Abnormalities in intracellular regulation in cystic fibrosis. Br Med Bull 1992;48:766.
3. Santis G, Geddes D. Recent advances in cystic fibrosis. Postgrad Med J 1994;70:247.
4. Ryley HC, Goodchild MC, Dodge JA. Cystic fibrosis: Screening for cystic fibrosis. Br Med Bull 1992;48:805.
5. Wilmott RW, Fiedler MA. Recent advances in the treatment of cystic fibrosis. Pediatr Clin North Am 1994;41:431.
6. Johnson SR, Varner MW, Yates SJ, et al. Diagnosis of maternal cystic fibrosis during pregnancy. Obstet Gynecol 1983;61:2S.
7. Di Sant' Agnese PA, Davis PB. Cystic fibrosis in adults. Am J Med 1979;66:121.
8. Littlewood JM. Cystic fibrosis: Gastrointestinal complications. Br Med Bull 1992;48:847.
9. Gaskin K, Gurwitz D, Durie P, et al. Improved respiratory prognosis in patients with cystic fibrosis with normal fat absorption. J Pediatr 1982;100:857.
10. Corkey CWB, Newth CJL, Corey M, et al. Pregnancy in cystic fibrosis: A better prognosis in patients with pancreatic function? Am J Obstet Gynecol 1981;140:737.
11. Kotloff RM, Stacey C, FitzSimmons SC, et al. Fertility and pregnancy in patients with cystic fibrosis. Clin Chest Med 1992;13:623.
12. Alton E, Caplen N, Geddes D, et al. Cystic fibrosis: New treatments for cystic fibrosis. Br Med Bull 1992;48:785.
13. Fiel SB. Clinical management of pulmonary disease in cystic fibrosis. Lancet 1993;341:1070.
14. Smyth RL, Higenbottam T, Scott J, et al. The current state of lung transplantation for cystic fibrosis. Thorax 1991;46:213.
15. Kraisinger M, Hochhaus G, Stecenko A, et al. Clinical pharmacology of pancreatic enzymes in patients with cystic fibrosis and in vitro performance of microencapsulated formulations. J Clin Pharmacol 1994;34:158.
16. Caplen NJ, Alton EW, Middleton PG, et al. Liposome-mediated CFTR gene transfer to the nasal epithelium of patients with cystic fibrosis. Nature Medicine 1995;1:39.
17. Canny GJ, Corey M, Livingstone RA, et al. Pregnancy and cystic fibrosis. Obstet Gynecol 1991;77:850.
18. Palmer J, Dillon-Baker C, Tecklin JS, et al. Pregnancy in patients with cystic fibrosis. Ann Intern Med 1983;99:596.
19. Howell PR, Kent N, Douglas MJ. Anaesthesia for the parturient with cystic fibrosis. Int J Obstet Anesth 1993;2:152.
20. Kent NE, Farquharson DF. Cystic fibrosis in pregnancy. Can Med Assoc J 1993;149:809.
21. Cohen LF, Di Sant-Agnese PA, Friedlander J. Cystic fibrosis and pregnancy. A national survey. Lancet 1980;2:842.
22. Novy MJ, Tyler JM, Shwachman H, et al. Cystic fibrosis and pregnancy. Report of a case with a study of pulmonary function and arterial blood gases. Obstet Gynecol 1967;30:530.
23. Geddes DM. Cystic fibrosis and pregnancy. J Roy Soc Med 1992;85:S36.
24. De Swiet M. Diseases of the respiratory system. In De Swiet (ed): Medical Disorders in Obstetric Practice, 2nd ed. Oxford, Blackwell Scientific Publications, 1989, p 1.
25. Shwachman H, Kylczychi LL. Long term study of one hundred five patients with cystic fibrosis. Am J Dis Child 1958;96:6.
26. Taussig LM, Kattwinkel J, Friedewald WT, et al. A new prognostic score and clinical evaluation system for cystic fibrosis. J Pediatr 1973;82:380.
27. Cole BNL, Seltzer MH, Kassabian J, et al. Parenteral nutrition in a pregnant cystic fibrosis patient. J Parenteral Enteral Nutrition 1987;11:205.
28. Valenzuela GJ, Comunale FL, Davidson BH, et al. Clinical management of patients with cystic fibrosis and pulmonary insufficiency. Am J Obstet Gynecol 1988;159:1181.
29. Morgan B, Bulpitt CJ, Clifton P, et al. Effectiveness of pain relief in labour: Survey of 1000 mothers. Br Med J 1982;285:689.
30. Carstoniou J, Levytam S, Norman P, et al. Nitrous oxide in early labor. Anesthesiology 1994;80:30.
31. Camann WR. Patient-controlled analgesia for the treatment of obstetric pain: Labor. In Ferrante FM, Ostheimer GW, Covino BG (eds): Patient-controlled Analgesia. Boston, Blackwell Scientific Publications, 1990 p 114.
32. Hyde NH, Harrison DM. Intrathecal morphine in a parturient with cystic fibrosis. Anesth Analg 1986;65:1357.
33. Collis RE, Baxandall ML, Srikantharajah ID, et al. Combined spinal-epidural (CSE) analgesia: Technique, management and outcome of 300 mothers. Int J Obstet Anesth 1994;3:75.
34. Hagerdal M, Morgan CW. Summer AE, et al. Minute ventilation and oxygen consumption during labor with epidural analgesia. Anesthesiology 1983;59:425.
35. Shnider SM, Abboud TK, Artal R, et al. Maternal catecholamine decrease during labor after lumbar epidural anesthesia. Am J Obstet Gynecol 1983;147:13.
36. Friedman AJ, Haseltine FP, Berkowitz RL. Pregnancy in a patient with cystic fibrosis and idiopathic thrombocytopenic purpura. Obstet Gynecol 1980;55:511.
37. Eisenach JC. Patient-controlled analgesia for the treatment of obstetric pain: Post-cesarean delivery. In Ferrante FM, Ostheimer GW, Covino BG (eds): Patient-controlled Analgesia. Boston, Blackwell Scientific Publications, 1990, p 122.
38. Luthman J, Kay NH, White JB. The morphine sparing effect of diclofenac sodium following caesarean section under spinal anaesthesia. Int J Obstet Anesth 1994;3:82.
39. Shiffman ML, Searle TW, Flux M, et al. Breast milk composition in women with cystic fibrosis: report of two cases and a review of the literature. Am J Clin Nutr 1989;49:612.
40. Tsang V, Hodson ME, Yacoub MH. Cystic fibrosis: Lung transplantation for cystic fibrosis. Br Med Bull 1992;48:949.
41. Edenborough FP, Stableforth DE, Mackenzie WE. Pregnancy in women with cystic fibrosis. Br Med J 1995;311:822.
42. Hou S: Pregnancy in organ transplant recipients. Med Clin North Am 1989;73:667.
43. Durie PR, Pencharz PB. Cystic fibrosis: Nutrition. Br Med Bull 1992;48:823.
44. Anonymous. Dornase alfa for cystic fibrosis. Drugs Ther Bull 1995;33:15.

ACUTE SEVERE ASTHMA

Paul R. Howell, M.B.

The natural course of asthma in pregnancy appears variable, with conflicting reports in the literature.[1-10] A significant proportion of patients experience a deterioration in symptoms, whereas others improve during pregnancy. Approximately two thirds of women show the same pattern in their asthma from one pregnancy to the next.[1] Status asthmaticus is a relatively uncommon occurrence in pregnancy, although a high proportion of pregnant asthmatic adolescents may require emergency room treatment of acute exacerbations.[2]

Early studies in the 1970s showed that asthma is associated with an increase in perinatal mortality, preterm labor, and intrauterine growth retardation, and that these problems increase with the severity of the asthma.[3, 4] Although this is still true when asthma control is poor, particularly if there are episodes of status asthmaticus in pregnancy,[1, 5-7] reports suggest a brighter picture if the asthma is well treated.[8, 9] Babies of mothers with severe asthma are more prone to hypoglycemia (possibly due to maternal treatment with steroids).[8]

The incidence of pre-eclampsia is increased in asthmatic mothers,[10, 11] although one report suggests that theophylline treatment may provide some protection.[12] The mechanism behind this relationship is not known. Cesarean section is more likely in asthmatics.[8, 9, 13] In patients with severe status asthmaticus (intubated and ventilated in an intensive therapy unit [ITU]) delivery of the baby may be necessary before there is improvement in the respiratory condition.[14]

ASTHMA TREATMENT IN PREGNANCY

Undertreatment is the single most important failing in the management of asthma during pregnancy.[1, 10] Pregnant women and their physicians should be reassured that most of the regularly prescribed drugs (including albuterol, terbutaline, epinephrine, methylxanthine, cromolyn, oral steroids, and inhaled beclomethasone) have been used widely for many years without any evidence of teratogenicity. There is less experience with some of the newer agents such as budesonide and ipratropium, but both appear safe.[1] Whenever possible, the inhaled route for drugs should be used in preference to the parenteral because the inhaled route greatly reduces systemic side effects.

Asthma may be lethal, and maternal mortality figures from the United Kingdom (UK) (1988–1990) show that acute asthma caused the deaths of two women and was contributory to the deaths of two others.[15] The risk to the fetus from failing to treat asthma appropriately is far greater than any perceived risk from the drug.[1, 10] Pregnant asthmatic women should be aware of this and should be regularly reviewed by a specialist respiratory physician who can optimize therapy and encourage drug compliance.

MANAGEMENT OF STATUS ASTHMATICUS IN PREGNANCY

General

Careful assessment of the patient's condition must be made after admission and frequently reviewed (Table 8–1). Treatment goals include minimizing hypoxemia, hypercarbia, or alkalosis, which reduce fetal oxygenation. Appropriate drugs for the treatment of asthma, and particularly in acute exacerbations, should not be withheld for fear of toxic effects on the fetus. In

TABLE 8–1. ASSESSMENT AND MONITORING

Level of consciousness (N.B. drowsiness)
Respiratory effort—accessory muscles
Respiratory rate
Temperature
Chest auscultation (N.B. "silent chest")
Pulse rate (N.B. bradycardia)
SaO_2 (N.B. <92%)
Blood pressure—pulsus paradoxus (N.B. hypotension)
PEFR/FEV_1
Blood gases (arterial PO_2, PCO_2, pH)
ECG—dysrhythmias
Chest radiography—infection (N.B. pneumothorax)
Fetal heart rate

TABLE 8–2. **MANAGEMENT OPTIONS OF STATUS ASTHMATICUS**

Drug	Route	Dose	Comments
Oxygen	Face mask	40–60%	Humidification important
β$_2$ adrenergic agonists			
Terbutaline	neb	10 mg	
Terbutaline[18]	s/c	0.25 mg	Repeat after 15–30 min, beware of hypotension
Albuterol	neb	5 mg	
Epinephrine[40]	s/c	0.3 mg	Repeat after 20 mins × 2
Steroids			
Methylprednisolone	IV	60–125 mg	Steroids ↑ gestational diabetes + fetal hypoglycemia
Hydrocortisone	IV	100–200 mg	Cover stressful events (e.g., delivery)
Prednisone/prednisolone	O	30–60 mg daily	
Methylxanthine			
Theophylline	IV (slowly)	5 mg/kg loading dose	↓ if previous doses or on theophylline
	Infusion	0.2–0.9 mg · kg^{-1} · hr^{-1}	Check plasma theophylline levels
			? Therapeutic range—see controversies
Anticholinergic			
Ipratropium	neb	0.5 mg	Works best in combination therapy[32]

neb = nebulized; s/c = subcutaneous; IV = intravenous; O = oral

general, standard emergency guidelines (e.g., British Thoracic Society Guidelines on the Management of Asthma[16]) should be followed. Therapeutic options are summarized in Table 8–2.

First-line therapy includes high-concentration, humidified oxygen followed by one of the β$_2$ adrenergic agonist agents by nebulized, intravenous, or subcutaneous injection routes. The subcutaneous route is not commonly used in the UK. Intravenous steroids are also given. The use of theophylline is controversial but commonplace, and a loading dose should be followed by a continuous infusion. Nebulized atropine or ipratropium may also be added. Cromolyn has no place in treating acute exacerbations. Any possible underlying infection should be treated aggressively with antibiotics.

Certain points are related particularly to pregnant patients:

1. Avoid aortocaval compression; the woman must never be allowed to lie supine without a lateral uterine tilt.
2. Reflux esophagitis is common in pregnancy and may aggravate asthma, so treat aggressively. The concomitant use of H$_2$ antagonists, however, may increase plasma theophylline levels.
3. Theophylline clearance may be reduced in the third trimester, so check plasma levels regularly.[17]
4. Intravenous albuterol, terbutaline, and ritodrine have well-known tocolytic effects; these agents are frequently given therapeutically in preterm labor. There is no evidence that these drugs interfere with the course of term labor when administered by the inhaled or subcutaneous routes, however.
5. Hypotension has been reported following the use of subcutaneous terbutaline in pregnancy.[18]

Intubation and Ventilation

If the patient fails to show improvement or fulfills any of the criteria listed in Table 8–3, she should be referred to the ITU and considered for endotracheal intubation and ventilation. *A rising arterial P$_{CO_2}$ (>38 mm Hg) is an ominous sign and must be taken seriously at levels that are considered normal in a nonpregnant woman.*

If intubation is considered appropriate, aortocaval occlusion must be avoided, and induction of anesthesia should include precautions against aspiration of gastric contents. Thiopentone, etomidate, and ketamine have all been administered as induction agents, but the marked bronchodilator properties of ketamine make it an obvious choice. Seizure-like extensor spasms have been reported, however, following the administration of ketamine to patients who have received theophylline, and caution is necessary.[19] The risk of histamine release from succinylcholine is outweighed by the excellent intubating conditions achieved. Intravenous lidocaine 1 mg/kg has been advocated to minimize further bronchospasm,[20] although the mechanism of action is unclear. In nonpregnant patients, nasal intubation is preferred, although the poor condition of the patient may necessitate rapid oral intubation. Nasal intubation in the pregnant patient may lead to marked epistaxis due to nasopharyngeal congestion. An inhalational induction with halothane is unlikely to be smooth or easy and it increases the risk of pulmonary aspiration; therefore, it is not recommended.

Once intubation has been performed, bronchodilation may be achieved with halothane. Experience with

TABLE 8–3. **INDICATIONS FOR ENDOTRACHEAL INTUBATION AND VENTILATION**

Clinical exhaustion	Hypotension
Reduced level of consciousness	Bradycardia
"Silent chest"—absent breath sounds	Worsening dysrhythmias
Pa$_{CO_2}$ rising, >38 mm Hg	Complications
Pa$_{O_2}$ falling, <50 mm Hg	Pneumothorax
pH <7.35	Pneumomediastinum
PEFR <70 l/min	

PEFR = peak expiratory flow rate

enflurane and isoflurane is still limited, but halothane is widely considered the superior agent, despite reducing the threshold for epinephrine-induced ventricular dysrhythmias. Hypotension may require inotropic support.[21]

Muscle relaxation should be provided by nondepolarizing agents that do not release histamine (e.g., vecuronium). Peak airway pressures are likely to be high, and careful manipulation of ventilator settings is required to minimize the risk of barotrauma (pneumothorax and pneumomediastinum). Normal physiologic (*pregnant*) values for arterial PO_2 and PCO_2 should be the aim. The use of positive end-expiratory pressure (PEEP) is controversial.

Labor and Delivery

Epidural analgesia markedly reduces the work and physiologic stress of labor[22, 23] and is strongly recommended for asthmatic parturients. A weak bupivacaine-opioid solution produces minimal motor block, avoiding respiratory embarrassment.[24] A combined spinal-epidural technique (CSE) may also provide rapid onset of good quality analgesia with minimal motor block.[25] Meningitis has been reported following CSE,[26] however, and high-dose steroids theoretically may increase the risk of this complication. Paracervical and pudendal blocks may be used for the first and second stages of labor when epidural/spinal analgesia is unsuitable, but these must be done by an experienced operator to maximize their effectiveness. Elective assisted delivery (forceps or vacuum extraction) minimizes maternal stress and effort and is recommended.

There are very clear advantages of epidural analgesia, but if relative contraindications exist, careful assessment of the risk-benefit ratio must be made. If regional anesthesia is still considered inappropriate, opioids (preferably intravenous ± a patient-controlled technique; or via intrathecal routes) may be administered to provide rather less effective analgesia, particularly for the second stage of labor. Histamine release is common with some opioids (e.g., I.V. morphine), and meperidine (or a derivative) is preferable. Careful assessment must be made of the effects of opioid analgesia on respiratory function.

Cesarean Section

When cesarean section is necessary in severely asthmatic patients, regional anesthesia is the clear first choice because it minimizes airway stimulation. Acute bronchospasm has been precipitated by spinal anesthesia in pregnancy, although the etiology is unclear.[27] It is postulated that high sensory blockade causes a fall in adrenal epinephrine output,[27] but this is unlikely to be of serious consequence or enough reason to avoid regional anesthesia. The rapidity of onset of spinal anesthesia provides the main indication for its use, but the greater control with an epidural technique generally makes it preferable. Whenever possible, the block is established slowly to minimize the risk of respiratory embarrassment. The block must be high enough to provide good quality analgesia (above T6 sensory level), because intraoperative pain and distress may aggravate bronchospasm. The addition of an epidural opioid (e.g., fentanyl, sufentanil) improves the quality of the sensory block and is recommended. Epidural epinephrine (still controversial in obstetric anesthesia) should be avoided to reduce the risk of potentially additive effects with other β_2 adrenergic agonists, particularly subcutaneous epinephrine. Many anesthesiologists, however, still prefer to give epinephrine in the initial test dose.

When the patient's condition is too poor to tolerate a regional technique (i.e., she is restless, dyspneic, and unable to lie supine), general anesthesia is required. The management of intubation is as described earlier. Nitrous oxide may increase the degree of air trapping; it reduces the maximum oxygen concentration and probably adds little of value to the anesthetic technique. Fetal oxygenation may be superior when 100% oxygen is used.[28] Anesthesia is maintained with a halogenated inhalation agent at a concentration high enough to avoid "light" anesthesia, which aggravates bronchospasm. Excessive blood loss due to uterine atony is unlikely to be a significant problem with the use of halothane 0.75%, enflurane 1.7%, or isoflurane 1.2% in oxygen following a short period of overpressure.[28]

Oxytocin should be given routinely after delivery, by infusion if the uterus does not contract well. Ergometrine and prostaglandin $F_{2\alpha}$ may both produce bronchospasm and are contraindicated in asthmatics.[1] Cautious administration may be necessary, however, when continual hemorrhage from uterine hypotonia occurs despite oxytocin. Other drugs to be avoided are listed in Table 8-4. When patients have recently received glucocorticoids and may have a suppressed pituitary-adrenal axis, additional doses of steroids (e.g., hydrocortisone) are commonly given for the stress of delivery or cesarean section.

Whatever anesthetic technique is selected, these women require high-dependency nursing care after delivery. Particularly when general anesthesia has been required, intensive care admission is advised because

---

TABLE 8-4. ANESTHETIC AND OBSTETRIC DRUGS TO AVOID

Prostaglandin $F_{2\alpha}$
Prostaglandin E_2
Ergometrine
Aspirin and other NSAIDs
Histamine-releasing drugs (e.g., atracurium, tubocurare)

it allows delayed extubation and optimization of respiratory and cardiovascular factors. In view of their potential to aggravate bronchospasm, nonsteroidal analgesic drugs (NSAIDs) are avoided and postoperative analgesia is provided by continuous regional anesthesia or parenteral opioids.

CONTROVERSIES

1. Subcutaneous epinephrine in pregnancy.

   Some recommend subcutaneous epinephrine for status asthmaticus in pregnancy.[29] Others consider inhaled terbutaline to be preferable, because it has been shown to be equally effective and may have less risk of reducing uterine blood flow.[30] This is not a significant problem with the subcutaneous route, however, and fetal compromise from undertreatment of the asthma is more likely than from a direct negative impact of therapy on uterine blood flow.

2. Bronchoalveolar lavage.

   Two case reports suggest that in the intubated severe asthmatic patient, bronchoalveolar lavage and suction down a flexible bronchoscope with saline alone[31] or metaproterenol and saline[32] may effect a gradual improvement in lung function. Prospective studies are needed to assess whether these findings were a result of fortuitous timing or therapeutic intervention.

3. H$_2$ antagonists in asthmatics.

   The use of H$_2$ antagonists to reduce gastric content and acidity is increasingly prevalent in perinatal practice. Despite an isolated report that these drugs may aggravate bronchospasm,[33] there is little clinical evidence to withhold them. Indeed, their clinical benefit in reducing the risk of pulmonary aspiration and reducing reflux esophagitis–aggravated asthma suggests that they be considered essential.

4. Theophylline in status asthmaticus.

   Although intravenous theophylline is recommended by many (to supplement β$_2$ adrenergic agonists),[10,34–36] there is little evidence that it adds benefit to patients already receiving combination therapy.[37–39] It is still often given in the acute situation, however.

5. Therapeutic range of theophylline in pregnancy.

   Reduced plasma protein binding of theophylline in pregnancy increases the availability of free (active) drug, and some consider the normal nonpregnant therapeutic range (10–20 μg/ml) excessive, increasing the risk of toxicity. Recommended plasma therapeutic ranges in pregnancy are between 5 to 12 μg/ml[35] and 8 to 15 μg/ml.[40]

TABLE 8–5. ALTERNATIVE DRUG NAMES

US		UK
Albuterol	=	Salbutamol
Isoproterenol	=	Isoprenaline
Epinephrine	=	Adrenaline
Metaproterenol	=	Orciprenaline
Cromolyn sodium	=	Sodium cromoglycate

6. Isoproterenol in status asthmaticus.

   Although evidence suggests that inhaled isoproterenol produces superior bronchodilation in the acute situation,[41] this drug has fallen from common practice. Concerns over its safety, following reports of myocardial dysfunction and sudden death, and the availability of other effective, apparently safer, β$_2$ adrenergic agonists make it difficult to recommend.

   Table 8–5 provides a listing of equivalent drug names in the US and UK.

CONCLUSIONS

It cannot be stressed enough that the greatest risk to an asthmatic mother and her baby arises from inadequate treatment of acute asthma. All the drugs commonly employed to treat an acute exacerbation are reliable and safe in pregnancy. They should not be withheld from the mother on the basis of potential, unproven, and unlikely toxic effects on the fetus.

References

1. Moore-Gillon JC. Pregnancy and the asthmatic (editorial). Respir Med 1991;85:451.
2. Apter AJ, Greenberger PA, Patterson R. Outcomes of pregnancy in adolescents with severe asthma. Arch Intern Med 1989; 149:2571.
3. Sims CD, Chamberlaine GVP, de Swiet M. Lung function tests in bronchial asthma during and after pregnancy. Br J Obstet Gynaecol 1976;83:434.
4. Bahna SL, Bjerkedal T. The course and outcome of pregnancy in women with bronchial asthma. Acta Allergologica 1972;27:397.
5. Schatz M, Zeiger RS, Hoffman CP, et al. Intrauterine growth is related to gestational pulmonary function in pregnant asthmatic women. Chest 1990;98:389.
6. Greenberger PA, Patterson R. The outcome of pregnancy complicated by severe asthma. Allergy Proc 1988;9:539.
7. Fitzsimons R, Greenberger PA, Patterson R. Outcome of pregnancy in women requiring corticosteroids for severe asthma. J Allergy Clin Immunol 1986;78:349.
8. Stenius-Aarniala B, Piirila P, Teramo K. Asthma and pregnancy: A prospective study of 198 pregnancies. Thorax 1988;43:12.
9. Coutts II, White RJ. Asthma in pregnancy. J Asthma 1991;28:433.
10. Clark SL. Asthma in pregnancy. Obstet Gynecol 1993;82:1036.
11. Lehrer S, Stone J, Lapinski R, et al. Association between pregnancy induced hypertension and asthma during pregnancy. Am J Obstet Gynecol 1993;168:1463.
12. Dombrowski MP, Bottoms SF, Boike GM, et al. Incidence of preeclampsia among asthmatic patients lower with theophylline. Am J Obstet Gynecol 1986;155:265.

13. Perlow JH, Montgomery D, Morgan MA, et al. Severity of asthma and perinatal outcome. Am J Obstet Gynecol 1992;167:963.
14. Gelber M, Sidi Y, Gassner S, et al. Uncontrollable life-threatening status asthmaticus—an indicator for termination of pregnancy by cesarean section. Respiration 1984;46:320.
15. Department of Health. Report on confidential enquiries into maternal deaths in the United Kingdom 1988–90. London, Her Majesty's Stationery Office (HMSO), 1994.
16. Guidelines on the management of asthma. Thorax 1993;48:S1.
17. Carter BL, Driscoll CE, Smith GD. Theophylline clearance during pregnancy. Obstet Gynecol 1986;68:555.
18. Margulies JL, Kallus L. Terbutaline-induced hypotension in a pregnant asthmatic patient. Am J Emerg Med 1986;4:218.
19. Hirshman CA, Krieger W, Littlejohn G, et al. Ketamine-aminophylline induced decrease in seizure threshold. Anesthesiology 1982;56:464.
20. Fung DL. Emergency anesthesia for asthma patients. Clin Rev Allergy 1985;3:127.
21. Rosseel P, Lauwers LF, Baute L. Halothane treatment in life-threatening asthma. Intensive Care Med 1985;11:241.
22. Hagerdal M, Morgan CW, Summer AE, et al: Minute ventilation and oxygen consumption during labor with epidural analgesia. Anesthesiology 1983;59:425.
23. Shnider SM, Abboud TK, Artal R, et al. Maternal catecholamines decrease during labor after lumbar epidural anesthesia. Am J Obstet Gynecol 1983;147:13.
24. Younker D, Clark R, Tessem J, et al. Bupivacaine-fentanyl epidural analgesia for a parturient in status asthmaticus. Can J Anaesth 1987;34:609.
25. Collis RE, Baxandall ML, Srikantharajah ID, et al: Combined spinal epidural (CSE) analgesia: Technique, management and outcome of 300 mothers. Int J Obstet Anesth 1994;3:75.
26. Harding SA, Collis RE, Morgan BM. Meningitis after combined spinal-extradural anaesthesia in obstetrics. Br J Anaesth 1994;73:545.
27. Mallampati SR. Bronchospasm during spinal anesthesia. Anesth Analg 1981;60:839.
28. Piggott SE, Bogod DG, Rosen M, et al. Isoflurane with either 100% oxygen or 50% nitrous oxide in oxygen for Caesarean section. Br J Anaesth 1990;65:325.
29. Greenberger PA, Patterson R. Management of asthma during pregnancy. N Engl J Med 1985;312:897.
30. Uden DL, Goetz DR, Kohen DP, et al. Comparison of nebulized terbutaline and subcutaneous epinephrine in the treatment of acute asthma. Ann Emerg Med 1985;14:229.
31. Munakata M, Abe S, Fujimoto S, et al. Bronchoalveolar lavage during third trimester pregnancy in patients with status asthmaticus: A case report. Respiration 1987;51:252.
32. Schreier L, Cutler RM, Saigal V. Respiratory failure in asthma during the third trimester: Report of two cases. Am J Obstet Gynecol 1989;160:80.
33. Nathan RA, Segall N, Glover GC, et al. The effects of H1 and H2 antihistamines on histamine inhalation challenges in asthmatic patients. Am Rev Respir Dis 1979;120:1251.
34. Mawhinney H, Spector SL. Optimum management of asthma in pregnancy. Drugs 1986;32:178.
35. Schatz M. Asthma during pregnancy: Interrelationships and management. Ann Allergy 1992;68:123.
36. McDonald AJ. Asthma. Emerg Med Clin North Am 1989;7:219.
37. Fanta CH, Rossing TH, McFadden ER. Emergency room treatment of asthma. Am J Med 1982;72:416.
38. Siegel D, Sheppard D, Gelb A, et al. Aminophylline increases the toxicity but not the efficacy of inhaled beta-adrenergic agonist in the treatment of acute exacerbations of asthma. Am Rev Respir Dis 1985;132:283.
39. Self TH, Abou-Shala N, Burns R, et al. Inhaled albuterol and oral prednisone therapy in hospitalized adult asthmatics. Does aminophylline add any benefit? Chest 1990;98:1317.
40. Greenberger PA. Asthma in pregnancy. Clin Chest Med 1992;13:597.
41. Fanta CH, Rossing TH, McFadden ER. Treatment of acute asthma. Is combination therapy with sympathomimetics and methylxanthines indicated? Am J Med 1986;80:5.

PNEUMOTHORAX AND PNEUMOMEDIASTINUM

■ ■ ■ ■ ■ ■ ■

Paul R. Howell, M.B.

PNEUMOTHORAX

Pneumothorax may present as an acute life-threatening emergency that requires rapid alleviation and appropriate management of pregnancy or delivery. It is rare in pregnancy but may occur in all three trimesters and may be bilateral.[1, 2] Approximately half of the reported cases develop at term as antepartum events,[2] however. Although generally considered to occur in parturients with risk factors following expulsive efforts in labor[3, 4] (Table 9–1), there are several documented cases wherein spontaneous pneumothorax has occurred in the absence of pre-existing pulmonary pathology.[5–7] Antecedent viral upper respiratory tract infection in pregnancy has been implicated in two cases.[1, 8] A review of the literature revealed that more than 50% of patients developing spontaneous pneumothorax during pregnancy had experienced a prior or recurrent pneumothorax.[2]

The clinical diagnosis should be confirmed with chest radiography unless cardiovascular embarrassment is present or tension pneumothorax is suspected, at which point treatment should be initiated immediately. Clinical presentation and radiography allow differentiation from pneumomediastinum (Table 9–2), although both conditions may coexist.[4] Provided that appropriate management is expedited, good fetal outcome is expected. The risk of recurrent pneumothorax and other maternal pulmonary complications, however, is high.[1]

PNEUMOMEDIASTINUM

Pneumomediastinum is more common in pregnancy than is pneumothorax, with an estimated incidence ranging between 1:2000 and 1:100,000.[9] It is generally less serious and usually presents in the second stage of labor, accompanied by surgical emphysema.[10] Pneumomediastinum may occur spontaneously in healthy individuals,[11] but there is frequently a history of predisposing pulmonary or bronchial disease or traumatic injury.[10] It is thought to occur as a result of air escaping through ruptured alveoli, tracking down the sheaths of pulmonary vessels into the mediastinum and then into the subcutaneous tissues. Pneumopericardium has been reported, although this condition rarely appears to be of cardiovascular significance.[12] Some patients with the syndrome of pneumomediastinum and surgical emphysema may demonstrate Hamman's sign: characteristic "crackles, bubbles or churning sounds" heard on auscultation at the left sternal edge synchronous with the heart beat.[13] Apart from surgical emphysema, the patient may be asymptomatic or may complain of pleuritic chest pain and dyspnea.

The diagnosis should always be suspected in parturients who develop surgical emphysema and should be

TABLE 9–1. **CAUSES OF PNEUMOTHORAX**

Idiopathic
Viral upper respiratory tract infection
Asthma
Emphysema and chronic bronchitis
Bullous lung disease
Pneumonia
Tuberculosis
Histoplasmosis
Lymphangiomyomatosis
Carcinoma of lung
Chest trauma
Iatrogenic (e.g., central venous pressure line insertion)
Barotrauma (intermittent positive-pressure ventilation and PEEP)

TABLE 9–2. **CLINICAL DIAGNOSIS**

	Pneumothorax	Pneumomediastinum
Surgical emphysema	−	+ +
Chest pain	+	+
Dyspnea	+ / + +	+
Cyanosis	+	Rare
Venous congestion	+	Rare
Hypotension	+ / + +	Rare
Neck swelling	−	+
Tracheal deviation	+	−

confirmed by chest radiography, because pneumothorax may also accompany the condition.[4, 9, 13] Posteroanterior radiographic views may show a sharply defined translucency along the upper left border of the heart, and streaks of air in mediastinal tissues between the heart and chest wall may be visible in lateral views.[14] Because increases in intrathoracic pressure may aggravate the condition, elective assisted delivery is recommended. Patients and clinicians should be reassured, however, in the knowledge that pneumomediastinum is usually self-limited and requires no specific treatment.[4]

MANAGEMENT

Acute Episodes

Management of both conditions requires rapid assessment and treatment, followed by avoidance of aggravating factors. The potential risk of fetal compromise due to maternal cardiovascular instability or hypoxemia suggests that all patients be admitted to the hospital for initial assessment (regardless of the size of initial pneumothorax), nursed in an (obstetric) high-dependency area, and receive continuous fetal heart monitoring. Maternal oxygen requirement is increased during pregnancy and maximal during labor; therefore oxygen is administered to all patients and minimal monitoring is established (including oxygen saturation, SaO2).

Needle aspiration of a moderate-sized pneumothorax is an effective technique associated with a low morbidity and is recommended in stable nonobstetric patients.[15] In the peripartum period, however, the risks of recurrence or hemorrhage and destabilization during delivery probably indicate tube thoracostomy. When hypotension is present, tension pneumothorax or pneumopericardium must be considered. If tension pneumothorax is suspected (tracheal shift, hypotension, cyanosis, absent air entry), relief should be obtained immediately through insertion of a large-bore needle cannula, followed by formal drainage using local anesthesia with an underwater seal or Heimlich valve. Tube drainage is indicated when more than 25% of the lung is thought to be collapsed (from radiographic evidence), or when increasing symptoms or size of pneumothorax is observed. Rarely, a malignant form of pneumomediastinum may occur that requires needle aspiration, skin incision, or even sternotomy to release trapped air and alleviate airway obstruction.[13, 14] Serial arterial blood gas analysis may be useful in plotting the progress of respiratory embarrassment and effectiveness of therapeutic intervention.

Pleuritic chest pain may require treatment with opioid analgesic drugs. Nonsteroidal anti-inflammatory drugs (NSAIDs) can be given when clinically indicated

for short-term use, because there is a paucity of evidence that they are harmful in pregnancy. Epidural or intrathecal opioids (e.g., fentanyl, sufentanil) given with regional anesthesia for labor may also provide some alleviation of symptoms, particularly if weak solutions of local anesthetic are employed, allowing safe extension of the sensory block to include the thoracic nerve roots.

LABOR AND DELIVERY

The patient's respiratory condition and proposed peripartum management are discussed at an early stage by the anesthesiologist, the chest physician, and obstetrician (Table 9–3). The risk of a "crash" cesarean section scenario should be minimized and the option of elective delivery considered. If vaginal delivery is chosen, the patient is not allowed to push in the second stage of labor, because increased intrapulmonary pressure (including Valsalva maneuver) raises the risk of air leakage and recurrence. An elective assisted delivery is recommended.

The analgesic technique of choice for labor is an epidural (or combined spinal/epidural), because it provides excellent analgesia and dramatically reduces maternal oxygen demand.[16] The sensory block may also be extended to cover operative delivery as necessary. Regional analgesia is encouraged at an early stage in labor, therefore, with care to ensure that it is working properly. Nitrous oxide mixed with equal parts of oxygen (e.g., Entonox) is avoided because it increases the size of gas-containing compartments, aggravates surgical emphysema, and increases the risk of further bronchopleural leaks. Regular aspiration prophylaxis (e.g., ranitidine) is recommended in labor and before operative delivery.

TABLE 9–3. SUMMARY OF PERIPARTUM MANAGEMENT

Do
Administer oxygen
Encourage patient to sit up
Monitor SaO2, ECG, and noninvasive blood pressure (as minimum)
Check chest radiograph
Consider chest drainage
Discuss respiratory condition with chest physician
Discuss peripartum management with obstetrician
Consider elective cesarean section
Avoid "crash" cesarean section
Use epidural analgesia in labor (and insert early)
Perform assisted delivery (if vaginal delivery)
Use regional anesthesia for assisted delivery/cesarean section
Use minimal inflation pressures for IPPV if general anesthesia
Nurse in (?obstetric) high-dependency area
Arrange postpartum follow-up by respiratory physician
Do Not
Use nitrous oxide or Entonox (equal parts N2O plus O2)
Use general anesthesia (especially IPPV) unless essential
Allow patient to push or strain

General anesthesia should be avoided if at all possible. Close monitoring of the mother's regional block and the fetal heart rate or fetal scalp capillary pH should allow adequate warning of imminent need for cesarean section, providing time for an epidural top-up or alternative regional technique to be used for all but the most unexpected of crash cesarean sections. When general anesthesia is unavoidable, rapid-sequence induction and intubation are usual. Positive-pressure ventilation increases the risk of tension pneumothorax if a chest drain is not present. In the presence of a continued bronchopleural leak, increased minute volumes may be required to maintain adequate ventilation. Peak and mean airway pressures, however, should be kept as low as possible and coughing avoided to minimize air leak. In the extreme and rare situation of a large lung leak, endobronchial intubation (e.g., using a double-lumen tube) may be necessary to isolate and ventilate the "good" lung.

LONG-TERM FOLLOW-UP

Following drainage and resolution of the pneumothorax, careful follow-up by a chest physician is important because the risk of recurrence is high.[1] Once the initial pneumothorax has been treated, residual air leak; incomplete lung expansion; or the risks of hemorrhage, infection, and recurrence may indicate pleural surgery via thoracotomy. The considerably less invasive technique of thoracoscopy has been shown to be both safe and effective for the diagnosis and treatment of spontaneous pneumothorax. It is considered by some to be the management of choice, allowing endoscopic pleurodesis; pleurectomy; and resection, clipping, and cauterization of small bullae and blebs.[17–19] Both thoracotomy and thoracoscopy have been reported in the management of spontaneous pneumothorax in pregnancy,[2, 20] but the advantages of thoracoscopic treatment, whenever possible, seem considerable.

References

1. Farall SJ. Spontaneous pneumothorax in pregnancy: A case report and review of the literature. Obstet Gynecol 1983;62:43S.
2. Van Winter JT, Nichols FC, Pairolero PC, et al. Management of spontaneous pneumothorax during pregnancy: Case report and review of the literature. Mayo Clin Proc 1996;71:249.
3. Burgener L, Solmes JG. Spontaneous pneumothorax and pregnancy. Can Med Assoc J 1979;120:19.
4. De Swiet M. Diseases of the respiratory system. In De Swiet (ed): Medical Disorders in Obstetric Practice, 2nd ed. London, Blackwell Scientific Publications, 1989.
5. Stewart B. Spontaneous pneumothorax and pregnancy. Can Med Assoc J 1979;121:25.
6. Najafi JA, Guzman LG. Spontaneous pneumothorax in labor: Case report. Mil Med 1978;143:341.
7. Jonas G. Spontaneous pneumothorax at term: Report of a case. Obstet Gynecol 1964;23:799.
8. Brantley WM, DelValle RA, Schoenbucher AK. Pneumothorax, bilateral, spontaneous, complicating pregnancy: Case report. Am J Obstet Gynecol 1961;81:42.
9. Reeder SR. Subcutaneous emphysema, pneumomediastinum and pneumothorax in labor and delivery. Am J Obstet Gynecol 1986;154:487.
10. Karson EM, Saltzman D, Davis MR. Pneumomediastinum in pregnancy: Two case reports and a review of the literature, pathophysiology and management. Obstet Gynecol 1984;64:39S.
11. Jayran-Nejad Y. Subcutaneous emphysema in labour. Anaesthesia 1993;48:139.
12. Luby BJ, Georgiev M, Warren SG, et al. Postpartum pneumopericardium. Obstet Gynecol 1983;62:46S.
13. Hamman L. Mediastinal emphysema. JAMA 1945;128:1.
14. Gray JM, Hanson GC. Mediastinal emphysema: Aetiology, diagnosis and treatment. Thorax 1966;21:325.
15. Light RW. Management of spontaneous pneumothorax. Am Rev Respir Dis 1993;148:245.
16. Hagerdal M, Morgan CW, Sumner AE, et al: Minute ventilation and oxygen consumption during labor with epidural analgesia. Anesthesiology 1983;59:425.
17. Boutin C, Astoul P, Rey F, et al. Thoracoscopy in the diagnosis and treatment of spontaneous pneumothorax. Clin Chest Med 1995;16:497.
18. Jacques LF. Videothoracoscopic operations for bullous lung disease. Chest Surg Clin North Am 1995;5:751.
19. Naunheim KS, Mack MJ, Hazelrigg SR, et al. Safety and efficacy of video-assisted thoracic surgical techniques for the treatment of spontaneous pneumothorax. J Thorac Cardiovasc Surg 1995;109:1198.
20. Brodsky JB, Eggen M, Cannon WB. Spontaneous pneumothorax in early pregnancy: Successful management by thoracoscopy. J Cardiothorac Vasc Anesth 1993;7:585.

PULMONARY EMBOLISM

. . . . . .

Shiv K. Sharma, M.B., and Girish P. Joshi, M.B.

Pulmonary embolism is a leading cause of maternal mortality.[1] An embolus is a detached intravascular mass (solid or gaseous) that is carried by the blood to a site distant from its point of origin. Emboli may consist of thrombus, air, or amniotic fluid, and rarely of fat, tumor, sickle cell, or infectious material. Each one of these emboli differs in incidence, clinical presentation, and outcome. For example, amniotic fluid embolism (AFE) is a rare entity with usually catastrophic outcome.[2] In contrast, venous air embolism (VAE) occurs commonly but is associated with a less severe clinical course.[3–7]

Prevention, early recognition, and correct management are necessary to reduce the morbidity and mortality associated with pulmonary embolism. Pulmonary embolism is one of the many causes of peripartum cardiopulmonary decompensation (Table 10–1).

THROMBOEMBOLISM

Pulmonary thromboembolism (PTE) is a complication of venous thrombosis. The majority of pulmonary emboli originate in the deep venous system of the lower extremities or pelvis. Half of the cases of PTE and venous thrombosis in women of childbearing years occur during pregnancy or puerperium.[8] In addition to PTE we discuss the clinical presentation, diagnostic technique, and treatment of venous thromboses.

Incidence

Superficial vein thrombosis is common in the antepartum and the postpartum period with an incidence of 1 in 700 pregnancies.[9] Deep vein thrombosis (DVT) occurs in 1:5000 to 1:300 of all pregnancies,[9–12] and the incidence is more common in the postpartum period. Puerperal ovarian and pelvic vein thrombosis occurs in the early postpartum period with an incidence of 1:4000 to 1:1000 of all pregnancies.[9, 13] Pulmonary thromboembolism mostly occurs as a result of DVT and rarely from superficial, pelvic, or ovarian vein

thromboses.[9] Pulmonary thromboembolism complicates 1 in 2000 pregnancies.[9] Approximately 13 to 24% of pregnant patients with untreated DVT experience PTE.[9, 14, 15] Although the incidence of maternal mortality from PTE has declined owing to improved management in the last two decades, PTE still accounts for approximately 12 to 25% of direct maternal mortality.[16–20]

Etiology

In pregnant women the risk of thromboembolism increases by five- to sixfold compared with the risk in nonpregnant women.[14] Increased venous stasis, the hypercoagulable state of pregnancy, and vascular injury associated with delivery all contribute to the increased frequency of DVT and thromboembolic disease.

The uterus extends into the abdomen as pregnancy progresses and may compress the inferior vena cava, which results in venous stasis in the pelvis and lower extremities. In pregnancy blood becomes hypercoagulable, in that several of the factors involved in the coagulation cascade (e.g., fibrinogen; factors V, VII, VIII, IX, X, XII; and von Willebrand) increase, whereas naturally occurring anticoagulants (antithrombin III, proteins C and S) decrease.[21, 22] The increased platelet reactivity, as a result of enhanced thromboxane A_2 (TXA_2) production, further contributes to the hypercoagulability during the third trimester of normal pregnancy.[23] The hypercoagulable state in normal parturients has also been confirmed by thromboelastography, which is a whole blood coagulation monitor.[24] As a result of the hypercoagulability, pregnancy accelerates compensatory fibrinolytic activity.[25, 26] Following delivery, fibrinolytic activity decreases in the first 48 hours,[26] and thus coagulation activity increases relative to fibrinolysis. The risk of thromboembolism is therefore even higher during the postpartum period.

Vascular trauma during cesarean section (CS) and vaginal delivery and separation of the placenta may initiate a series of physiologic events leading to an

TABLE 10–1. CAUSES OF PERIPARTUM CARDIOPULMONARY DECOMPENSATION

Pulmonary embolism	Acute cardiac failure
Hemorrhagic shock	■ Acute myocardial infarction
■ Uterine atony	■ Cardiomyopathy
■ Retained placenta	■ Valvular heart disease
■ Placenta previa	■ Tocolytic therapy
■ Placental abruption	Anaphylaxis
■ Uterine rupture	Aspiration pneumonitis
Eclampsia	Total spinal anesthesia
Intracranial hemorrhage	Local anesthetic toxicity
Septic shock	

acceleration of coagulation activity and increased risk of thromboembolism. The risks of DVT and PTE are five to fifteen times higher after cesarean delivery than after vaginal delivery.[8, 27] The presence of other coexisting coagulation abnormalities, such as anticardiolipin antibodies, deficiency of coagulation factors, dysfibrinogenemia, and previous history of thromboembolism, further increases the risk of thromboembolism during pregnancy.[8, 28]

Pathophysiology

The severity of the hemodynamic consequences of pulmonary embolism not only depends on the extent of the occlusion but also on the cardiovascular status of the patient. Pulmonary thromboembolism leads to obstruction of the pulmonary arterial tree, which results in physiologic changes in the pulmonary vasculature. The acute reduction in the pulmonary vascular cross-sectional area increases pulmonary vascular resistance and right ventricular afterload, which can lead to right ventricular failure.

Massive PTE acutely increases right ventricular afterload and enlarges the right ventricle, resulting in a shift of the ventricular septum to the left. This sequence may cause left ventricular failure because of poor left ventricular filling and decreased cardiac output. Disruption of the normal capillary integrity may also be associated with PTE. Consequently, the increase in hydrostatic pressure and disruption of the normal capillary integrity predispose the patient to pulmonary edema. In the presence of underlying cardiac or respiratory disease, the risk of cardiorespiratory decompensation in PTE is further increased.

Pulmonary complications of PTE result from the direct effects of vascular occlusion and from the released vasoactive and bronchoactive mediators. Pulmonary thromboembolism causes an increase in ventilation/perfusion ($\dot{V}/\dot{Q}$) mismatching, especially an increase in the alveolar dead space, leading to arterial hypoxemia.[29] A decrease in cardiac output in patients with right ventricular failure causes a decrease in mixed-venous oxygen content and further increases the effects of $\dot{V}/\dot{Q}$ mismatching.[29] Other mechanisms of hypox-

emia following PTE are impairment of pulmonary hypoxic vasoconstriction and decreased surfactant production, which further increase $\dot{V}/\dot{Q}$ mismatching. In 85 to 95% of patients with PTE, PaO_2 remains lower than 85 mm Hg.[30] One in six patients with PTE may have a normal PaO_2, however. Hypocarbia results from compensatory tachypnea due to an increase in the alveolar dead space; when associated with hypoxemia, hypocarbia is suggestive of a pulmonary embolism.

Clinical Presentation

Deep Vein Thrombosis

Pulmonary emboli occur in 50% of patients with documented DVT. Half of the patients with documented DVT are asymptomatic.[31] Most clinically significant emboli arise from thrombi in the deep veins of the thigh. Calf vein thromboses rarely produce large emboli. Common signs and symptoms of DVT are swelling of calf muscles (with 2-cm difference in leg circumference at the mid-calf between the affected and unaffected legs), pain, tenderness, positive Homans sign (painful passive dorsiflexion of the foot), change in limb color, and palpable cord due to associated thrombophlebitis. Rarely, a thrombosed iliofemoral vein may produce marked swelling, cyanosis, impairment of arterial blood flow with diminished pulses, and a cold extremity. Puerperal ovarian vein and pelvic vein thromboses may appear in the postpartum period with fever lasting more than 72 hours that is unresponsive to antibiotic therapy. Patients with these disorders may also have concurrent DVT; they present with leg pain, tenderness, and edema.[28] They may not complain of pelvic pain; neither may they have a palpable pelvic mass.[13, 28]

Pulmonary Thromboembolism

The clinical diagnosis of PTE is difficult to make because the presenting signs and symptoms may be nonspecific and may mimic other cardiopulmonary complications of pregnancy. Most cases are asymptomatic and not life-threatening. The common presentations of PTE are dyspnea, tachypnea, palpitations, chest pain (pleuritic or secondary to infarction), hemoptysis, and hemodynamic collapse. The classic triad of dyspnea, pleuritic pain, and hemoptysis is present in only 25% of patients. Examination of the cardiovascular system reveals tachycardia and signs of right ventricular failure (e.g., split second heart sound, jugular venous distension, parasternal heave, and hepatic enlargement). Low-grade fever, cyanosis, diaphoresis, altered mental status, wheezing, and clinical signs of DVT may also be present. Rarely, patients experience abdominal pain due to referred pain from an impinging infarcted lung on the diaphragm. Disseminated intravascular coagulation is another rare presentation of extensive venous thrombosis.

Diagnosis

Deep Vein Thrombosis

The objective tests for DVT are either invasive or noninvasive, and each has its advantages and disadvantages. The invasive tests are more sensitive and specific than noninvasive tests but have added risk. Doppler ultrasound is best at detecting proximal thrombosis, with 90% of popliteal, femoral, and iliac lesions diagnosed.[32] Thrombi that either completely occlude proximal veins or are not large enough to obstruct blood flow may be missed. In addition, 50% of small calf thrombi may be missed because of collateral circulation. Compression ultrasonography and color flow Doppler imaging may substitute for contrast venography in the diagnosis of symptomatic DVT.[10, 33]

Impedance plethysmography measures volume changes within the leg. Although sensitivity of plethysmography is high (90%) for proximal thrombosis, it is low for distal thrombosis.[34] Furthermore, thrombotic and non-thrombotic occlusion cannot be differentiated by plethysmography. Therefore, compression of the common iliac vein and/or the vena cava by the gravid uterus may yield false-positive results.

Ascending venography is the most accurate test for diagnosis of DVT; however, it is not useful for the evaluation of the pelvic vasculature. Inaccurate results occur owing to poor technique, poor interpretation, or chemical phlebitis. Approximately 3% of patients with a negative venogram reading have a positive isotope scanning result following venography.

Isotope scanning is an effective method of diagnosing DVT. It involves the use of ^{125}I-labeled fibrinogen and its detection as it is incorporated into the developing thrombus. Because this method involves systemic injection of radioactive isotope of iodine, which may cross the placenta and affect the fetus, its use is contraindicated during pregnancy. Computerized axial tomography and magnetic resonance imaging have been shown to be sensitive diagnostic tools that can be employed to follow the clinical resolution of puerperal ovarian vein and septic pelvic vein thromboses.[13, 35]

Pulmonary Thromboembolism

A decrease in SaO_2 and end-tidal carbon dioxide reflects the abnormal $\dot{V}/\dot{Q}$ relationship and increased physiologic dead space that can result from PTE.

Electrocardiography may show signs of right ventricular strain, right axis shift, P pulmonale, supraventricular dysrhythmias, and S1, Q3, T3 pattern. The most

TABLE 10–2. CAUSES OF ST-SEGMENT DEPRESSION DURING PREGNANCY

Tachycardia	Hyperventilation
Myocardial ischemia	Mitral valve prolapse
Coronary vasospasm	Exogenous drugs
Acute hypervolemia	Pulmonary embolism
Hyperdynamic circulation	

common electrocardiographic finding, however, is ST-segment changes—phenomena commonly seen in patients undergoing CS using both regional and general anesthesia.[36–38] ST-segment depression during regional anesthesia may result from diminished cardiac sympathetic tone,[39] but there are other proposed mechanisms (Table 10–2).

The chest radiograph is neither specific nor sensitive,[9, 30] because similar findings are observed in other conditions (Table 10–3). In approximately 25 to 40% of patients with pulmonary embolism, the chest radiograph shows a normal appearance[9, 30] but chest radiographs may help rule out other conditions such as pneumonia and pneumothorax, which can mimic PTE.

Invasive hemodynamic monitoring with central venous catheter or pulmonary artery catheter may reveal increased central venous pressure (CVP), raised mean pulmonary arterial pressure, and normal or low pulmonary artery occlusion pressure (PAOP).[30] Monitoring of PAOP and cardiac output helps guide administration of fluids and inotropic drugs.

A definite diagnosis can be made with $\dot{V}/\dot{Q}$ scan if there is a high clinical suspicion; the scan shows high-probability readings for PTE if there is normal ventilation with a segmental perfusion defect.[30] The probability of PTE is only 10 to 40% if the perfusion defect is subsegmental.[30] Normal perfusion displayed on lung scan excludes the diagnosis of PTE, but multiple perfusion defects and $\dot{V}/\dot{Q}$ mismatch suggest a high probability of a pulmonary embolus. If the scan reveals low probability of pulmonary embolus but clinical suspicion is high, pulmonary angiography should be considered. Angiography also is helpful in excluding a hypoplastic pulmonary artery, which is an unusual congenital malformation that mimics PTE both clinically and radiologically.[40]

Echocardiography is useful in the detection of a pulmonary embolus after cesarean section.[41] Although early therapeutic intervention is possible if pulmonary embolism is diagnosed by echocardiography, it does not replace pulmonary angiography.

TABLE 10–3. CHEST RADIOGRAPHIC FINDINGS IN PULMONARY THROMBOEMBOLISM

Atelectasis
Pleural effusion
Elevated hemidiaphragm
Peripheral segmental or subsegmental infiltration

Small amounts of fetal radiation exposure increase the risk of childhood cancer to a limited degree,[42] and a higher incidence of teratogenesis occurs only when fetal radiation exposure exceeds 5 rads.[42, 43] Although the total fetal radiation exposure is less than 60 mrads with the use of chest radiography, lung scan, and pulmonary angiography,[43] physicians should limit unnecessary fetal radiation exposure.

Management

Deep Vein Thrombosis

The clinician should have a high index of suspicion for DVT, and before therapy is started a definitive diagnosis must be established. An algorithm for diagnosis and management of DVT and pulmonary embolism has been proposed (Fig. 10–1).[44] Heparin therapy should be started immediately after the diagnosis of DVT to prevent the occurrence of PTE. The loading dose of heparin is 100 U/kg followed by an initial infusion rate of 1000 U/hr.[28] During pregnancy, dose requirements may be increased as a result of hypercoagulability. The adequacy of anticoagulation should be monitored by performing serial partial thromboplastin times (PTT), which should be maintained between 1.5 and 2.0 times normal for 7 to 10 days.[28] After therapeutic PTT values are maintained for 2 days, subcutaneous administration can be substituted for intravenous administration because the subcutaneous route decreases the incidence of bleeding complications.[9]

Heparin therapy may be discontinued when the patient begins active labor[28] or 4 to 6 hours before CS. The baseline anticoagulant activity should be assessed by performing a PTT level immediately after discontinuing the heparin therapy. For surgical hemostasis, protamine in incremental doses up to a calculated dose of 1 mg protamine per 100 U heparin should be considered.

Heparin therapy can be reinstituted in the postpartum period if the patient's condition is stable. Warfarin can be administered concurrently, while monitoring anticoagulation by the prothrombin time (PT). Once a therapeutic PT level is achieved, heparin can be discontinued. Anticoagulation is maintained for 3 months postpartum.[9] Prophylaxis with heparin may be considered for a pregnant woman with a history of thromboembolic disease. The optimal management regimen of pregnant women at risk of thromboembolism, however, is controversial[45]

Pulmonary Thromboembolism

The successful management of a patient with PTE requires prompt diagnosis and rapid institution of appropriate therapy (Table 10–4). The first hour after a PTE is most critical, and approximately 10% of all affected patients die during that period.[46]

TABLE 10–4. **MANAGEMENT OF PULMONARY THROMBOEMBOLISM**

Cardiopulmonary support
Anticoagulation therapy
Venous interruption
Fibrinolytic therapy
Surgical embolectomy

Initial supportive management of PTE consists of maintaining oxygenation, ventilation, and hemodynamic status. Hypoxemia should be treated with supplemental oxygen, which may not be adequate because of severe $\dot{V}/\dot{Q}$ mismatching and decreased mixed-venous oxygen tension. Mechanical ventilation is necessary in patients with hemodynamic instability and severe hypoxemia. Improved oxygenation reduces right ventricular afterload and improves hemodynamic status. Volume resuscitation with colloids or crystalloids improves cardiac output and arterial blood pressure. In patients with poor right ventricular compliance, however, fluid administration may decrease cardiac output and increase central venous pressure. If inotropic support for the right ventricle is required, dobutamine may be preferable to dopamine because it reduces ventricular afterload.

Heparin therapy should be started immediately. An intravenous bolus dose of 100 U/kg should be followed by a continuous infusion of 1000 U/hr to maintain the PTT at twice normal values.[9, 30] Heparin improves oxygenation and hemodynamic status not only by reducing pulmonary artery obstruction but also by preventing the further release of vasoactive and bronchoconstrictive mediators from platelets and thrombin, thus reducing pulmonary vascular resistance.

Inferior vena caval interruption with either ligation or filter should be considered in patients who experience recurrent emboli while on anticoagulation therapy or in those who cannot be anticoagulated.[47] The insertion of an inferior vena caval filter in nonpregnant patients reduces the recurrence rate of lethal emboli to less than 1%.

Patients with massive pulmonary embolus and acute decompensation may respond to thrombolytic therapy.[30, 48–50] Although urokinase and streptokinase have been used successfully in pregnancy,[48–51] urokinase is considered less antigenic. A thrombolytic agent, recombinant tissue plasminogen activator (rt-PA), has been administered successfully in a pregnant patient with massive pulmonary embolism.[52] The rt-PA is associated with minimal bleeding complications; because it does not induce systemic fibrinolysis, it is active only when it binds to thrombin and it is clot-specific.[52] Thrombolytic therapy should be monitored by thrombin time, which should not be greater than five times normal. Thrombolytic therapy in a pregnant patient is associ-

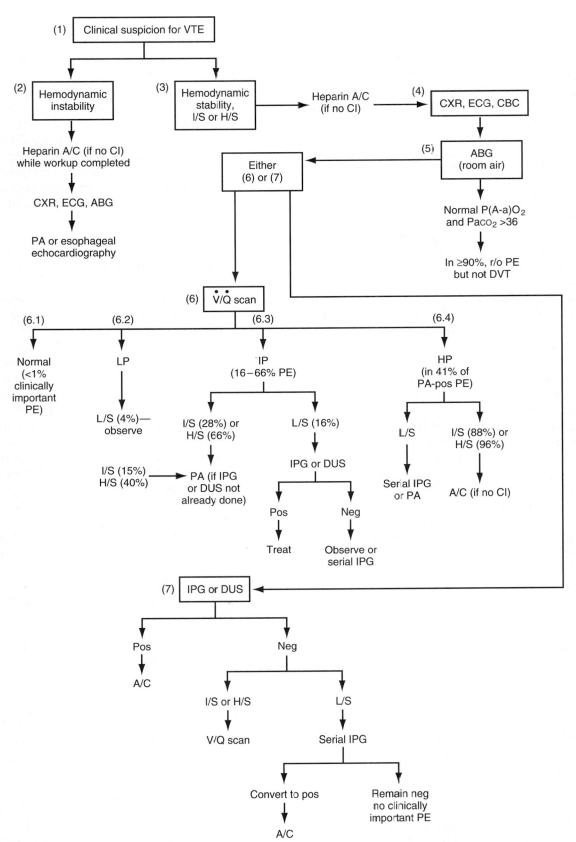

Figure 10–1. An algorithmic approach to diagnosis and management of venous and pulmonary thromboembolism. VTE = venous thromboembolism; I/S = intermediate stability; H/S = high stability; A/C = anticoagulation; CI = contraindication; CXR = chest radiograph; ECG = electrocardiogram; CBC = complete blood count; PA = pulmonary angiography; PE = pulmonary embolus; LP = low probability; IP = intermediate probability; HP = high probability; L/S = low stability; IPG = impedence plethysmography; DUS = duplex ultrasonography. (From Rosenow EC: Venous and pulmonary thromboembolism: An algorithmic approach to diagnosis and management. Mayo Clin Proc 1995;70:45.)

ated with the risk of maternal bleeding and abruptio placentae.[28, 48, 49] Thus, this therapy should be used cautiously after consultation with a hematologist. Surgical embolectomy is associated with a high mortality rate and should be a last measure in those patients showing rapid clinical deterioration.[14] The procedure has been described in pregnant women.[53, 54]

In anticoagulated patients requiring regional anesthesia, the risk of epidural hematoma formation must be considered and balanced against the risk of PTE. The incidence of epidural vessel puncture during epidural placement is higher in pregnant patients than in nonpregnant patients. An epidural hematoma can occur, however, in anticoagulated patients without epidural anesthesia.[55] The risk of general anesthesia in the anticoagulated patient includes that of airway bleeding. Heparin should be discontinued and PTT should be in a normal range before elective CS is performed. Protamine may be administered in selected patients who require emergency CS. Regional anesthesia should be avoided for both labor analgesia and CS in patients with abnormal PTT. If the patient has received epidural anesthesia, the catheter should be removed before reinstitution of anticoagulation therapy to avoid the risk of venous disruption and epidural hematoma. Epidural anesthesia is also contraindicated in patients receiving concomitant fibrinolytic therapy, because of the risk of epidural hematoma formation.[56]

All patients who receive regional anesthesia after anticoagulation or fibrinolytic therapy should be followed for signs and symptoms of a developing epidural hematoma (Table 10-5). Magnetic resonance imaging (MRI) or computerized tomography (CT) scan can be helpful if the diagnosis of epidural hematoma is in doubt. Early spinal cord decompression reduces the risk of permanent neurologic deficits.[56]

VENOUS AIR EMBOLISM

Venous air embolism (VAE) is a common occurrence during CS[4-7] and vaginal delivery.[57] VAE can occur, however, in the antepartum and postpartum periods.[58, 59] The severity of VAE depends on the volume, rate, and duration of air entrainment and the patient's general medical condition.

TABLE 10-5. **SIGNS AND SYMPTOMS OF EPIDURAL HEMATOMA**

Severe persistent backache
Neurologic deficit, including decreased lower limb movements
Tenderness over the spinous process
Unexplained fever

Incidence

The actual incidence of VAE is unknown because routine monitoring for VAE is not carried out during CS. Furthermore, a small embolus may go undetected, and the clinical manifestations of a large embolus may mimic cardiopulmonary and cerebrovascular dysfunction from other causes.[60] The incidence during CS as detected by precordial Doppler monitoring has been reported to be 10 to 60%.[3-7] Although maternal morbidity has been reported,[61-63] the mortality rate is not very high. VAE accounts for approximately 1% of all maternal deaths in the US.[1]

Etiology and Pathophysiology

For VAE to occur there must be vascular access and a gradient between the incisional area and right side of the heart. A subatmospheric venous pressure allows air to be entrained into the venous circulation. A gradient as small as 5 cm H_2O may result in entrainment of large amounts of air. The higher the pressure gradient the greater the risk of air entrainment and fatal air embolism. The pressure gradient increases with the height of the venous site above the level of the heart.

The volume and rate of air entrainment and the site of embolization determine the outcome from VAE. Other factors that modify outcome include body position, ventilation depth, and central venous pressure. In one animal study, slow venous air infusion (0.01–2 ml·kg^{-1}·min^{-1}) resulted in increased central venous and pulmonary artery pressures, decreased peripheral resistance, and compensatory increased cardiac output.[64] A bolus of air (25–200 ml), however, caused an air lock in the right ventricle, resulting in a severe fall in systemic blood pressure.[64] Another animal study reported acute increases in pulmonary vascular resistance and right ventricular pressures following VAE, which led to a decrease in cardiac output and arterial blood pressure.[65] Pulmonary edema can develop as a result of increased capillary permeability and/or increased hydrostatic pulmonary pressure.[66, 67] Hypoxemia occurs invariably in clinically significant air embolism primarily as a result of increased $\dot{V}/\dot{Q}$ mismatching. Hypercarbia can occur owing to an increased alveolar dead space. In humans, large volumes (more than 3 ml/kg) of air may obstruct the pulmonary artery and can be fatal,[59, 68] whereas smaller volumes may result in a $\dot{V}/\dot{Q}$ mismatch, hypoxemia, dysrhythmia, and hypotension. There is a compensatory increase in minute volume during spontaneous ventilation. There may be a reflex gasp, which is probably mediated by pulmonary stretch receptors.

The open uterine vessels during CS allow easy access of air into the venous circulation. The risk of VAE (as suggested by Doppler studies) during CS further increases with exteriorization of the uterus.[7, 69] In addition, left uterine displacement, Trendelenburg position, and hemorrhage all increase the pressure gradient and thus increase the risk of VAE during CS.[70]

The influence of maternal position on the incidence is controversial. Some investigators have suggested that the incidence is reduced to 1% when patients are placed in a 5° reverse Trendelenburg position during CS.[71] In contrast, another group of investigators did not observe any reduction in the frequency of VAE with 5° head-up tilt.[5]

In paradoxical air embolism (arterial air embolus via a patent foramen ovale or microvascular intrapulmonary shunts), as little as 0.025 ml of air entering the coronary or cerebral circulation can lead to severe cardiovascular and neurologic sequelae.[72-74] Rarely, during the antepartum period, air can be forced through the vagina and can travel through the cervical canal to pass beneath the fetal membranes and enter the circulation via subplacental sinuses, resulting in severe VAE.[58]

Clinical Presentation

Depending on its severity, VAE may go unrecognized or may appear as cardiopulmonary dysfunction (see Fig. 10–1). Chest pain and/or dyspnea occurs in approximately 50% of cases, and SaO_2 falls in 25% of cases.[3-7] Other physical findings include hypotension, heart rate alteration (both tachycardia and bradycardia), and signs of elevated right-sided pressures. In addition, wheezing and râles due to acute bronchospasm and pulmonary edema may occur. A patient with massive air embolism can present with cardiovascular collapse.[61, 62]

Diagnosis

Clinical diagnosis of VAE may be difficult because it often mimics other acute cardiopulmonary and cerebrovascular events. Thus, the diagnosis of VAE requires a high level of clinical suspicion. VAE should be suspected when patients complain of chest pain and/or dyspnea and when they develop hypotension, low SaO_2, and dysrhythmias.

Electrocardiographic changes include bradycardia or tachycardia, premature ventricular contractions, heart block, and ST-segment depression. One study, however, found no association between the occurrence of VAE and ST-segment depression.[36] A decrease in SaO_2 and end-tidal carbon dioxide levels reflects the abnormal $\dot{V}/\dot{Q}$ relationship and increased physiologic dead space that can result from clinically significant VAE. A rise in end-tidal concentration of nitrogen (as detected by RASCAL monitors) is specific for air embolism. A transient "mill wheel" murmur, heard during continuous monitoring with an esophageal or precordial stethoscope, is specific. This murmur is described as a rhythmic, churning sound produced by the movement of air bubbles in the right ventricle and heard throughout the cardiac cycle.

In high-risk patients, such as patients with intracardiac shunts and hypovolemia, precordial Doppler monitoring is recommended. Precordial, low-frequency Doppler monitoring is a highly sensitive and readily available method that can detect air bubbles as small as 0.1 ml.[75-77] The Doppler transducer is usually placed over the third to sixth intercostal space to the right of the sternum. Transesophageal echocardiography (TEE) is most sensitive in detecting air embolism; however, it requires expensive equipment and an anesthesiologist experienced in its use. In addition, TEE is not well accepted by awake patients.[36]

Chest radiography can demonstrate an air fluid level in the pulmonary vessels and is pathognomonic for VAE.[78] In an animal study, following injection of air in the pulmonary artery, there was significant increase in end-tidal oxygen content and decrease in dynamic lung compliance as measured by side-stream spirometry.[79] The investigators in this study recommend continuous monitoring of end-tidal oxygen concentration and side-stream spirometry for the detection of VAE in high-risk patients.[79]

Central venous or pulmonary artery catheters may help in the diagnosis and management of VAE as central venous and pulmonary artery pressures increase and cardiac output decreases. Abrupt elevations in pulmonary artery pressure (PAP) accompanied by a fall in end-tidal carbon dioxide (CO_2) level is indicative. The sensitivity of PAP with respect to VAE, however, is similar to that of the end-tidal CO_2. Aspiration of air from the right atrium via the central venous catheter also indicates the occurrence of VAE and may be therapeutic. Arterial blood gas analysis often shows hypoxemia and hypercarbia.[66, 75] Sensitivity of the detection parameters for venous air embolism with increasing air volume is shown in Figure 10–2.

Management

Prompt recognition of VAE and rapid initiation of therapy are necessary to reduce the associated morbidity and mortality. The management is outlined in Table 10–6. Positioning the patient in the left lateral position with 5° head-down tilt places the heart in a dependent position, minimizing the possibility of developing an air lock and improving venous return. In patients with delayed emergence from anesthesia, CT scan or MRI should be considered to exclude the presence of intracerebral air.

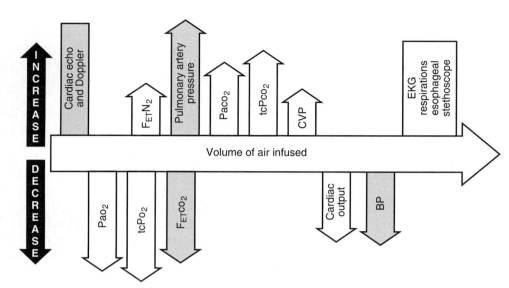

Figure 10–2. Sensitivity of the detection parameters for venous air embolism with increasing air volume. (From Black S, Cucchiara RF: Tumor surgery. In Cucchiara RF, Michenfelder JD (eds): Clinical Neuroanesthesia. New York, Churchill Livingstone, 1990, p 285.)

AMNIOTIC FLUID EMBOLISM

Amniotic fluid embolism (AFE) is a rare but catastrophic complication of pregnancy. Patients present with sudden hypoxemia, hypotension, and coagulopathy. The syndrome was first described in 1926 by Meyer, who reported the presence of constituents of amniotic fluid in the pulmonary vasculature of a young woman who suffered fatal cardiopulmonary collapse during pregnancy.[80] In 1941, Steiner and Lushbaugh detailed the clinical and pathologic features of a series of women who died of sudden shock during labor.[81]

Incidence

Since its initial description, over 300 cases have been documented in the literature. The exact incidence of this condition has been difficult to establish because the definitive cause is assigned only after autopsy, and many cases of minor embolism may pass unnoticed. The reported incidence varies from 1 in 8000 to 1 in 80,000 pregnant women.[81] The overall mortality rate of clinically recognized AFE is reported to be up to 86%,[82] with cardiopulmonary collapse in 63 to 75% of cases.[83] Approximately 25 to 50% of the patients die within the first hour of clinical presentation.[84, 85] Overall, AFE accounts for approximately 10% of all maternal deaths.

TABLE 10–6. MANAGEMENT OF VENOUS AIR EMBOLISM AT CESAREAN BIRTH

Flood surgical field with saline
Position patient 5° head-down and left lateral
Discontinue nitrous oxide
Administer 100% oxygen
Support circulation with intravenous volume expansion and vasopressor drugs
Aspirate air through a multiorifice CVP line

With decreasing fatality from sepsis and eclampsia, however, its rate may increase.[83, 86] The incidence of hematologic abnormalities with AFE have been reported to be about 40%,[87] and these are the presenting manifestations in 10 to 15% of cases.[82, 84, 88]

Etiology and Pathophysiology

The pathogenesis of the AFE is not completely understood. There seems to be a significant interspecies difference in the physiologic response to experimental AFE. The hemodynamic and hematologic responses are not consistent after intravenous injection of amniotic fluid in primates.[87] Amniotic fluid access to the maternal circulation is essential to its pathogenesis. The disruption of the integrity of fetal membranes, open uterine or cervical veins, and concomitant pressure gradient between the amnion and the uterine and cervical veins, sufficient to drive the amniotic fluid into the maternal circulation, facilitate amniotic fluid access to the maternal circulation. No correlation exists between the presence of amniotic fluid in the circulation and the onset of clinical symptoms.[87]

Various proposed mechanisms may produce the clinical picture of AFE (Table 10–7). Pulmonary edema is a common (70%) presentation in humans, but is absent in other primates.[87] Left heart failure is a major physiologic aberration,[89–91] but it may be preceded by right heart failure. The speculation that mechanical obstruction is fundamental to the pathogenesis of AFE has been discounted by autopsy studies that have shown a poor correlation between the amount of particulate matter and clinical findings.[92, 93] Clark[87] proposed that AFE is a maternal type I hypersensitivity response. It was hypothesized that amniotic fluid triggers the release of maternal endogenous mediators, which results in a clinical response similar to anaphylaxis.[87]

The coagulopathy associated with AFE is also incompletely understood. Animal studies have been inconsistent in demonstrating coagulopathy. Some in vitro studies have shown that amniotic fluid has a thromboplastin-like effect that decreases whole blood clotting time, induces platelet aggregation, and is associated with the release of platelet factor III and activation of complement and factor X–activating factor.[94–96] Others have concluded that the amount of procoagulant in clear amniotic fluid is insufficient to cause significant intravascular coagulation.[97] The presence of active tissue factor in amniotic fluid[98] and circulating trophoblast[87] may be responsible for the hemostatic alterations. In addition, uterine atony caused by the myometrial depressant effect of amniotic fluid[94] may result in massive hemorrhage and contribute to coagulopathy.

Metabolites of arachidonic acid (prostaglandins and leukotrienes) produce similar hemodynamic and hematologic effects as in patients with clinical AFE.[87] The clinical course may be attributable to the metabolites of arachidonic acid,[99] because the concentration of these metabolites in amniotic fluid increases during labor.[100] In an animal study, Hankins and coworkers observed a pressor response consistent with a potent vasoconstrictor, decreased oxygen saturation, and transient left ventricular dysfunction after intravascular meconium injection.[101] It was suggested that the presence of a pressor agent in meconium potentiates the cardiopulmonary responses to an infusion of amniotic fluid.[101]

The summation of many of these findings led Clark to propose a biphasic model for the pathogenesis of AFE that reconciles human and animal data.[85] The model describes the release of amniotic fluid containing vasoactive substances leading to an initial phase I response, which lasts for 15 to 30 minutes and involves hypoxemia, dyspnea, pulmonary hypertension, cor pulmonale, and left ventricular injury. A secondary phase II response includes left ventricular failure, adult respiratory distress syndrome, and consumptive coagulopathy (Fig. 10–3).

TABLE 10–7. PATHOPHYSIOLOGY OF AMNIOTIC FLUID EMBOLISM

Mechanical obstruction of pulmonary vasculature by
  particulate matter
- Fetal squamous epithelium
- Mucin
- Lanugo hair

Pulmonary edema due to
- Alveolar capillary leak
- Microvascular embolic insult

Left ventricular dysfunction secondary to
- Arterial hypoxia
- Decreased coronary blood flow
- Circulatory myocardial depressants

Release of vasoactive substances eliciting a hemodynamic
  response
- Pulmonary hypertension

Anaphylactic shock

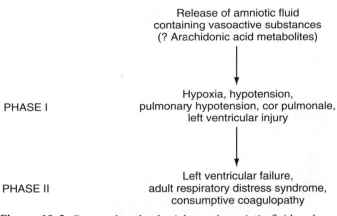

Figure 10–3. Proposed pathophysiology of amniotic fluid embolism. (From Clark SL: Amniotic fluid embolism. Crit Care Clin 1991;7:877.)

Clinical Presentation

Most cases of AFE have been reported to occur during labor.[87] This syndrome has occurred during first and second trimester abortions,[102, 103] however, and as late as 48 hours post partum.[104]

The clinical presentation is often dramatic, with abrupt onset of hypoxemia (oxygen desaturation), dyspnea, and hypotension with rapid progression to cardiopulmonary arrest. Pulmonary edema has been observed in 24 to 70% of cases.[85] In 40% of cases, pulmonary edema is followed by varying degrees of consumptive coagulopathy. Coagulopathy may be the presenting manifestation in 10 to 15% of patients. Central nervous system hypoxia may lead to alterations in mental status with seizures in 10 to 20% of cases.[82]

Amniotic fluid embolism may be complicated by myocardial ischemia and infarction, renal failure, liver damage, and neurologic deficits. Superimposed renal failure worsens the prognosis. Occlusion of retinal arterioles by amniotic fluid emboli has been reported in one patient who survived an episode of AFE.[105] These dramatic features may be heralded by nonspecific symptoms of shivering, anxiety, coughing, vomiting, a sensation of bad taste in the mouth, and a sense of impending doom.[106]

Diagnosis

The initial diagnosis is based on the clinical presentation. The definitive cause is learned at autopsy with the finding of fetal debris in the maternal pulmonary vasculature, generally in the arterioles (Fig. 10–4) and capillaries,[84] but occasionally in the large vessels as well.[93] Routine hematoxylin-eosin staining may be insufficient to demonstrate the fetal elements, and special stains such as acid mucopolysaccharide may be required.

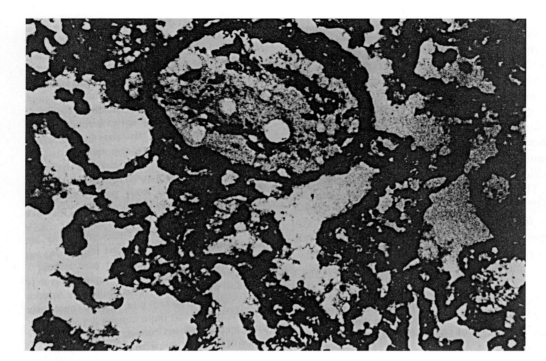

Figure 10–4. Alcian blue stain (original magnification × 200) demonstrating mucin in a small pulmonary arteriole of patient with amniotic fluid embolism (AFE). (From Dudney TM, Elliott CG: Pulmonary embolism from amniotic fluid, fat, and air. Prog Cardiovasc Dis 1994;36:447.)

A number of noninvasive methods for the antemortem diagnosis of AFE have been suggested, including the use of antibodies to human keratin,[107] of zinc coproporphyrin levels in maternal plasma,[108] and of monoclonal antibodies to an amniotic fluid-specific antigen.[109] The sensitivity, specificity, and positive and negative predictive values of these methods of diagnosis remain poorly defined. In addition, there may be no time to perform these tests, because of the catastrophic nature of this syndrome.

Electrocardiographic changes include nonspecific ST-segment and T-wave changes, atrial or ventricular rhythm disturbances, right ventricular abnormalities, such as right bundle branch block, right atrial strain, and right axis deviation. Chest radiographic changes include infiltrate, pleural infusion, atelectasis, or elevation of a hemidiaphragm due to pneumoconstriction. Arterial blood gas measurements may show hypoxemia with a mixed metabolic acidosis and respiratory alkalosis.

Coagulation abnormalities include decreased fibrinogen and increased levels of fibrin degradation products (FDP), prolonged PT, PTT, and thrombocytopenia. $\dot{V}/\dot{Q}$ scans may be useful to estimate the probability of embolism based on the size of perfusion defect and the presence or absence of matching ventilation scan and chest radiographic abnormalities.

Patients surviving to receive invasive hemodynamic monitoring generally demonstrate left ventricular dysfunction accompanied by moderate or severe elevations in pulmonary artery occlusion pressure (PAOP), pulmonary artery pressure (PAP), and pulmonary vascular resistance (PVR), with depressed left ventricular stroke work index.[91, 92] In addition, the systemic vascular resistance (SVR) may be decreased.

Masson and coworkers[110] proposed using pulmonary microvascular cytology (PMVC) on samples obtained with pulmonary artery catheter in the wedge position to identify amniotic fluid debris. The presence of anucleate squamous epithelial cells in the pulmonary microvascular circulation is supportive of AFE. This feature is no longer considered pathognomonic, however, because some investigators have observed squamous cells in the pulmonary vasculature of both pregnant[111, 112] and nonpregnant[113, 114] patients with no clinical evidence of amniotic fluid embolism. The additional findings of mucin, hair, or fat may add credence to the diagnosis of AFE.

Management

Treatment of AFE is primarily supportive and directed toward oxygenation, maintenance of cardiac output and peripheral perfusion, and management of coagulopathy. Aggressive cardiopulmonary resuscitation is imperative due to the catastrophic nature of AFE (see Chapter 3). Supplemental oxygen should be provided to treat hypoxemia. If supplemental oxygen is insufficient, high concentrations of oxygen with continuous positive airway pressure (CPAP) increase functional residual capacity. Mechanical ventilation is usually necessary because of inadequate maternal PaO_2 and hemodynamic instability. If pulmonary edema ensues, PEEP should be considered, but it may decrease venous return. PEEP may also shift the ventricular septum to the left, increase right ventricular wall stress, and decrease the cardiac output, producing hemodynamic deterioration in an already decompensated patient.

It is important to maintain left uterine displacement to avoid aortocaval compression by the gravid uterus during cardiopulmonary resuscitation (CPR). If there is no response to advanced CPR within 5 minutes, cesarean section should be performed to optimize the outcome for both mother and baby.[115]

Hypotension following AFE should be treated initially with rapid-volume fluid administration to increase cardiac preload. In cases of persistent hypotension, fluid administration should be titrated to central venous pressure measurements. Placement of a pulmonary artery catheter is helpful in fluid management and drug therapy in those patients who develop pulmonary edema.[89] Central venous pressure in severe AFE may be high; however, fluid administration should be continued as long as the cardiac index continues to improve. Vasopressors such as ephedrine and epinephrine may be necessary for severe hemodynamic collapse. Although drugs with alpha adrenergic activity may compromise uterine blood flow, the effect on uterine blood flow may not be an issue, considering the catastrophic presentation of this syndrome.

Coagulopathy associated with AFE may be severe but is usually self-limiting. Administration of blood components (fresh-frozen plasma, platelets, packed red blood cells) is often successful. Esposito and coworkers[116] reported the successful use of cardiopulmonary bypass and pulmonary artery embolectomy for treatment of postpartum shock caused by AFE. Continuous arteriovenous hemofiltration (CAVH) has been successful in a patient who developed AFE complicated by renal failure after CS.[117] Continuous arteriovenous hemofiltration allows slower removal of fluids and substances that cause left ventricular and respiratory dysfunction. Patients who receive regional anesthesia before the onset of AFE should be monitored for the development of epidural hematoma. The indwelling epidural catheter should be removed only after correction of the coagulopathy.[118, 119]

MISCELLANEOUS EMBOLI

Fat, sickle cell, tumor, and infectious foci are rare causes of pulmonary embolism. These disorders share some of the common clinical presentations, which include respiratory distress, chest pain, hypoxemia, and elevated central venous pressure. Not all patients with these disorders exhibit clinical signs of pulmonary embolism.

Fat Embolism

Pulmonary fat embolism is a pathologic entity characterized by occlusion of pulmonary blood vessels with fat globules that are too large to pass through the capillary bed. Unlike other types of embolism, vascular occlusion in fat embolism is often temporary or incomplete because the fat globules are deformable. Despite the extensive work performed on the subject, many aspects of fat embolism remain poorly understood, and controversies about its etiology, pathophysiology, diagnosis, and treatment persist. A pregnant patient who sustains skeletal trauma or develops acute fatty liver or sickle cell crisis is susceptible to pulmonary fat embolism.

Incidence and Pathophysiology

Not all patients with fat embolization to the lungs manifest the clinical picture of fat embolism syndrome (FES). The reported incidence of post-traumatic FES in the literature ranges from 19 to 29%,[120–122] with a mortality rate of 10 to 20%.[123, 124] The prognosis in patients with cerebral manifestations of fat embolism is very poor.

Entry of fat globules into the circulation occurs following skeletal trauma, particularly that involving the lower extremity long bones.[125, 126] Fat is detected in pulmonary arterial samples of up to 70% of patients with long-bone and pelvic fractures.[127] The events that promote entry of marrow contents into the circulation following a fracture include movement of unstable bone fragments and reaming of the medullary cavity with internal fixation devices. Both of these events produce distortion and pressure increase in the medullary cavity, permitting entry of marrow fat into torn venous channels. Multiple fractures release a greater amount of fat into the marrow vessels than a single fracture, increasing the amount of substrate available to develop FES.

Other causes of fat embolism include burns, subcutaneous adipose tissue injury, and acute pancreatitis. Sickle cell crisis during pregnancy may be associated with bone marrow infarction and release of fat globules into the circulation, with subsequent FES.[128] In acute fatty liver of pregnancy, increased release of fat into the circulation may cause pulmonary fat embolism.[129]

The pulmonary complications of fat embolism result from two mechanisms: (1) physical obstruction of the pulmonary vasculature with embolized fat, and (2) direct toxicity of circulating free fatty acids on pneumocytes and capillary endothelium, causing interstitial hemorrhage, edema, and clinical pneumonitis.[123]

Clinical Presentation

Patients with pulmonary fat embolism initially present with tachypnea, dyspnea, and cyanosis. Pulmonary vascular obstruction and pulmonary hypertension lead to acute cor pulmonale, severe respiratory distress, hypoxemia, hypotension, anginal pain, dysrhythmia, and elevated central venous pressure. Other manifestations include temperature elevation (>37.8° C), tachycardia (>100 beats/min), change in level of consciousness, and retinopathy (cotton wool–like spots and flame-like hemorrhages). Petechial rashes that appear on the upper anterior portion of the body, including the chest, neck, upper arm, axillae, shoulders, oral mucous membranes, and conjunctivae, are considered a pathognomonic sign of fat embolism, and their presence establishes the diagnosis.[130] These petechiae result from occlusion and distension of dermal capillaries by fat globules. Patients may show mild to severe oozing from the gums and arteriovenous cannulation sites, as a result of thrombocytopenia or disseminated intravascular coagulation.

Diagnosis and Treatment

The diagnosis of pulmonary fat embolism is based on the history and physical examination but requires confirmation with laboratory findings. Arterial blood gas analysis initially reveals hypoxemia with PaO_2 below 60 mm Hg and respiratory alkalosis. Cytologic examination of urine, blood, and sputum after Sudan or oil red O staining may permit detection of fat globules, either free or in macrophages. Coagulation abnormalities include thrombocytopenia, prolonged PT and PTT, and elevated levels of FDP.

Chest radiography shows diffuse, evenly distributed fleck-like shadows. Dilatation of the right heart may occur if cor pulmonale develops. $\dot{V}/\dot{Q}$ scans show subsegmental perfusion defects. The electrocardiogram may show a pattern of acute cor pulmonale or myocardial ischemia.

A specific therapy with proven efficacy is lacking. Early surgical fixation of fractures and improvement in supportive treatment, however, may reduce the mortality rate. Supportive therapy includes prompt attention to hypotension using fluids and inotropes, administration of platelets and cryoprecipitate to correct coagulation defects, optimization of renal function, and reduction of brain edema. Mechanical ventilation, preferably with PEEP, must be instituted to maintain adequate arterial oxygenation. There is no specific therapy for fat embolism, although alcohol, heparin, aprotinin, hypertonic glucose, and corticosteroids have all been used.[131]

Sickle Cell Embolism

Maternal mortality due to sickle cell anemia is as high as 1%, mainly as a result of pulmonary embolism and infection.[132] In sickle cell disease, erythrocytes undergo sickling when deoxygenated. The sickled cells are elongated and crescent-shaped and have a tendency to form aggregates. The sickling mainly depends on the presence of abnormal hemoglobin (HbS), which is a hemoglobin variant (valine replaces glutamic acid in the sixth position of the beta-chain). Increased sickling occurs when more than 50% of hemoglobin is the HbS type. Other factors that affect sickling include vascular stasis, hypothermia, hypovolemia, and acidosis.

The sickle cells aggregate in the circulation, which can lead to pulmonary vascular obstruction and pulmonary infarction. Common with other embolic disorders, patients with sickle cell embolism present with respiratory distress, chest pain, hypoxemia, $\dot{V}/\dot{Q}$ mismatch, and pulmonary hypertension. Anesthetic management includes maintenance of oxygenation and avoidance of dehydration, acidosis, and vascular stasis.[133] Avoidance of aortocaval compression is essential even in patients with sickle cell trait. One patient died following release of aortocaval compression at the time of delivery.[134] This was likely the result of sudden return of acidotic, hypoxic blood and sickled red blood cells to the heart and pulmonary circulation.

Tumor Embolism

Pulmonary tumor emboli to the lung usually arise from malignancies of the breast, stomach, kidney, or uterus. They vary in size and number and appear with varying degrees of severity. Only half of the patients with tumor pulmonary emboli are symptomatic.[135] The most common symptoms are dyspnea, cough, hemoptysis, and pleuritic chest pain.[136] On examination there may be a pleural friction rub, decreased breath sounds, and dullness to percussion. Hypoxemia occurs as a result of $\dot{V}/\dot{Q}$ mismatch and intrapulmonary shunting. Cardiac examination may reveal tachycardia, jugular venous distension secondary to elevated right heart pressure and pulmonary hypertension. Radionuclide $\dot{V}/\dot{Q}$ scans may show subsegmental perfusion defects. Treatment of tumor emboli generally involves removal of the primary source. Anesthesia may be complicated by the patient's pulmonary dysfunction, cachexia, and chemotherapy. Tumor embolism, however, has not yet been reported in pregnancy.

Infectious Embolism

Infectious emboli may complicate infection anywhere in the body. Even a minor infection may produce a major embolic event. The most common foci are the pelvis, tricuspid and pulmonic valves, abdomen, veins of the extremities, and skin and subcutaneous tissues.[137, 138] Gram-positive, gram-negative, and anaerobic organisms may be involved and produce somewhat different signs and symptoms. Patients with septic emboli may exhibit similar pulmonary dysfunction as described for tumor emboli. For treatment to be successful, the source of infection must be removed. Thus, the patient requires aggressive perioperative treatment of the infection and of septic shock if it is present. Intravenous-drug users can develop subacute bacterial endocarditis and seed to the cerebral circulation, creating mycotic aneurysms that require surgical clipping. When pregnant, such a patient requires all the anesthetic considerations of managing a parturient with an intracranial lesion (see Chapter 16).

CONCLUSIONS

Pulmonary embolism should be suspected in a pregnant woman presenting with acute cardiopulmonary decompensation. With an increased incidence of DVT in pregnant women, anesthesiologists need to be aware that these patients are prone to PTE. Evidence has shown that many women who develop DVT during pregnancy have a high prevalence of a mutation of Arg 506 in the Factor V gene (i.e., Factor V Leiden).[139] These women have a resistance to protein C, an important factor in neutralizing thrombin. Some advocate screening for all pregnant women,[140] since the risk of thromboembolic disease is ten-fold in heterozygotes and one hundred-fold in homozygotes. Knowledge of the signs and symptoms of PTE is important for early diagnosis and management. Anticoagulation with heparin is the standard management; however, this may increase the risk of bleeding in the peripartum period.

The entrainment of small quantities of air into the vascular compartment is a relatively common occurrence that rarely produces clinically detectable effects. Larger volumes of air with sufficiently rapid intravascular entrainment, however, can result in functional compromise. Patients undergoing CS using regional anesthesia, with the uterus exteriorized, who develop hypovolemia are at a high risk of VAE. Continuous monitoring of end-tidal oxygen concentration and dynamic lung compliance with side-stream spirometry may be useful in detecting VAE in high risk patients.

Although our understanding of AFE syndrome has increased, it still remains an unpredictable and unpreventable event with high maternal mortality. AFE is usually heralded by a sudden onset of oxygen desaturation, respiratory distress, and cardiovascular collapse. Consumptive coagulopathy and respiratory distress syndrome are the most common complications observed in patients who survive acute AFE. Clinicians must retain a high degree of suspicion, particularly in clinical settings in which the risk of embolism is high. Current diagnostic and monitoring techniques allow objective evaluation of cardiac function and make it possible for rational treatment and precise interpretation of the response to therapy. Early recognition, invasive monitoring, and aggressive management should improve the outcome.

References

1. Kaunitz AM, Hughes JW, Grimes DA, et al. Causes of maternal mortality in the United States. Obstet Gynecol 1985;65:605.
2. Resnik R, Swartz WH, Plumer MH, et al. Amniotic fluid embolism with survival. Obstet Gynecol 1976;47:295.
3. Malinow AM, Naulty JS, Hunt CO, et al. Precordial ultrasonic monitoring during cesarean delivery. Anesthesiology 1987; 66:816.
4. Fong J, Gadalla F, Pierri MK, Druzin M. Are Doppler detected venous emboli during cesarean section air emboli? Anesth Analg 1990;71:254.
5. Karuparthy VR, Downing JW, Husain FJ, et al. Incidence of venous air embolism during cesarean section is unchanged by the use of a 5–10° head-up tilt. Anesth Analg 1989;69:620.
6. Vartikar JV, Johnson MD, Datta S. Precordial Doppler monitoring and pulse oximetry during cesarean delivery: detection of venous air embolism. Reg Anesth 1989;14:145.
7. Handler JS, Bromage PR. Venous air embolism during cesarean delivery. Reg Anesth 1990;15:170.
8. Bonnar J. Venous thromboembolism and pregnancy. Clin Obstet Gynecol 1981;8:455.
9. Weiner CP. Diagnosis and management of thromboembolic disease during pregnancy. Clin Obstet Gynecol 1985;28:107.
10. Polak JF, Wilkinson DL. Ultrasonographic diagnosis of symptomatic deep venous thrombosis in pregnancy. Am J Obstet Gynecol 1991;165:625.
11. Rothbard MJ, Gluck D, Stone ML. Anticoagulation therapy in antepartum pulmonary embolism. N Y State J Med 1976;76:582.
12. Friend JR, Kakkar VV. The diagnosis of deep vein thrombosis in the puerperium. J Obstet Gynecol Br Common 1970;77:820.
13. Brown CEL, Lowe TW, Cunningham FG, Weinreb JC. Puerperal pelvic thrombophlebitis: Impact on diagnosis and treatment using x-ray computed tomography and magnetic resonance imaging. Obstet Gynecol 1986;68:789.
14. Bolan JC. Thromboembolic complications of pregnancy. Clin Obstet Gynecol 1983;26:913.
15. Villasanta U. Thromboembolic disease in pregnancy. Am J Obstet Gynecol 1965;93:142.
16. Rochat RW, Koonin LM, Atrash HK, Jewitt JF. Maternal Mortality in the United States: Report from the Maternal Mortality Collaborative. Obstet Gynecol 1988;72:91.
17. Abrams ME, Metters JS (eds). Report on Confidential Enquiries into Maternal Deaths in the United Kingdom 1985–1987. London, HMSO, 1991.
18. Sachs BP, Brown DAJ, Driscoll SC, et al. Maternal mortality in Massachusetts. N Engl J Med 1987;316:667.
19. Gabel HD. Maternal mortality in South Carolina from 1970–1984: An analysis. Obstet Gynecol 1987;69:307.
20. Franks AL, Atrash HK, Lawson HW, Colberg KS. Obstetrical pulmonary embolism mortality: United States 1970–1985. Am J Public Health 1990;80:720.
21. Stirling Y, Woolf L, North WRS, Seghatchian MJ, Meade TW. Haemostasis in normal pregnancy. Thromb Haemostas 1984; 52:176.
22. Weiner CP, Kwaan H, Hauck WW, et al. Fibrin generation in normal pregnancy. Obstet Gynecol 1984;64:46.
23. Norris LA, Sheppard BL, Bonnar J. Increased whole blood platelet aggregation in normal pregnancy can be prevented in vitro by aspirin and dazmergel (UK 38485). Br J Obstet Gynaecol 1992;99:253.
24. Sharma SK, Wallace DH, Sidawi JE, et al. Thromboelastography with disposable cups and pins: Normal measurements in nonpregnant, pregnant and postpartum women (abstract). Anesth Analg 1995;80:S432.
25. Gerbasi FR, Bottoms S, Farag A, Mammen EF. Increased intravascular coagulation associated with pregnancy. Obstet Gynecol 1990;75:385.
26. Gerbasi FR, Bottoms S, Farag A, Mammen EF. Changes in hemostatic activity during delivery and the immediate postpartum period. Am J Obstet Gynecol 1990;162:1158.

27. Bergqvist A, Bergqvist D, Hallbook T. Acute deep vein thrombosis (DVT) after cesarean section. Acta Obstet Gynecol Scand 1979;58:473.

28. Sipes SL, Weiner CP. Venous thromboembolic disease in pregnancy. Semin Perinatol 1990;14:103.

29. Gal TJ. Causes and consequences of impaired gas exchange. In Benumof J, Saidman L (eds). Anesthesia and Perioperative Complications. St. Louis, CV Mosby, 1992, p 203.

30. Spence TH. Pulmonary embolization syndrome. In Civetta JM, Taylor RM, Kirby RR (eds): Critical Care. Philadelphia, JB Lippincott, 1988, p 1091.

31. Kakkar VV, Howe CT, Flanc C, Clarke MB. Natural history of post-operative deep vein thrombosis. Lancet 1969;2:230.

32. Kakkar VV, Sasahara AA. Diagnosis of venous thrombosis and pulmonary embolism. In Bloom AL, Thomas DP (eds): Haemostasis and Thrombosis. Edinburgh, Churchill Livingstone, 1987, p 779.

33. Greer IA, Barry J, Mackon N, Allan PL. Diagnosis of deep venous thrombosis in pregnancy a new role for diagnostic ultrasound. Br J Obstet Gynaecol 1990;97:53.

34. Hull R, van Aken WG, Hirsh J, et al. Impedance plethysmography using the occlusive cuff technique in the diagnosis of venous thrombosis. Circulation 1976;53:696.

35. Mintz MC, Levy DW, Axel L, et al. Puerperal ovarian vein thrombosis: MR diagnosis. Am J Radiol 1987;149:1273.

36. Matthew JP, Fleisher LA, Rinehouse JA, et al. ST segment depression during labor and delivery. Anesthesiology 1992;77:635.

37. Palmer CM, Norris MC, Giudici MC, et al. Incidence of electrocardiographic changes during cesarean delivery under regional anesthesia. Anesth Analg 1990;70:36.

38. McLinte AJ, Pringle SD, Lilley S, et al. Electrocardiographic changes during cesarean section under regional anesthesia. Anesth Analg 1992;74:51.

39. Eisenach JC, Tuttle R, Stein A. Is ST segment depression of the electrocardiogram during cesarean section merely due to cardiac sympathetic block? Anesth Analg 1994;78:287.

40. Vohra N, Alvarez M, Abramson AF, Lockwood CJ. Hypoplastic pulmonary artery: An unusual entity mimicking pulmonary embolism during pregnancy. Obstet Gynecol 1992;80:483.

41. Rosenberg JM, Lefor AT, Kenien G, et al. Echocardiographic diagnosis and surgical treatment of postpartum pulmonary embolism. Ann Thorac Surg 1990;49:667.

42. Ginsberg JS, Hirsh J, Rainbow AJ, Coates G. Risks to the fetus of radiologic procedures used in the diagnosis of maternal venous thromboembolic diseases. Thromb Haemost 1989;61:189.

43. Mossman KL, Hill LT. Radiation risks in pregnancy. Obstet Gynecol 1982;60:237.

44. Rosenow III EC. Venous and pulmonary thromboembolism: An algorithmic approach to diagnosis and management. Mayo Clin Proc 1995;70:45.

45. Barbour LA, Pickard J. Controversies in thromboembolic disease during pregnancy: A critical review. Obstet Gynecol 1995;86:621.

46. Dalen JE, Alpert JS. Natural history of pulmonary embolism. Prog Cardiovasc Dis 1975;17:259.

47. Jones TK, Barnes RW, Greenfield J. Greenfield vena caval filter: Rationale and current indications. Ann Thorac Surg 1986;42:S48.

48. Declos GL, Davila F. Thrombolytic therapy for pulmonary embolism in pregnancy: A case report. Am J Obstet Gynecol 1986;155:375.

49. Fagher B, Ahlgren M, Astedt B. Acute massive pulmonary embolism treated with streptokinase during labor and the early puerperium. Acta Obstet Gynecol Scand 1990;69:659.

50. Hall RJC, Young C, Sutton GC, Cambell S. Treatment of acute massive pulmonary embolism by streptokinase during labor and delivery. Br Med J 1972;4:647.

51. Kramer WB, Belfort M, Saade GR, et al. Successful urokinase treatment of massive pulmonary embolism in pregnancy. Obstet Gynecol 1995;86:660.

52. Flossdorf T, Breulmann M, Hopf HB. Successful treatment of massive pulmonary embolism with recombinant tissue type plasminogen activator (rt-PA) in a pregnant woman with intact gravidity and preterm labour. Intensive Care Med 1990;16:454.

53. Blegvad S, Lund O, Nielsen TT, Guldholt I. Emergency embolectomy in a patient with massive pulmonary embolism during second trimester pregnancy. Acta Obstet Gynecol Scand 1989;68:267.

54. Splinter WM, Dwane PD, Wigle RD, McGrath MJ. Anaesthetic management of emergency cesarean section followed by pulmonary embolectomy. Can J Anaesth 1989;36:689.

55. Harik J, Raichle ME, Reis DJ. Spontaneously remitting spinal epidural hematoma in a patient on anticoagulants. N Engl J Med 1971;284:1355.

56. Dickman CA, Shedd SA, Spetzler RF, et al. Spinal epidural hematoma associated with epidural anesthesia: Complications of systemic heparinization in patients receiving peripheral vascular thrombolytic therapy. Anesthesiology 1990;72:947.

57. Flanagan J, Slimack J, Black D, et al. The incidence of venous air embolism in the parturient (abstract). Reg Anesth 1990;15:A10.

58. Hill BF, Jones JS. Venous air embolism following orogenital sex during pregnancy. Am J Emerg Med 1993;11:155.

59. Nelson PK. Pulmonary gas embolism in pregnancy and the puerperium. Obstet Gynecol Surv 1960;15:449.

60. O'Quin RJ, Lakshminarayan S. Venous air embolism. Arch Intern Med 1982;142:2173.

61. Younker D, Rodriguez V, Kavanagh J. Massive air embolism during cesarean section. Anesthesiology 1986;65:77.

62. Fong J, Gadalla F, Gimbel AA. Precordial Doppler diagnosis of haemodynamically compromising air embolism during caesarean section. Can J Anaesth 1990;37:262.

63. Steiner PE, Lushbaugh CC. Maternal pulmonary embolism by amniotic fluid. JAMA 1941;117:1245.

64. Adornato DC, Gildenberg PL, Ferrario CM, et al. Pathophysiology of intravenous air embolism in dogs. Anesthesiology 1978;49:120.

65. Butler BD, Hills BA. Transpulmonary passage of venous air emboli. J Appl Physiol 1985;59:543.

66. Clark MC, Flick MR. Permeability pulmonary edema caused by venous air embolism. Am Rev Respir Dis 1984;129:633.

67. Ohkuda K, Nakahara K, Weidner WJ, et al. Lung fluid exchange after uneven pulmonary artery obstruction in sheep. Circ Res 1978;43:152.

68. Richardson HF, Coles BC, Hall GE. Experimental gas embolism: I. Intravenous air embolism. Can Med Assoc J 1937;36:584.

69. Bromage PR, Hohman WA. Uterine posture and incidence of venous air embolism (VAE) during cesarean section (abstract). Reg Anesth 1991;15:S29.

70. Skerman JH, Huckaby T, Otterson WN. Emboli in pregnancy. In Datta S (ed): Anesthetic and Obstetrical Management of High-Risk Pregnancy. St. Louis, Mosby-YearBook, 1991, p 495.

71. Fong J, Gadalla F, Druzin M. Venous emboli occurring during cesarean section: The effect of patient position. Can J Anaesth 1991;38:191.

72. Durant TM, Long J, Oppenheimer MJ. Pulmonary (venous) air embolism. Am Heart J 1947;33:269.

73. Gronert GA, Messick JM, Cucchiara RF, Michenfelder JD. Paradoxical air embolism from a patent foramen ovale. Anesthesiology 1979;50:548.

74. Michel L, Pokanzer DC, Mckusick KA, et al. Fatal paradoxical air embolism to the brain: Complication of central venous catheterization. J Parenter Enteral Nutr 1982;6:68.

75. English JB, Westenskow D, Hodges MR, Stanley TH. Comparison of venous air embolism monitoring methods in supine dogs. Anesthesiology 1978;48:425.

76. Chang JL, Albin MS, Bunegin L, et al. Analysis and comparison of venous air embolism detection methods. Neurosurgery 1980;7:135.

77. Albin MS, Carroll RG, Marron JC. Clinical considerations concerning detection of venous air embolism. Neurosurgery 1978;3:380.

78. Peters SG. Mediastinal air-fluid level and respiratory failure. Chest 1988;94:1063.

79. Kytta J, Randell T, Tanskanen P, et al. Monitoring lung compliance and end-tidal oxygen content for the detection of venous air embolism. Br J Anaesth 1995;75:447.

80. Meyer JR. Embolis pulmonar-caseosa. Braz J Med Biol Res 1926;1:301.

81. Steiner PE, Lushbaugh CC. Maternal pulmonary embolism by amniotic fluid as a cause of obstetric shock and unexpected death in obstetrics. JAMA 1941;117:1341.

82. Morgan M. Amniotic fluid embolism. Anaesthesia 1979;34:20.

83. Peterson EP, Taylor HB. Amniotic fluid embolism—an analysis of 40 cases. Obstet Gynecol 1970;35:787.

84. Courtney LD. Amniotic fluid embolism. Obstet Gynecol Survey 1974;29:169.
85. Clark SL. Amniotic fluid embolism. Crit Care Clin 1991;7:877.
86. Guha-Ray DK. Maternal mortality in an urban hospital. A fifteen-year study. Obstet Gynecol 1976;47:430.
87. Clark SL. New concepts of amniotic fluid embolism: A review. Obstet Gynecol Surv 1990;45:360.
88. Clark SL. Amniotic fluid embolism. Clin Perinatol 1986;13:801.
89. Clark SL, Cotton DB, Gonik B, et al. Central hemodynamic alterations in amniotic fluid embolism. Am J Obstet Gynecol 1988;158:1124.
90. Clark SL, Montz FJ, Phelan JP. Hemodynamic alterations associated with amniotic fluid embolism: A reappraisal. Am J Obstet Gynecol 1985;151:617.
91. Girard P, Mal H, Laine JF, et al. Left heart failure in amniotic fluid embolism. Anesthesiology 1986;64:262.
92. Reis RL, Pierce WS, Behrendt DM. Hemodynamic effects of amniotic fluid embolism. Surg Gynecol Obstet 1969;129:45.
93. Liban E, Raz S. A clinicopathologic study of fourteen cases of amniotic fluid embolism. Am J Clin Pathol 1969;51:477.
94. Courtney LD. Coagulation failure in pregnancy. Br Med J 1970;1:691.
95. Ratnoff OD, Vosburgh GJ. Observations of the clotting defect in amniotic fluid embolism. N Engl J Med 1952;247:970.
96. Bellar FK, Douglas GW, Debrovner CH, Robinson R. The fibrinolytic system in amniotic fluid embolism. Am J Obstet Gynecol 1963;87:48.
97. Phillips LL, Davidson EC. Procoagulant properties of amniotic fluid. Am J Obstet Gynecol 1972;113:911.
98. Lockwood CJ, Bach R, Guha A, et al. Amniotic fluid contains tissue factor, a potent initiator of coagulation. Am J Obstet Gynecol 1991;165:1335.
99. Azegami M, Mori N. Amniotic fluid embolism and leukotrienes. Am J Obstet Gynecol 1986;155:1119.
100. Karim SMM, Devlin J. Prostaglandin content of amniotic fluid during pregnancy and labour. J Obstet Gynaecol Br Cwlth 1967;74:230.
101. Hankins GDV, Snyder RR, Clark SL, et al. Acute hemodynamic and respiratory effects of amniotic fluid embolism in the pregnant goat model. Am J Obstet Gynecol 1993;168:1113.
102. Cromey MG, Taylor PJ, Cumming DC. Probable amniotic fluid embolism after first trimester pregnancy termination. J Reprod Med 1983;28:209.
103. Meier PR, Bowes WA. Amniotic fluid embolus-like syndrome presenting in the second trimester of pregnancy. Obstet Gynecol 1983;61:31S.
104. Mallory GK, Blackburn N, Sparling J, Nickerson DA. Maternal pulmonary embolism by amniotic fluid. Report of three cases and discussion of the literature. N Engl J Med 1950;243:583.
105. Chang M, Herbert WNP. Retinal arteriolar occlusions following amniotic fluid embolism. Ophthalmology 1984;91:1634.
106. Ricou B, Reper P, Sutur PM. Rapid diagnosis of amniotic fluid embolism causing severe pulmonary failure. Intensive Care Med 1989;15:129.
107. Garland IWC, Thompson WD. Diagnosis of amniotic fluid embolism using an antiserum to human keratin. J Clin Pathol 1983;36:625.
108. Kanayama N, Yamazaki T, Naruse H, et al. Determining zinc coproporphyrin in maternal plasma—a new method for diagnosing amniotic fluid embolism. Clin Chem 1992;38:526.
109. Kobayashi H, Ohi H, Terao T. A simple, noninvasive, sensitive method for diagnosis of amniotic fluid embolism by monoclonal antibody TKH-2 that recognizes NeuAca2-6 GalNAc. Am J Obstet Gynecol 1993;168:848.
110. Masson RG, Ruggieri J, Siddiqui MM. Pulmonary microvascular cytology. A new diagnosis application of the pulmonary artery catheter. Chest 1985;88:908.
111. Lee W, Ginsburg KA, Colton DB, et al. Squamous and trophoblastic cells in the maternal pulmonary circulation identified by invasive hemodynamic monitoring during the peripartum period. Am J Obstet Gynecol 1986;155:999.
112. Plauche WC. Amniotic fluid embolism. Am J Obstet Gyncecol 1983;147:982.
113. Clark SL, Pavlova A, Greenspoon J, et al. Squamous cells in the maternal pulmonary circulation. Am J Obstet Gynecol 1986;154:104.
114. Giampaolo C, Schnider V, Kowalski BH, et al. The cytologic diagnosis of amniotic fluid embolism: A critical reappraisal. Diagn Cytopathol 1987;3:126.
115. Oates S, Williams GL, Rees GAD. Cardiopulmonary resuscitation in late pregnancy. Br Med J 1988;297:404.
116. Esposito RA, Grossi EA, Coppa G, et al. Successful treatment of postpartum shock caused by amniotic fluid embolism with cardiopulmonary bypass and pulmonary artery thromboembolectomy. Am J Obstet Gynecol 1990;163:572.
117. Weksler N, Ovadia L, Stav A, et al. Continuous arteriovenous hemofiltration in the treatment of amniotic fluid embolism. Int J Obstet Anesth 1994;3:92.
118. Sprung J, Cheng SY, Patel S. When to remove an epidural catheter in a parturient with disseminated intravascular coagulation. Reg Anesth 1992;17:351.
119. Sprung J, Rakic M, Patel S. Amniotic fluid embolism during epidural anesthesia for cesarean section. Acta Anaesth Belg 1991;42:225.
120. Gurd AR, Wilson RI. The fat embolism syndrome. J Bone Joint Surg 1974;56B:408.
121. Lindeque BGP, Schoeman HS, Dommisse GF, et al. Fat embolism and the fat embolism syndrome. A double-blind therapeutic study. J Bone Joint Surg 1987;69B:128.
122. Riska EB, Myllynen P. Fat embolism in patients with multiple injuries. J Trauma 1982;22:891.
123. Levy D. The fat embolism syndrome. Clin Orthop 1990;261:81.
124. Peltier LF. Fat embolism. A current concept. Clin Orthop 1969;66:241.
125. ten Duis HJ, Nijsten MW, Klasen JH, Binnendijk B. Fat embolism in patients with an isolated fracture of the femoral shaft. J Trauma 1988;28:383.
126. Fabian TC, Hoots AV, Stanford DS, et al. Fat embolism syndrome: Prospective evaluation in 92 fracture patients. Crit Care Med 1990;18:42.
127. Lozman J, Deno C, Feustel PJ, et al. Pulmonary and cardiovascular consequences of immediate fixation or conservative management of long-bone fractures. Arch Surg 1986;121:992.
128. Shapiro MP, Hayes JA. Fat embolism in sickle cell disease. Report of a case with brief review of the literature. Arch Intern Med 1984;144:181.
129. Jones MB. Pulmonary fat emboli associated with acute fatty liver of pregnancy (Letters to the Editor). Am J Gastroenterol 1993;88:791.
130. Pazell JA, Peltier LF. Experience with sixty-three patients with fat embolism. Surg Gynecol Obstet 1972;135:77.
131. Capan LM, Miller SM, Patel KP. Fat embolism. Anesth Clin North Am 1993;2:25.
132. Poddar D, Maude GH, Plant MJ, et al. Pregnancy in Jamaican women with homozygous sickle cell disease: Fetal and maternal outcome. Br J Obstet Gynaecol 1986;93:727.
133. Esseltine DW, Baxter MRN, Bevan JC. Sickle cell states and the anaesthetist. Can J Anaesth 1988;35:385.
134. Dunn A, Davies A, Eckert G, et al. Intraoperative death during cesarean section in a patient with a sickle-cell trait. Can J Anaesth 1987;34:67.
135. Winterbaur RH, Elfenbein IB, Ball WC. Incidence and clinical significance of tumor embolization to the lungs. Am J Med 1968;45:271.
136. Starr DS, Lawrie GM, Morris GC. Unusual presentation of bronchogenic carcinoma. Case report and review of the literature. Cancer 1981;47:398.
137. Griffith GL, Maull KI, Sachatello CR. Septic pulmonary embolism. Surg Gynecol Obstet 1977;144:105.
138. Louria DB. Embolic infections of the lungs. In Baum GL, Wolinsky E (eds): Textbook of Pulmonary Diseases, 3rd ed. Boston, Little, Brown, 1983, p 501.
139. Thomas DP. Venous thrombosis revisited (editorial). Blood Coag Fibrinol 1996;7:583.
140. Vandenbroucke JP, van der Meer FJ, Helmerhorst FM, Rosendaal FR. Factor V Leiden: should we screen oral contraceptive users and pregnant women? Br Med J (Clin Res Ed) 1996;313:1127.

11

TRANSPLANTATION

Kerri M. Robertson, M.D.

Transplantation is recognized as a life-saving therapy for individuals suffering from end-stage organ failure. Currently, the transplant community accepts both severity-of-disease and quality-of-life indications for transplant eligibility. For many young women and children coping with major organ failure, transplantation allows them the opportunity to attain normal reproductive capacity, with the choice of subsequent childbearing. The most extensive experience with pregnancy in the post-transplant parturient has been in renal recipients, with isolated cases and small series reported after liver, heart, heart-lung, and pancreas-kidney transplantation. Despite the inherent increased maternal, fetal, and graft risks, a successful outcome in such pregnancies is achievable.

This chapter reviews the literature concerning pregnancy after kidney, pancreas-kidney, liver, heart, and lung transplantation including historical overview; registry data; risks for the mother, fetus, and graft during pregnancy; pregnancy physiology and impact on graft function; immunosuppressive therapy; and specific anesthetic considerations and controversies, with suggestions for management of labor and delivery.

HISTORICAL OVERVIEW: PAST TO PRESENT

The hallmarks for a successful pregnancy reported in a transplant recipient occurred in 1958 (twin-twin kidney donor),[1] 1966 (living related kidney donor),[2] 1970 (cadaver kidney donor: azathioprine),[3] 1976 (liver: azathioprine),[4] 1983 (cadaver kidney donor: cyclosporine [CyA]),[5] 1986 (pancreas-kidney),[6] 1988 (heart),[7] 1988 (liver: CyA, azathioprine),[8] 1989 (heart-lungs),[9] and 1992 (ABO-incompatible kidney).[10] In addition, parturients have successfully undergone more than one pregnancy, including the delivery of twins and triplets. Most of the earlier reports described post-transplant pregnancy and lactation with azathioprine and prednisone immunosuppression. The introduction of CyA in 1978 and FK506 in 1986 has led to significant improve-

ments in patient and graft survival rates, making childbearing a realistic consideration.

Statistics

Advances in the past two decades in donor and recipient surgical techniques, organ preservation, immunosuppression, detection of rejection and rejection treatment have resulted in an ever-expanding pool of female patients who, following organ transplantation, are healthy and have an excellent chance of survival during and beyond their reproductive years. Table 11–1 shows data provided by the United Network for Organ Sharing (UNOS) summarizing the number of organ transplants performed in the United States for females

TABLE 11–1. **UNITED NETWORK FOR ORGAN SHARING; NUMBER OF ORGAN TRANSPLANTS PERFORMED ON FEMALES LESS THAN 34 YEARS: 1988–1993**

Organ	Donor Type	1988 N	1989 N	1990 N	1991 N	1992 N	1993 N
Kidney	Cadaveric	971	988	996	951	911	928
	Living	436	440	498	550	507	565
	Total	1407	1428	1494	1501	1418	1493
Liver	Cadaveric	353	388	414	406	398	419
	Living	0	2	10	11	17	22
	Total	353	390	424	417	415	441
Pancreas	Cadaveric	51	102	94	102	122	140
	Living	1	1	2	0	1	0
	Total	52	103	96	102	123	140
Heart	Cadaveric	111	113	146	165	170	161
	Living	0	0	2	0	0	1
	Total	111	113	148	165	170	162
Lung	Cadaveric	4	11	32	67	69	77
	Living	0	0	1	4	0	6
	Total	4	11	33	71	69	83
Heart/ Lung	Cadaveric	22	21	12	14	12	27
	Living	0	0	0	0	0	0
	Total	22	21	12	14	12	27
Total	Cadaveric	1512	1623	1694	1705	1682	1752
	Living	437	443	513	565	525	594
	Total	1949	2066	2207	2270	2207	2346

Based on UNOS OPTN data as of August 14, 1995.
Data subject to change based on future data submission or correction.

TABLE 11–2. **UNITED NETWORK FOR ORGAN SHARING; PATIENT SURVIVAL RATES FOR ORGAN TRANSPLANTS IN FEMALES: 10/01/87–12/31/93 WHERE RECIPIENT WAS UNDER 34 YEARS OLD**

Organ	1-Year Survival			3-Year Survival		
	N	*%*	*Std Err*	*N*	*%*	*Std Err*
Kidney	17,558	96.63	0.13	10,251	93.62	0.19
Liver	3801	79.98	0.61	2661	75.53	0.69
Pancreas	1075	91.51	0.80	642	84.82	1.15
Heart	2109	79.22	0.85	1530	71.12	1.01
Lung	422	71.71	2.11	254	52.87	2.88
Heart/Lung	187	63.09	2.46	144	52.05	3.83

N = number of cases with follow-up at the given interval.
Based on UNOS Scientific Registry data as of August 14, 1995.
Data subject to change based on future data submission or correction.

TABLE 11–4. **UNITED NETWORK FOR ORGAN SHARING; NUMBER OF REGISTRATIONS ON WAITING LIST AT YEAR END 1993 FOR FEMALES UNDER 34 YEARS OLD**

Organ	Number of Registrations
Kidney	3205
Liver	372
Pancreas	39
Kidney-pancreas	170
Heart	110
Lung	206
Heart-lung	71
Total	4173

Based on UNOS OPTN data as of August 16, 1995.
Data subject to change based on future data submission or correction.

under age 34 years, by organ and donor type, for 1988 to 1993. Tables 11–2 and 11–3 indicate the 1- and 3-year patient and graft survival statistics for the corresponding recipient groups. Table 11–4 is the number of registrations for females under age 34 years on the UNOS waiting list at 1993 year's end.

Conception

Following kidney transplantation and resolution of uremia, endocrine and menstrual function is restored within 1 to 14 months (mean 4.2 months), correlating closely with the level of renal function and pattern of rejection episodes.[11] Resumption of normal menstrual function and fertility following liver transplantation also frequently occurs, with reports of a median period of 8 weeks[12] and overall interval of 10 months[13] in women with prior nonalcoholic chronic liver disease. Conception, followed by an uncomplicated pregnancy, has been reported as early as 3 weeks following liver transplantation[14] and 4 months after heart transplantation.[15]

An understanding of the optimal criteria for consideration of pregnancy in transplant recipients will alert the physician to those patients who, not satisfying these prerequisites, may anticipate a prohibitively high-risk antenatal and peripartum course (Tables 11–5,[16] 11–6,[17] and 11–7[18]).

Kidney and Pancreas-Kidney

Although the incidence of pregnancy in reproductive-age women on long-term hemodialysis is estimated as 1 in 200, there is high fetal wastage at all stages of pregnancy, with a live birth outcome rate of 19%, at best.[16] Fifteen years ago it was estimated that about 1 in 50 women of childbearing age with a functioning renal transplant became pregnant,[19] with an average interval from surgery to conception of 35 months (4 weeks to 13 years). In reviewing single-center studies, the incidence of post-transplant parenthood has been reported as high as 20%. This has accounted for more than 5000 pregnancies reported worldwide in the past 30 years.

The recommended waiting period of 2 years before considering pregnancy after kidney transplantation is

TABLE 11–3. **UNITED NETWORK FOR ORGAN SHARING; GRAFT SURVIVAL RATES FOR ORGAN TRANSPLANTS IN FEMALES: 10/01/87–12/21/93 WHERE RECIPIENT WAS UNDER 34 YEARS OLD**

Organ	1-Year Survival			3-Year Survival		
	N	*%*	*Std Err*	*N*	*%*	*Std Err*
Kidney	18,377	84.09	0.26	12,688	72.99	0.34
Liver	4503	66.88	0.68	3494	59.66	0.74
Pancreas	1168	72.27	1.27	828	61.41	1.49
Heart	2153	77.51	0.87	1590	68.67	1.03
Lung	434	69.51	2.14	273	49.05	2.85
Heart/Lung	189	62.36	3.46	148	50.30	3.81

N = number of cases with follow-up at the given interval.
Based on UNOS Scientific Registry data as of August 14, 1995.
Data subject to change based on future data submission or correction.

TABLE 11–5. **CRITERIA FOR CONSIDERATION OF PREGNANCY IN KIDNEY AND PANCREAS-KIDNEY TRANSPLANT RECIPIENTS**

1. Good general health
2. Elapsed time from transplant surgery 24 months, possibly 1 year for a living donor recipient
3. Minimal or no proteinuria
4. Hypertension, if present, minimal and easily controlled
5. No clinical or laboratory evidence of graft rejection in the preceeding 6 to 12 months
6. Mild renal dysfunction with a serum creatinine of less than 1.8 μmol/l (2 mg/dl) or preferably less than 1.25 μmol/l (1.4 mg/dl)
7. Stable maintenance level of immunosuppressive therapy
   Prednisone alternate-days or 15 mg/day or less
   Azathioprine 2 mg•kg^{-1}•day^{-1} or less
   With or without CyA 5 mg•kg^{-1}•day^{-1} or less
8. No pelvicalyceal distension on a recent intravenous pyelogram
9. Stature compatible with good obstetric outcome

TABLE 11–6. CRITERIA FOR CONSIDERATION OF PREGNANCY IN LIVER TRANSPLANT RECIPIENTS

1. Pregnancy avoided for at least the first 6 months and preferably 9 to 12 months after transplantation
2. Evidence of stabilization of liver function and recovery from surgical complications
3. Completion of post-transplant prophylactic treatment of opportunistic infections, with no evidence of active viral infection
4. Maintenance immunosuppressive therapy
5. No evidence of acute rejection

based on evidence suggesting that at this time, stable renal function indicates a high probability of graft survival at 5 years (80% with cadaver kidneys). In addition, with minimal immunosuppressive therapy, the incidence of premature deliveries and low-birth-weight infants may be reduced.[20, 21] Marushak and coworkers[22] found that women who did not meet this criteria had a two-to threefold increase in the rates of pre-eclampsia, prematurity, and intrauterine growth retardation.

These guidelines are largely based on experience with azathioprine and prednisone maintenance therapy in patients receiving cadaver donor kidneys (see Table 11–5). A significantly greater proportion of CyA-treated women have prepregnancy hypertension, diabetes, elevated serum creatinine levels, and shorter transplant-to-pregnancy intervals, which may put them at even greater risk for delivery of low-birth-weight infants or graft loss.[23–25]

Liver

Consideration of pregnancy in liver transplant recipients coincides with avoiding periods when cytomegalovirus (CMV) infection is most likely, because poor maternal outcome and neonatal death may result.[26] *Listeria* or cryptococcal infections occur at any time after transplantation, whereas CMV, toxoplasmosis, and opportunistic infections usually occur in the first 6 months.[27] Most graft dysfunction and complications occur in the first year postoperatively, leading to the

TABLE 11–7. CRITERIA FOR CONSIDERATION OF PREGNANCY IN HEART AND HEART-LUNG TRANSPLANT RECIPIENTS

1. Pregnancy is generally not recommended in the first year after heart transplantation, and ideally not for 2 years post-transplant, to allow for recovery from primary and secondary disease processes
2. Asymptomatic, normal exercise tolerance, New York Heart Association Functional Class I
3. Well-preserved ventricular function (echocardiography and cardiac catheterization)
4. No evidence of coronary atherosclerosis by angiography
5. Stable immunosuppressive regimen
6. No evidence of rejection on endomyocardial biopsy
7. Normal or near-normal renal function

recommendation of postponing pregnancy for 12 months and in some programs for at least 2 years after liver transplantation.[28]

Heart and Heart-Lung

Myocardial rejection is most likely to occur in the first 90 days after transplantation and is rare beyond 1 year. Nevertheless, surveillance endomyocardial biopsies are often performed on a regular basis, indefinitely.[29] Limitations for the detection of rejection may be imposed by the concern of a potential teratogenic risk of performing right ventricular endomyocardial biopsies or coronary angiography under radiographic guidance.[15] Before pregnancy is considered, there should be no biopsy evidence of rejection, and cardiac catheterization should indicate normal cardiac performance (normal cardiac index, normal coronary vasculature, and absence of ventricular wall motion abnormalities).

Sterilization had once routinely been advised for female heart transplant recipients of childbearing age. An assessment of the predictive "risk" of pregnancy for the mother and fetus is based on reviewing an isolated number of single case reports of pregnancies after heart and heart-lung transplantation. Extrapolation from outcome studies of pregnancies in immunosuppressed renal transplant recipients is then done. An individual's decision to take this risk must also include consideration of the uncertainty of their life expectancy following transplantation (12-year heart transplantation survival <40%, 10-year heart-lung transplantation survival <20%, and 4-year single and bilateral/double lung transplantation survivals <40%[30]).

PREGNANCY AND RISKS FOR THE MOTHER

Despite good preconceptual and peripartum graft function with minimal patient morbidity from immunosuppressive therapy and the coexistence of other diseases, pregnancy should be considered high risk, and a number of potential complications anticipated.

Kidney and Pancreas-Kidney

The age range of renal transplant patients who have completed successful pregnancies is 18 to 41 years.[31] It is estimated that 12% of women with renal grafts develop new long-term medical problems after pregnancy. This rate doubles if uncontrolled hypertension, renal deterioration, or rejection occurs before 28 weeks. It is difficult to know whether such problems are pregnancy-induced or whether they follow the natural time course for graft recipients.[32]

Hypertension and pre-eclampsia are common and frequently severe in pregnant transplant recipients. A blood pressure greater than 140/90 mm Hg in women with renal transplants should be treated early and aggressively.[33] Maintaining the diastolic pressure between 80 and 85 mm Hg may preserve renal function and prevent life-threatening hypertensive crisis or eclampsia. Hypertension, particularly before 28 weeks' gestation, is associated with adverse perinatal outcome.[34] Antihypertensive medications considered relatively safe during pregnancy include methyldopa, beta adrenergic antagonists, clonidine, hydralazine, nifedipine, and diuretics.[31, 35] Delivery of the infant, regardless of gestational age, should be considered when the patient develops a hypertensive crisis, seizures, or diastolic blood pressure over 110 mm Hg that is refractory to maximal therapy, and when no reversible aggravating factor can be elicited.[36]

There is an increased incidence of pre-eclampsia of 25 to 40% in the transplant patient, compared with 8% in the nontransplant patient.[16, 37, 38] Diagnosis of pre-eclampsia is difficult without a renal biopsy, because edema, proteinuria, hypertension, and increased serum uric acid levels may indicate exacerbation of pre-existing renal disease, cyclosporine toxicity, or acute rejection.[33] Abnormalities in the platelet count or in liver function tests may be consistent with pre-eclampsia or drug-induced changes in an otherwise uncomplicated pregnancy. The patients may be treated with low-dose aspirin to prevent the development of pre-eclampsia and fetal growth retardation.[39]

An increased incidence of bacterial infections of the genitourinary tract (as high as 40%) and, less frequently, opportunistic viral and fungal infections are seen as a result of chronic immunosuppression and exposure to blood products during years on hemodialysis. Diagnosis and treatment are dictated by verification of infection with culture and sensitivity and/or serologic monitoring, because uncommon organisms are frequently seen. Potential hazards to the mother and fetus include pulmonary, liver, and renal dysfunction; spontaneous abortion; intrauterine and perinatal infections producing a wide spectrum of pathology; intrauterine growth retardation; and preterm delivery. Cesarean birth is indicated if a cervical culture is positive for herpes simplex virus (HSV) at term, because the incidence of neonatal infection resulting from vaginal delivery is at least 50%. With premature rupture of membranes, waiting for greater fetal maturity may not be desirable in view of this enhanced susceptibility to infection.

After kidney transplantation, persistent hypercalcemia due to hyperparathyroidism frequently occurs in up to 20% of women, with the possibility of exacerbation at the beginning of the third trimester. This finding is associated with an increase in 1,25-dihydroxy vitamin D of placental origin.[40] Patients with moderate hypercalcemia (total serum calcium level 11.5–13 mg/dl) may show symptoms of lethargy, hypotension from polyuria, and/or nausea and vomiting with hypovolemia. A total serum calcium level exceeding 14 mg/dl represents a medical emergency because serious complications including hypertension, arrhythmias, complete heart block, severe neuromyopathic symptoms, and renal failure may result.[41]

Causes of maternal death include infection, renal failure, uterine rupture, gastroenteritis, and cerebrovascular and cardiac disease. Few deaths have been reported during or shortly after pregnancy; the majority occur 6 to 8 years later. In several small series, from 5 to 30% of renal transplant recipient mothers died during their offspring's childhood.[31, 42] This raises the concern of the advisability of childbearing, given the uncertainty of the quality of life and life expectancy of transplant recipients.

Physiologic Adaptations and Coexisting Systemic Disease

Residual physiologic alterations of end-stage renal disease (Table 11–8) potentially affect obstetrical outcome. Successful pregnancies have been reported in a number of transplant patients with coexisting systemic disease that renders them at high risk, in addition to their transplant-related considerations. The most common conditions include juvenile-onset diabetes mellitus, systemic lupus erythematosus (SLE), scleroderma, type 1 primary hyperoxaluria, sickle cell disease, and Wegener and Goodpasture syndromes.

In the patient with juvenile-onset diabetes, there is a twofold increase in the complication rate over other pregnant renal recipients. This is likely to be related to the vascular complications seen with severe longstanding diabetes.[6, 43, 44] In addition, immunosuppression adds to the complexity of the pregnancies with its increased risk of infection, potentially poor diabetic control, exacerbation of pre-existing hypertension, and thromboembolism. Fractures in these patients may be associated with steroid-induced osteoporosis, neuropathy, and vascular insufficiency compounded by increased calcium requirements and weight gain during pregnancy. It appears from isolated reports that the outlook for pregnancy in women with diabetic nephropathy may be better after combined pancreas-kidney transplantation.[45]

In the nontransplant parturient, although fasting and postprandial blood glucose levels frequently remain within the normal range, pregnancy results in a diabetogenic state.[46] The risk of developing gestational diabetes in nondiabetic women has been reported to be in the range of 0.15 to 12.3%, depending on the diagnostic criteria.[45] Glucosuria is a common finding, resulting

TABLE 11–8. PHYSIOLOGIC ALTERATIONS IN END-STAGE RENAL DISEASE

Neurologic	Central: lethargy, seizures, personality traits Peripheral: Sensory and motor neuropathy, autonomic dysfunction
Respiratory	Hypocarbia Pleural effusion, edema, pneumonitis, infection
Cardiovascular	Indeterminate volume status, susceptible to fluid overload High cardiac output Hypertension, left ventricular hypertrophy Accelerated peripheral and coronary atherosclerosis Tachycardia, arrhythmias, and conduction disorders Attenuated reactivity of the sympathetic nervous system Reduced oxygen-carrying capacity, increased peripheral extraction of O_2 Pericarditis, cardiac tamponade
Endocrine	Electrolyte disorders (hyperkalemia, hyperphosphatemia, hypermagnesemia, hypercalcemia, hyponatremia) Metabolic acidosis Secondary hyperparathyroidism Glucose intolerance
Gastrointestinal	Delayed gastric emptying and increased volume and acidity of gastric contents, aspiration risk
Musculoskeletal	Osteodystrophy, muscle wasting
Hematologic	Chronic anemia, right shift of hemoglobin dissociation curve Platelet dysfunction, coagulopathy Increased susceptibility to infection, carrier state for hepatitis B antigen and HIV
Altered drug effects	Reduced serum protein and abnormal binding Decreased drug or metabolic clearance Abnormal electrolyte and acid-base status Altered permeability of the blood-brain barrier Increased sensitivity to CNS depressants Reduced serum cholinesterase level Altered end-organ sensitivity or response or both Altered volume of distribution

from an increase in the filtered glucose load (increased GFR) and less efficient tubular reabsorption.

A segmental pancreas graft contains only 50% of the normal islet mass, and if the beta-cells cannot increase insulin secretion, hyperglycemia results. Therefore, the beta-cell mass may be the critical determinant of whether gestational diabetes occurs after total pancreatectomy and autologous islet transplantation.[47] Hyperglycemia following vascularized pancreatic transplantation may result from ischemia, rejection, steroids, CyA, or FK506. Surprisingly, transplanted islets, per se, are not associated with a high risk for gestational diabetes or insulin dependency post partum.[31]

Liver

A review of case reports and small patient series of pregnancies in liver transplant recipients treated with CyA or FK506 and prednisone identifies several problems previously discussed in recipients of renal allografts. Obstetric and medical complications include renal insufficiency, pre-eclampsia, anemia, hyperbilirubinemia, and CMV infection. The incidence of clinical toxemia in pregnant orthotopic liver transplant recipients is 10 to 20%,[48] and is more frequent in women with pre-existing renal dysfunction.

Physiologic Adaptations and Coexisting Systemic Disease

End-stage liver disease is associated with unique systemic physiologic alterations (Table 11–9). Factors contributing to hyperdynamic circulation in patients with chronic liver disease are summarized in Table 11–10.[49] Liver transplantation does not fully correct these splanchnic and systemic hemodynamic changes. Total liver blood flow is increased, despite the return of portal pressures to normal, with persistence of portal-systemic collaterals evident 4 years after transplantation.[50] Portal venous inflow is still under the influence of the normal vasomotor tone of the superior mesenteric artery, whereas the hepatic artery is denervated, which may be the main cause of the increase in hepatic perfusion. The potential long-term effect of persistently elevated liver blood flow on various metabolic pathways in the liver or disposition of high-hepatic-extraction drugs (i.e., lidocaine) is unknown.[51] Clinical implications of the loss of neural control of the hepatic vasculature may include an inability to vasoconstrict and shunt blood centrally in response to systemic hypotension, resulting in an increased susceptibility to hemorrhagic shock.[52]

Reported changes in the systemic hemodynamic status appear more controversial. Arterial hypertension and increased total systemic vascular resistance are consistent findings, but cardiac index has been observed to remain high in the presence of good liver function[53] and subsequently return to a more normal value.[50, 52, 54, 55] Compounding variables that may account for this difference in reporting include rejection, liver dysfunction, or immunosuppressive and antihypertensive therapy.[51] Insufficient data are available on the hemodynamic changes associated with pregnancy and delivery following liver transplantation.

The persistence of a high-output state generally is well tolerated. Significant increases in peripheral vascular resistance, due to the combined effect of the liver graft reversing the vasodilation in portal hypertension and to the vasoconstrictor effect of cyclosporine, may be physiologically detrimental in patients with evidence of coexisting cardiomyopathy or valvular insufficiency. Myocardial ischemia may occur in patients with underlying coronary artery disease or in those with coronary spasm or accelerated arteriosclerotic disease secondary to CyA and steroid therapy. The same hypercoagulable state contributing to hepatic artery thrombosis after liver transplantation may cause intracoronary thrombosis and myocardial ischemia in the absence of significant coronary disease.[56] CMV is the most common opportunistic viral infection following liver transplantation and, although frequently asymptomatic, may be associated with serious complications,

TABLE 11–9. CARDIOVASCULAR, PULMONARY, AND RENAL COMPLICATIONS OF ADVANCED CIRRHOSIS

Cardiovascular

"Hyperdynamic circulation"
  High cardiac index and stroke volume
  Low systemic vascular resistance
  Low-to-normal mean arterial pressure (widened pulse pressure)
  Mild tachycardia
Central hypovolemia
  Increased total blood volume
  Decreased effective plasma volume
  Increased sympathetic tone
Hyporesponsiveness of the vasculature to pressor therapy
Flow-dependent oxygen consumption
Hepatic and splanchnic vasculature
  Portal hypertension
  Portal-systemic collateral circulation
  Decreased hepatic blood flow

Pulmonary

Arterial hypoxemia (PaO_2 <70 mm Hg)
  Intrapulmonary vascular abnormalities
    Intrapulmonary shunting (precapillary or arteriovenous intrapulmonary vascular dilatations)
    Portal-pulmonary or pleural shunting
    Ventilation/perfusion mismatch (pleural effusions, ascites and diaphragm dysfunction, increased closing capacities, and/or aspiration pneumonitis)
    Diffusion-perfusion defect (interstitial pneumonitis, fibrosis, or pulmonary hypertension)
    Impaired hypoxic pulmonary vasoconstriction
    Pulmonary hypertension
    Hepatopulmonary syndrome
  Parenchymal abnormalities
    Restrictive ventilatory pattern due to ascites limiting diaphragmatic excursion, pleural effusions, or chest wall deformity due to osteoporosis
    Obstructive airway disease, emphysema, bronchitis-bronchiectasis
    Interstitial lung disease (infection, pneumonitis, pulmonary edema)

Renal

Renin-angiotensin-aldosterone activation: impaired sodium handling, water excretion, potassium metabolism, and concentrating ability
Impaired renal acidification
Prerenal insufficiency (ascites or diuretics)
Acute renal failure (acute liver failure, biliary obstruction, sepsis)
Hepatorenal syndrome
Glomerulopathies

TABLE 11–10. POSTULATED CAUSES OF HYPERDYNAMIC CIRCULATION IN CHRONIC DISEASE OF THE LIVER

Hepatic structural
  Intrahepatic shunts
Hepatic functional
Pulmonary structural
  Pulmonary arteriovenous fistulas
Systemic structural
  Portacaval shunts
  Portopulmonary shunts
  Peripheral vasodilatation
Other
  Increased blood volume
  Anemia
  Shift of O_2 dissociation curve to right
Abnormal levels of vasodilator substances
  Hepatic vasodepressor
  Vasoactive polypeptides
  Prostacyclins
  Endotoxin
  Glucagon
  Endothelium-derived relaxing factor
  Nitric oxide
Impaired utilization of thiamine
Increased need for heat elimination

including pneumonitis, encephalitis, nephritis, hepatitis, and myocarditis.[57, 58]

A spectrum of pulmonary considerations affects the liver transplant candidate (see Table 11–9). The most common pulmonary complication following liver transplantation is infection, with no evidence of the significant airway obstruction or bronchiolitis obliterans seen in bone marrow transplant recipients and heart-lung patients. Pulmonary hypertension in association with cirrhosis occurs in 1% of patients receiving liver transplants.[59] Moderate pulmonary hypertension and normal left ventricular function increase the perioperative mortality rate, but resolution of the hypertensive state has been observed in survivors over a period of 13 months after liver transplantation.[60] Approximately 50% of all liver transplant candidates have some form of abnormal arterial oxygenation, frequently with a partial oxygen pressure less than 70 mm Hg. Hepatopulmonary syndrome (HPS) accounts for 13 to 47% of these patients, and it is defined as the triad of hepatic dysfunction, pulmonary vascular dilatation, and abnormal arterial oxygenation (frequently PaO_2 <50 mm Hg).[61, 62] A decade ago, the presence of HPS was considered an absolute contraindication to transplantation, but normalization in arterial PaO_2 at rest and exercise has been demonstrated from 1 to 9 months following transplantation in a select group of patients (response to 100% oxygen and type-1 angiographic pattern) with severe hypoxemia and intrapulmonary shunting.[63–65]

Progressive severe osteoporosis and low back pain with vertebral fractures, which is related to osteodystrophy of chronic liver disease and corticosteroid use, are frequent chronic problems in as many as 30 to 50% of patients following liver transplantation. Whether substantial recovery of bone mineral density occurs following transplantation is currently under investigation.

Heart and Heart-Lung

Limited information exists on the course and outcome of pregnancies after heart or heart-lung transplantation.[9, 15, 36, 42, 66–82] The largest multicenter survey and literature review series to date reports on 32 pregnancies in heart (n = 29) and heart-lung (n = 3) allograft recipients resulting in 29 successful deliveries.[80] The onset of pregnancy from the time of transplantation was 2.6 ± 0.3 years, with the age at conception ranging from 19 to 35 years. Hypertension (44%), pre-eclampsia (22%), worsening of ongoing chronic renal insufficiency (15%), infection (15%), cholestatic jaundice (15%), premature labor (30%), and premature delivery (41%) were the most frequent maternal complications. Six patients (22%) were successfully treated for acute rejection episodes, which were detected during prospective surveillance in the absence of clinical signs, with no peripartum or early postpartum maternal deaths. Three patients had a pretransplant diagnosis of peripartum cardiomyopathy (PPCM), but none had a recurrence. A widely held impression is that PPCM tends to recur with subsequent pregnancies. It remains unclear what effect, if any, cardiac transplantation and/or immunosuppressive therapy has on the recurrence rate of PPCM.[73]

Physiologic Adaptations and Coexisting Systemic Disease

The chronically denervated and nonrejecting heart has essentially normal ventricular contractile characteristics and cardiac reserve,[83] which suggests that the cardiovascular changes associated with pregnancy should be well tolerated by the heart transplant patient. The ejection fraction at rest is typically normal, with a low-normal cardiac output and a heart rate of 90 to 110 beats/min reflecting the intrinsic rate of depolarization at the donor sinoatrial node.[84] Although functionally much improved, the maximal exercise capacity of cardiac transplant recipients is typically reduced to 60 to 70% of predicted values compared with age- and sex-matched sedentary normal controls.[85]

In the absence of autonomic neural control, adaptive mechanisms responsible for increasing cardiac output during exercise or hemodynamic stress are initially dependent upon venous return. An increase in left ventricular end-diastolic volume mediates an increase in stroke volume and ejection fraction by means of the Frank-Starling mechanism, which is followed by an increase in heart rate and contractility in response to circulating catecholamines.[74, 86–88] Because this heart rate response may take 5 or 6 minutes to appear,[89] the patient may show exaggerated responses to hypovolemia, sudden changes in posture, or decreases in systemic vascular resistance. Denervation results in increased sensitivity to beta adrenergic receptor blocking agents, exogenous catecholamine stimulation, and adenosine.[88] In the absence of changing cardiac function, for example from acute rejection or the development of accelerated coronary artery disease (ACAD), intracardiac hemodynamics have been shown to be stable for at least 6 years post-transplantation.[90] A late, persistent, myocardial restrictive pattern has also been identified that requires volume loading to characterize. This pattern may reflect irreparable intrinsic myocardial damage.[91, 92]

Although there is no real histologic evidence for reinnervation of the cardiac allograft in humans,[93] functional reinnervation is clearly demonstrated by the reappearance of orthostatic cardiac acceleration and rapid heart rate deceleration at cessation of exercise, vasovagal reaction to head-up tilt, increase in heart rate variability, and evidence of cardiac stores of norepinephrine.[94–98]

Late after cardiac transplantation the heart may have mildly elevated intracardiac pressures, functional tricuspid regurgitation with right ventricular enlargement, unique "normal" physiologic alterations (Table 11–11), and accelerated atherosclerosis, all reflecting the effects of immunosuppressive therapy, as well as the normal adaptive intrinisic mechanisms of the graft myocardium.[102] Angiographic evidence of CAD is present in 10 to 20% of patients 1 year after transplantation and in up to 50% by 5 years,[103] the etiology of which is likely multifactorial.[104] The consequences of ACAD include myocardial infarction, congestive heart failure, and sudden death occurring at a rate of 1.9% per

---

TABLE 11–11. PATHOPHYSIOLOGY OF THE TRANSPLANTED HEART: GENERAL CONSIDERATIONS

1. Preload-dependent with normal to mildly elevated filling pressures
2. Afterload: CyA-induced systemic hypertension, delayed or blunted blood pressure response
3. Sinus tachycardia, decrease in heart rate variability, delayed and attenuated heart rate response
   Beta adrenergic and cholinergic supersensitivity
4. ECG: "two P waves," some degree of right bundle branch block in up to 70% of cases,[99] increased incidence of atrial and ventricular dysrhythmias,[100] sinus node dysfunction requiring permanent pacemaker insertion (implantation rates 4–29%[48]), nonspecific ST segment abnormalities, and T wave inversion[101]
5. Low-normal cardiac output, normal intrinsic contractility and reserve
6. Coronary circulation: autoregulation intact in the absence of rejection or CAD, accelerated atherosclerotic coronary artery disease (ACAD), silent ischemia
7. Normalization of pulmonary artery pressure and pulmonary capillary wedge pressure

patient year after the first year post-transplantation and accounting for more than one third of late deaths.[105] The danger of ACAD lies in its frequently asymptomatic nature due to disruption of the afferent limb of the sympathetic nervous system that conveys the pain impulses of ischemia. Angina pectoris, however, occurs in as many as one third of patients who present late after cardiac transplantation with proximal or mid-vessel CAD.[106]

Transplantation of the lungs en bloc results in the loss of pulmonary innervation, bronchial arterial supply, and pulmonary lymphatic drainage. Clinicians can anticipate being unable to elicit a carinal cough reflex or to induce bronchoconstriction with stimulation distal to the site of bronchial anastomosis. These factors and impaired lymphatic and mucociliary clearance mechanisms result in increased susceptibility of the donor lungs to the deleterious effects of noxious stimuli or fluid overload. Reinnervation of the lungs[107] and re-establishment of lymphatic drainage has been demonstrated in the canine model,[108] but there is no good evidence of this finding in humans.

The hemodynamic indices between isolated cardiac and combined heart-lung transplant patients are strikingly similar.[92] At 1 year follow-up, patients undergoing heart-lung transplantation have normal resting pulmonary artery pressure (PAP), pulmonary vascular resistance (PVR), and cardiac output, but they have elevated blood pressure and systemic resistance.[109] After single lung transplant for pulmonary hypertension, PVR and pulmonary pressures dramatically decrease and remain stable over a 3-year follow-up, with significant improvement in right ventricular function.[110, 111] In patients with end-stage pulmonary parenchymal disease, the donor lung is often perfused preferentially by virtue of its lesser vascular resistance compared with the remaining diseased lung.[112]

The extent and time course of improvement in pulmonary function following transplantation is dependent on the disease treated and single versus bilateral lung replacement.[113] Determinants of new lung function include a history of pulmonary edema at the time of implantation, postoperative infection, chronic rejection, and mechanical effects of tamponade from the native lung if obstructive airway disease is present.[114] The absence of pulmonary afferent nerves does not appear to be important for the control of respiration,[115] with a return of FEV_1 and FVC to near-normal predicted preoperative values by 6 months in patients receiving bilateral lung replacement and single lung transplant for pulmonary hypertension.[113, 116] The resting blood gas values in a well patient are usually normal, but the patient may also have compensated respiratory acidosis with hypercarbia.[114] Maximal oxygen consumption and indices of exercise capacity are significantly improved, but they remain markedly below normal values.[113] The prevalence of bronchiolitis

obliterans in long-term survivors is between 20 and 50%, usually commencing from 6 months to 2 years following transplantation, and is characterized by airflow limitation in small airways manifested by decreasing FEV_1.[113] Progressive pulmonary failure from obliterative bronchiolitis and infection are the commonest causes of death in patients more than 100 days after transplantation.[117]

PREGNANCY AND RISKS FOR THE GRAFT

Kidney and Pancreas-Kidney

Most studies conclude that pregnancy does not have an adverse long-term effect on patient survival or on renal allograft function or survival in renal transplant recipients, if GFR is well preserved and the patient is normotensive.[31, 118–120] Contrary to these findings, one report indicates that pregnancy carries an increased risk of reduced renal function and a significantly shorter 10-year graft survival rate, when compared with matched never-pregnant post-transplant control patients.[121] The overall risk of graft loss or permanent renal impairment from all causes is estimated at 7 to 15%.[19, 31, 32]

Adaptations of the kidney to pregnancy are paralleled by the denervated renal graft, although to a lesser degree. A sustained increase in GFR and renal plasma flow (RPF) is seen in the first and second trimester, with a transient decrease of no more than 30% during the third trimester, and a return to normal by 8 to 12 weeks post partum, without permanent sequelae.[36] The better the renal function before pregnancy, the greater the increase in GFR during pregnancy,[122] but there is evidence that the normal increases in GFR and RPF induced with amino acid infusions may be blunted.[123] Proteinuria, frequently more than 500 mg per 24 hours and as remarkable as 2 to 3 g per 24 hours,[19] is seen in the third trimester in 30 to 40% of patients.[124] In the absence of hypertension or renal dysfunction, however, proteinuria is not significant and usually resolves spontaneously post partum.[122]

The estimated incidence of serious rejection episodes (9%) is identical in recipients with pregnancies lasting into the third trimester and nonpregnant transplant patients.[31, 37] This finding is not in keeping with the notion that pregnancy is an immunologically "privileged" state, when theoretically the graft should be protected from acute rejection,[125] with a possible "rebound" increase in rejection seen post partum.[74] In contrast, the mother may become allosensitized by the fetus, producing an augmented immune response during pregnancy.[80] In 1994, the National Transplantation Pregnancy Registry (NTPR) data base reported a significantly increased incidence of rejection during preg-

TABLE 11–12. HALLMARKS OF CLINICAL REJECTION IN THE TRANSPLANTED KIDNEY

Fever
Diminishing urine output
Fluid retention
Hypertension
Worsening renal function (i.e., increased BUN, creatinine, beta-2 microglobulins)
Enlargement and tenderness of the ectopic kidney

nancy and up to 3 months post partum in CyA- (14.5%) versus azathioprine-treated (5.7%) recipients.[24] In a review of 197 pregnancies in 141 CyA-treated female kidney transplant recipients, a slightly lower rejection rate of 11% was found.[23]

No factors are consistently predictive of which patients will develop acute rejections during pregnancy or in the puerperium. The diagnosis may be difficult (Table 11–12), and the influence of pregnancy in this process remains undefined. Previous pregnancies or a history of the donor or recipient having been breast-fed may decrease the risk of acute rejection.[126, 127] Subclinical chronic rejection may be a problem in all recipients. If a deterioration in renal function occurs at any stage of pregnancy, treatable causes should be excluded (Table 11–13). Graft dysfunction and rejection are both strongly associated with graft loss within 2 years of pregnancy.[24]

Tyden and coworkers[45] reported one case of a successful pregnancy in a 27-year-old woman with juvenile-onset diabetes mellitus treated with kidney-pancreas transplantation 2.5 years before conception. She developed acute pancreas-graft rejection immediately after delivery, with subsequent loss of the graft 10 weeks' post-delivery. With surgical placement of the pancreatic graft in the pelvis, the potential exists for compression-induced injury by the enlarging uterus. This fear, although not substantiated, has been heightened by a report of pancreatic graft failure after pelvic examination.[129]

Liver

A discussion of liver abnormalities during pregnancy includes the effects of normal pregnancy on maternal liver function, liver diseases specifically related to pregnancy, and effects of pregnancy on pre-existing liver disease, including the impact on liver graft function.

The biochemical alterations in liver function inherent in normal pregnancy are summarized in Table 11–14.[130] All changes in liver function are maximum in the third trimester except the decrease in albumin/total serum protein levels and increase in fibrinogen occurring in the second trimester. Serum glutamic pyruvic transaminase (ALT or SGPT) and glutamic oxaloacetic transaminase (AST or SGOT) are considered the standard serologic markers and most sensitive indicators of liver damage during pregnancy. Physical examination may reveal spider angiomata or palmar erythema in as many as 66% of pregnant women, which is not diagnostic for the presence of chronic liver disease.[131] During pregnancy, liver blood flow is essentially unchanged as the increase in blood volume and cardiac output is balanced by a decrease in the proportion of cardiac output directed to the liver.[132] Alterations in drug distribution and metabolism are attributable to changes in protein binding, increases in plasma volume, presence of extracellular water and adipose tissue mass, as well as competitive inhibitory effect of estrogen on liver enzyme systems.

TABLE 11–13. CAUSES OF FUNCTIONAL IMPAIRMENT OF THE TRANSPLANTED KIDNEY DURING PREGNANCY

Functional stress of pregnancy (glomerular hyperfiltration and sclerosis)[128]
Accelerated progression of an underlying disease process
Pre-eclampsia
CyA nephrotoxicity
Rejection (acute or chronic)
Hypertension

TABLE 11–14. BIOCHEMICAL ALTERATIONS IN LIVER FUNCTION IN NORMAL PREGNANCY

Alkaline phosphatase	Increases up to 200% (placental >fetal bone isoenzymes)
Gamma glutamyl transpeptidase	Normal or increased, reduced response to hepatocellular injury
Aminotransferases (AST, ALT)	No change with slight increase, usually within the normal range, near term
Lactate dehydrogenase (LDH)	Increased
Bilirubin	Unchanged, or mild decrease or increase, rarely greater than 2 mg/dl
Total protein	Mild progressive decline
Alpha and beta globulins	Tend to increase
Gamma globulins	Tend to decrease
Albumin	Decrease 20–50%
Albumin-to-globulin ratio	Decreases
Triglyceride and cholesterol	Increase substantially (300% and 50–100%, respectively)
Ceruloplasmin	Gradually increased to term
Serum cholinesterase activity	Decreases by 30% at 3 days post partum, rarely clinically significant prolongation of succinylcholine
PT and PTT, bleeding time, platelet function	Unchanged
Fibrinolytic activity	Slightly reduced
Fibrinogen	Increases 50%, accounting for a hypercoagulable state
Factors VII, VIII, IX, and X	Increase
Platelet count	Decreases by 20% due to plasma volume expansion
Glucose	Fasting, decreased 10% or no change

Modified from Seifert RD, Kang Y. Obstetric patients with liver disease. In Park GR, Kang Y (eds): Anesthesia and Intensive Care for Patients With Liver Disease. Boston, Butterworth-Heinemann, 1995, p 165.

The incidence of pregnancy complicated by liver disease is relatively low. Icteric hepatic dysfunction during normal pregnancy varies from 1:1500 to 1:5000, with viral hepatitis accounting for 50% of cases.[133] Derangements in liver and biliary function that are specific to pregnancy include pre-eclampsia/eclampsia with HELLP syndrome and rarely hepatic infarction or rupture, acute fatty liver, intrahepatic cholestasis, and possibly increased incidence of acute cholelithiasis. Hyperemesis gravidarum may result in a mild transient hyperbilirubinemia and abnormal liver test results in up to 50% of patients, which resolve with supportive care and are not associated with chronic sequelae. In general, pregnancy does not appear to hasten the natural course of pre-existing chronic liver disease, unless metabolic decompensation occurs early in the pregnancy.[130] Following liver transplantation, recurrence of the original disease is possible for Budd-Chiari syndrome; malignancy; and hepatitis B, A, and C. Recurrence of primary biliary cirrhosis and primary sclerosing cholangitis are still controversial. In patients with cirrhosis and portal hypertension, massive variceal bleeding in pregnancy is considered a significant risk, accounting for the majority of maternal deaths. Others suggest that, with no evidence of raised portal pressure, pregnancy does not alter the risk of variceal bleeding in women with known esophageal varices that have not yet bled.[134] The incidence of premature delivery, placental insufficiency, and perinatal mortality is increased.

Because limited information is available regarding the impact of pregnancy on graft function in the liver transplant patient, close surveillance of liver function is imperative. Graft rejection is not accelerated by pregnancy,[17, 28, 48] although mild to moderate increases in liver transaminase levels, progressive chronic rejection, and acute rejection episodes are documented (Table 11–15[48]). In the largest reported single-center series, the incidence of elevated hepatic enzymes during the course of the pregnancy was 35%. This was not consistent with rejection, and greater than 80% of those cases not treated resolved spontaneously.[135] The cause of persistently abnormal liver function tests, unrelated to rejection, may reflect the known hepatotoxicity of CyA or azathioprine. A successful response has been seen to steroid pulse therapy or adjustments in the antirejection regimen for rejection episodes during pregnancy. Graft loss for chronic rejection 6 months following delivery has been successfully treated with retransplantion.[82]

Heart and Heart-Lung

Histologic analysis of endomyocardial samples obtained by biopsy is considered the standard method of rejection surveillance in heart transplant patients. This surveillance raises the issue of possible radiation exposure to the fetus, with adverse sequelae, especially during the first two trimesters. Myocardial biopsies in the third trimester may be technically difficult owing to symptomatic aortocaval compression from supine positioning, which is aggravated by the weight of the lead apron needed to screen the fetus from radiation exposure.[73] This potential risk is preventable using echocardiographic visualization of the right ventricle for biopsy. Rejection historically caused symptoms of allograft dysfunction including fever, malaise, and symptoms of congestive heart failure. The clinical presentation of rejection has changed in the post-CyA era such that most rejection is asymptomatic and is not associated with significant allograft dysfunction except in cases of advanced rejection.[88] Routine 12-lead electrocardiogram (ECG) findings of bradyarrhythmias, small ECG complexes, ischemia, or, in particular, sustained ventricular tachycardia, ventricular fibrillation, or atrial flutter seem to be correlated with cardiac allograft rejection.[136]

Detecting rejection of a transplanted lung can often be difficult, because signs and symptoms of fatigue, dyspnea, gas exchange impairment, mild pyrexia, leukocytosis, and infiltrate seen on chest radiographs may mimic those of infection.[112] The majority of acute rejection episodes occur in the first 3 months after transplant. The diagnosis is made utilizing bronchoalveolar lavage and transbronchial lung biopsy. In heart-lung allografts, differential rejection may occur, and therefore each organ must be monitored independently.

The actual physiologic adaptations that occur in the transplanted heart and heart-lungs under the influence of pregnancy have not been described. Although beyond the scope of this chapter, the reader should refer to several excellent comprehensive reviews of the physiologic cardiorespiratory alterations that occur during normal pregnancy and implications for anesthetic care of the parturient.[137–139] The changes in the cardiovascular and respiratory systems during pregnancy are summarized in Tables 11–16 and 11–17.

Recognition of cardiac decompensation may be difficult because pregnancy is frequently associated with signs and symptoms suggestive of heart disease includ-

TABLE 11–15. HALLMARKS OF CLINICAL REJECTION IN THE TRANSPLANTED LIVER

Clinical signs	Jaundice
	Tenderness of the right upper quadrant of the abdomen
	Asterixis
Biologic parameters	Increased aminotransferases, alkaline phosphatase, bilirubin levels
	Decreased serum albumin, coagulation factors
Liver biopsy	Perivascular lipid accumulation
	Periportal fibrosis
	Cholestasis

TABLE 11–16. CHANGES IN CARDIOVASCULAR SYSTEM DURING PREGNANCY AT TERM

Variable	Direction of Change	Average Change
Blood volume	↑	+35%
Plasma volume	↑	+45%
Red blood cell volume	↑	+20%
Cardiac output	↑	+40%
Stroke volume	↑	+30%
Heart rate	↑	+15%
Femoral (uterine?) venous pressure	↑	+15 mm Hg
Total peripheral resistance	↓	−15%
Mean arterial blood pressure	↓	−15 mm Hg
Systolic blood pressure	↓	−0–15 mm Hg
Diastolic blood pressure	↓	−10–20 mm Hg
Central venous pressure	↔	No change

ing early fatigability; dyspnea; peripheral edema; syncope; grade I or II systolic murmur or third heart sound; benign dysrhythmias; and reversible ST, T, and Q wave changes on the ECG.[67] These normal findings must be differentiated from those indicating heart disease, which include (1) systolic murmur greater than grade III; (2) any diastolic murmur; (3) severe dysrhythmias; and (4) unequivocal cardiac enlargement on radiographic examination (see Chapter 1).[140, 141]

For the normal, healthy patient, changes in blood volume and hemodynamics that place an increased workload on the heart occur during pregnancy. Although volume expansion, increased cardiac output, and decreased peripheral vascular resistance are apparently well tolerated in the normal parturient, the poten-

TABLE 11–17. CHANGES IN THE RESPIRATORY SYSTEM DURING PREGNANCY AT TERM

Variable	Direction of Change	Average Change
Minute ventilation	↑	+50%
Alveolar ventilation	↑	+70%
Tidal volume	↑	+40%
Respiratory rate	↑	+15%
Arterial P_{O_2}	↑	+10 mm Hg
Inspiratory lung capacity	↑	+5%
Oxygen consumption	↑	+20%
Dead space	↔	No change
Lung compliance (alone)	↔	No change
Arterial pH	↔	No change
Vital capacity	↔	No change
FEV_1	↔	No change
Diffusing capacity	↔	No change
Maximal breathing capacity	↔	No change
Closing volume	↔ or ↓	No change
Airway resistance	↓	−36%
Total pulmonary resistance	↓	−50%
Total compliance	↓	−30%
Chest wall compliance (alone)	↓	−45%
Arterial P_{CO_2}	↓	−10 mm Hg
Serum bicarbonate	↓	−4 mEq/l
Total lung capacity	↓	−0–5%
Functional residual capacity	↓	−20%
Expiratory reserve volume	↓	−20%
Residual volume	↓	−20%

tial risk of these hemodynamic changes, if any, to the cardiac transplant recipient and fetus remains unknown. One may anticipate that problems complicating these high-risk pregnancies are more likely to be related to the coexistence of other morbidity and the potential adverse effects of immunosuppressive therapy.[42, 80] There is no evidence that theoretical concerns regarding the possibility of atrial, pulmonary, or aortic suture line disruption during pregnancy have any basis.

In a lung transplant patient with compromised lung function and limited respiratory reserve, the decrease in functional residual capacity, increase in oxygen consumption at rest and during stress, and increase in supine alveolar-arterial gradient during pregnancy make the patient more vulnerable to hypoxia.[142] Airway compromise from bronchomalacia and stenosis of the bronchial anastomosis may be exacerbated by mucosal engorgement, laryngeal edema associated with pre-eclampsia, volume overload, and upper respiratory tract infections.[143–145] Lung volumes and lung capacities are essentially unchanged by pregnancy; therefore, a decrease in the patient's FEV_1 by 10 to 20% may indicate significant pulmonary dysfunction.[113, 117] A vital capacity of 1 liter has been suggested as the minimal functional requirement necessary to maintain a successful pregnancy.[146] There is little objective support for this particular value, because a successful pregnancy has been reported in a patient pretransplant with a vital capacity of 800 ml.[147] In patients with residual pulmonary hypertension, elevations of cardiac output and pulmonary blood volume or sudden increases in venous return from evacuation of the uterus and caval decompression may precipitate acute right ventricular failure and cardiovascular collapse.

PREGNANCY AND RISKS FOR THE FETUS AND NEWBORN

There is uniform agreement regarding an increased incidence of premature and low-birth-weight infants in female transplant recipients. Numerous factors can account for this finding, including drug therapy (immunosuppressive therapy, antihypertensive medications), persistent hypertension, renal insufficiency, or vascular changes associated with an underlying systemic illness. Fears regarding gross physical or developmental abnormalities in these children attributable to intrauterine exposure to low baseline therapeutic levels of immunosuppressive drugs have not been substantiated. Continued long-term surveillance and evaluation of these offspring are needed (Table 11–18).

Kidney and Pancreas-Kidney

Pregnancy loss during the first trimester is estimated at 35% and may be attributable to spontaneous abor-

TABLE 11–18. **RISKS OF INTRAUTERINE EXPOSURE TO IMMUNOSUPPRESSIVE THERAPY**

Azathioprine	Susceptibility to infection Transient germ cell chromosomal abnormalities Abnormal liver function study results Bone marrow toxicity (lymphopenia, thrombocytopenia, anemia) Intrauterine growth retardation, low birth weight
Steroids	Adrenal insufficiency Thymic hypoplasia Depressed hematopoiesis Lymphocytopenia Premature rupture of membranes
CyA	Intrauterine growth retardation, low birth weight Prematurity

tion (8.7–14%; similar to that of the general population), ectopic pregnancy (0.5–1%; possibly increased by intraperitoneal adhesions), and therapeutic termination (12–20%). Of the pregnancies that continue past the first trimester, greater than 80% of patients deliver successfully with an overall complication rate estimated at 49%. If complications occur before 28 weeks' gestation, successful obstetric outcome occurs in 70%, compared with 93% when pregnancy is trouble-free before 28 weeks.[32]

In CyA recipients, the NTPR reported a complication rate of 61% for newborns weighing less than 2500 g, compared with 12% for newborns weighing more than 2500 g. The overall newborn complication rate was 21.7% in the CyA group compared with 29.6% in the azathioprine group.[24] Prepregnancy factors that appear to increase the risk of prematurity (45–60%), birth weight less than 2500 g (20–50%), or perinatal complications are maternal drug-treated hypertension, diabetes, and serum creatinine greater than 1.5 mg/dl. Prepregnancy chronic hypertension or hypertension before 28 weeks appears to be the most significant clinical marker of perinatal complications and adverse pregnancy outcome.[34]

Liver

The majority of neonates are generally healthy. Analysis of outcomes from 48 pregnancies in 34 female liver transplant recipients indicates an overall favorable outcome with a high rate of preterm delivery (39%) and low-birth-weight infants (31%), which was associated with drug-treated hypertension, pre-eclampsia, and preterm premature rupture of membranes.[148] Congenital CMV sepsis in the setting of primary maternal CMV infection or rejection necessitating increased immunosuppression is primarily responsible for fatalities in preterm infants following delivery.[17] Exposure of the fetus to acyclovir during the first trimester of pregnancy is not associated with an increase in congenital abnormalities or spontaneous abortion.[149]

Heart and Heart-Lung

Prematurity (41%) and low birth weight (17%) are the most common neonatal complications, occurring more frequently when compared with the general population (5–10% and 10%, respectively).[80] The incidence of early spontaneous abortions caused by fetal anomalies is unknown. Wagoner and coworkers[80] reported no fetal anomalies or neonatal deaths in 29 successful pregnancy outcomes, with all children observed to be in good health at 3.4 ± 0.4 years of age. Liljestrand and Lindstrom reported a pregnancy complicated by worsening premature ventricular contractions and infections, with the vaginal delivery of a 2680-g infant at 39 weeks. The newborn subsequently developed a cardiomyopathy at 12 months of age, the etiology of which was attributed to hereditary factors, teratogenic effects, or maternal infections during pregnancy.[76] Patients who have undergone cardiac transplant for cardiomyopathic conditions should be made aware of the risk of recurrence to the fetus of 50% for familial types and 25% for sporadic types.[78]

IMMUNOSUPPRESSIVE THERAPY

Immunosuppressive protocols for pregnant allograft patients generally include varying combinations of prednisone, azathioprine, CyA, and FK506, with individual tailoring according to rejection episodes and side effects. The short-term effects of corticosteroids and azathioprine in pregnancy are well described from pregnancies in renal transplant recipients and in patients suffering from connective tissue disorders. The first successful pregnancy in a CyA-treated kidney recipient was reported in 1983, and in 1993 in an FK506-treated liver transplant patient.[150, 151] Limited information is therefore available for these drugs on peripartum dosing requirements and drug effects during the course of pregnancy or maternal and neonatal outcome. To gather, analyze, and disseminate this information the NTPR was established in 1991 to study pregnancy outcomes in transplant recipients on CyA and non-CyA regimens before and during pregnancy.

Although pregnancy is considered a state of immunologic tolerance, there is no evidence that episodes of rejection of any organ occur less frequently or that lower doses of immunosuppressants are necessary during pregnancy.[17] Immunosuppressive agents must be continued during pregnancy, with consideration given to general recommendations listed in Table 11–19.

Cyclosporine

Cyclosporine is the drug of choice for long-term maintenance immunosuppression and for treatment of

TABLE 11–19. RECOMMENDATIONS FOR IMMUNOSUPPRESSIVE THERAPY DURING PREGNANCY

1. Maintain immunosuppressive therapy at prepregnancy levels unless signs of toxicity or acute rejection mandate changes
2. Monitor patient for adverse effects attributable to specific drugs
3. Consider all patients susceptible to life-threatening infections; aseptic technique and the adminstration of prophylactic antibiotics before any invasive procedure are necessary
4. Breast-feeding should be discouraged in patients taking CyA, FK506 and/or azathioprine owing to the transfer of these drugs to breast milk, and the uncertainty of drug exposure in the newborn[152]
5. Steroid supplementation is required for the stress of labor and delivery
6. Adjustments in the dose of azathioprine may be indicated if there is evidence of acute rejection, a decrease in maternal leukocyte or platelet counts, or abnormal liver function test results
7. Close monitoring of CyA doses is crucial; there are considerable discrepancies regarding requirements, especially in the third trimester and the immediate postdelivery period
8. Patient noncompliance with medications must be detected early or may result in severe deterioration or loss of graft function

acute rejection in solid-organ transplantation. CyA is an 11 amino acid–cyclic polypeptide molecule extracted from soil fungus that inhibits lymphokine production and release (macrophage IL-1 and helper T lymphocyte IL-2). It selectively inhibits helper and cytotoxic T cells by blocking antigen-induced T-cell

activation, without bone marrow suppression (Fig. 11–1).[153, 154] A safe fetal dose for CyA has not been established.

Prepregnancy therapeutic levels should be maintained, keeping the daily dose low, preferably at 2 to 4 mg·kg⁻¹·day⁻¹ for renal transplant patients. Blood concentrations of CyA are measured regularly, with the aim of maintaining a therapeutic trough concentration of 100 to 300 ng/l. A possible fetotoxic effect of the drug in human pregnancy has been postulated, and in the rat such an effect seems to be dose-related.[155] Monitoring drug concentrations is essential because overdosing may precipitate the enhanced systemic toxicity, increased neoplastic and infection risk, and altered graft function seen with excessive immunosuppression.

Formulations of CyA include soft gelatin capsule, oral solution, and concentrate for intravenous infusion. Potential risks include lipid necrosis of the lung with aspiration of the oral forms and hypersensitivity reactions. Intravenous CyA contains the solvent polyoxyethylated castor oil, which together have been linked to anaphylactoid reactions (incidence <1:1000 cases), histamine release, nephrotoxicity, cholestasis, and interaction with nondepolarizing muscle relaxants.[156–158] Central venous administration of CyA may result in hyperkalemia, coronary vasoconstriction, and adult

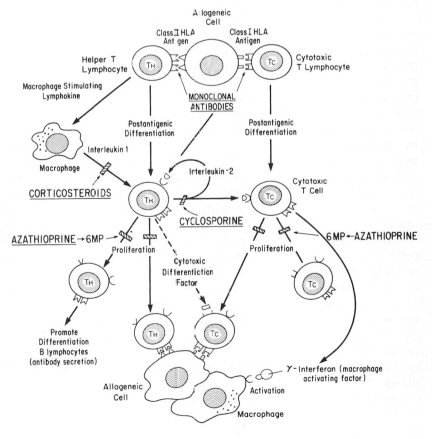

Figure 11–1. Schematic representation of graft rejection and the sites of action of the currently used immunosuppressive agents: azathioprine, corticosteroids, cyclosporine, and monoclonal antibodies. (*From* Flye MW. Immunosuppressive therapy. *In* Flye MW (ed): Principles of Organ Transplantation. Philadelphia, WB Saunders, 1989, pp 155–175.)

GRAFT REJECTION

respiratory distress syndrome of the lung.[159, 160] Limiting intravenous infusion rates to 2 mg/kg over a period of 1 hour is recommended.[159]

CyA dose requirements may increase during pregnancy, which is likely a result of decreased bioavailability, altered tissue distribution, and increased metabolism.[31, 161–163] These effects may be offset by increased concentrations of circulating sex steroids, which may inhibit liver microsomes (cytochrome P450 IIIA) and impair hepatic clearance of CyA.[163] Interpatient variability in CyA pharmacokinetics following oral administration may account for reports of no appreciable change in the patient's dosing schedules.[164] Possible effects of the normal physiologic changes of pregnancy on drug distribution, metabolism, and clearance have been summarized elsewhere.[165]

CyA readily crosses the placenta with fetal levels ranging from 10 to 50% of maternal levels.[161] Concerns regarding fetal outcome appear to be dose-dependent; they include an increased incidence of intrauterine growth retardation, prematurity, and low birth weight. Overall, the pregnancy success rate with CyA appears comparable to that with azathioprine.[21, 24] Evidence of detrimental effects of CyA on endothelial cell function, lipoprotein metabolism, placental and umbilical cord vascular prostanoid production, and platelet function, in conjunction with longstanding hypertension, may contribute to placental insufficiency and may account for an estimated 30% incidence of pre-eclampsia.[166, 167]

Nephrotoxicity and hypertension complicate CyA therapy in virtually every patient. Three etiologic mechanisms have been postulated, including increased proximal renal tubular pressure, decreased filtration coefficient, and vasoconstriction.[168, 169] Nephrotoxicity is manifested as a dose-dependent reduction in maternal GFR with decreased creatinine clearance, increased blood urea nitrogen (BUN) and creatinine, hyperkalemia, hyperuricemia, hypertension, and hyperkalemic hyperchloremic renal tubular acidosis. Renal function and fluid and electrolyte balances should be monitored closely. Concomitant administration of drugs known to have nephrotoxic potential and those dependent on renal elimination should be avoided.

Additional complications of CyA include mild hepatic dysfunction, pancreatobiliary problems, hypochromic anemia, fatigue, hypertrichosis, gum hyperplasia, predisposition to thromboembolic phenomena, and rarely a hemolytic-uremic–like syndrome. Glucose intolerance and hyperinsulinemia, which may progress to overt diabetes mellitus, are associated with an increased risk of atherosclerosis, which is a leading cause of death in long-term survivors of solid organ transplants.[170–172]

Various neurologic sequelae have been reported in 15 to 40% of patients treated with CyA, including tremor, seizures, cerebellar dysfunction, encephalopathy, neuropathy, and motor deficit syndromes.[173, 174] Par-

esthesia of the distal extremities (especially hands) is a more common finding than focal weakness, although evidence of combined demyelination and axonal damage has been reported.[175] Most neurotoxic side effects of CyA are completely reversible with drug withdrawal.[174]

In considering the advisability of regional anesthesia, documentation of any existing neurologic deficit is prudent, as is prevention of hypomagnesemia, which potentiates CyA-induced neurotoxicity. Care with patient positioning must be taken. An additional concern is the possibility of a concurrent viral or opportunistic central nervous system (CNS) infection, frequently presenting with few clinical findings and reported in approximately 5 to 10% of transplant patients.[176] Neurologic complications of organ transplantation may also result from a progression of the underlying disease process, from a complication of the surgical procedure or from a unique feature of a specific transplant type.[174]

The possibility exists of interactions between CyA and any drug that is a substrate for cytochrome P450.[177–179] A potential for drug interactions with CyA has been described for macrolide antibiotics, azole antifungal drugs, calcium channel blockers (excluding nifedipine), histamine H_2-receptor antagonists, nonsteroidal anti-inflammatory agents, and any nephrotoxic drugs. Agents commonly used in clinical practice that may demonstrate modified pharmacodynamic action include benzodiazepines, neuromuscular blocking agents, opioids, antibiotics, and propofol. A few animal and human studies of possible drug interactions between CyA and anesthetic agents, including isoflurane, nondepolarizing muscle relaxants, fentanyl, and pentobarbital, have appeared in the literature. Isoflurane decreases the rate of absorption of CyA by reducing gastric emptying and absorption from the proximal small bowel.[180] Oral doses should be given 4 to 7 hours preoperatively, because the formulation contains olive oil, castor oil, or corn oil, and represents a significant risk if regurgitation and aspiration occur. In addition, the desired therapeutic blood levels may not be achieved if given outside of this time interval.[181]

Cyclosporine has been shown to prolong nondepolarizing neuromuscular blockade,[157, 158, 182–185] which is thought to be secondary to a combined effect of the parent drug causing inhibition of calcium entry into the muscle cell. In addition, polyoxethylated castor oil, which nonspecifically interferes with drug binding, effectively increases the concentration of nondepolarizing drug at the neuromuscular junction. The interaction between CyA and depolarizing muscle relaxants has not been studied in humans. CyA has been reported to increase analgesia produced by fentanyl in a dose-dependent manner and to increase pentobarbital hypnosis.[186] Insufficient corroborating data exist to determine the clinical significance of these findings.

It is essential to appreciate the potential interactions

between CyA and anesthetic agents because many of these drugs cause liver enzyme induction, which may alter CyA levels, evident 7 to 10 days later, or potentiate CyA-related side effects.

Azathioprine

Azathioprine in combination with prednisone had been the conventional regimen for immunosuppressive therapy in transplant recipients from 1961 until the introduction of CyA in 1978. The normal maintenance dose is 1 to 2 mg/kg, with a reduction required if bone marrow depression or liver toxicity occurs. Additional maternal effects include rashes, gastrointestinal manifestations, pancreatitis, and increased risk of neoplasm and infection. Reversible interstitial pneumonitis has been reported as a hypersensitivity reaction.[187] Azathioprine crosses the placenta, achieving fetal blood concentrations that are 63 to 93% of those seen in maternal blood.[188] Theoretically, the fetus should be protected from the effects of azathioprine during the period of organogenesis because the fetal liver lacks the enzyme iosinate pyrophosphorylase, which is required for conversion of the parent drug to its active metabolites. Fetal and neonatal effects include bone marrow toxicity (lymphopenia, thrombocytopenia, megaloblastic anemia); intrauterine growth retardation; sepsis; transient lymphocyte chromosomal damage and theoretical concerns of developing malignancies; congenital anomalies; and infertility in the next generation. An overall malformation rate estimated at 3% does not exceed that of the general population. Evidence exists that azathioprine potentiates succinylcholine-induced muscle relaxation in the cat model[189] and antagonizes nondepolarizing neuromuscular blockade in both animal and human studies by presynaptic inhibition of the motor nerve terminal.[189–191]

Steroids

Prednisone is a synthetic 17-hydroxyglucocorticoid with potent anti-inflammatory activity, which was introduced in 1963 for prophylactic immunosuppressive therapy against graft rejection. Maternal side effects include hypertension, salt and water retention, obesity and cushingoid features, hyperglycemia, hypokalemia, skin fragility, nausea and vomiting, gastric ulceration and hemorrhage, myopathy, "steroid psychosis," pancreatitis, increased susceptibility to infection, and poor wound healing.[192] Osteoporosis with compression fractures and aseptic necrosis of the hip, knee, shoulder, and elbow with proximal muscle weakness necessitates careful positioning. Dose-limiting strategies are useful in preventing the growth retardation seen in as many as 60% of pediatric patients undergoing renal trans-

plantation. With maturity and subsequent pregnancy, short stature may necessitate surgical delivery owing to cephalopelvic disproportion. Patient compliance and cooperation may be hampered by psychological effects ranging from slight mood changes to fulminant psychosis. Patients may be at risk for exaggerated postpartum depression. Hypercholesterolemia is one possible mechanism contributing to corticosteroid-induced vascular damage and increased incidence of accelerated coronary atherosclerosis seen in heart and renal transplant recipients.[193]

Corticosteroid therapy during pregnancy in animal studies has shown runting, and anomalies such as cleft lip and palate, and a reduction in litter sizes. No similar effects of prednisone or its active metabolite prednisolone have been confirmed in humans. Reports of fetal growth retardation and low-birth-weight neonates are common for azathioprine and CyA regimens (containing prednisone), with the individual contributory effect of each drug undetermined.[194, 195] Complications in infants born to mothers on steroid therapy include thymic hypoplasia, depressed hematopoiesis, lymphocytopenia, and rarely adrenal insufficiency. Prednisone readily crosses the placenta; however, the fetus is unable to convert prednisone to prednisolone, which accounts for fetal levels only 10% of those seen in the mother. Maternal doses of less than 15 mg/day are insufficient to accelerate fetal lung maturation, with the subsequent risk of respiratory distress syndrome in the premature infant. A high incidence of preterm delivery associated with premature rupture of membranes has been attributed to long-term steroid therapy.[37] Weakening of connective tissue may also predispose the mother to uterine rupture.

Steroid therapy is continued during pregnancy at prepregnancy dosing, with high-dose therapy indicated for treatment of episodes of acute rejection. Augmenting steroids post partum to cover "rebound immunoresponsiveness" is a controversial issue.[124, 196] With little evidence of beneficial effect, the current practice is to continue baseline therapy post partum. There is a longstanding debate regarding whether a history of exogenous steroid administration, followed by surgical stress with no supplementation, precipitates acute adrenal insufficiency. Recommendations for perioperative steroid coverage take into consideration the route of administration, total dose, interval from last dose to surgery, duration of therapy, magnitude of perceived surgical stress, and presence of glucose intolerance.

There is evidence in an animal model study of hemodynamic instability and higher mortality rates from documented adrenal insufficiency due to adrenal suppression from steroid administration and subsequent surgical stress with no replacement therapy.[197] In reality, few patients with suppressed adrenal function and no steroid supplement develop hypotension following surgery. The diagnosis of adrenal insufficiency is primarily one of exclusion. There is agreement among experts, however, that supplemental high-dose steroid therapy has little associated morbidity and should be administered during labor and delivery to cover maximal stress requirements equivalent to cortisol 200 to 500 mg/day. Essential monitoring includes vital signs, temperature, and serum glucose and electrolyte levels. An adrenal crisis is life-threatening, and many of the symptoms are masked by similiar complaints of nausea and vomiting, abdominal or back pain, dizziness, fainting, low-grade fever, headache, and lethargy during normal labor.

A reduction of plasma cholinesterase activity by 50% in patients on long-term prednisone therapy may prolong the duration of action of succinylcholine.[198] Antagonism of pancuronium-induced blockade by interaction between the steroid-based pancuronium nucleus and corticosteroids, or modulation of choline uptake presynaptically, has been reported.[199-201]

FK506

FK506 is the newest macrolide immunosuppressive agent. It was introduced into clinical trials in April, 1990. The drug's immunosuppressive properties are due to an inhibitory effect on the synthesis of IL-2 and other lymphokines and T-cell activation and proliferation.[202, 203] Its pharmacokinetic profile is similar to that of CyA with P450 liver enzyme metabolism, but it does not require bile acids for solubilization and absorption. Therapeutic advantages over CyA include greater potency; hepatotrophic effect; increased steroid-sparing; and lower incidence of hypertension, hypercholesterolemia, hyperuricemia, and serious infection. The incidence of new-onset diabetes mellitus, nephrotoxicity, and gastrointestinal tract complaints with FK506 is similar to that of CyA.[204] Neurologic complications, including seizures and central pontine myelinolysis with dysarthria and motor disturbances, resolve with dose reduction.[205] Headache and insomnia are common complaints that are dose related. Of concern, animals immunosuppressed with FK506, when compared with CyA, have been shown to develop more significant coronary artery disease over a relatively short interval of 4 weeks in the transplanted and native heart.[206] FK506 crosses the placenta, and umbilical blood concentrations are approximately 50% of maternal concentrations.[151] Transient unexplained hyperkalemia, normalizing spontaneously within 24 to 48 hours, is reported in newborns of liver transplant recipients taking FK506 during pregnancy.[150] As with the other immunosuppressive agents, therapeutic dosing of FK506 has demonstrated no significant teratogenic activity in humans. In a limited number of published reports, birth weights were normal for gestational age, which

may result from the effect of steroid withdrawal or may represent an intrinsic property of FK506.[150, 151]

ANESTHETIC CONSIDERATIONS DURING THE MANAGEMENT OF LABOR AND DELIVERY

Collaboration of a multidisciplinary team is essential to the antenatal assessment and peripartum management of the transplant recipient. The patient should be seen in consultation by an attending anesthesiologist early in the third trimester, because preterm labor and delivery is common. The evaluation should consist of a thorough history and physical examination and a review of the patient's medical records and personal diary with special attention given to assessment of maternal antenatal problems, immunosuppressive therapy, graft function, and fetal surveillance (Table 11-20). Spontaneous onset of labor with vaginal delivery is the ultimate goal, with cesarean section reserved for obstetric indications only. In patients in whom the transplanted kidney or pancreatic graft is placed in the pelvis close to the uterus, there is no evidence to substantiate the fear of organ injury during vaginal delivery or dysfunction from compression by the enlarging uterus. Dystocia is a rare complication.[207] The patient should be encouraged to deliver in a hospital-based setting that is equipped with a high-risk maternal and fetal monitoring unit and an intensive care facility.

Tocolytic therapy for managing preterm labor includes magnesium, nifedipine, and beta agonists (terbutaline and ritodrine). These medications are probably safe in renal and liver transplant recipients.[208] There are no case reports discussing beta agonists in the cardiac transplant recipient, but they are probably not safe and should not be used in this population.[208] Indomethacin should be avoided because it may potentiate cyclosporine nephrotoxicity.[209] It is vital to maintain a good urine output perioperatively, because further renal insults from drugs or periods of low cardiac output

TABLE 11-20. ANTENATAL ASSESSMENT OF THE TRANSPLANT RECIPIENT

Maternal problems	Pregnancy (hypertension/pre-eclampsia, gestational diabetes, infection, renal dysfunction)
	Coexisting systemic disease process
	Transplant surgery-related
Immunosuppressive therapy	Drug levels
	Complications, toxicities, adverse reactions
	Drug interactions
Graft function	Detection of acute/chronic rejection, ischemia, or failure
	Physiologic adaptations to pregnancy
	Laboratory and diagnostic studies
Fetal surveillance	

may be additive and can cause the patient to become rapidly anuric.[210]

It is generally recommended that attention to aseptic technique, with handling of all intravascular and airway equipment with sterile gloves, and use of prophylactic antibiotics are essential to protect the patient from nosocomial infection. Invasive procedures, such as fetal monitoring with a scalp electrode, intrauterine pressure monitoring, and placement of a Foley catheter or central venous or arterial cannula, carry an increased risk of infection in transplant recipients. One researcher has observed, however, that there are no reports in the literature suggesting an increased risk of infectious complications in the immunosuppressed pregnant patient.[74] One must therefore clearly weigh the risk-benefit ratio. Intubation via the orotracheal route is preferable given the possibility of technical difficulty from nasal mucosal edema, risk of inducing epistaxis, and potential of infection by diphtheroids and staphylococcal commensals from the nasopharynx and skin.

Transfusion practices should take into consideration the Rhesus titer and CMV status of the patient. Institutional practices vary from (1) administering only CMV-negative blood products to all transplanted patients or administering them exclusively to the CMV-negative recipient who has received a CMV-negative organ, (2) white-cell filtering the blood and platelets to prevent transmission of CMV carried in the leukocytes, and (3) irradiation to destroy T cells, which provoke graft versus host disease.

General considerations for management of the transplant recipient during labor and delivery include the following:

1. Mandatory strict adherence to aseptic techniques
2. Steroid augmentation for labor-induced stress
3. Minimize invasive monitoring techniques
4. Essential antibiotic prophylaxis for all invasive monitoring and instrumentation
5. Assessment and optimization of graft function
6. Anticipation of altered physiologic and pharmacologic responses in the denervated organ
7. Continuation of immunosuppressive therapy, with monitoring for signs of toxicity or acute rejection. For patients not permitted oral intake, the oral to intravenous conversion factors for immunosuppressive drugs are prednisone po: methylprednisolone IV—1:0.8; azathioprine po: azathioprine IV—1:1; and CyA po bid: CyA IV—1:0.25, infused over 6 hours twice daily.[159]
8. Maintain surveillance and optimization of renal function
9. Identify maternal problems related to the pregnancy, immunosuppressive therapy, transplant surgery, or coexisting systemic illness.

Virtually all anesthetic techniques have been utilized successfully in transplant recipients for labor analgesia and forceps-assisted or surgical delivery. Anesthetic technique depends on obstetric considerations, evidence of graft dysfunction, use of drugs and techniques minimizing additional insult or physiologic trespass to the transplanted organ, presence of absolute or relative contraindications for regional anesthesia, and individual preference. Continuation of aspirin, azathioprine, and dipyridamole in the peripartum period can affect platelet adhesiveness. In the absence of evidence of overt platelet dysfunction, however, most clinicians do not consider use of these drugs a contraindication for regional anesthesia. Routine immunosuppressive therapy should be continued, with monitoring for signs of toxicity or acute rejection. The problems of anesthetizing patients on long-term steroid, azathioprine, CyA, or FK506 therapy are summarized in Table 11–21.

Kidney and Pancreas-Kidney

In addition to monitoring (see Table 11–12) and optimizing graft function (Table 11–22), while avoiding potential nephrotoxins and ischemic injury in the kidney transplant recipient, coexisting systemic disease and residual physiologic alterations of end-stage renal disease may have a pronounced impact on anesthetic management (see Table 11–8). Deterioration of renal function may necessitate hemodialysis, with its inherent complications. Patients with a history of chronic renal failure have a high incidence of viral hepatitis (types B, C, and human immunodeficiency virus), which is a blood-borne infectious disease risk to the health care team. These infections may ultimately result in hepatic dysfunction in the recipient. There is a potential for significant accumulation and prolongation of the effect of anesthetic agents, which is dependent on renal metabolism and elimination. Caution should be exercised in the use of succinylcholine for intubation in a patient with peripheral neuropathy or hyperkalemia resulting from renal insufficiency or CyA and terbutaline administration. Atracurium 0.5 mg/kg is an alternate choice, with no adverse neonatal effects at this intubating dose. Hypercalcemia should be corrected, if possible, before administration of anesthesia with monitoring of ionized serum calcium, potassium, and magnesium; volume status; and renal and cardiac function. Metabolic or respiratory acidosis must be avoided since it raises the ionized calcium concentration even further. Responses to anesthetic agents are not predictable.

Liver

Specific perianesthetic considerations for patients with liver disease and the pregnant patient with significant hepatic dysfunction are reviewed in detail elsewhere.[130, 211]

In the liver transplant patient, analgesia for labor and delivery or anesthesia for cesarean section can be administered as in the healthy parturient if liver function is stable and coagulation is within normal limits. The "healthy" transplanted liver is no more susceptible

TABLE 11–21. COMPLICATIONS AND ANESTHETIC CONSIDERATIONS OF IMMUNOSUPPRESSIVE THERAPY

Cyclosporine	Neurologic sequelae (tremor, seizures, cerebellar dysfunction, encephalopathy, neuropathy, motor deficit syndromes, fatigue)
	ARDS
	Aspiration pneumonitis
	Hypertension, vasoconstriction
	Accelerated atherosclerosis, hypercholesterolemia
	Nephrotoxicity and enhanced susceptibility to renal insults
	Hyperkalemic hyperchloremic renal tubular acidosis
	Hemolytic-uremic-like syndrome
	Glucose intolerance
	Hyperkalemia, hypomagnesemia
	Hepatic dysfunction and pancreatobiliary complications
	Hypertrichosis, gum hyperplasia
	Predisposition to thromboembolic phenomena
	Increased neoplastic and infection risk
	Hypersensitivity reactions, histamine release
	Drug interactions (P450 IIIA microsomal enzymes)
	Prolongs nondepolarizing neuromuscular blockade
	Increases fentanyl analgesia
FK506	Neurologic sequelae (seizures, central pontine myelinolysis, headache, insomnia)
	Hypertension, accelerated atherosclerosis, hypercholesterolemia
	Glucose intolerance
	Nephrotoxicity
	Gastrointestinal tract complaints, hepatotrophic effect
	Infection and neoplastic risk
	Hyperkalemia
Azathioprine	Bone marrow depression (lymphopenia, thrombocytopenia, anemia) and synergy with other marrow suppressants
	Hepatic dysfunction and jaundice
	Hypersensitivity reactions, rashes
	Gastrointestinal manifestations, pancreatitis
	Infection and neoplastic risk
	Drug interactions
	Potentiation of depolarizing and antagonism of nondepolarizing neuromuscular blockade
Prednisone	Psychological effects (mood changes to psychosis)
	Hypertension, salt and water retention, accelerated atherosclerosis
	Obesity and cushingoid features
	Adrenal insufficiency
	Hyperglycemia, hypokalemia
	Osteoporosis, compression fractures, aseptic necrosis, skin fragility, short stature
	Proximal myopathy
	Peptic ulcer disease, nausea and vomiting, pancreatitis
	Poor wound healing
	Increased susceptibility to infection
	Drug interactions
	Reduction of plasma cholinesterase activity
	Antagonism of pancuronium effects

TABLE 11–22. ACHIEVING OPTIMAL FUNCTION OF THE TRANSPLANTED KIDNEY

1. Homeostatic environment (fluids, electrolytes, acid-base status, hematocrit)
2. Cardiovascular stability (systolic blood pressure 120–140 mm Hg)
3. Intravascular volume expansion to a CVP of 12–15 mm Hg
4. Drug therapy: dopamine 2.5–5 $\mu g \cdot kg^{-1} \cdot min^{-1}$, mannitol 25 g, furosemide 40–400 mg
5. Avoidance of nephrotoxic agents
6. Anticipation of alterations in drug pharmacokinetics and pharmacodynamics
7. Recognition and treatment of rejection, infection, or acute tubular necrosis

to potentially hepatotoxic drugs (i.e., halothane) than the liver in a normal patient.[212]

Continuing evidence of portal hypertension, and the possible presence of large venous collaterals, may be a relative contraindication for placement of a catheter in the epidural space, with increased risk of vessel penetration and possible hematoma formation.[212] Mild to severe graft dysfunction from acute or chronic rejection, recurrence of hepatitis, or malignancy may lead to altered drug distribution, coagulopathy, and portal hypertension. Additional anesthetic considerations include the potential for variceal bleeding with Valsalva maneuver or insertion of a nasogastric tube and decreased anesthetic requirements. Maintenance of hepatic blood flow and avoidance of potential hepatotoxins are essential.

The disposition and pharmacologic effects of drugs in patients with chronic liver disease and the ability of the newly transplanted liver to metabolize and eliminate drugs are poorly described. Caution should be exercised in the administration of all agents, because the pharmacokinetic and pharmacodynamic properties of each drug depend on a composite of different factors, including altered graft function (rejection, recurrence of the primary disease process, nonspecific hepatocellular damage or cholestasis), persistent pathophysiologic changes characteristic of end-stage liver disease, and drug interactions or toxic effects of the immunosuppressive therapy. Possible effects of the normal physiologic changes of pregnancy on drug distribution, metabolism, and clearance have been summarized elsewhere.[165]

Hepatic extraction of morphine, fentanyl, and vecuronium is well handled by the newly transplanted liver.[213] In a study aimed at quantifying morphine use and comparing the analgesic efficacy and side effect profiles of intravenous patient-controlled analgesia morphine following liver transplantation (OLTx) and liver resection, we found that morphine use was significantly decreased in the OLTx group at 6, 12, 24, 48, and 72 postoperative hours. No differences occurred in pain or sedation scores. With no evidence of primary nonfunction or significant rejection in these patients, factors likely to account for this difference include altered pain perception (steroids, cerebral spinal fluid endorphins, low-grade encephalopathy, liver denervation, CyA, personality traits) or persistent pharmacokinetic and pharmacodynamic changes inherent in end-stage liver disease. We have not yet determined whether this significant difference persists long-term.[214] Accumulation of active morphine metabolites with prolonged narcosis should be anticipated in patients with impaired renal function.[215]

Clinically, the pharmacokinetics of propofol in patients 48 hours following liver transplantation are identical with data obtained in patients with no evidence of hepatic disease who received a prolonged infusion of propofol.[216] In contrast, the human cytochrome P450 mono-oxygenase system is suppressed by propofol in vitro. This suggests that potential drug interactions may exist between propofol and substrates, such as CyA, using cytochrome P450 for drug metabolism.[217]

Because bupivacaine is eliminated almost entirely by hepatic metabolism, impairment of hepatic function in conjunction with repeated drug doses can result in drug accumulation, with the risk of CNS and cardiovascular toxicity. Repeated bilateral intercostal injections of bupivacaine have been given immediately following liver transplantation to provide analgesia, limiting the need for the systemic administration of narcotics. Pharmacokinetic studies reveal prolonged elimination of both enantiomers of bupivacaine with no tendency for accumulation, even upon repeated dosing.[218]

During the reperfusion phase of liver transplantation, there is progressive recovery of cytochrome P450-dependent microsomal enzyme activity starting immediately after unclamping the portal vein and inferior vena cava.[219] Therefore, neuromuscular blocking agents that are eliminated by the liver (e.g., vecuronium, rocuronium, pipecuronium) are suitable for use in patients with normal liver graft function.[219, 220] Plasma concentrations and neuromuscular effects of atracurium are not influenced by the absence of hepatic function or circulation, although an accumulation of its metabolite laudanosine has been reported.[221, 222]

In all liver transplant patients, large bore intravenous access is essential for the rapid administration of fluids and blood products, as required. The patient may be at risk for intraoperative hemorrhage from excessive surgical blood loss due to the presence of residual portal-systemic collaterals, mild to moderate coagulopathy, and clinical impression of a decreased capacity of the denervated hepatic vasculature to compensate for systemic hypotension.

Heart and Heart-Lung

In the patient with a heart or heart-lung transplant, invasive hemodynamic monitoring may be helpful to assess the balance between peripheral vasodilatation and volume loading. Indications include a suspicion of cardiac decompensation during an acute rejection episode, pre-existing marginal cardiac reserve from chronic rejection, myocardial ischemia, or anticipated large fluid volume shifts. Additional indications include oliguria unresponsive to fluids, respiratory compromise, and need for short-acting vasoactive medications (e.g., sodium nitroprusside).[208] In most instances, a minimal amount of monitoring is needed.[223] The left internal jugular, antecubital, or subclavian vein is preferred for central venous cannulation to keep the right side of the neck available for the rejection surveillance of serial endomyocardial biopsies.[210] Radial artery lines are preferable to femoral artery lines, whenever possible.[114] Transesophageal echocardiography may provide the least invasive method to evaluate ventricular filling and contractility. Infective endocarditis is a rare complication[224]; however, routine administration of standard endocarditis prophylaxis according to the American Heart Association guidelines is recommended on the basis of the immunocompromised condition of the patients and theoretical risk of suture line infection.[88]

In the absence of reflex vasocontriction following hypovolemia, patients are exquisitely sensitive to changes in preload and thus require attention to left-sided uterine displacement and volume loading. Before instituting spinal or epidural anesthesia for cesarean section, a preload of a colloid solution in the "compromised" patient may be more efficacious than a crystalloid preload in preventing hypotension.[208] Cautious titration of drugs is imperative, with the avoidance or judicious use of myocardial depressants. The anesthetized patient with a heart transplant may show exaggerated responses to hypovolemia, orthostatic hypotension, or systemic vascular resistance decreases.[112] Treatment of hypotension includes adequate volume loading and availability of an infusion of isoproterenol, epinephrine, or dobutamine to increase the heart rate rapidly and improve cardiac contractility. Most reports indicate that despite both direct and indirect cardiac effects, the clinical actions of ephedrine and dopamine are apparently unchanged.[225–227] Depth of anesthesia or responses to noxious stimuli may be difficult to assess owing to a normally elevated baseline heart rate and delayed cardiac output and heart rate responses. Blood pressure responses, therefore, may provide a more accurate guide to anesthetic requirements. Both atrial and ventricular dysrhythmias are common findings in the recently transplanted heart patient, in the presence of coronary artery disease, during episodes of acute rejection, and as, an incidental finding, in the long-term heart transplant patient. Ventricular dysrhythmias may be due to a lack of suppressant vagal tone, increased endogenous catecholamine concentrations, and/or hypersensitivity to catecholamines.[210, 228] Supraventricular dysrhythmias occur frequently, possibly because of surgical trauma to the sinoatrial node, ischemia, or rejection.[229] These dysrhythmias respond to treatment with standard antidysrhythmic drugs, cardioversion if appropriate, and correction of an underlying rejection episode with large doses of immunosuppressive drugs.[100] For treatment of tachydysrhythmias, evidence suggests adenosine supersensitivity of the denervated heart.[230]

Only direct-acting pharmacologic agents have predictable inotropic or chronotropic responses. Any maneuver or drug that relies solely on reflex autonomic neural pathways for its chronotropic effect does not produce a change in heart rate with administration. Examples are M-(muscarinic)1 and M2 agonist (fentanyl, phenylephrine); M1 and M2 antagonist (atropine, glycopyrrolate, demerol); M2 antagonist (pancuronium) or cholinergic; M2 agonist (neostigmine, edrophonium, pyridostigmine). Peripheral actions on vascular tone, however, are maintained.[231]

Sodium thiopentone may produce greater hypotension than expected, because of its intrinsic myocardial depressant action and absence of reflex increases in heart rate. Opioids may not be as effective in the treatment of "light anesthesia" because of their inability to decrease heart rate and blood pressure via vagal mechanisms.[232] Nitrous oxide can produce unanticipated hypotension because of the lack of its sympathetic stimulating properties to offset its direct myocardial depressant effect.[233] Isoflurane can also produce exaggerated hypotension owing to an absence of reflex increase in heart rate in response to vasodilatation.[232] Reflex tachycardia, which is often seen with vasodilator drugs used to treat pregnancy-induced hypertension (hydralazine, nitroglycerin, and sodium nitroprusside), is absent and hypotension may be exaggerated.[112] Caution should be exercised in the administration of ergonovine or prostaglandin $F_{2\alpha}$ for uterine hypotonia. Although no cases of angina pectoris have been reported in a pregnant transplant patient, ECG monitoring for coronary ischemia during labor and delivery is essential. Three years after heart transplant, at least 30% of patients have significant single- or multivessel coronary artery disease.[102]

A choice of muscle relaxant with minimal histamine-releasing and ganglionic-blocking properties is preferable.[232] Neostigmine has been reported to produce bradycardia and sinus arrest in heart transplant patients, which can be explained by cholinergic receptor hypersensitivity; direct activation of cardiac ganglionic cells; vagal reinnervation; or sinus node dysfunction from surgical trauma, ischemia, or rejection.[234–236] If muscle relaxants are required, recommendations include administration of short- or intermediate-acting agents (atracurium, mivacurium). Assisted ventilation of the lungs is performed until spontaneous recovery of muscular function occurs without attempting reversal with anticholinesterases and a muscarinic antagonist.[234]

Both external and internal pacemakers, atropine, and beta adrenergic agonists (isoproterenol or epinephrine) should always be readily available to treat bradydysrhythmias in heart transplant patients undergoing general anesthesia.[236]

The immediate sympathetic response to laryngoscopy and intubation should be absent. Other maneuvers such as externalization of the uterus, producing vagal stimulation and reflex bradycardia with hypotension, is not expected.[208]

Epidural anesthesia may be the preferred technique for labor analgesia and delivery because incremental injection of local anesthetics and titration of the level of sympathetic blockade allow time for volume loading and physiologic compensation by the patient. Clinicians should be cognizant of the additional infection risk to the CNS when choosing epidural and spinal anesthesia.[86] The epidural catheter should not be left in situ for more than 2 days, because the incidence of infection increases after this time.[212] Complete sympathetic denervation implies that levels of regional anesthesia above T4 are not expected to result in bradycardia.[70] Epidural injection of an epinephrine-containing local anesthetic in a patient with a transplanted heart can produce a profound tachycardia, with the risk of precipitating myocardial ischemia. The proposed mechanism for this exaggerated response is systemic absorption of epinephrine in the presence of an exquisite sensitivity of the transplanted heart to beta adrenergic agonists.[70] Others report intact alpha and beta adrenoreceptors in the denervated heart responding normally to circulating catecholamines without evidence of hypersensitivity to exogenous and endogenous catecholamines.[225, 237] Suggested techniques for general and regional anesthesia for heart transplant patients are summarized in Tables 11–23 and 11–24.

Postpartum monitoring includes assessment of cardiovascular and renal status, temperature, fluid balance; ventricular function with serial ECGs, echocardiograms, and cardiac isoenzyme levels; and cardiac biopsy, if an acute rejection is suspected.

All equipment applied directly on patients with heart-lungs or lung transplants should be sterile, and a disposable circuit with a bacterial filter should be on the anesthetic machine.[212] Careful placement of the endotracheal tube with monitoring of FiO_2, arterial blood gases (by pulse oximetry, capnography, or invasive monitoring), peak airway pressures, and fluid infusion should minimize the risk of (1) oxygen toxicity, (2) barotrauma, (3) stress on the tracheal/bronchial anastomosis, (4) excessive increases in PVR, and (5) volume overload of the lungs. Excessive secretions with sputum retention and ventilation/perfusion mismatch can be minimized with antisialogues, suctioning, and humidification of inspiratory gases. Although 60 to 80% of both ventilation and perfusion are to the new lung in single-lung recipients, the patient should be extubated with the native lung (or the least important lung during an episode of rejection or infection) in the dependent position.[114] In the absence of a cough reflex, the patient is extubated when fully awake, as early as possible to minimize the risk of bacterial pneumonia. Expectoration is encouraged from the transplanted lung by postural drainage and physiotherapy.[112]

Despite denervation of vagal efferents, bronchoconstriction has been described in a patient with a transplanted lung that subsequently was rejected[238] and in another following implantation of apparently normal lungs.[239] The response to bronchodilators such as isoprenaline, aminophylline, and epinephrine was poor. Some heart-lung transplant patients have an increased Pa_{CO_2} in the postoperative period, which decreases to within normal limits in time.[112] Concerns have been raised that drugs that depress ventilation may further obtund the response to carbon dioxide.[238] The clinical significance of this observation is not clear.

Volatile agents are well tolerated[223]; their use is preferable to long-acting muscle relaxants, high-dose narcotics, or benzodiazepines, which may preclude early extubation.[114] Although an intravenous crystalloid is acceptable for heart recipients, this practice in lung

---

TABLE 11–23. GENERAL ANESTHESIA FOR CESAREAN SECTION: A SUGGESTED TECHNIQUE FOR HEART TRANSPLANT PATIENTS

External and internal pacemakers, atropine, and beta-adrenergic agonists such as isoproterenol or epinephrine should always be readily available.
1. Administer aspiration, steroid, and antibiotic prophylaxis
2. Volume preload with dextrose-free crystalloid (or colloid) solution, preferably two indwelling intravenous catheters
3. Position supine (left uterine displacement, LUD), surgical preparation and draping
4. Noninvasive monitors: ECG, automatic blood pressure cuff, pulse oximetry, neuromuscular blockade (invasive monitoring for renal, respiratory, or cardiac compromise)
5. Preoxygenation (O_2 >6 l/min)
6. Assistant readiness to apply cricoid pressure, surgeon poised
7. Rapid-sequence induction with cricoid pressure: thiopental 4 mg/kg and succinylcholine 1.5 mg/kg, careful intubation of trachea within 60 seconds, verify cuffed endotracheal tube placement with end-tidal CO_2 monitor and chest auscultation before releasing cricoid pressure. Do not precurarize the patient because of interaction potential of magnesium, CyA, and nondepolarizing muscle relaxants.
8. Maintenance: nitrous oxide 50%, isoflurane <0.75%. Choice of muscle relaxants: no additional relaxant, mivacurium, or atracurium (do not administer reversal dose of neostigmine and atropine, document sustained head lift for 5 seconds before extubation and again in recovery room)
9. Hypotension (systolic blood pressure <100 mm Hg or decreased by 30%): determine etiology, ensure LUD, administer fluids, ephedrine 5 to 15 mg IV, isoproterenol (avoid maternal hyperventilation and high peak inspiratory pressures)
10. With delivery of the baby, deepen anesthesia with narcotics and benzodiazepines, continue isoflurane <0.50%/N_2O/O_2, limit FiO_2 to 40% in heart-lung transplant patients
11. Extubate with the patient fully awake; demonstrate adequate ventilation, oxygenation, and recovery from residual muscle relaxant

---

TABLE 11–24. REGIONAL ANESTHESIA FOR CESAREAN SECTION: SUGGESTED TECHNIQUES FOR HEART TRANSPLANT PATIENTS

1. Administer aspiration prophylaxis
2. Volume load with 1 to 2 liters of dextrose-free crystalloid (or colloid) solution
3. Administer supplemental oxygen, apply hemodynamic monitors (blood pressure cuff, ECG, pulse oximetry), and position patient

Resuscitation equipment and drugs must be readily available for use.

Epidural Anesthesia

Local anesthetic solutions
1. 0.5% bupivacaine
2. 1.5 to 2% lidocaine
3. 3% chloroprocaine

Addition of epinephrine to a concentration of 1:200,000 for the test dose (15 μg) and fractionated incremental doses up to 20 ml is controversial. Availability of a titratable infusion of esmolol and observation of heart rate with ECG monitoring is essential.

Adjustment for rapid onset with sodium bicarbonate (8.4%): 1 ml:10 ml with lidocaine or chloroprocaine and 0.1 ml:10 ml with bupivacaine.

Addition of epidural narcotics for intraoperative analgesia recommended (fentanyl 50 to 100 μg) and morphine 3 mg following delivery.

4. Position patient supine with LUD
5. Monitor arterial blood pressure every minute until delivery of the baby, then every 5 minutes for the duration of the block
6. Anxiety or "patchy" anesthesia may be treated with fentanyl 1 mg/kg, ketamine 0.25 mg/kg, midazolam 1–2 mg with additional intravenous narcotic following delivery

Spinal Anesthesia

Local anesthetic solutions

1. Bupivacaine 10.5 to 12.5 mg (0.75% with 8.25% dextrose solution)
2. Tetracaine 7 to 10 mg (tetracaine 1% and equal volumes of 10% dextrose in water)

Avoid hyperbaric lidocaine solutions.
Optional addition of intrathecal narcotics including fentanyl 10 to 25 μg or preservative-free morphine 0.1 to 0.25 mg for postoperative pain relief

---

transplant patients may severely damage the organs, owing to their extreme sensitivity to pulmonary leakage.[114] Monitoring of right ventricular function is essential if there is evidence of residual pulmonary hypertension or cardiac decompensation.

CONCLUSIONS

During the past two decades organ transplantation has become widely accepted as an established therapeutic option for patients suffering from end-stage organ failure. The ultimate goal for these patients is not purely survival at all costs, but rather the resumption of a normal lifestyle, which for many young women includes childbearing. Important advancements in organ preservation and immunosuppressive therapy have drastically improved patient and graft survival.

It is inevitable that with increasing frequency, the anesthesiologist will be requested to participate in the care of the pregnant transplant recipient during labor and delivery. This chapter has been compiled from a review of the literature, discussion among colleagues, and personal experience as a transplant anesthesiologist to help our readers address this challenge.

References

1. Murray JE, Reid DE, Harrison JH, Merrill JP. Successful pregnancies after human renal transplantation. N Engl J Med 1963; 269:341.
2. Hume DM, Lee HM, Williams GM, et al. Comparative results of cadaver and related donor renal homografts in man and immunologic implications of the outcome of second and paired transplants. Ann Surg 1966;164:352.
3. Caplan RM, Dossetor JB, Maughan GB. Pregnancy following cadaver kidney homotransplantation. Am J Obstet Gynecol 1970;106:644.
4. Walcott WO, Derick DE, Jolley JJ, Snyder DL. Successful pregnancy in a liver transplant patient. Am J Obstet Gynecol 1978;132:340.
5. Lewis GJ, Lamont CA, Lee HA, Slapak M. Successful pregnancy in a renal transplant recipient taking cyclosporin A. Br Med J (Clin Res Ed) 1983;286:603.
6. Castro LA, Boltzer U, Hillebrand G, et al. Pregnancy in juvenile diabetes mellitus under cyclosporine treatment after combined kidney and pancreas transplantation. Transplant Proc 1986;18:1780.
7. Lowenstein BR, Vain NW, Perrone SV, et al. Successful pregnancy and vaginal delivery after heart transplantation. Am J Obstet Gynecol 1988;158:589.
8. Haagsma EB, Visser GH, Klompmaker IJ, et al. Successful pregnancy after orthotopic liver transplantation. Obstet Gynecol 1989;74:442.
9. Rose ML, Dominguez M, Learer N, et al. Analysis of T cell subpopulations and cyclosporine levels in the blood of two neonates born to immunosuppressed heart-lung transplant recipients. Transplantation 1989;48:223.
10. Takahashi K, Sonda K, Okuda H, et al. The first report of a successful delivery in a woman with an ABO-incompatible kidney transplantation. Transplantation 1993;56:1288.
11. Norton PA, Scott JR. Gynecologic and obstetric problems in renal allograft recipients. In Buchsbaum HJ, Schmidt JD (eds): Gynecologic and Obstetric Urology, 3rd ed. Philadelphia, WB Saunders, 1993, p 657.
12. de Koning ND, Haagsma EB. Normalization of menstrual pattern after liver transplantation: Consequences for contraception. Digestion 1990;46:239.
13. Cundy TF, O'Grady JG, Williams R. Recovery of menstruation and pregnancy after liver transplantation. Gut 1990;31:337.
14. Laifer SA, Darby MJ, Scantlebury VP, et al. Pregnancy and liver transplantation. Obstet Gynecol 1990;76:1083.
15. Ahner R, Kiss H, Zuckerman A, et al. Pregnancy and spontaneous delivery 13 months after heart transplantation. Acta Obstet Gynecol Scand 1994;73:511.
16. Davison JM. Dialysis, transplantation and pregnancy. Am J Kidney Dis 1991;17:127.
17. Laifer SA, Guido RS. Reproductive function and outcome of pregnancy after liver transplantation in women. Mayo Clin Proc 1995;70:388.
18. Lindheimer MD, Katz AI. Pregnancy in the renal transplant patient. Am J Kidney Dis 1992;19:173.
19. Penn I, Makowski EL, Harris P. Parenthood following renal transplantation. Kidney Int 1980;18:221.
20. Cunningham RJ, Buszta CC, Braun WE, et al. Pregnancy in renal allograft recipients and long-term follow-up of their offspring. Transplant Proc 1983;15:1067.
21. Ahlswede KM, Armenti VT, Mokritz MJ, et al. Premature births in female renal transplant recipients: Degree and effect of immunosuppressive regiment. Surg Forum 1992;43:524.
22. Marushak A, Weber T, Bock J, et al. Pregnancy following kidney transplantation. Acta Obstet Gynecol Scand 1986;65:557.
23. Armenti VT, Ahlswede KM, Ahlswede BA, et al. Variables affecting birthweight and graft survival in 197 pregnancies in cyclosporine-treated female kidney transplant recipients. Transplantation 1995;59:476.
24. Armenti VT, Ahlswede KM, Ahlswede BA, et al. National Transplantation Pregnancy Registry—Outcomes of 154 pregnancies in cyclosporine-treated female kidney transplant recipients. Transplantation 1994;57:502.
25. Armenti VT, Ahlswede BA, Moritz MJ, et al. National Transplantation Pregnancy Registry: Analysis of pregnancy outcomes of female kidney recipients with relation to time interval from transplant to conception. Transplant Proc 1993;25:1036.
26. Laifer SA, Ehrlich GD, Huff DS, et al. Congenital cytomegalovirus infection in offspring of liver transplant recipients. Clin Infect Dis 1995;20:52.
27. Dummer JS, Hardy A, Poorsattar A, et al. Early infections in kidney, heart and liver transplant recipients on cyclosporine. Transplantation 1983;36:259.
28. Baruch Y, Weiner Z, Enat R, et al. Pregnancy after liver transplantation. Int J Gynecol Obstet 1993;41:273.
29. White JA, Guirandan C, Pflugfelder PW, et al. Routine surveillance myocardial biopsies are unnecessary beyond 1 year after heart transplantation. J Heart Lung Transplant 1995;14:1052.
30. Hosenpud JD, Novick RJ, Breen TJ, et al. The Registry of the International Society for Heart and Lung Transplantation: Eleventh official report—1994. J Heart Lung Transplant 1994;13:561.
31. Bumgardner GL, Matas AJ. Transplantation and pregnancy. Transplantation Rev 1992;6:139.
32. Davison JM. Pregnancy in renal allograft recipients: Problems, prognosis and practicalities. Baillieres Clin Obstet Gynaecol 1994;8:501.
33. Sims CJ. Organ transplantation and immunosuppressive drugs in pregnancy. Clin Obstet Gynecol 1991;34:100.
34. Sturgiss SN, Davison JM. Perinatal outcome in renal allograft recipients: Prognostic significance of hypertension and renal function before and during pregnancy. Obstet Gynecol 1991;78:573.
35. Cunningham FG, MacDonald PC, Gant NF, et al (eds). Drugs and Medications During Pregnancy. In Williams Obstetrics, 19th ed. Norwalk, Connecticut, Appleton & Lange, 1993, p 959.
36. Hou S. Pregnancy in organ transplant recipients. Med Clin North Am 1989;73:667.
37. Rudolph JE, Schweizer RT, Bartus SA. Pregnancy in renal transplant patients: A review. Transplantation 1979;27:26.
38. Fine RN. Pregnancy in renal allograft recipients. Am J Nephrol 1982;2:117.
39. Dekker GA, Sibai BM. Low-dose aspirin in the prevention of preeclampsia and fetal growth retardation: Rationale, mechanisms, and clinical trials. Am J Obstet Gynecol 1993;168:214.
40. Fromm GA, Labarrere CA, Ramirez J, et al. Hypercalcaemia in pregnancy in a renal transplant recipient with secondary hyperparathroidism: Case report. Br J Obstet Gynaecol 1990; 97:1049.
41. Zaloga GP, Prough DS. Fluids and electrolytes. In Barash PG, Cullen BF, Stoelting RK (eds): Clinical Anesthesia, 2nd ed. Philadelphia, JB Lippincott, 1992, p 226.
42. Kirk EP. Organ transplantation and pregnancy: A case report and review. Am J Obstet Gynecol 1991;164:1629.
43. Vinicor F, Golichowski A, Filo R, et al. Pregnancy following renal transplantation in a patient with insulin-dependent diabetes mellitus. Diabetes Care 1984;7:280.
44. Ogburn PL Jr, Kitzmiller JL, Hare JW, et al. Pregnancy following renal transplantation in class T diabetes mellitus. JAMA 1986;255:911.
45. Tyden G, Brattstrom C, Bjorkman U, et al. Pregnancy after combined pancreas-kidney transplantation. Diabetes 1989;38:43.
46. Kalkhoff RK, Kissebah AH, Kim HJ. Carbohydrate and lipid metabolism during normal pregnancy: Relationship to gestational hormone action. Semin Perinatol 1978;2:291.
47. Wahoff DC, Leone JP, Farney AC, et al. Pregnancy after total pancreatectomy and autologous islet transplantation. Surgery 1995;117:353.
48. Ville Y, Fernandez H, Samuel D, et al. Pregnancy in liver trans-

plant recipients: Course and outcome in 19 cases. Am J Obstet Gynecol 1993;168:896.

49. Abelmann WH. Hyperdynamic circulation in cirrhosis: a historical perspective (editorial). Hepatology 1994;20:1356.

50. Chezmar JL, Redvanly RD, Nelson RC, et al. Persistence of portosystemic collaterals and splenomegaly on CT after orthotopic liver transplantation. Am J Roentgenol 1992;159:317.

51. Henderson JM. Abnormal splanchnic and systemic hemodynamics of end-stage liver disease: What happens after liver transplantation? (editorial). Hepatology 1993;17:514.

52. Navasa M, Feu F, Garcia-Pagan JC, et al. Hemodynamic and humoral changes after liver transplantation in patients with cirrhosis. Hepatology 1993;17:355.

53. Hadengue A, Lebrec D, Moreau R, et al. Persistence of systemic and splanchnic hyperkinetic circulation in liver transplant patients. Hepatology 1993;17:175.

54. Textor SC, Wiesner RH, Wilson DJ, et al. Reversal of systemic vasodilation and hyperdynamic cardiac output during four weeks after liver transplantation. Hepatology 1992;16:290A.

55. Gadano A, Hadengue A, Widmann JJ, et al. Hemodynamics after orthotopic liver transplantation: Study of associated factors and long-term effects. Hepatology 1995;22:458.

56. Rubin DA, Schulman DS, Edwards TD, et al. Myocardial ischemia after orthotopic liver transplantation. Am J Cardiol 1994;74:53.

57. Ho M. Cytomegalovirus. In Mandell GL, Douglas RG, Bennet JE (eds): Principles and Practices of Infectious Diseases, 3rd ed. Edinburgh, Churchill Livingstone, 1990, p 1159.

58. Stack WA, Mulcahy HE, Fenelon L, et al. Cytomegalovirus myocarditis following liver transplantation. Postgrad Med J 1994;70:658.

59. Hamdani R, Chelluri R, Selby R, et al. Sudden death in patients with pulmonary hypertension undergoing liver transplantation (abstract). Hepatology 1991;14:282A.

60. Koneru B, Ahmed S, Weisse AB, et al. Resolution of pulmonary hypertension of cirrhosis after liver transplantation. Transplantation 1994;58:1133.

61. Krowka MJ, Cortese DA. Hepatopulmonary syndrome: An evolving perspective in the era of liver transplantation. Hepatology 1990;11:138.

62. Lange PA, Stoller JK. The hepatopulmonary syndrome. Ann Intern Med 1995;122:521.

63. Dimand RJ, Heyman MB, Lavine JE, et al. Hepatopulmonary syndrome: Response to hepatic transplantation. Hepatology 1991;14:55A.

64. McCloskey JJ, Schleien C, Schwarz K, et al. Severe hypoxemia and intrapulmonary shunting resulting from cirrhosis reversed by liver transplantation in a pediatric patient. J Pediatr 1991;118:902.

65. Krowka MJ. Clinical management of hepatopulmonary syndrome. Semin Liver Dis 1993;13:414.

66. Lopes P, Petit T, Quentin M, et al. Grossesse et accouchement chez une transplantee cardiaque. Presse Med 1988;17:869.

67. Kossoy LR, Herbert CM 3d, Wentz AC. Management of heart transplant recipients: Guidelines for the obstetrician-gynecologist. Am J Obstet Gynecol 1988;159:490.

68. Lowenstein BR, Vain NW, Perrone SV, et al. Successful pregnancy and vaginal delivery after heart transplantation. Am J Obstet Gynecol 1988;158:589.

69. Key TC, Resnik R, Dittrich HC, et al. Successful pregnancy after heart transplantation. Am J Obstet Gynecol 1989;160:367.

70. Camann WR, Goldman GA, Johnson MD, et al. Cesarean delivery in a patient with a transplanted heart. Anesthesiology 1989;71:618.

71. Hedon B, Montoya F, Cabrol A. Twin pregnancy and vaginal birth after heart transplantation. Lancet 1990;335:476.

72. Darbois Y, Seebacher J, Vauthier-Brouzes D, et al. Transplantations cardiaques: Repercussions sur la fecondite feminine. Bull Acad Natl Med 1991;175:531.

73. Camann WR, Jarcho JA, Mintz KJ, et al. Uncomplicated vaginal delivery 14 months after cardiac transplantation. Am Heart J 1991;121:939.

74. Hunt SA. Pregnancy in heart transplant recipients: A good idea? J Heart Lung Transplant 1991;10:499.

75. Carvalho AC, Almeida D, Cohen M, et al. Successful pregnancy, delivery and puerperium in a heart transplant patient with previous peripartum cardiomyopathy. Eur Heart J 1992;13:1589.

76. Liljestrand J, Lindstrom B. Childbirth after post partum cardiac insufficiency treated with cardiac transplant. Acta Obstet Gynecol Scand 1993;72:406.

77. Scott JR, Wagoner LE, Olsen SL, et al. Pregnancy in heart transplant recipients: Management and outcome. Obstet Gynecol 1993;82:324.

78. Baxi LV, Rho RB. Pregnancy after cardiac transplantation. Am J Obstet Gynecol 1993;169:33.

79. Laifer SA, Yeagley CJ, Armitage JM. Pregnancy after cardiac transplantation. Am J Perinatol 1994;11:217.

80. Wagoner LE, Taylor DO, Olsen SL, et al. Immunosuppressive therapy, management and outcome of heart transplant recipients during pregnancy. J Heart Lung Transplant 1993;12:993.

81. Chinayon P, Sakornpant P. Successful pregnancy after heart-lung transplantation: A case report. Asia Oceania J Obstet Gynaecol 1994;20:275.

82. Radomski JS, Ahlswede BA, Jarrell BE, et al. Outcomes of 500 pregnancies in 335 female kidney, liver, and heart transplant recipients. Transplant Proc 1995;27:1089.

83. Borow KM, Neumann A, Areumsman FW, Yacoub MH. Left ventricular contractility and contractile reserve in human heart, after cardiac transplantation. Circulation 1985;71:866.

84. Scott CD, Dark JH, McComb JM. Sinus node function after cardiac transplantation. J Am Coll Cardiol 1994;24:1334.

85. Kao AC, Vantright P 3rd, Shaeffer-McCall GS, et al. Allograft diastolic dysfunction and chronotropic incompetence limit cardiac output response to exercise two to six years after heart transplantation. J Heart Lung Transplant 1995;14:11.

86. Bricker SR, Sugden JC. Anaesthesia for surgery in a patient with a transplanted heart. Br J Anaesth 1985;57:634.

87. Gilbert EM, Eiswirth CC, Mealey PC et al. Beta-adrenergic supersensitivity of the transplanted human heart is presynaptic in origin. Circulation 1989;79:344.

88. Taylor AJ, Bergir JD. Cardiac transplantation for the cardiologist not trained in transplantation. Am Heart J 1995;129:578.

89. Schroeder JS. Hemodynamic performance of the human transplanted heart. Transplant Proc 1979;11:304.

90. von Scheidt W, Ziegler U, Kemkes BM, Evelmann E. Heart transplantation: Hemodynamics over a five-year period. J Heart Lung Transplant 1991;10:342.

91. Skowronski EW, Epstein M, Ota D, et al. Right and left ventricular function after cardiac transplantation. Changes during and after rejection. Circulation 1991;84:2409.

92. Young JB, Leon CA, Short HD 3rd, et al. Evolution of hemodynamics after orthotopic heart and heart-lung transplantation: Early restrictive patterns persisting in occult fashion. J Heart Transplant 1987;6:34.

93. Rowan RA, Billingham ME. Myocardial innervation in long-term heart transplant survivors: A quantitative ultrastructural survey. J Heart Transplant 1988;7:448.

94. Rudas L, Pflugfelder PW, Menkis AH, et al. Evolution of heart rate responsiveness after orthotopic cardiac transplantation. Am J Cardiol 1991;68:232.

95. Rudas L, Pflugfelder PW, Kostuk WJ. Vasodepressor syncope in a cardiac transplant recipient: A case of vagal re-innervation? Can J Cardiol 1992;8:403.

96. Fallen EL, Kamath MV, Ghista DN, et al. Spectral analysis of heart rate variability following human heart transplantation: Evidence for functional innervation. J Auton Nerv Syst 1988;23:199.

97. Fitzpatrick AP, Banner N, Cheng A, et al. Vasovagal reactions may occur after orthotopic heart transplantation. J Am Coll Cardiol 1993;21:1132.

98. Stark RP, McGinn AL, Wilson RF. Chest pain in cardiac-transplant recipients. Evidence of sensory reinnervation after cardiac transplantation. N Engl J Med 1991;324:1791.

99. Gao SZ, Hunt SA, Wiederhold V, et al. Characteristics of serial electrocardiograms in heart transplant recipients. Am Heart J 1991;122:771.

100. Schroeder JS, Berke DK, Graham AF, et al. Arrhythmias after cardiac transplantation. Am J Cardiol 1974;33:604.

101. Babuty D, Aupart M, Cosnay P, et al. Electrocardiographic and electrophysiologic properties of cardiac allografts. J Cardiovasc Electrophysiol 1994;5:1053.

102. Mendelson MA. Pregnancy after cardiac transplantation. In Gleicher N (ed): Principles and Practice of Medical Therapy in Pregnancy, 2nd ed. Norwalk, Connecticut, Appleton & Lange, 1992, p 841.

103. Uretsky BF, Murali S, Reddy PS, et al. Development of coronary artery disease in cardiac transplant patients receiving immunosuppressive therapy with cyclosporine and prednisone. Circulation 1987;76:827.

104. Miller LW. Long-term complications of cardiac transplantation. Prog Cardiovasc Dis 1991;33:229.

105. Uretsky BF, Kormos RL, Zerbe TR, et al. Cardiac events after heart transplantation: Incidence and predictive value of coronary arteriography. J Heart Lung Transplant 1992;11:545.

106. Keogh AM, Valantine HA, Hunt SA, et al. Impact of proximal or midvessel discrete coronary artery stenoses on survival after heart transplantation. J Heart Lung Transplant 1992;11:892.

107. Popovitch B, Mihm FG, Hilberman M, et al. Reinnervation of the lungs after transplantation. Anesthesiology 1982;57:A491.

108. Ruggiero R, Muz J, Fietsam R Jr, et al. Reestablishment of lymphatic drainage after canine lung transplantation. J Thorac Cardiovasc Surg 1993;106:167.

109. Dawkins KD, Jamieson SW, Hunt SA, et al. Long-term results, hemodynamics, and complications after combined heart and lung transplantation. Circulation 1985;71:919.

110. Pasque MK, Kaiser LR, Dresler CM, et al. Single lung transplantation for pulmonary hypertension: Technical aspects and immediate hemodynamic results. J Thorac Cardiovasc Surg 1992;103:475.

111. DeHoyos A, Patterson GA, Maurer JR, et al. Pulmonary transplantation: Early and late results. The Toronto Lung Transplant Group. J Thorac Cardiovasc Surg 1992;103:295.

112. Shaw IH, Kirk AJ, Conacher ID. Anesthesia for patients with transplanted hearts and lungs undergoing non-cardiac surgery. Br J Anaesth 1991:67:772.

113. Davis RD, Pasque MK. Pulmonary transplantation. Ann Surg 1995;221:14.

114. Boscoe M. Anesthesia for patients with transplanted lungs and heart and lungs. Int Anesthesiol Clin 1995;33:21.

115. Jamieson SW, Ogunnaike HO. Cardiopulmonary transplantation. Surg Clin North Am 1986;66:491.

116. Theodore J, Jamieson SW, Burke CM, et al. Physiologic aspects of human heart-lung transplantation. Pulmonary function status of the post-transplanted lung. Chest 1984;86:349.

117. Bando K, Paradis IL, Komatsu K, et al. Analysis of time-dependent risks for infection, rejection, and death after pulmonary transplantation. J Thorac Cardiovasc Surg 1995;109:49.

118. First MR, Combs CA, Weiskittel P, et al. Lack of effect of pregnancy on renal allograft survival or function. Transplantation 1995;59:472.

119. Sturgiss SN, Davison JM. Effect of pregnancy on long-term function of renal allograft. Am J Kidney Dis 1992;19:167.

120. Rizzoni G, Ehrich JH, Broyer M, et al. Successful pregnancies in women on renal replacement therapy: Report from the EDTA Registry. Nephrol Dial Transplant 1992;7:279.

121. Salmela K, Kyllonen L, Holmberg C, et al. Influence of pregnancy on kidney graft function. Transplant Proc 1993;25:1302.

122. Davison JM. The effect of pregnancy on kidney function in renal allograft recipients. Kidney Int 1985;27:74.

123. Sturgiss SN, Wilkinson R, Davison JM. Pregnancy alternates renal haemodynamic reserve (RHR) in women with renal allografts. Hypertension in Pregnancy 1993;12:275.

124. Lau RJ, Scott JR. Pregnancy following renal transplantation. Clin Obstet Gynecol 1985;28:339.

125. Davison JM. Renal transplantation and pregnancy. Am J Kidney Dis 1987;9:374.

126. Assellin BL, Lawrence RA. Maternal disease as a consideration in lactation management. Clin Perinatol 1987;14:71.

127. Fauchet R, Wattelet J, Goneter B, et al. Role of blood transfusions and pregnancies in kidney transplantation. Vox Sang 1979;37:222.

128. Feehally J, Harris KP, Bennett SE, et al. Is chronic renal transplant rejection a nonimmunological phenomenon? Lancet 1986; 2:486.

129. Tyden G, Groth CG. Pancreatic graft failure due to pelvic examination. Lancet 1987;1:812.

130. Seifert RD, Kang Y. Obstetric patients with liver disease. In Park GR, Kang Y (eds): Anesthesia and Intensive Care for Patients with Liver Disease, 1st ed. Boston, Butterworth-Heinemann, 1995, p 163.

131. Bean WB, Cogswell R, Dexter M, et al. Vascular changes of the skin in pregnancy. Surg Gynecol Obstet 1949;88:739.

132. Haemmerli UP, Wyss HI. Recurrent intrahepatic cholestasis of pregnancy. Report of six cases and review of the literature. Medicine 1967;46:299.

133. Haemmerli UP. Jaundice during pregnancy with special emphasis on recurrent jaundice during pregnancy and its differential diagnosis. Acta Med Scand 1966;179:S444.

134. Gray JR, Bouchier IAD. Pregnancy and the liver. In Calder AA, Dunlop W (eds): High-risk Pregnancy. Oxford, Butterworth-Heinemann 1992, p 210.

135. Scantlebury V, Gordon R, Tzakis A, et al. Childbearing after liver transplantation. Transplantation 1990;49:317.

136. Scott CD, Dark JH, McComb JM. Arrhythmias after cardiac transplantation. Am J Cardiol 1992;70:1061.

137. Cheek TA, Gutsche BB. Maternal physiologic alterations during pregnancy. In Shnider SM, Levinson G (eds): Anesthesia for Obstetrics, 3rd ed, Baltimore, Williams & Wilkins, 1993, p 3.

138. Camann WR, Ostheimer GW. Physiological adaptations during pregnancy. Int Anesthesiol Clin 1990;28:2.

139. Weinberger SE, Weiss ST. Pulmonary diseases. In Burrow GN, Ferris TF (eds): Medical Complications During Pregnancy, 4th ed. Philadelphia, WB Saunders, 1995, p 439.

140. Metcalf J, McAnulty JH, Ueland K. Physiology and management. In Burwell and Metcalfe's Heart Disease and Pregnancy: Physiology and Management, 2nd ed. Boston, Little, Brown, 1986, p 25.

141. Elkayam U, Gleicher N. Hemodynamics and cardiac function during normal pregnancy and the puerperium. In U Elkayam, N Gleicher (eds): Diagnosis and Management of Maternal and Fetal Disease: Cardiac Problems in Pregnancy, 2nd ed. New York, Alan R Liss, 1990, p 5.

142. Prowse CM, Gaensler EA. Respiratory acid base changes during pregnancy. Anesthesiology 1965;26:381.

143. MacKenzie AI: Laryngeal oedema complicating obstetric anaesthesia (correspondence). Anaesthesia 1978;33:271.

144. Procter AJ, White JB. Laryngeal oedema in pregnancy (letter). Anaesthesia 1983;38:167.

145. Heller PJ, Scheider EP, Marx GF. Pharyngolaryngeal edema as a presenting symptom in pre-eclampsia. Obstet Gynecol 1983;62:523.

146. Novy MJ, Edwards MJ. Respiratory problems in pregnancy. Am J Obstet Gynecol 1967;99:1024.

147. Hung CT, Pelosi M, Langer A, et al. Blood gas measurements in the kyphoscoliotic gravida and her fetus: Report of a case. Am J Obstet Gynecol 1975;121:287.

148. Radomski JS, Moritz MJ, Munoz SJ, et al. National Transplantation Pregnancy Registry: Analysis of pregnancy outcomes in female liver transplant recipients. Hepatology 1994;20:142A.

149. Andrews EB, Yankaskas BC, Cordero JF, et al. Acyclovir in pregnancy registry: Six years experience. The Acyclovir in Pregnancy Registry Advisory Committee. Obstet Gynecol 1992;79:7.

150. Jain A, Venkataramanan R, Lever J, et al. FK506 and pregnancy in liver transplant patients. Transplantation 1993;56:1588.

151. Winkler ME, Neisert S, Ringe B, et al. Successful pregnancy in a patient after liver transplantation maintained on FK506. Transplantation 1993;56:1589.

152. Huynh LA, Min DI. Outcomes of pregnancy and the management of immunosuppressive agents to minimize fetal risks in organ transplant patients. Ann Pharmacother 1994;28:1355.

153. Kahan BD. Cyclosporine. N Engl J Med 1989;321:1725.

154. Shaefer M, Williams L. Nursing implications of immunosuppression in transplantation. Nurs Clin North Am 1991;26:291.

155. Mason RJ, Thomson AW, Whitney PH, et al. Cyclosporine-induced fetotoxicity in the rat. Transplantation 1985;39:9.

156. Yee GC. Dosage forms of cyclosporine. Pharmacotherapy 1991;11:149S.

157. Crosby E, Robblee JA. Cyclosporine-pancuronium interaction in a patient with a renal allograft. Can J Anaesth 1988;35:300.

158. Wood GG. Cyclosporine-vecuronium interaction. Can J Anaesth 1989;36:358.

159. Dash A. Anesthesia for patients with a previous heart transplant. Int Anesthesiol Clin 1995;33:1.

160. Powell-Jackson PR, Carmichael FJL, Calne RY, et al. Adult respiratory distress syndrome and convulsions associated with administration of cyclosporine in liver transplant recipients. Transplantation 1984;38:341.

161. Biesenbach G, Zazgornik J, Kaiser W, et al. Cyclosporin requirement during pregnancy in renal transplant recipients. Nephrol Dial Transplant 1989;4:667.

162. Haugen G, Fauchald P, Sodal G, et al. Pregnancy outcome in renal allograft recipients: Influence of cyclosporin A. Eur J Obstet Gynecol Reprod Biol 1991;39:25.

163. Roberts M, Brown AS, James OF, et al. Interpretation of cyclosporine A levels in pregnancy following orthotopic liver transplantation. Br J Obstet Gynaecol 1995;102:570.

164. Bourget P, Fernandez H, Quinquis V, et al. Pharmacokinetics of cyclosporin A during pregnancy; monitoring of treatment and specific assays of cyclosporine, based on five liver transplant patients. J Pharm Biomed Anal 1993;11:43.

165. Witter FR. Clinical pharmacokinetics in the treatment of rheumatoid arthritis in pregnancy. Clin Pharmacokinet 1993;25:444.

166. Rosenthal RA, Chukwuogo NA, Ocasio VH, et al. Cyclosporine inhibits endothelial cell prostacyclin production. J Surg Res 1989;46:593.

167. Begnigni A, Morigi M, Perico N, et al. The acute effect of FK506 and cyclosporine on endothelial cell function and renal vascular resistance. Transplantation 1992;54:775.

168. Kahan BD. Immunosuppressive therapy with cyclosporine for cardiac transplantation. Circulation 1987;75:40.

169. Textor SC, Canzanello VJ, Taler SJ, et al. Cyclosporine-induced hypertension after transplantation. Mayo Clin Proc 1994;69:1182.

170. Schneider DJ, Nordt TK, Sobel BE. Attenuated fibrinolysis and accelerated atherogenesis in type II diabetic patients. Diabetes 1993;42:1.

171. Raine AEG. Cardiovascular complications after renal transplantation. In Morris PJ (ed): Kidney Transplantation: Principles and Practice. Philadelphia, WB Saunders, 1988, p 575.

172. Jindal RM. Posttransplant diabetes mellitus—a review. Transplantation 1994;58:1289.

173. Stein DP, Lederman RJ, Vogt DP, et al. Neurological complications following liver transplantation. Ann Neurol 1992;31:644.

174. Patchell RA. Neurological complications of organ transplantation. Ann Neurol 1994;36:688.

175. Amato AA, Barohn RJ, Sahenk Z, et al. Polyneuropathy complicating bone marrow and solid organ transplantation. Neurology 1993;43:1513.

176. Conti DJ, Rubin RH. Infection of the central nervous system in organ transplant recipients. Neurol Clin 1988;6:241.

177. Yee GC, McGuire TR. Pharmacokinetic drug interactions with cyclosporin (part I). Clin Pharmacokinet 1990;19:310.

178. Yee GC, McGuire TR. Pharmacokinetic drug interactions with cyclosporin (part II). Clin Pharmacokinet 1990;19:400.

179. Lake KD, Nolen JG, Slaker RA, et al. Over-the-counter medications in cardiac transplant recipients: Guidelines for use. Ann Pharmacother 1992;26:1566.

180. Gelb AW, Freeman D, Robertson KM, et al. Isoflurane alters the kinetics of oral cyclosporine. Anesth Analg 1991;72:801.

181. Brown MR, Brajtbord D, Johnson DW, et al. Efficacy of oral cyclosporine given prior to liver transplantation. Anesth Analg 1989;69:773.

182. Lepage JY, Malinowsky JM, de Dieuleveult C. Interaction cyclosporine atracurium et vecuronium. [Interactions of cyclosporine with atracurium and vecuronium.] Ann Fr Anesth Reanim 1989;8:R135.

183. Gramstad L, Gjerlow JA, Hysing ES, et al. Interaction of cyclosporin and its solvent, Cremophor, with atracurium and vecuronium. Studies in the cat. Br J Anesth 1986;58:1149.

184. Sharpe MD, Gelb AW. Cyclosporin potentiates vecuronium blockade and prolongs recovery time in humans. Can J Anaesth 1992;39;A126.

185. Sidi A, Kaplan RF, Davis RF. Prolonged neuromuscular blockade and ventilatory failure after renal transplantation and cyclosporine. Can J Anaesth 1990;37:543.

186. Cirella VN, Pantuck CB, Lee YJ, et al. Effects of cyclosporine on anesthetic action. Anesth Analg 1987;66:703.

187. Bedrossian CW, Sussman J, Conklin RH, et al. Azathioprine-associated interstitial pneumonitis. Am J Clin Pathol 1984;82:148.

188. Saarikoski SA, Seppala M. Immunosuppression during pregnancy: Transmission of azathioprine and its metabolites from mother to the fetus. Am J Obstet Gynecol 1973;115:1100.

189. Dretchen KL, Morgenroth VH 3rd, Standaert FG, et al. Azathioprine: Effects on neuromuscular transmission. Anesthesiology 1976;45:604.

190. Gramstad KL. Atracurium, vecuronium and pancuronium in end-stage renal failure. Dose-response properties and interactions with azathioprine. Br J Anaesth 1987;59:995.

191. Vetten KB. Immunosuppressive therapy and anaesthesia. S Afr Med J 1973;47:767.

192. Cameron DE, Traill TA. Complications of immunosuppressive therapy. In Baumgartner WA, Reitz BA, Achuff SC (eds): Heart and Heart-lung Transplantation. Philadelphia, WB Saunders, 1990, p 237.

193. Maxwell SR, Moots RJ, Kendall MJ. Corticosteroids: Do they damage the cardiovascular system? Postgrad Med J 1994;70:863.

194. Reinisch JM, Simon NG, Karow WG, Gandelman R. Prenatal exposure to prednisone in humans and animals retards intrauterine growth. Science 1978;202:436.

195. Scott JR. Potential immunopathological pregnancy problems. Semin Perinatol 1977;1:149.

196. Penn I. Pregnancy following renal transplantation. In Andreucci VE (ed): The Kidney in Pregnancy. Boston, Martinus Nijhoff, 1986, p 195.

197. Udelsman R, Ramp J, Gallucci WT, et al. Adaptation during surgical stress. A reevaluation of the role of glucocorticoids. J Clin Invest 1986;77:1377.

198. Foldes FF, Arai T, Gentsch HH, Zarday Z. The influence of glucocorticoids on plasma cholinesterase. Proc Soc Exp Biol Med 1974;146:918.

199. Meyers EF. Partial recovery from pancuronium neuromuscular blockade following hydrocortisone administration. Anesthesiology 1977;46:148.

200. Laflin MJ. Interaction of pancuronium and corticosteroids. Anesthesiology 1977;47:471.

201. Leeuwin RS, Veldesema-Currie RD, van Wilgenburg H, et al. Effects of corticosteroids on neuromuscular blocking actions of d-tubocurarine. Eur J Pharmacol 1981;69:165.

202. Kino T, Hatanaka H, Miyata S, et al. FK-506, a novel immunosuppressant isolated from Streptomyces. II. Immunosuppressive effect of FK-506 in vitro. J Antibiot 1987;40:1256.

203. Bierer BE, Hollander G, Fruman D, et al. Cyclosporin A and FK 506: Molecular mechanisms of immunosuppression and probes for transplantation biology. Curr Opin Immunol 1993;5:763.

204. First MR. Transplantation in the nineties. Transplantation 1992;53:1.

205. Cillo V, Alleniami M, Fun GJ, et al. Major adverse effect of FK 506 used as an immunosuppressive agent after liver transplantation. In Abstracts of the XIVth International Congress of the Transplantation Society, Paris, August, 1992, p 68.

206. Shibata T, Ogawa N, Kayama I, et al. Does FK-506 accelerate the development of coronary artery disease in the transplanted heart as well as the native heart? Transplant Proc 1993;25:1145.

207. Davison JM. Towards long-term graft survival in renal transplantation: Pregnancy. Nephrol Dial Transplant 1995;10:S85.

208. Riley ET. Obstetric management of patients with transplants. Int Anesthesiol Clin 1995;33:125.

209. Sturrock ND, Lang CC, Struthers AD. Indomethacin and cyclosporin together produce marked renal vasoconstriction in humans. J Hypertens 1994;12:919.

210. Grebenik CR, Robinson PN. Cardiac transplantation at Harefield. A review from the anaesthetist's standpoint. Anaesthesia 1985;40:131.

211. Brown BR Jr. Anesthesia in Hepatic and Biliary Tract Disease. Philadelphia: FA Davis, 1988.

212. Black AE. Anesthesia for pediatric patients who have had a transplant. Int Anesthesiol Clin 1995;33:107.

213. Kelley SD, Cauldwell CB, Fisher DM, et al. Recovery of hepatic drug extraction after hypothermic preservation. Anesthesiology 1995;82:251.

214. Robertson KM, Gan TJ, Parrillo S, et al. Comparison of postoperative opiate following liver transplantation and liver resection. Anesth Analg 1996;82:S381.

215. Shelly MP, Cory EP, Park GR. Pharmacokinetics of morphine in

two children before and after liver transplantation. Br J Anaesth 1986;58:1218.

216. Debruyne D, Albessard TF, Samba D, et al. Clinical pharmacokinetics of propofol in postoperative sedation after orthotopic liver transplantation. Clin Drug Invest 1995;9:8.

217. Chen TL, Ueng TH, Chen SH, et al. Human cytochrome P450 mono-oxygenase system is suppressed by propofol. Br J Anaesth 1995;74:558.

218. Mather LE, McCall P, McNicol PL. Bupivacaine enantiomer pharmacokinetics after intercostal neural blockade in liver transplantation patients. Anesth Analg 1995;80:328.

219. Pittet JF, Morel DR, Mentha G, et al. Vecuronium neuromuscular blockade reflects liver function during hepatic autotransplantion in pigs. Anesthesiology 1994;81:168.

220. Magorian T, Wood P, Caldwell J, et al. The pharmacokinetics and neuromuscular effects of rocuronium bromide in patients with liver disease. Anesth Analg 1995;80:754.

221. Pittet JF, Tassonyi E, Schopfer C, et al. Plasma concentrations of laudanosine, but not of atracurium, are increased during the anhepatic phase of orthotopic liver transplantation in pigs. Anesthesiology 1990;72:145.

222. Robertson KM, Mimeault RE, Freeman DJ, et al. A pharmacokinetic study of atracurium in anhepatic pigs. Anesth Analg 1990;70:S325.

223. Melendez JA, Delphin E, Lamb J. Noncardiac surgery in heart transplant recipients in the cyclosporine era. J Cardiothorac Vasc Anesth 1991;5:218.

224. Counihan PJ, Yelland A, de Belder MA, et al. Infective endocarditis in a heart transplant recipient. J Heart Lung Transplant 1991;10:275.

225. Kanter SF, Samuels SI. Anesthesia for major operations on patients who have transplanted hearts. A review of 29 cases. Anesthesiology 1977;46:65.

226. Cooper DK, Becerra EA, Novitzky D, et al. Surgery in patients with heart transplants. Anaesthetic and operative considerations. S Afr Med J 1986;70:137.

227. Eisenkraft JB, Dimich I, Sachdev VP. Anesthesia for major non-cardiac surgery in a patient with a transplanted heart. Mt Sinai J Med 1981;48:116.

228. Cheng DC, Ong DD. Anaesthesia for non-cardiac surgery in heart-transplanted patients. Can J Anaesth 1993;40:981.

229. MacKintosh AF, Carmichael DJ, Wren C, et al. Sinus node dysfunction in first three weeks after cardiac transplantation. Br Heart J 1982;48:584.

230. Ellenbogen KA, Thames MD, DiMarco JP, et al. Electrophysiological effects of adenosine in the transplanted human heart. Evidence of supersensitivity. Circulation 1990;81:821.

231. Leachman RD, Cokkinos DV, Cabrera R, et al. Response of the transplanted, denervated human heart to cardiovascular drugs. Am J Cardiol 1971;27:272.

232. Bailey DL, Stanley TH. Anesthesia for patients with a prior cardiac transplant. J Cardiothorac Anesth 1990;4:38.

233. Ebert TJ, Kampine JP. Nitrous oxide augments sympathetic outflow: Direct evidence from 3 human peroneal nerve recordings. Anesth Analg 1989;69:444.

234. Backman SB, Ralley FE, Fox GS. Neostigmine produces bradycardia in a heart transplant patient. Anesthesiology 1993;78:777.

235. Backman SB, Bachoo M, Polosa C. Mechanism of the bradycardia produced in the cat by the anticholinesterase neostigmine. J Pharmacol Exp Ther 1993;265:194.

236. Beebe DS, Shumway SJ, Maddock R. Sinus arrest after intravenous neostigmine in two heart transplant recipients. Anesth Analg 1994;78:779.

237. Demas K, Wyner J, Mihm FG, et al. Anaesthesia for heart transplantation. A retrospective study and review. Br J Anaesth 1986;58:1357.

238. Finch EL, Jamieson SW. Anesthesia for combined heart and lung transplantation. Contemp Anesth Pract 1987;10:109.

239. Casella ES, Humphrey LS. Bronchospasm after cardiopulmonary bypass in the heart-lung recipient. Anesthesiology 1988;69:135.

12

MYOPATHIES

Chantal Crochetière, M.D.

Myopathies are primarily diseases of striated muscles. This chapter discusses hereditary myopathies (Table 12–1); metabolic, inflammatory, endocrine, and toxic myopathies are mentioned in the corresponding chapters. Pregnant women with myopathies have specific needs. Exacerbation of muscle weakness is common because labor and delivery can be like a marathon. Pregnancy may also uncover a disease that was previously asymptomatic.

HEREDITARY MYOPATHIES

Muscular Dystrophy

Muscular dystrophy is a major cause of progressive weakness and wasting of the musculature of the limbs and trunk. It can be differentiated from neuropathies by the involvement of the proximal muscle groups, absence of sensory disturbances, electromyography (EMG), muscle biopsy, and more recently, by deoxyribonucleic acid (DNA) studies. Muscular dystrophies are the result of a primary genetic defect specific to each type. Inheritance is due to a dominant, recessive, or sex-linked gene or to a mutation. Classification is based on historical descriptions or clinical similarities. Duchenne, Becker, and Emery-Dreifuss muscular dystrophies are sex-linked disorders affecting males. These three diseases are amenable to carrier detection and prenatal diagnosis by DNA analysis. Female carriers usually manifest no clinical signs but may on occasion manifest minor features or even varying degrees of weakness.[3–5] Symptomatic female carriers for Duchenne muscular dystrophy may be difficult to distinguish clinically from those with limb-girdle muscular dystrophy.[6] Because oculopharyngeal dystrophy has an onset in the fifth or sixth decade, it is not discussed here.

Myotonic Dystrophy

Myotonic dystrophy is the most frequently inherited muscular disorder among adults.[7] The incidence of the gene is 13.5 in 100,000 and the prevalence of the disease is 5 in 100,000.[8] It is an autosomal dominant transmitted disease with a great variety of expression. Although myotonic dystrophy (dystrophia myotonica = myotonia atrophica = dystrophy) usually begins in early adult life, a congenital form is well described. Prevalence is equal between the sexes, but pathologic changes may be more obvious in males.[9]

Progressive distal limb muscle weakness and wasting, failure of muscles to relax after a forceful contraction (myotonic handshake), and weakness of facial muscles[10] are the major distinguishing features. Myotonia is the most common finding on physical examination, but it is often a relatively insignificant component in relation to the other features of the syndrome. Per-

TABLE 12–1. HEREDITARY MYOPATHIES

Muscular dystrophy
  Myotonic
  Facioscapulohumeral
  Limb girdle
  Distal
  Scapuloperoneal
  Congenital

Congenital myopathies
  Central core
  Mini core
  Nemaline
  Myotubular

Metabolic myopathies
  Carnitine deficiency
  Carnitine-palmitoyl-transferase deficiency
  Complex III deficiency

Myotonia
  Congenita
  Paramyotonia congenita

Periodic paralysis
  Hypokalemic
  Hyperkalemic

Data from Griggs RC, Bradley WG. Disorders of nerve and muscle: Approach to the patient with neuromuscular disease. In Isselbacher KJ, Braunwald E, Wilson JD, et al (eds): Harrison's Principles of Internal Medicine, 13th ed. New York, McGraw-Hill, 1994, p 2359.[1] Mendell JR, Griggs RC. Inherited, metabolic, endocrine, and toxic myopathies. In Isselbacher KJ, Braunwald E, Wilson JD, et al (eds): Harrison's Principles of Internal Medicine, 13th ed. New York, McGraw-Hill, 1994, p 2383.[2]

cussion myotonia may be present when the grasp response is not found. Severe atrophy of the temporalis and sternocleidomastoid muscles appears early and leads to the typical facies.[11] Diagnosis is made by family history and physical examination and confirmed by electromyography and muscle biopsy findings. Myotonic dystrophy is a multisystem disease (Table 12–2) and involves smooth as well as striated muscle.

Myotonic Dystrophy and Pregnancy

Many case reports have been described during pregnancy.[10, 11, 15–26] Fertility in women is not reduced except in those severely affected.[27] Pregnancy does not usually affect the long-term course of the disease.[28] Temporary exacerbation of myotonia and muscle weakness may occur during the third trimester,[10, 24, 25] with rapid improvement after delivery. Deterioration may be related to progesterone levels[25, 29] or may be attributed partly to inactivity.[10, 22, 25] In many women, symptoms are first noticed during pregnancy[21, 29] or the disease is diagnosed only after the birth of a child with the congenital form.[11, 21, 22, 29]

Some[24, 30] have described inadequate uterine contractions in the first stage of labor, whereas others[19, 29] observed a normal or shorter course of labor with normal response to oxytocin. The prospective mother with myotonic dystrophy has a high incidence of ob-

TABLE 12–2. CLINICAL FEATURES OF MYOTONIC DYSTROPHY

Mild mental retardation

Alopecia

Blepharoconjunctivitis

Cataract

Nasal voice

Dysarthria

Respiratory system
    Atrophy of respiratory muscles
    Central sleep apnea[12]
    Aspiration pneumonia

Cardiac system
    Cardiac conduction defects
    Atrial dysrhythmias
    Relative hypotension[13]
    Cardiomyopathy

Digestive system
    Dysphagia
    Incoordination of upper esophageal sphincter
    Decreased tone in the lower esophageal sphincter
    Dilated stomach and delayed gastric emptying
    Intestinal pseudo-obstruction[14]

Endocrine system
    Abnormalities of glucose metabolism
    Gonadal atrophy in male

TABLE 12–3. MYOTONIC DYSTROPHY—OBSTETRIC COMPLICATIONS

Spontaneous abortion
Polyhydramnios
Premature labor
Abnormal presentation
Cesarean delivery
Prolonged first stage (?)
Inability to bear down
Uterine atony
Retained placenta
Placenta previa and accreta
Increased incidence of neonatal death

stetric complications that may require anesthetic assistance (Table 12–3). Premature labor is very common. Ritodrine and other β_2 receptor stimulants may precipitate myotonia from any cause,[31] not only myotonic dystrophy.[32] This effect is reversible and can be improved by phenytoin.[33] If other measures (bed rest, hydration, sedation, indomethacin) fail to halt premature labor, ritodrine can be used.[33] Use of magnesium sulfate, however, has potential problems.

Harper has reported a reduced frequency of pre-eclampsia in myotonic pregnancies,[34] quoting an incidence of 2% in myotonic patients compared with 7% in a control group (statistically insignificant). The incidence of pre-eclampsia in the general population is between 3 and 7%.[35] Pre-eclampsia complicating myotonic dystrophy does raise an interesting question: Is the use of magnesium sulfate contraindicated? Magnesium in therapeutic dosage is associated with abnormal neuromuscular transmission,[36] and an overdose can lead to maternal weakness, respiratory insufficiency, and cardiac failure.[37] Phenytoin should be given first if there are no cardiac conduction problems. If magnesium is used, blood levels should be assessed frequently and kept close to the lowest therapeutic level (2 mmol/l). The patient must be examined more frequently for increased weakness.

Congenital Myotonic Dystrophy

Congenital myotonic dystrophy is the most severe form of the disease, and it has a high mortality rate.[38] It is transmitted solely by an affected mother[39] who may be asymptomatic.[27] The risk of having an affected child with the congenital form is 10%, increasing to 40% if a previous child was affected.[40] Older women have more severely affected children.[41] The most characteristic symptoms during pregnancy are reduced fetal movements and hydramnios caused by impaired fetal swallowing.[38, 42] It also is associated with nonimmune hydrops fetalis.[43, 44] The neonate has severe generalized hypotonia and weakness without myotonia and difficulties in breathing, sucking, and swallowing.[29, 45–47] A gradual improvement occurs after the neonatal period. Unfortunately, children who survive are mentally retarded and later develop the underlying disease, which is gradually progressive. Genetic counseling of affected individuals before pregnancy is most important. The finding of the abnormal gene, localized to chromosome 19,[27, 48–50] indicates a carrier state and prenatal detection can now be performed.[27, 51–54] Subsequent generations manifest the disease more severely and at earlier ages. This phenomenon, called *anticipation*, is a unique feature of myotonic dystrophy.[55, 56]

Myotonic Dystrophy, Pregnancy, and Anesthesia

Interesting case reports have been described in the obstetric anesthesia literature.[57–65] Patients with established myotonic dystrophy may not be the ones at greatest risk; rather, risks are higher for mildly affected or undiagnosed patients.[66] These patients may fail to mention or may be unaware of their muscle symptoms.[67]

Respiratory and cardiac involvement should be carefully assessed. Many patients have serious cardiac involvement.[68] Most cardiac problems are due to involvement of conducting tissue. The conduction abnormalities include first-degree atrioventricular (AV) block, interventricular conduction defects, and bundle branch block. Dilated cardiomyopathy is uncommon.[69–71] Cardiac decompensation resulting from anesthesia[72] or pregnancy occasionally occurs.[73, 74] Preoperative investigation should include an electrocardiogram

TABLE 12–4. MYOTONIC DYSTROPHY, PREGNANCY, AND ANESTHETIC CONSIDERATIONS

Airway
  Malocclusion
  Temporomandibular dislocation

Respiratory
  Increased sensitivity to any respiratory depressant
  Decreased cough reflex, potential for pneumonia
    and atelectasis
  Postoperative respiratory failure

Cardiac
  Conduction problems
  Dysrhythmia

Digestive
  Aspiration

Obstetric
  Prolonged labor
  Hemorrhage
  More frequent cesarean delivery
  Neonatal resuscitation

Myotonic crisis (see Tables 12–5 and 12–6)

TABLE 12–5. MYOTONIC CRISIS PREVENTION

Warming of
  Patient
  Delivery room
  IV fluids

Avoidance of
  Succinylcholine
  Shivering

Gentle handling of muscles

(ECG), even in the asymptomatic patient, Holter monitoring, echocardiogram, chest radiograph, pulmonary function tests, and blood gas analysis. A vital capacity of 1 l is the minimal functional requirement necessary to maintain successful pregnancy.[75] Invasive intraoperative monitoring depends on the patient's physical status. Anesthetic considerations are summarized in Table 12–4. Abnormalities of the airway have been described, but difficult intubation has not been reported.[64, 76]

Myotonic crisis is a unique complication in which the patient develops marked, generalized contracture of skeletal muscles that can last 2 to 3 minutes. Spontaneous and controlled ventilation can be severely compromised.[77] Crisis is not relieved by neuromuscular, regional, or peripheral nerve block or even by general anesthesia. A generalized and localized contracture should be prevented by prewarming of the delivery room and intravenous (IV) fluids, warming blankets, strict avoidance of succinylcholine, anesthetic technique that diminishes shivering, and gentle handling of muscles during surgery (Table 12–5). Medication for treatment should be readily available (Table 12–6).

Epidural is the method of choice for analgesia during labor, for forceps delivery, or for cesarean section. Spinal deformities are very rare in myotonic dystrophy. Spinal anesthesia may be used, but it is relatively contraindicated for cesarean section if the respiratory system is severely compromised. Case reports suggest a reduced respiratory complication rate with regional anesthesia.[57, 60, 61, 64] Two case reports have described successful combined spinal-epidural anesthesia for cesarean delivery in women with myotonic dystrophy.[78, 79] The benefits were rationalized as the ability to give the lowest possible dose of intrathecal bupivacaine to avoid excessively high dermatomal levels, with an epi-

TABLE 12–6. TREATMENT OF MYOTONIC CRISIS

For generalized myotonic contracture
  Procainamide, quinine (careful, if conduction defects)
  Dantrolene
  Diphenylhydantoin

For localized myotonic contracture
  Direct injection of local anesthetic in muscle

TABLE 12–7. MUSCULAR DYSTROPHY—OTHER FORMS[2, 27, 98-101]

	Onset	Clinical Course	Muscular Involvement	Respiratory Involvement	Cardiovascular Involvement	Anesthesia Problems	Obstetric Problems	Specific References	Prenatal Diagnosis
Facioscapulo-humeral—dominant	Adolescence or early adulthood	Very slow, arrest of progression is common	Face first then neck, shoulder, and pelvic girdle	Atrophy of accesssory muscles of respiration predispose to infection. Respiratory failure is rare	Labile hypertension common One case of atrial paralysis	Hyperkalemia with succinylcholine Exagerated lordosis Postoperative respiratory problems		102, 103	Yes
Limb girdle—recessive	10 to 30 years old	Variable	Pelvic first then shoulder girdle	Respiratory failure after 30 years or more of disease	Occasional conduction anomalies, dysrhythmias, and cardiomyopathy	Hyperkalemia with succinylcholine, lumbar lordosis	Prolonged second stage	104, 105, 106, 107, 108	Soon
Distal (includes 3 variants). The most frequent form is recessive	Third decade	Slow	Legs, hands		Cardiomyopathy in the dominant form with late onset	Hyperkalemia with succinylcholine		109, 110	
Scapuloperoneal—dominant	Late childhood or early adulthood	Very slow, arrest of progession is common	Shoulder girdle, legs, then pelvic girdle	Uncommon		Hyperkalemia with succinylcholine		102	Yes
Congenital (includes more than one disorder)—recessive	Birth	Non-progressive or very slowly progressive or improves	Generalized, proximal more than distal. Swallowing difficulties, diaphragmatic involvement	Respiratory failure may occur much later		Hyperkalemia with succinylcholine, kyphoscoliosis		111	

dural catheter in situ to provide further anesthesia, incrementally, as required. In addition, epidural fentanyl reduces shivering. General anesthetic drugs, which increase the risk of perioperative muscle weakness and aspiration, are avoided.

If regional anesthesia fails or is contraindicated, general anesthesia can be performed safely, keeping in mind the anesthetic considerations of pregnancy and myotonic dystrophy. Respiratory depressant drugs should be administered cautiously,[9] with a preference for short-acting drugs.[80, 81] Halothane is relatively contraindicated because of the depression of cardiac conduction and postoperative shivering.[82] Nondepolarizing neuromuscular blocking agents appear to behave normally,[83, 84] but the effect of a small amount of residual muscle weakness, usually not clinically apparent in normal patients, may cause postoperative respiratory failure. Some investigators[85, 86] suggest that neostigmine may precipitate myotonic crisis, but others[82, 33, 87] have used it safely and report a normal response. It may be prudent to use short-acting muscle relaxants that do not require antagonism[88, 89] and that have no residual effects. *Malignant hyperthermia is not associated with myotonic dystrophy.*[90–94]

The postoperative period is critical.[95–97] Patients should be monitored for dysrhythmias and airway obstruction, preferably in an intensive care unit setting. Physiotherapy should begin as soon as possible; morbidity and mortality are usually due to respiratory problems such as aspiration pneumonia[22] or cardiac failure. Analgesia is best achieved by regional blockade or neuraxial opioids. Systemic opioids should be administered with caution.

Muscular Dystrophy (Other Forms)

Other forms of muscular dystrophy are all very slowly progressive diseases (Table 12–7). Women of childbearing age are usually not much affected; many do not know the exact name of their disease. Very few case reports exist. Unlike myotonic dystrophy, the smooth muscle is never involved. Each parturient should be treated on an individual basis. Management should be determined after consultation with a neurologist or an internist. Succinylcholine should always be avoided because of the risk of hyperkalemia and rhabdomyolysis. Regional anesthesia is always preferred, when feasible.

Congenital Myopathies (Sarcoplasmic Myopathies)

Congenital myopathies are a group of rare diseases characterized by the presence of specific abnormalities in the muscle biopsy (Table 12–8). Muscle biopsy is the only way of making an accurate diagnosis. Serum enzyme levels and EMG are usually normal. In most, a pattern of inheritance has been defined. The congenital myopathies possess a number of common characteristics. Profound weakness and hypotonia are present at birth but are usually nonprogressive. Muscle wasting and weakness are associated with secondary skeletal changes or dysmorphic features. Difficulties in tracheal intubation and in regional anesthesia may occur. Succinylcholine is contraindicated, as in every primary mus-

TABLE 12–8. **CONGENITAL MYOPATHIES**[2, 93, 99, 112, 113]

	Clinical Course	Muscular Involvement	Respiratory Involvement	Cardiovascular Involvement	Anesthesia Problems	Obstetric Problems	Specific References
Central core—dominant with variable expression	Nonprogressive	Mild, symmetric, proximal, face and legs	Some		Airway (mandibular hypoplasia, short neck), kyphoscoliosis, malignant hyperthermia, lumbar lordosis		114, 115, 116, 117, 118
Minicore (multicore)—recessive	Slowly progressive or nonprogressive	Proximal, mild, trunk, face and extremities, swallowing difficulties	Recurrent chest infections secondary to kyphoscoliosis, diaphragmatic weakness and chronic aspiration. Nocturnal hypoventilation	Cardiomyopathy (rare)	Kyphoscoliosis	See Chapter 14	119
Nemaline (rod body) 4 forms, most common form is—recessive	Slowly progressive or nonprogressive	Mild, generalized, symmetric, proximal, swallowing difficulties	Chronic aspiration, microatelectasis secondary to diaphragmatic involvement. Nocturnal hypoventilation	Cardiomyopathy, congenital heart disease (rare)	Airway (high-arched palate, prognathism), kyphoscoliosis, lumbar lordosis, and other dysmorphic features, aspiration	Dystocia	120–124
Myotubular (centrilobular)—dominant or sex-linked	May or may not be progressive	Generalized		Cardiomyopathy (rare)	Airway (high-arched palate), kyphoscoliosis		

TABLE 12–9. METABOLIC MYOPATHIES (MITOCHONDRIAL MYOPATHIES)[2, 27, 98, 99, 125-127]

	Onset	Clinical Course	Muscular Involvement	Respiratory Involvement	Cardiovascular Involvement	Anesthesia Problems	Obstetrical Problems	Specific References
Carnitine deficiency, systemic form—recessive	Childhood	Progressive weakness, death secondary to irreversible coma. Treatment: carnitine supplement and carbohydrate	Proximal, improved with carnitine supplement in some cases	Possible	Rare cardiomyopathy	Avoid fasting, succinylcholine, shivering, hypoglycemia, metabolic acidosis; recurrent hepatic encephalopathy	Postpartum rapid progression of weakness; if no treatment, death	128, 129, 130, 131
Carnitine deficiency, myopathic form—recessive	Childhood	Slowly progressive. Treatment: Carnitine supplement and diet	Proximal, can affect pharyngeal muscles	Progress to respiratory failure	Cardiomyopathy	Rhabdomyolysis		132
Carnitine-palmitoyl-transferase deficiency—recessive	Childhood	Normal strength between attacks. Treatment: High carbohydrate and low fat diet	Weakness is induced by fasting and exercise and may be severe and generalized. Muscle cramps	May require respiratory assistance during episode of weakness		Rhabdomyolysis precipitated by fasting, exercise, succinylcholine, NSAID. Avoid shivering, give glucose Malignant hyperthermia?	Rhabdomyolysis in labor; normal uterine muscle tone despite abnormal muscle biopsy	133–136
Complex III deficiency	Childhood	Slowly progressive	Mild generalized weakness, muscle cramps, exercise intolerance	Decreased O_2 consumption, increased CO_2 production	Wolff-Parkinson-White syndrome in one case report	Severe lactic acidosis, prevent shivering	Preterm labor; avoid labor; elective cesarean section	137

cle disease. A normal response to nondepolarizing neuromuscular blocking agents may be present. *A strong association exists between malignant hyperthermia and central core myopathy* supported by clinical and laboratory evidence, including the proximity of the two genes on chromosome 19.[92, 94]

Metabolic Myopathies (Mitochondrial Myopathies)

Mitochondrial myopathies are a heterogenous group of uncommon diseases in which mitochondrial metabolism is defective, with predominantly skeletal muscle involvement (Table 12–9). The most practical classification is based on the area of mitochondrial metabolism specifically affected (Table 12–10). Obstetric case reports reveal defects of substrate transport; one report identified a defect of the respiratory chain.

Other mitochondrial disorders have a multisystemic involvement that predominantly affects the brain; no cases have been reported in obstetrics.

Because both carnitine-palmitoyl-transferase (CPT) deficiency and malignant hyperthermia can cause rhabdomyolysis, some believe there is an association between the two.[138] Clinicians may consider the possibility of malignant hyperthermia, avoiding triggering drugs and monitoring temperature.

Myotonia

Myotonia is a clinical sign or symptom that occurs in many disorders. Myotonic dystrophy is the most severe and most common form of myotonia. Myotonia congenita and paramyotonia congenita are two other diseases in which myotonia is prominent. The term describes a persistent contraction of a muscle observed after cessation of voluntary contraction.[139] Although it is difficult to interpret caffeine-halothane contracture test results in myotonic patients, most believe that myotonias are not associated with susceptibility to malignant hyperthermia.[140–143]

TABLE 12–10. MITOCHONDRIAL MYOPATHIES[123]

Defects of substrate transport (lipid metabolism disorders)
• Carnitine deficiency
• Carnitine-palmitoyl-transferase deficiency
Defects of substrate utilization
Defects of the Krebs cycle
Defects of oxidation-phosphorylation coupling
Defects of the respiratory chain (complex III deficiency)

Myotonia Congenita (Thomsen Disease)

Myotonia congenita is a rare inherited autosomal dominant disease. Symptoms may be present from birth, but they usually appear later on. This rather mild, nonprogressive, disease is characterized by generalized painless myotonia and muscular hypertrophy. The patient's main complaint is stiffness. Stiffness on initiating voluntary movement is relieved by exercise ("warm-up" phenomenon). There is no muscular weakness and no involvement of other organs. Smooth muscles are never affected, and uterine contractions are normal. Temporary worsening of the myotonia can occur in the second half of pregnancy.[144] Treatment is with an oral lidocaine-like antiarrhythmic agent. Several variants of this condition have been described,[145] including the more severe autosomal recessive form (Becker).

Epidural, spinal, or general anesthesia can be given safely as long as precipitation of a myotonic crisis is prevented, as described previously (see Table 12–5). Treatment is readily available (see Table 12–6); response to nondepolarizing muscle relaxants is normal.[83]

Paramyotonia Congenita

Paramyotonia congenita is the rarest of the myotonic syndromes. It is transmitted as an autosomal dominant characteristic. The myotonia is termed *paradoxical* because the muscular stiffness is exacerbated by exercise.[139] Paramyotonia congenita is a nonprogressive illness, and for most patients the symptoms are more of a nuisance than a handicap. As in myotonia congenita there is a tendency to hypertrophy of the musculature. It affects mostly the face, tongue, neck, and hand muscles, and occasionally the leg muscles. The disease is commonly induced or aggravated after exercise or exposure to cold. Usually, symptoms respond rapidly to warming, but episodes of flaccid paralysis lasting several hours after the muscles have rewarmed may be present. Pretreatment with tocainide prevents or improves the symptoms in all patients.[146] No other system appears to be involved.

Doubt has arisen as to whether paramyotonia congenita and hyperkalemic periodic paralysis are separate entities.[139, 147] There is increasing evidence to suggest that they are allelic disorders, the locus having been traced to chromosome 17.[148] The predominant feature of paramyotonia congenita is the *myotonia*, whereas in hyperkalemic periodic paralysis the main clinical symptom is the *muscle weakness*.[149] In severely affected women, symptoms may be worse during pregnancy.[146, 149] A case report suggested that a cold-temperature–induced abdominal wall contraction led

TABLE 12–11. DYSKALEMIC PERIODIC PARALYSIS[149, 153]

	Onset	Muscular Involvement	Provocation of Attacks	Duration of Attacks	Respiratory Involvement
Hypokalemic— dominant	Late first or second decade, males more severely affected	Proximal limbs progressing to trunk and neck, rarely bulbar or respiratory muscles	Rest after exercise, high sodium or carbohydrate meal, bicarbonate, glucose, insulin, adrenalin, corticosteroid, cold temperature, stress, infection, trauma, menstruation	2 to 4 hrs to days	Rarely respiratory distress can be fatal
Hyperkalemic— dominant	Infancy and childhood	Proximal limbs progressing to trunk and face	Fasting, cold, rest after exercise, KCl, corticosteroid	2 to 3 hrs	Mild weakness

to premature labor and delivery.[150] Subsequently, the same patient had another pregnancy with a normal delivery and epidural anesthesia without any problem.[151] Anesthetic considerations are the same as for myotonia congenita.

Dyskalemic Periodic Paralysis

In the past few years, advances in knowledge have helped in classifying many syndromes under the term *ion channel disorders*. The syndromes involved include dyskalemic periodic paralysis, myotonia congenita, paramyotonia, and cystic fibrosis.[149]

Dyskalemic periodic paralysis causes transient paralysis of muscles. There are two main forms: hypokalemic and hyperkalemic. The most frequent form is the hypokalemic; some cases occur in association with thyrotoxicosis in Asian races.[152] The hyperkalemic form is rarer, less severe, and never fatal. Three clinically different subtypes of the hyperkalemic form have been described: with myotonia, without myotonia, and with paramyotonia. Periodic paralysis is amenable to treatment, and progressive weakness can be prevented. *Neither form is associated with malignant hyperthermia.*[143] Clinical features, prevention, treatment, anesthesia, and obstetric problems are summarized in Table 12–11.

TUMORS AND MASSES

Myositis Ossificans Progressiva

Myositis ossificans progressiva is a rare, autosomal dominant disease characterized by extraskeletal ossifi-

cation involving muscle connective tissue.[163] The illness usually starts in early childhood and is progressively debilitating. Patients develop diffuse lesions that may be exacerbated by attempts at excision. Disodium ethane 1-hydroxy-1, 1-disphosphate (EHDP) halts the progression of the disease, but well-formed ossifications do not regress.[164] As the disease progresses, patients develop severe limitation in chest motion with the potential for secondary respiratory and cardiac failure.[99] Fertility is reduced, and early pregnancy loss is common. The first reported case of a pregnancy associated with myositis ossificans progressiva was an induced abortion at 10 weeks' gestation.[163] The only case report of a successful pregnancy was by Fox and coworkers, who described a cesarean section performed using local anesthesia and sedation for delivery of a 26-week viable infant.[165] Intubation of these patients may be impossible, even with a fiberoptic bronchoscope because of a fixed and flexed position of the neck. Tracheostomy may be difficult because of extensive calcification of the tracheal rings. Regional anesthesia depends on the extent of any associated kyphoscoliosis. Anesthetic and obstetric considerations are summarized in Table 12–12.

TABLE 12–12. MYOSITIS OSSIFICANS PROGRESSIVA—ANESTHETIC CONSIDERATIONS

Airway
Difficult intubation (fixed neck and jaw)
Calcification of tracheal rings, preventing rapid tracheotomy

Musculoskeletal
Kyphoscoliosis

Respiratory
Restrictive syndrome secondary to a fixed rib cage

Obstetric
Fixed hip joints
Cesarean delivery
Tissue calcification in the wound

TABLE 12–11. **DYSKALEMIC PERIODIC PARALYSIS** *Continued*

Cardiac Involvement	Treatment	Anesthesia Problems	Obstetric Problems	Case Reports	Prenatal Diagnosis
Fluid retention, bradycardia, dysrhythmia, cardiac failure	Acute: KCl, prevention: acetazolamide + KCl	Avoid: hypokalemia, succinylcholine, glucose load, alkalosis, monitor ECG, K^+ and glucose, keep warm, nondepolarizing muscle relaxants are safe	PIH More frequent and worse crises	154–159	
Dysrhythmia	Acute: glucose and insulin or calcium gluconate Prevention: acetazolamide, frequent meals	Avoid: fasting, succinylcholine, KCl, monitor ECG, K^+, glucose, give glucose, keep warm, nondepolarizing muscle relaxants are safe	PIH More frequent and worse crises	160–162	Possible

References

1. Griggs RC, Bradley WG. Disorders of nerve and muscle: Approach to the patient with neuromuscular disease. In Isselbacher KJ, Braunwald E, Wilson JD, et al (eds): Harrison's Principles of Internal Medicine, 13th ed. New York, McGraw-Hill, 1994, p 2359.
2. Mendell JR, Griggs RC. Inherited, metabolic, endocrine, and toxic myopathies. In Isselbacher KJ, Braunwald E, Wilson JD, et al (eds): Harrison's Principles of Internal Medicine, 13th ed. New York, McGraw-Hill, 1994, p 2383.
3. Dubowitz V. The Muscular Dystrophies. In Dubowitz V (ed): Muscle Disorders in Childhood, 2nd ed. London, WB Saunders, 1995, p 61.
4. Harper PS. The differential diagnosis of myotonic dystrophy: Other dystrophies and myotonic disorders. In Harper PS (ed): Myotonic Dystrophy, 2nd ed. London, WB Saunders, 1989, p 43.
5. Barkhaus PE, Gilchrist JM. Duchenne muscular dystrophy manifesting carriers. Arch Neurol 1989;46:673.
6. Boylan K. Duchenne muscular dystrophy manifesting carriers (letter). Arch Neurol 1990;47:951.
7. Harper PS. Muscle pathology in myotonic dystrophy. In Harper PS (ed): Myotonic Dystrophy, 2nd ed. London, WB Saunders, 1989, p 228.
8. Harper PS. The genetic basis of myotonic dystrophy. In Harper PS (ed): Myotonic Dystrophy. London, WB Saunders, 1989, p 318.
9. Speedy H. Exaggerated physiological responses to propofol in myotonic dystrophy. Br J Anaesth 1990;64:110.
10. Jaffe R, Mock M, Abramowicz J, et al. Myotonic dystrophy and pregnancy: A review. Obstet Gynecol Surv 1986;41:272.
11. Sun SF, Binder J, Streib E, et al. Myotonic dystrophy: Obstetric and neonatal complications. South Med J 1985;78:823.
12. Stoelting RK. Skin and musculoskeletal diseases. In Stoelting RK, Dierdorf SF (eds): Anesthesia and Co-existing Disease, 3rd ed. New York, Churchill Livingston, 1993, p 437.
13. O'Brien T, Harper PS, Newcombe RG. Blood pressure and myotonic dystrophy. Clin Genet 1983;23:422.
14. Brunner HG, Hamel BC, Rieu P, et al. Intestinal pseudo-obstruction in myotonic dystrophy. J Med Genet 1992;29:791.
15. Freeman RM. Placenta accreta and myotonic dystrophy. Two case reports. Br J Obstet Gynaecol 1991;98:594.
16. Paris G, Laframboise R, Bouchard J-P. La mère et l'enfant atteints de dystrophie myotonique de Steinert. Can J Neurol Sci 1989;16:104.
17. Chung HT, Tam AYC, Wong V, et al. Dystrophia myotonica and pregnancy—an instructive case. Postgrad Med J 1987;63:555.
18. Ditlev F, Gjerstad L. Obstetric complications as the first sign of myotonic dystrophy. Case report. Acta Obstet Gynecol Scand 1986;65:667.
19. Arulkumaran S, Rauff M, Ingemarsson I, et al. Uterine activity in myotonia dystrophica. Case report. Br J Obstet Gynaecol 1986;93:634.
20. Monnier JC, Patey P, Vansteenberghe F, et al. Maladie de Steinert et grossesse. J Gynecol Obstet Biol Reprod 1984;13:541.
21. Webb D, Muir I, Faulkner J, et al. Myotonia dystrophica: Obstetric complications. Am J Obstet Gynecol 1978;132:265.
22. Hilliard GD, Harris RE, Gilstrap III LC, et al. Myotonic muscular dystrophy in pregnancy. South Med J 1977;70:446.
23. Dunn LJ, Dierker LJ. Recurrent hydramnios in association with myotonia dystrophica. Obstet Gynecol 1973;42:104.
24. Shore RN, MacLachlan TB, et al. Pregnancy with myotonic dystrophy. Course, complications and management. Obstet Gynecol 1971;38:448.
25. Hopkins A, Wray S. The effect of pregnancy on dystrophia myotonica. Neurology 1967;17:166.
26. Walpole AR, Ross AW. Acute cord prolapse in an obstetric patient with myotonia dystrophica. Anaesth Intensive Care 1992;20:526.
27. Gilchrist JM. Muscle disease in the pregnant woman. In Devinsky O, Feldmann E, Hainline B (eds): Neurological Complications of Pregnancy. New York, Raven Press, 1994, p 193.
28. Harper PS. Endocrine abnormalities in myotonic dystrophy. In Harper PS (ed): Myotonic Dystrophy. London, WB Saunders, 1989, p 127.
29. Sarnat HB, O'Connor T, Byrne PA. Clinical effects of myotonic dystrophy on pregnancy and the neonate. Arch Neurol 1976;33:459.
30. Sciarra JJ, Steer CM. Uterine contractions during labor in myotonic muscular dystrophy. Am J Obstet Gynecol 1961;82:612.
31. Sholl JS, Hughey MJ, Hirschmann RA. Myotonic muscular dystrophy associated with ritodrine tocolysis. Case report. Am J Obstet Gynecol 1985;151:83.
32. Ricker K, Haass A, Glötzner F. Fenoterol precipitating myotonia in a minimally affected case of recessive myotonia congenita. J Neurol 1978;219:279.
33. Streib EW, Sun SF. Myotonic muscular dystrophy associated with ritodrine tocolysis. Am J Obstet Gynecol 1985;153:593.
34. Harper PS. Endocrine abnormalities in myotonic dystrophy. In Harper PS (ed): Myotonic Dystrophy. London, WB Saunders, 1989, p 129.
35. Gutsche BB, Cheek TG. Anesthetic considerations in preeclampsia-eclampsia. In Shnider SM, Levinson G (eds): Anesthesia for Obstetrics, 3rd ed. Baltimore, Williams & Wilkins, 1993, p 305.
36. Ramanathan J, Sibai BM, Pillai R, et al. Neuromuscular transmission studies in preeclamptic women receiving magnesium sulfate. Am J Obstet Gynecol 1988;158:40.
37. Gutsche BB, Cheek TG. Anesthetic considerations in preeclampsia-eclampsia. In Shnider SM, Levinson G (eds): Anesthesia for Obstetrics, 3rd ed. Baltimore, Williams & Wilkins, 1993, p 315.
38. Hageman ATM, Gabreëls FJ, Liem KD, et al. Congenital myotonic dystrophy; a report on thirteen cases and a review of the literature. J Neurol Sci 1993;115:95.
39. Harper PS, Dyken PR. Early-onset dystrophia myotonica. Evidence supporting a maternal environmental factor. Lancet 1972;2:53.

40. Koch MC, Grimm T, Harley HG, et al. Genetic risks for children of women with myotonic dystrophy. Am J Hum Genet 1991;48:1084.

41. Andrews PI, Wilson J. Relative disease severity in siblings with myotonic dystrophy. J Child Neurol 1992;7:161.

42. Levine AB, Eddleman KA, Chitkara U, et al. Congenital myotonic dystrophy: An often unsuspected cause of severe polyhydramnios. Prenat Diagn 1991;11:111.

43. Afifi AM, Bhatia AR, Eyal F. Hydrops fetalis associated with congenital myotonic dystrophy. Am J Obstet Gynecol 1992;166:929.

44. Stratton RF, Patterson RM. DNA confirmation of congenital myotonic dystrophy in non-immune hydrops fetalis. Prenat Diagn 1993;13:1027.

45. Wesström G, Bensch J, Shollin J. Congenital myotonic dystrophy. Incidence, clinical aspects and early prognosis. Acta Paediatr Scand 1986;75:849.

46. Pearse RG, Höweler CJ. Neonatal form of dystrophia myotonica. Five cases in preterm babies and a review of earlier reports. Arch Dis Child 1979;54:331.

47. Harper PS. Myotonic dystrophy in infancy and childhood. In Harper PS (ed): Myotonic Dystrophy. London, WB Saunders, 1989, p 195.

48. Harley HG, Brook JD, Rundle SA, et al. Expansion of an unstable DNA region and phenotypic variation in myotonic dystrophy. Nature 1992;355:545.

49. Buxton J, Shelbourne P, Davies J, et al. Detection of an unstable fragment of DNA specific to individuals with myotonic dystrophy. Nature 1992;355:547.

50. Aslanidis C, Jansen G, Amemiya C, et al. Cloning of the essential myotonic dystrophy region and mapping of the putative defect. Nature 1992;355:548.

51. Brook JD, McCurrach ME, Harley HG, et al. Molecular basis of myotonic dystrophy: Expansion of a trinucleotide (CTG) repeat at the 3' end of a transcript encoding a protein kinase family member. Cell 1992;68:799.

52. Fu YH, Pizzuti A, Fenwick RG, et al. An unstable triplet repeat in a gene related to myotonic muscular dystrophy. Science 1992;255:1256.

53. Mahadevan M, Tsilfidis C, Sabourin L, et al. Myotonic dystrophy mutation: An unstable CTG repeat in the 3' untranslated region of the gene. Science 1992;255:1253.

54. Caskey CT, Pizzuti A, Fu YH, et al. Triplet repeat mutations in human disease. Science 1992;256:784.

55. Abeliovich D, Lerer I, Pashut-Lavon I, et al. Negative expansion of the myotonic dystrophy unstable sequence. Am J Hum Genet 1993;52:1175.

56. Tsilfidis C, MacKenzie AE, Mettler G, et al. Correlation between CTG trinucleotide repeat length and frequency of severe congenital myotonic dystrophy. Nat Genet 1992;1:192.

57. Hook R, Anderson EF, Noto P. Anesthetic management of a parturient with myotonia atrophica. Anesthesiology 1975;43:689.

58. Wheeler AS, James III FM. Local anesthesia for laparoscopy in a case of myotonia dystrophica. Anesthesiology 1979;50:169.

59. Harris MNE. Extradural analgesia and dystrophia myotonica. Anaesthesia 1984;39:1032.

60. Paterson RA, Tousignant M, Skene DS. Caesarean section for twins in a patient with myotonic dystrophy. Can Anaesth Soc J 1985;32:418.

61. Cope DK, Miller JN. Local and spinal anesthesia for cesarean section in a patient with myotonic dystrophy. Anesth Analg 1986;65:687.

62. Blumgart CH, Hughes DG, Redfern N. Obstetric anaesthesia in dystrophia myotonica. Anaesthesia 1990;45:26.

63. Camann WR, Johnson MD. Anesthetic management of a parturient with myotonia dystrophica: A case report. Reg Anesth 1990;15:41.

64. Stevens JD, Wauchob TD. Dystrophia myotonica—Emergency caesarean section with spinal anaesthesia. Eur J Anaesthesiol 1991;8:305.

65. Campbell AM, Thompson N. Anaesthesia for Caesarean section in a patient with myotonic dystrophy receiving warfarin therapy. Can J Anaesth 1995;42:409.

66. Aldridge LM. Anaesthetic problems in myotonic dystrophy. Br J Anaesth 1985;57:1119.

67. Harper PS. Cardiorespiratory problems. In Harper PS (ed): Myotonic Dystrophy. London, WB Saunders, 1989, p 114.

68. Towbin JA, Roberts R. Cardiovascular diseases due to genetic abnormalities. In Schlant RC, Alexander RW (eds): Hurst's the Heart: Arteries and Veins, 8th ed. New York, McGraw-Hill, 1996, p 1739.

69. Hawley RJ, Milner MR, Gottdiener JS, et al. Myotonic heart disease: A clinical follow-up. Neurology 1991;41:259.

70. Perloff JK, Stevenson WG, Roberts NK, et al. Cardiac involvement in myotonic muscular dystrophy (Steinert's disease): A prospective study of 25 patients. Am J Cardiol 1984;54:1074.

71. Harper PS. Cardiorespiratory problems. In Harper PS (ed): Myotonic Dystrophy. London, WB Saunders, 1989, p 100.

72. Meyers MB, Barash PG. Cardiac decompensation during enflurane anesthesia in a patient with myotonia atrophica. Anesth Analg 1976;55:433.

73. Fall LH, Young WW, Power JA, et al. Severe congestive heart failure and cardiomyopathy as a complication of myotonic dystrophy in pregnancy. Obstet Gynecol 1990;76:481.

74. Dodds TM, Haney MF, Appleton FM. Management of peripartum congestive heart failure using continuous arteriovenous hemofiltration in a patient with myotonic dystrophy. Anesthesiology 1991;75:907.

75. Novy MJ, Edwards MJ. Respiratory problems in pregnancy. Am J Obstet Gynecol 1967;99:1024.

76. Müller H, Punt-van Manen JA. Maxillo-facial deformities in patients with dystrophia myotonica and the anaesthetic implications. J Maxillofac Surg 1982;10:224.

77. Stoelting RK. Skin and musculoskeletal diseases. In Stoelting RK, Dierdorf SF (eds): Anesthesia and Co-existing Disease, 3rd ed. New York, Churchill Livingstone, 1993, p 438.

78. O'Connor PJ, Caldicott LD, Braithwaite P. Urgent caesarean section in a patient with myotonic dystrophy: A case report and review. Int J Obstet Anesth 1996;5:272.

79. Driver IK, Broadway JW. Dystrophia myotonica: Combined spinal-epidural anaesthesia for caesarean section. Int J Obstet Anesth 1996;5:275.

80. White DA, Smyth DG. Continuous infusion of propofol in dystrophia myotonica. Can J Anaesth 1989;36:200.

81. Pollard BJ, Young TM. Anaesthesia in myotonia dystrophica (letter). Anaesthesia 1989;44:699.

82. Ravin M, Newmark Z, Saviello G. Myotonia dystrophica—an anesthetic hazard: Two case reports. Anesth Analg 1975;54:216.

83. Mitchell MM, Ali HH, Savarese JJ. Myotonia and neuromuscular blocking agents. Anesthesiology 1978;49:44.

84. Castano J, Pares N. Anaesthesia for major abdominal surgery in a patient with myotonia dystrophica. Br J Anaesth 1987;59:1629.

85. Azar I. The response of patients with neuromuscular disorders to muscle relaxants: A review. Anesthesiology 1984;61:173.

86. Buzello W, Krieg N, Schlickewei A. Hazards of neostigmine in patients with neuromuscular disorders. Report of two cases. Br J Anaesth 1982;54:529.

87. Rosenberg H. Neuromuscular diseases, myopathies and anesthesia. Curr Rev Clin Anesth 1983;3:99.

88. Nightingale P, Healy TEJ, McGuinness K. Dystrophia myotonica and atracurium. A case report. Br J Anaesth 1985;57:1131.

89. Boheimer N, Harris JW, Ward S. Neuromuscular blockade in dystrophia myotonica with atracurium besylate. Anaesthesia 1985;40:872.

90. Britt BA, Kalow W. Malignant hyperthermia: A statistical review. Can Anaesth Soc J 1970;17:293.

91. Harper PS. Cardiorespiratory problems. In Harper PS (ed): Myotonic Dystrophy. London, WB Saunders, 1989, p 117.

92. Brownell AKW. Malignant hyperthermia: Relationship to other diseases. Br J Anaesth 1988;60:303.

93. Lehmann-Horn F, Knorr-Held S. Muscle diseases relevant to the anaesthetist. Acta Anaesth Belg 1990;41:113.

94. Wedel DJ. Review article: Malignant hyperthermia and neuromuscular disease. Neuromusc Disord 1992;2:157.

95. Mudge BJ, Taylor PB, Vanderspek AF. Perioperative hazards in myotonic dystrophy. Anaesthesia 1980;35:492.

96. Moore JK, Moore AP. Postoperative complications of dystrophia myotonica. Anaesthesia 1987;42:529.

97. Branthwaite MA. Myotonic dystrophy and respiratory function (letter). Anaesthesia 1990;45:250.

98. Miller JD, Lee C. Muscle diseases. In Katz J, Benumof JL, Kadis

LB (eds): Anesthesia and Uncommon Diseases, 3rd ed. Philadelphia, WB Saunders, 1990, p 590.

99. Duncan PG. Neuromuscular diseases. In Katz J, Steward DJ (eds): Anesthesia and Uncommon Pediatric Diseases, 2nd ed. Philadelphia, WB Saunders, 1993, p 672.

100. Harper PS. The differential diagnosis of myotonic dystrophy: Other dystrophies and myotonic disorders. In Harper PS (ed): Myotonic Dystrophy, 2nd ed. London, WB Saunders, 1989, p 37.

101. Dubowitz V. The muscular dystrophies. In Dubowitz V (ed): Muscle Disorders in Childhood, 2nd ed. London, WB Saunders, 1995, p 34.

102. Munsat TL. Facioscapulohumeral dystrophy and the scapuloperoneal syndrome. In Engel AG, Banker BQ (eds): Myology, vol II. New York, McGraw-Hill, 1986, p 1251.

103. Baldwin BJ, Talley RC, Johnson C, et al. Permanent paralysis of the atrium in a patient with facioscapulohumeral muscular dystrophy. Am J Cardiol 1973;31:649.

104. Shields RW Jr. Limb girdle syndromes. In Engel AG, Banker BQ (eds): Myology, vol II. New York, McGraw-Hill, 1986, p 1349.

105. Jackson CE, Strehler DA. Limb-girdle muscular dystrophy: Clinical manifestations and detection of preclinical disease. Pediatrics 1968;41:495.

106. Antonio JH, Diniz MC, Miranda D. Persistent atrial standstill with limb-girdle muscular dystrophy. Cardiology 1978;63:39.

107. Ville Y, Barbet JP, Pompidou A, et al. Myopathie des ceintures et grossesse: Un cas. J Gynecol Obstet Biol Reprod 1991;20:973.

108. Ekblad U, Kanto J. Pregnancy outcome in an extremely small woman with muscular dystrophy and respiratory insufficiency. Acta Anaesth Scand 1993;37:228.

109. Markesbery WR, Griggs RC. Distal myopathies. In Engel AG, Banker BQ (eds): Myology, vol II. New York, McGraw-Hill, 1986, p 1313.

110. Tomoda A, Zhao J, Ohtani Y, et al. Two patients with distal muscular dystrophy and autonomic nerve dysfunction. Brain Dev 1994;16:65.

111. Banker BQ. Congenital muscular dystrophy. In Engel AG, Banker BQ (eds): Myology, vol II. New York, McGraw-Hill, 1986, p 1367.

112. Dubowitz V. The congenital myopathies. In Muscle Disorders in Childhood, 2nd ed. London, WB Saunders, 1995, p 134.

113. Banker BQ. The congenital myopathies. In Engel AG, Banker BQ (eds): Myology, vol II. New York, McGraw-Hill, 1986, p 1527.

114. Denborough MA, Dennett X, Anderson RM. Central-core disease and malignant hyperpyrexia. Br Med J 1973;1:272.

115. Harriman DGF, Ellis FR. Central-core disease and malignant hyperpyrexia (letter). Br Med J 1973;1:545.

116. Otsuka H, Komura Y, Mayumi T, et al. Malignant hyperthermia during sevoflurane anesthesia in a child with central core disease. Anesthesiology 1991;75:699.

117. Calore EE, Cavaliere MJ, Perez NM, et al. Hyperthermic reaction to haloperidol with rigidity associated to central core disease. Acta Neurol (Napoli) 1994;16:157.

118. Islander G, Henriksson KG, Ranklev-Twetman E. Malignant hyperthermia susceptibility without central core disease (CCD) in a family where CCD is diagnosed. Neuromuscul Disord 1995;5:125.

119. Gordon CP, Litz S. Multicore myopathy in a patient with anhidrotic ectodermal dysplasia. Can J Anaesth 1992;39:966.

120. Heard ST, Kaplan RF. Neuromuscular blockade in a patient with nemaline myopathy. Anesthesiology 1983;59:588.

121. Cunliffe M, Burrows FA. Anaesthetic implications of nemaline rod myopathy. Can Anaesth Soc J 1985;32:543.

122. Asai T, Fujise K, Uchida M. Anaesthesia for cardiac surgery in children with nemaline myopathy. Anaesthesia 1992;47:405.

123. Pourmand R, Azzarelli B. Adult-onset of nemaline myopathy associated with cores and abnormal mitochondria. Muscle Nerve 1994;17:1218.

124. Stackhouse R, Chelmow D, Dattel BJ. Anesthetic complications in a pregnant patient with nemaline myopathy. Anesth Analg 1994;79:1195.

125. Morgan-Hughes JA. The mitochondrial myopathies. In Engel AG, Banker BQ (eds): Myology, vol II. New York, McGraw-Hill, 1986, p 1709.

126. Dubowitz V. Metabolic myopathies. II. Lipid disorders, mitochondrial disorders. In Muscle Disorders in Childhood, 2nd ed. London, WB Saunders, 1995, p 211.

127. Schapira AH Mitochondrial myopathies: Mechanisms now better understood (letter). Br Med J 1989;298:1127.

128. Boudin G, Mikol J, Guillard A, et al. Fatal systemic carnitine deficiency with lipid storage in skeletal muscle, heart, liver and kidney. J Neurol Sci 1976;30:313.

129. Cornelio F, Di Donato S, Peluchetti D, et al. Fatal cases of lipid storage myopathy with carnitine deficiency. J Neurol Neurosurg Psychiatry 1977;40:170.

130. Angelini C, Govoni E, Bragaglia MM, et al. Carnitine deficiency: Acute postpartum crisis. Ann Neurol 1978;4:558.

131. Rowe RW, Helander E. Anesthetic management of a patient with systemic carnitine deficiency. Anesth Analg 1990;71:295.

132. Beilin B, Shulman D, Schiffman Y. Anaesthesia in myopathy of carnitine deficiency. Anaesthesia 1986;41:92.

133. Katsuya H, Misumi M, Ohtani Y, et al. Postanesthetic acute renal failure due to carnitine palmitoyl transferase deficiency. Anesthesiology 1988;68:945.

134. Zierz S, Schmitt U. Inhibition of carnitine palmitoyltransferase by malonyl-CoA in human muscle is influenced by anesthesia. Anesthesiology 1989;70:373.

135. Berkowitz K, Monteagudo A, Marks F, et al. Mitochondrial myopathy and preeclampsia associated with pregnancy. Am J Obstet Gynecol 1990;162:146.

136. Dreval D, Bernstein D, Zakut H. Carnitine palmitoyl transferase deficiency in pregnancy. A case report. Am J Obstet Gynecol 1994;170:1390.

137. Roseag OP, Morrison S, MacLeod JP. Clinical report: Anaesthetic management of labour and delivery in the parturient with mitochondrial myopathy. Can J Anaesth 1996;43:403.

138. Allen GC. Malignant hyperthermia in musculoskeletal disorders. In Kirby RR, Brown DL (eds): Problems in Anaesthesia, vol V. Philadelphia, JP Lippincott, 1991, p 146.

139. Russell SH, Hirsch NP. Anaesthesia and myotonia. Br J Anaesth 1994;72:210.

140. Harper PS. Cardiorespiratory problems. In Harper PS (ed): Myotonic Dystrophy. London, WB Saunders, 1989, p 116.

141. Heiman-Patterson T, Martino C, Rosenberg H, et al. Malignant hyperthermia in myotonia congenita. Neurology 1988;38:810.

142. Haberer JP, Fabre F, Rose E. Malignant hyperthermia and myotonia congenita (Thomsen's disease). Anaesthesia 1989;44:166.

143. Lehmann-Horn F, Iaizzo PA. Are myotonias and periodic paralyses associated with susceptibility to malignant hyperthermia? Br J Anaesth 1990;65:692.

144. Schwartz IL, Dingfelder JR, O'Tuama L, et al. Recessive congenital myotonia and pregnancy. Int J Gynaecol Obstet 1979;17:194.

145. Ptacek LJ, Ziter FA, Roberts JW, et al. Evidence of genetic heterogeneity among the nondystrophic myotonias. Neurology 1992;42:1045.

146. Streib EW. Paramyotonia congenita. Semin Neurol 1991;11:249.

147. De Silva SM, Kuncl RW, Griffin JW, et al. Paramyotonia congenita or hyperkalemic periodic paralysis? Clinical and electrophysiological features of each entity in one family. Muscle Nerve 1990;13:21.

148. Ptacek JJ, Tarwil R, Griggs RC, et al. Linkage of atypical myotonia to a sodium channel locus. Neurology 1992;42:431.

149. Dubowitz V. Metabolic myopathies. III. Ion channel disorders. In Muscle Disorders in Childhood, 2nd ed. London, WB Saunders, 1995, p 266.

150. Chitayat D, Etchell M, Wilson RD. Cold-induced abortion in paramyotonia congenita. Am J Obstet Gynecol 1988;158:435.

151. Howell PR, Douglas MJ. Lupus anticoagulant, paramyotonia congenita and pregnancy. Can J Anaesth 1992;39:992.

152. Richey SD, Wendel GD. Thyrotoxic hypokalemic periodic paralysis following second-trimester prostaglandin-induced abortion. Obstet Gynecol 1993;82:696.

153. Engel AG. Periodic paralysis. In Engel AG, Banker BQ (eds): Myology, vol II. New York, McGraw-Hill, 1986, p 1843.

154. Bashford AC. Case report: Anaesthesia in familial hypokalaemic periodic paralysis. Anaesth Intensive Care 1977;5:74.

155. Rooney RT, Shanahan EC, Sun T, et al. Atracurium and hypokalemic familial periodic paralysis. Anesth Analg 1988;67:782.

156. Fukuda K, Ogawa S, Yokozuka H, et al. Long-standing bidirectional tachycardia in a patient with hypokalemic periodic paralysis. J Electrocardiol 1988;21:71.

157. Lema G, Urzua J, Moran S, et al. Successful anesthetic manage-

ment of a patient with hypokalemic familial periodic paralysis undergoing cardiac surgery. Anesthesiology 1991;74:373.

158. Laurito CE, Becker GL, Miller PE. Atracurium use in a patient with familial periodic paralysis. J Clin Anesth 1991;3:225.

159. Neuman GG, Kopman AFP. Dyskalemic periodic paralysis and myotonia. Anesth Analg 1993;76:426.

160. Johnstone FD, Greer IA. Hyperkalaemic periodic paralysis and HELLP syndrome: An unusual combination. Scot Med J 1989;34:530.

161. Aarons JJ, Moon RE, Camporesi EM. General anesthesia and hyperkalemic periodic paralysis. Anesthesiology 1989;71:303.

162. Ashwood EM, Russell WJ, Burrow DD. Hyperkalaemic periodic paralysis and anaesthesia. Anaesthesia 1992;47:579.

163. Davidson BN, Bowerman RA, La Ferla JJ. Myositis ossificans progressiva and pregnancy. A therapeutic dilemma. J Reprod Med 1985;30:945.

164. Banker BQ. Other inflammatory myopathies. In Engel AG, Banker BQ (eds): Myology, vol II. New York, McGraw-Hill, 1986, p 1501.

165. Fox S, Khoury A, Mootabar H, et al. Myositis ossificans progressiva and pregnancy. Obstet Gynecol 1987;69:453.

Case Reports

A. Weston LA, DiFazio CA. Labor analgesia and anesthesia in a patient with spinal muscular atrophy and vocal cord paralysis: A rare and unusual case report. Reg Anesth 1996;21:350.

B. Pash MP, Balaton J, Eagle C. Anaesthetic management of a parturient with severe muscular dystrophy, lumbar lordosis and a difficult airway. Can J Anaesth 1996;43:403.

PARTURIENTS OF SHORT STATURE

· · · · · · ·

Emily F. Ratner, M.D., and Sheila E. Cohen, M.B.

Dwarfism is defined as failure to achieve a height of 4 feet 10 inches (148 cm) at adulthood.[1] Short stature is a clinical entity that has numerous etiologies. These conditions can be of genetic, constitutional, or metabolic origin. More than 100 different types of dwarfism exist, none of which is very common. The most common variety, achondroplasia, occurs in only 0.5 to 1.5 per 10,000 live births.[2, 3] Two major classifications of dwarfism are especially useful to the anesthesiologist: (1) patients with short stature who are proportionate and have normal trunk-to-limb ratio; and (2) patients who have disproportionate growth and have either short trunks in relation to their limbs or short limbs in relation to their trunks (Table 13–1).[2]

Since the formation of the Little People of America, which is a society for people of short stature, the opportunity for dwarfs to meet each other, socialize, and eventually procreate increases the likelihood that more pregnant dwarfs will present for medical care in the future.

PROPORTIONATE SHORT STATURE

This category of dwarfism refers to those people who have short stature with proportionate trunk-to-limb length ratio. Individuals may have proportionate short stature as a result of an endocrine deficiency, metabolic disorder, or long-standing cardiac, renal, neurologic, or gastrointestinal disease.[4] Although some of these patients are infertile or do not survive long enough to reach childbearing age,[4] those with an endocrinologic etiology are frequently capable of becoming pregnant. Two endocrine disorders that cause proportionate short stature and may be seen in pregnancy are isolated growth hormone deficiency and Laron dwarfism.

Isolated Growth Hormone Deficiency

Four types of isolated growth hormone deficiency exist. Patients vary in terms of mode of inheritance (autosomal dominant, autosomal recessive, X-linked)

as well as in degree of hormonal deficiency.[5] Although it is possible for other hormonal deficiencies to be present in conjunction with growth hormone deficiency (e.g., in patients with panhypopituitary disease, decreased levels of luteinizing hormone [LH], follicle-stimulating hormone [FSH], thyroid-stimulating hormone [TSH], and adrenocorticotropic hormone [ACTH] exist), puberty usually does not occur, and pregnancy is unlikely.[5] The other tropic hormones appear to be normal in the pregnant growth hormone–deficient patients.[6]

A common type of isolated growth hormone deficiency (individuals known as ateliotic dwarfs) carries an autosomal recessive gene that causes a decrease in human growth hormone production.[7] Infants typically are of normal weight and length at birth, but over the next few months of life have a much lower growth rate than unaffected infants. Their height rarely exceeds 130 cm, which is the height of a normal 8½-year-old.[1] Those who achieve sexual maturation, known as sexual ateliotics, may not reach puberty until the late second or third decade of life. In addition to having short stature, these persons have soft, prematurely wrinkled skin, high-pitched voices, and possibly mild micrognathia. Some patients also lack a normal lumbar lordosis.[1, 6]

Isolated growth hormone deficiency is not usually diagnosed by random blood samples of human growth hormone (hGH) alone, because these levels are normally low throughout most of the day. Provocative tests are more frequently used, and these include measuring hGH (after stimulation by exercise), L-dopa, insulin, arginine, clonidine, glucagon, or a combination of these.[5] Some growth hormone–deficient dwarfs have abnormal glucose metabolism or response to insulin, with glycosuria in early gestation progressing to gestational diabetes.[1] These patients should be thoroughly investigated in the antenatal period to detect and control glucose perturbations during pregnancy.

Laron Dwarfism

This is also an autosomal recessive disorder, which is clinically very similar to isolated growth hormone

TABLE 13–1. CLASSIFICATION OF DWARFISM

Proportionate short stature
  Endocrine etiology
    Isolated growth hormone deficiency
    Laron dwarfism
  Constitutional
  Chronic disease states
Disproportionate short stature
  Osteochondrodysplasias—abnormalities of cartilage
    ± bone growth and development
  Achondroplasia
  Pseudoachondroplasia
  Spondyloepiphyseal dysplasia congenita
  Spondyloepiphyseal dysplasia tarda
  Spondylometepiphyseal dysplasia
Primary metabolic abnormalities
  Calcium derangements
  Phosphorus derangements
  Complex carbohydrate derangements

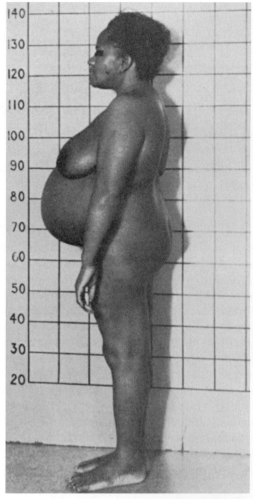

Figure 13–1. Patient L.L. An ateliotic dwarf in the twenty-eighth week of gestation. (From Tyson JE, Barnes AC, McKusick VA, et al. Obstetric and gynecologic considerations of dwarfism. Am J Obstet Gynecol 1970;108:688.)

deficiency. Laron dwarfs, however, have increased release but resistance to growth hormone, very low serum levels of insulin-like growth factor (IGF-I), and abnormal growth hormone receptors.[8] In addition to having a normally proportioned trunk and extremities, affected persons may have frontal bossing, saddle nose, acromicria (hypoplasia of the extremities of the skeleton—the nose, jaws, fingers, and toes),[9] high-pitched voice, and slow and sparse hair growth.[10]

Effects Of Pregnancy

The normal physiologic changes of pregnancy can have serious implications for maternal health in proportionate dwarfs. The most serious problem is cardiorespiratory embarrassment. The abdominal dimensions of these patients are markedly smaller than those of their normal-sized counterparts. For example, the average distance from xiphoid to symphysis is significantly less in ateliotic dwarfs than in normal-sized patients (Table 13–2). The uterus therefore becomes an intra-abdominal organ much earlier in gestation (Fig. 13–1). Additionally, these dwarfs may not have a lumbar lordosis, causing an effectively smaller intra-abdominal area. These factors may cause significant mechanical diaphragmatic dysfunction. The decrease in functional residual capacity (FRC) that normally occurs during pregnancy causes additional respiratory compromise.[11]

TABLE 13–2. VERTICAL AND HORIZONTAL ABDOMINAL MEASUREMENTS (cm)

	Achondroplasia	Ateliotic	SED and Diastrophic	Normal
Xiphoid to symphysis	29	25	24	33
Intercristal	21	24	25	30

From Tyson JE, Barnes AC, McKusick VA, et al. Obstetric and gynecologic considerations of dwarfism. Am J Obstet Gynecol 1970;108:688.

Pregnant dwarfs may suffer from decreased vital capacity, hypoxia, and acidosis. They may develop tachypnea and tachycardia to compensate for these physiologic derangements. Deterioration of pulmonary status may warrant immediate delivery of the fetus to improve maternal condition.[1]

Obstetric Management

Some believe that almost all pregnant patients of short stature should undergo cesarean section.[12] Others report ateliotic patients who have had successful vaginal deliveries but fail to give details concerning these deliveries.[1] The pelvic diameters of such patients are typically smaller than those of parturients of normal stature and are frequently sufficient only for delivery of a premature infant.[1] Cesarean section is thus performed frequently for cephalopelvic disproportion as well as for relief of maternal cardiopulmonary embarrassment.

Other complications of pregnancy include higher than normal rates of spontaneous abortion, stillbirth, and premature delivery.[1] It is unclear whether these abnormalities result from a mechanical, genetic, or hormonal problem; however, premature delivery is more likely when maternal respiratory embarrassment is present.[1] Early fetal loss may be due to some unknown physiologic actions of growth hormone in the first half of pregnancy, before placental production of a variant type of growth hormone.[13] Additionally, there is a higher incidence of premature births resulting from maternal indications.[1]

Anesthetic Considerations

No case reports concerning anesthesia for pregnant patients with proportionate short stature have been published, although one of us (EFR) is currently a coauthor of one such report. Preoperative consultation should include the usual history and physical examination with emphasis on the airway and anatomic landmarks relevant to regional anesthesia (Table 13–3). If respiratory compromise is present, arterial blood gas analysis, pulmonary function tests, and chest radiographs may be indicated. Measurement of oxyhemoglobin saturation using pulse oximetry, with the mother in the upright and Trendelenburg positions, is a useful screening test to detect potential deterioration with further decrease in FRC. No additional laboratory or radiologic studies are necessary in the absence of other complicating conditions. Routine noninvasive monitoring is all that is required during labor and delivery in patients without other complicating factors. If respiratory problems are present, intra-arterial catheter placement with monitoring of oxygenation, ventilation, and acid-base status may be prudent.

In those instances when a vaginal delivery is anticipated, intravenous or intramuscular opioids may be helpful. Epidural analgesia, however, provides superior pain relief without respiratory depression and is the technique of choice. The appropriate dose of a dilute local anesthetic, in combination with an opioid, can be titrated slowly to achieve adequate analgesia. If cesarean section is necessary, as is frequently the case, additional local anesthetic can be injected to provide surgical anesthesia. Careful titration is essential to avoid high epidural blockade with potential respiratory embarrassment. Precautions against aspiration are particularly important in pregnant dwarfs because the uterus causes additional impingement on intra-abdominal structures.[14, 15] For the same reason, supine hypotension may be even more problematic than in the normal parturient.

For patients undergoing planned cesarean sections, a continuous technique is preferable to a single-shot technique. We prefer continuous epidural anesthesia over continuous spinal anesthesia because of the lower incidence of headache and perhaps less potential for neurologic deficit. A continuous spinal anesthetic, however, can be used with slow titration of local anesthetic to provide adequate neural blockade. Although it is presumed that the spinal cord is proportionately reduced in size relative to the volume of the spinal canal, it is not known with certainty that smaller cord size is the case. If the spinal cord is large in relation to the size of the spinal canal, an increased risk of neurologic damage with regional anesthesia may be present.

As in individuals of normal size, a test dose can be given to identify unintentional epidural catheter placement in the subarachnoid space or in an epidural vein. It is unclear which dose is optimal for this purpose, but it is probably prudent to choose a reduced dose of local anesthetic. One of us (EFR) managed a proportionate dwarf who was 125 cm tall and weighed 35 kg with a continuous lumbar epidural anesthetic for a cesarean section. A 2-ml test dose of 2% lidocaine with 1:200,000 epinephrine was given, in the belief that this dose would be adequate to provide evidence of spinal blockade without producing a high or total spinal anesthetic. Our dose of 10 μg of epinephrine may have been inadequate for identification of intravenous placement of an epidural catheter, compared with the more commonly accepted 15-μg dose.[16] On a microgram per kilogram basis, our epinephrine dose was slightly greater than that normally used. Careful incremental injection of local anesthetic is critical to avoid risk of intravenous injection or high block.

TABLE 13–3. **ANESTHETIC CONSIDERATIONS FOR PROPORTIONATE DWARFS**

Dwarfism Characteristics	Anesthetic Implications
Upper airway	
Micrognathia possible	Possible difficult intubation
Smaller airway	May need smaller endotracheal tube
Short stature	Decreased dosage of local anesthetic for regional anesthesia
	Continuous regional technique is preferred
Small pelvis	High rate of cesarean section
Uterine impingement on intrathoracic structures	Respiratory compromise
	May not tolerate supine position or intravenous fluid administration
Uterine impingement on abdominal structures	Risk of supine hypotension
	Risk of aspiration

Although a single-dose spinal anesthetic can be performed, the appropriate dosage of local anesthetic may be difficult to predict because of the presence of a shortened spinal cord. Local anesthetic doses comparable to those in the pediatric population may be appropriate; however, no studies have been performed to confirm this observation. Problems with subarachnoid blockade include underdosage, resulting in inadequate anesthesia for cesarean section, as well as overdosage, resulting in high spinal anesthesia with the risk of airway control loss, respiratory arrest, hemodynamic instability, and cardiac arrest.

Although some investigators have advocated general anesthesia for all patients with nonproportional short stature,[12] no such recommendation exists for dwarfs with proportionate short stature. Because descriptions of such dwarfs have included micrognathia as a clinical feature, however, difficult intubation is a potential problem. Caution should be used in these patients. A thorough airway evaluation should be performed before induction of general anesthesia to avoid difficulties with airway management. Prediction of the appropriate size of endotracheal tube for proportionate dwarfs is difficult. Whereas age is usually the best guide to endotracheal tube size in children, weight was found to be a better guide in pediatric patients with proportionate small stature.[17]

Pain management after cesarean delivery can utilize epidural opioids, preferably in a reduced dosage, because no schedule for appropriate dosage of epidural opioids exists for dwarfs. In view of the potential risk for respiratory depression, we recommend a high level of postoperative monitoring including frequent vital signs and continuous pulse oximetry for 16 to 24 hours.

Neonatal Considerations

Infants born to mothers with isolated growth hormone deficiency are usually of normal birth weight and length.[6] The diagnosis is made either in infancy or in childhood, because growth does not progress at a normal rate. Laron dwarfs have birth lengths that are abnormally shorter than average, with a normal birth weight.[5] Considerations for immediate neonatal resuscitation are similar to those for other infants born to mothers with a small pelvis.

DISPROPORTIONATE SHORT STATURE

Etiologies of disproportionate short stature include the osteochondrodysplasias (abnormalities of cartilage and/or bone growth and development) and primary metabolic diseases that involve the skeleton.[2, 18] Patients with primary metabolic diseases frequently do not survive into adulthood, or they are infertile. Patients with disproportionate short stature have potentially a more complicated course from an anesthetic perspective than those with proportionate short stature.[19, 26]

Achondroplastic Dwarfism

Achondroplastic dwarfism is the most common type of dwarfism, with a prevalence rate of 0.5 to 1.5 per 10,000 births.[3] A summary of the anatomic and physical characteristics of achondroplasia is listed in Table 13–4. Short stature in this condition is a result of abnormal endochondral bone formation. These patients have normal truncal lengths, but shortened limbs, which are primarily responsible for their short stature. Achondroplastic dwarfs are usually no taller than 130 cm.[2] The mode of inheritance in this condition is autosomal dominance, although 80% of patients with achondroplasia reflect a result of spontaneous mutation.[19, 27]

Achondroplastic dwarfs are usually diagnosed at birth. They have numerous craniofacial abnormalities such as megalocephaly (large head size), megalencephaly (overgrowth of the brain), frontal bossing, and depressed nasal bridge (Fig. 13–2).[2, 9] Maxillary hypoplasia, a large mandible, and a large tongue may be present in these dwarfs,[28] indicating a potential for difficult airway management. In a series of 36 anesthetic procedures performed in 27 patients, Mayhew and coworkers[28] experienced no difficulty in airway management with either mask ventilation or direct laryngoscopy. Two reports of difficult intubation in achondroplastic patients attribute the problem to limited neck extension.[27, 29]

Numerous spinal anomalies can occur in achondroplastic dwarfs. Thoracolumbar stenosis and generalized spinal stenosis are frequent findings.[30–33] Additional abnormalities include lumbar hyperlordosis and/or thoracolumbar kyphosis, thoracic dystrophy, square ilia, narrow sciatic notch, and horizontal sa-

TABLE 13–4. ACHONDROPLASTIC DWARFS—ANATOMIC AND PHYSICAL FINDINGS

General	Spine/Skeletal
Normal trunk length	Generalized spinal stenosis
Short limbs	Abnormally shaped vertebrae
Craniofacial	Hyperplastic intervertebral
Megalocephaly—large head size	discs
	Lumbar hyperlordosis
Megalencephaly—large brain size	Thoracolumbar kyphosis
	Square ilia
Brachycephaly—short head	Narrow sciatic notch
Foramen magnum stenosis	Horizontal sacrum
Frontal bossing	**Respiratory/Cardiac**
Depressed nasal bridge	Chest deformities
Maxillary/facial hypoplasia	Thoracic dystrophy/kyphosis
Narrowed upper airways	Rib hypoplasia
Central nervous system	Upper airway obstruction
Hydrocephalus	Obstructive sleep apnea
Hypotonia	Cor pulmonale

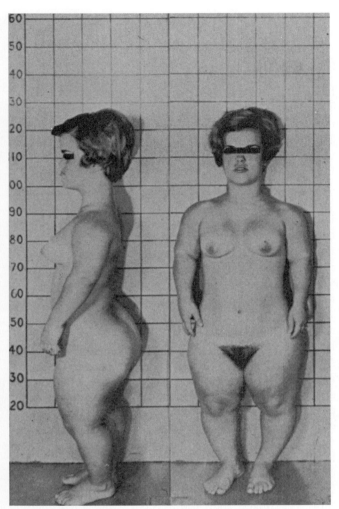

Figure 13–2. Achondroplasia associated with short limbs, characteristic facies, and contracted pelvis. (From Tyson JE, Barnes AC, McKusick VA, et al. Obstetric and gynecologic considerations of dwarfism. Am J Obstet Gynecol 1970;108:688.)

crum. Because of lumbar lordosis, the fifth lumbar vertebra seems to have a lower position relative to the ilia than that in the nondwarf population.[34]

Spinal canal stenosis can occur at any spinal level,[34] although the thoracolumbar and lumbar regions are the most commonly narrowed segments in achondroplastic dwarfs. Spinal cord compression can result from narrowing owing to abnormally shaped vertebrae or hyperplastic intervertebral discs.[30] The narrowing of the spinal canal from underdeveloped vertebral arches and shallow vertebral bodies results in a narrowing of the epidural and subarachnoid space,[35] which has anesthetic implications when regional anesthesia is attempted. Additionally, the abnormal intervertebral discs frequently bulge laterally and posteriorly and can cause neurologic deficits.[2, 36] Anatomic findings in one cadaveric achondroplastic spine revealed thickened pedicles, inferior facet encroachment, and nerve root stenosis in a patient who had suffered from nonvascular claudication symptoms.[37] These physical findings

were consistent with the symptomatology seen in this patient before death from an unrelated cause. Because symptoms of neurologic compromise can progress to paralysis,[30, 34, 37–42] it is critical for the anesthesiologist to be aware of and document neurologic symptoms before anesthetic intervention. In a series of 46 pregnant dwarfs, 4 of 26 achondroplastic patients had symptoms of nerve root compression consisting of numbness and tingling in the lower limbs.[12] No mention is made of the route of delivery, use of forceps, size of the infant, whether or not the patient received regional anesthesia or analgesia, duration of pushing while in stirrups, or other details of the obstetric course.

Foramen magnum stenosis due to bony hypertrophy is also a common finding in achondroplasia[2] and can result in medullary and upper cervical neurologic deficits. Care must be taken to limit hyperextension of the head to avoid exacerbating previous deficits, causing new cervical spinal cord injury.[31, 43–46] It is important for the anesthesiologist to question the patient regarding neurologic symptoms before institution of general anesthesia or performance of direct laryngoscopy and intubation.

Hypotonia and hydrocephalus are also features seen in achondroplasia, although hydrocephalus does not always require ventricular shunting.[2, 34] Progressive hydrocephalus with concomitant elevations in intracranial pressure may warrant shunting. The mechanism for hydrocephalus in these dwarfs is thought to be intracranial venous hypertension or cerebral spinal fluid flow obstruction at the level of the stenosed foramen magnum.[47–49]

In addition to the neurologic problems described earlier, respiratory complications occur commonly. In a survey conducted by Allanson and Hall,[12] 4 of 26 achondroplastic pregnant women had respiratory difficulties during the last 2 months of gestation. The etiologies include chest deformities, upper airway obstruction, sleep apnea, neurologic problems, and other unrelated pulmonary conditions.[3] Thoracic cage deformities, including rib hypoplasia and other rib deformities, can cause restrictive lung disease. Additionally, these mechanical problems may be associated with recurrent respiratory tract infections.[2, 50–52] As in nondwarfs, severe kyphoscoliosis can cause baseline hypoxemia and low lung volumes, which tend to worsen during sleep (or anesthesia).[53] In adult achondroplastic patients, Stokes[54] demonstrated that it is the shape of the adult thorax that differs most compared with the anatomy of nondwarf individuals. The expansion of the uterus to become an intra-abdominal organ very early in gestation limits respiratory mechanics more in dwarfs than in women of normal stature. The additional decrease in FRC that occurs in pregnancy can worsen respiratory status in individuals with significant kyphoscoliosis.[14, 23]

The mechanism of upper airway obstruction in

achondroplasia is unclear. It may be due to mechanical factors such as brachycephaly (short head),[9] flattened nasal bridge, facial hypoplasia, or narrowed upper airways.[50] Alternatively, obstruction may be the result of a functional problem such as hypotonia of airway muscles, which is seen in a generalized fashion in many achondroplastic patients.[50] Sleep apnea probably has an obstructive mechanical origin in these patients rather than a central etiology.[44] Other respiratory difficulties are related to the neurologic problems. For example, foramen magnum stenosis causing compression of a normal-sized medulla can cause apnea and respiratory embarrassment.[43] Increased intracranial pressure in an achondroplastic dwarf with hydrocephalus can also precipitate herniation through the abnormally small foramen magnum.[39, 50, 55]

Occasionally, cor pulmonale occurs as a consequence of these respiratory problems.[2, 50, 56, 57] Corrective procedures performed early in childhood may reverse this process, however. Stokes and coworkers[50] describe an achondroplastic child with upper airway obstruction who experienced resolution of right atrial and right ventricular enlargement after undergoing adenoidectomy and tracheostomy. Unfortunately, this problem is unlikely to be reversible in patients with long-standing chest deformities and pulmonary hypertension who present for treatment while pregnant.

The achondroplastic dwarf has a reduced xiphoid-to-symphysis length as well as a decreased intercristal diameter (see Table 13–2). These decreased pelvic measurements, as well as the hyperlordotic features of the achondroplastic patient, make the uterus an abdominal organ even before pregnancy. Uterine enlargement during pregnancy occurs in an exaggerated anterior and superior direction, compared with parturients of normal stature.[1] By the sixteenth week, these patients appear to be in their thirtieth week of pregnancy.[1]

Pseudoachondroplasia

Three cases of pregnancy with pseudoachondroplasia were noted in a survey of dwarfs.[12] No mention was made of anesthetic management or other complications encountered in these parturients. Patients with pseudoachondroplasia typically present in early childhood, with similar stature to achondroplastic dwarfs but no craniofacial abnormalities. They may have lumbar hyperlordosis, genu valgum (knock knees), genu varum (knees are abnormally separated and the lower extremities are bowed inwardly, that is, bow leg),[9] and scoliosis. As adults, they usually are less that 130 cm tall.[2]

Nonachondroplastic Dwarfism

A higher rate of spontaneous abortion, stillbirth, and premature delivery occurs in nonachondroplastic dwarfs, as with dwarfs of proportionate short stature.[1]

Spondyloepiphyseal Dysplasia

This is a rare form of dwarfism that is usually diagnosed at birth or in late childhood, depending on the variant form. It arises from a spontaneous mutation or from X-linked or autosomal dominant inheritance.[58] The patients have a short trunk with normal or shortened limb length and are usually less than 130 cm tall.[2] The spondyloepiphyseal dysplasia *congenita* variant usually is present at birth; the infant may have short limbs.[2, 58] The spondyloepiphyseal dysplasia *tarda* variant is diagnosed in late childhood. The child usually has normal limb length.[2] Deformities in these patients include progressive kyphoscoliosis, pectus carinatum (prominent sternum), platyspondyly (congenital flattening of the vertebral bodies), central anterior pointing of the vertebral bodies, genu valgum, talipes equinovarus (foot deformity with plantar flexion of the foot and an inward-turned heel), coxa vara (hip deformity with a decreased angle between the femoral head and neck and the axis of the femoral shaft), and odontoid hypoplasia.[2, 9, 26] They may also have visual problems, retinal detachment, deafness, and cleft palate.[2] Myer and Cotton[58] report the presence of laryngotracheal stenosis in two dwarfs with spondyloepiphyseal dysplasia. This is an important finding for the anesthesiologist if patients require general anesthesia with the need for mask ventilation, direct laryngoscopy, and intubation. Odontoid hypoplasia can cause anterior dislocation of the first cervical vertebra, producing spinal cord compression.[59] The pelvis of these dwarfs is more contracted than the pelvis of those with achondroplasia, with markedly reduced xiphoid-to-symphysis pubis and intercristal measurements (see Table 13–2).[1]

Spondylometepiphyseal Dysplasia

This is an extremely rare form of short trunk dwarfism with fewer than 20 patients diagnosed with this condition.[60] Features of concern include progressive kyphoscoliosis with spinal cord compression, pectus carinatum, coxa vara hip deformity, contracted pelvis with narrowing of the sacrosciatic notches, and odontoid hypoplasia. Additionally, these patients may have cleft palates, hemangiomas, inguinal hernias, congenital hydronephrosis, and mitral valve prolapses.[17] Although this is an extremely rare form of dwarfism, a case report exists of an obstetric patient with this disorder who received general anesthesia for cesarean section in the presence of hemorrhage and a marginal placenta previa.[17] A description of this case follows later in this chapter.

Effects of Pregnancy

Only some patients with osteochondrodysplasias survive into adulthood and are fertile. Many of the considerations are the same as those for proportionate dwarfs. Because of their abnormal upper airway and thoracic anatomy, however, disproportionate dwarfs also have a higher risk of cardiac and respiratory compromise earlier in gestation.

Obstetric Management

There is some literature discussing obstetric concerns in this population,[12] but few reports describe anesthesia for pregnant osteochondrodysplastic dwarfs other than that for achondroplastic patients.[25, 26] Osteochondrodysplastic dwarfs are likely to need cesarean sections, as do their proportionately short-statured counterparts. Because inadequate pelvic capacity and other abnormal pelvic configurations prevent the head from engaging, breech presentation is more common, making cesarean section an even more likely event.[1]

Anesthetic Considerations

A review of the literature reveals several descriptions of anesthetic management for achondroplastic dwarfs,[14, 15, 19-24] but only one case report each for patients with spondyloepiphyseal dysplasia congenita[25] and spondylometepiphyseal dysplasia.[17] Because disproportionate dwarfs are at such high risk for cesarean section, the anesthesia service should be contacted early in gestation so that appropriate examination can be performed and a plan developed before labor and delivery (Table 13–5). Some investigators have recommended general anesthesia for cesarean section, citing fears that regional techniques may damage the spinal cord.[12] The same investigators, however, acknowledge "a higher risk of complications compared with spinal and epidural anesthesia."[12]

In one survey of 70 pregnancies in dwarfs, 63 patients underwent cesarean section. The other seven patients, all of whom had a chondrodystrophy of unknown etiology, had vaginal deliveries. General anesthesia was used in the majority of surgical cases, although 23 patients received successful epidural anesthesia. Twelve of these patients were achondroplastic dwarfs.[12]

Because the uterus is an extrapelvic organ in these patients, its enlargement may increase the incidence and severity of supine hypotension.[14, 15] Left uterine displacement, vigorous prehydration, and appropriate pressor support are indicated. Because uterine enlargement also increases the risk for pulmonary aspiration, appropriate aspiration prophylaxis (metoclopramide, nonparticulate antacids, and H_2 histamine blocking drugs) should be included in the treatment regimen.

Some researchers have recommended that all chondrodysplastic dwarfs have cervical spine flexion and

TABLE 13–5. ANESTHETIC CONSIDERATIONS FOR DISPROPORTIONATE DWARFS

Dwarfism Characteristics	Anesthetic Implications
Large head, maxillary hypoplasia, large tongue, large mandible, limited neck extension, foramen magnum stenosis, odontoid hypoplasia, atlantoaxial instability	Possible difficult intubation, neurologic injury, upper airway obstruction, may need smaller endotracheal tube size
Spinal stenosis, lumbar hyperlordosis, thoracolumbar kyphosis, short stature	Technically difficult regional anesthesia, previous neurologic damage, ? more prone to neurologic injury, inadvertent dural puncture, smaller epidural space, decreased local anesthetic dosage for regional anesthesia
Chest deformities, hypoxia, hypercarbia, obstructive sleep apnea, cor pulmonale, uterine impingement on intrathoracic structures	Cardiac/respiratory compromise Risk of respiratory depression with parenteral and neuraxial opioids May not tolerate supine position or intravenous fluid administration
Small abnormally shaped pelvis	High risk of cesarean section
Uterine impingement on abdominal structures	Risk of supine hypotension Risk of aspiration

extension radiographs to exclude C1 instability before administration of anesthesia.[12] Certainly, *nonachondroplastic* disproportionate dwarfs should have these studies because a high percentage of them have atlantoaxial instability, and the majority also have myelopathy.[17, 27, 61]

Anesthesia for Achondroplastic Parturients

Both general and regional anesthesia pose potential hazards in these patients. A thorough history and physical examination are essential, paying special attention to head, neck, and airway anatomy; range of flexion and extension of the neck; presence of respiratory and neurologic signs and symptoms; and anatomic landmarks on the back. It is probably prudent to obtain flexion and extension radiographs of the neck because of the high incidence of atlantoaxial instability and other upper cervical vertebral anomalies.[12, 27]

If signs or symptoms of respiratory compromise are present, further investigations should be performed. Arterial blood gas analyses, pulmonary function tests, and chest radiographs may be helpful in prescribing appropriate therapy to optimize pulmonary condition. The tests are also helpful as baseline determinations for later in gestation and the postpartum period.[12, 17] Routine intraoperative monitoring is all that is necessary for those patients without pulmonary compromise. If respiratory embarrassment is present, an intra-arterial catheter assists in monitoring oxygenation, ventilation, and acid-base status. Two reports have mentioned difficulty with the accuracy of noninvasive blood pressure monitoring in achondroplastic dwarfs because of their short yet often obese arms.[15, 20] In one instance, intra-arterial catheter placement was necessary to accurately measure blood pressure in a previously hypertensive parturient.[20]

The choice between general and regional anesthesia in this condition should be specific to each patient. The factors that increase anesthetic risk are detailed in Table 13–6. If a general anesthetic is chosen, there is the increased aspiration risk present in all parturients undergoing general anesthesia as well as additional risk from uterine impingement on the abdominal contents.[62, 63]

A very serious concern is the risk of difficult intubation. The presence of a large head with facial hypoplasia and a large mandible, limited neck extension, and cervical instability is an important consideration.[28] Although two reports describe difficult intubation in achondroplastic patients,[27, 29] in other cases difficulties were not encountered.[27, 28] A high degree of caution regarding the airway is appropriate, and awake direct laryngoscopy and fiberoptic laryngoscopy are options to be considered when a general anesthetic is planned.

If a patient is suffering from pulmonary compromise before cesarean section, she may not be able to tolerate the supine position while awake. Additionally, the fluid loading administered routinely before institution of regional anesthesia may not be well tolerated. Patients with significant pulmonary insufficiency may

benefit from intubation and mechanical ventilation during surgery and the postpartum period.

As with proportionate dwarfs,[27] endotracheal tube size is thought to be best predicted in achondroplastic dwarfs by weight rather than age.[28] Most studies, however, are reviews primarily of pediatric patients. In the five adults intubated in the report by Mayhew and coworkers,[28] all patients over the age of 17 years were intubated with either a 7.0- or 7.5-mm cuffed endotracheal tube. In four case reports of general anesthesia for cesarean section in achondroplastic patients, a 6.5-mm endotracheal tube was used once, a 7.0-mm tube was used twice, and tube size was not reported in one case.[14, 20, 21, 23] It seems prudent to have numerous endotracheal tube sizes available for the parturient dwarf because the airway changes induced by pregnancy, including airway edema, may necessitate the use of a smaller tube.[11]

Regional anesthesia is a viable option in many achondroplastic patients, particularly if neurologic symptoms are absent. Because of their abnormal spinal anatomy, they have a higher likelihood of patchy blocks, dural puncture, technical difficulty, or spinal cord injury. Nevertheless, a regional anesthetic may be a better choice than general anesthesia for many patients.[12, 14] Walts and coworkers[27] reviewed a number of anesthetics for dwarfs and noted that eight achondroplastic dwarfs received six spinal or epidural anesthetics without neurologic sequelae, although technical difficulty was frequently encountered.

The details of five reports of continuous epidural anesthesia for cesarean section are outlined in Table 13–7. Although some technical difficulty occurred, all patients obtained successful epidural anesthesia without neurologic sequelae.[14, 15, 19, 22, 64] Some patients had multiple attempts at epidural placement, one patient had an unintentional dural puncture, and one patient had an intravascular catheter that was recognized and then replaced with some difficulty.[14, 15] All but one of these patients required a decreased dosage for appropriate surgical level of anesthesia compared with nondwarf parturients. A continuous regional technique is preferred to a single-shot technique for this reason, because no dosage guidelines are available for patients with short stature and abnormal spinal anatomy.

Epidural test doses given in the reported cases have been quite variable (Table 13–8).[14, 15, 19, 22] Although no guidelines exist for the optimal test dose, the amount of local anesthetic injected should be large enough to detect a subarachnoid catheter without inducing high or total spinal anesthesia.[19] Because the patients have abnormal spinal and epidural anatomy, it is not known what this dose is for any individual patient. Additionally, the optimal amount of epinephrine, if included in the test dose, is unknown. One patient received epinephrine, 5 μg, in the test dose.[19] Such a dose, however, may not be sufficient to produce the increase

TABLE 13–6. ANESTHETIC CONSIDERATIONS IN ACHONDROPLASIA

Airway
  Possible difficult mask airway/intubation
  Large head
  Maxillary hypoplasia
  Large tongue
  Large mandible
  Limited neck extension
  Narrow upper airways
  Upper airway obstruction
  Upper cervical spinal cord injury with neck extension
Pulmonary
  Compromised respiratory status
  Thoracic cage deformities
  Infection
  Cor pulmonale
  May not tolerate fluid administration before regional anesthesia
Supine hypotension
  Early intra-abdominal location of uterus
Aspiration risk
  Early intra-abdominal location of uterus
Skeletal anomalies
  Technical difficulty of regional anesthesia
  Inadvertent dural puncture
  Uncertain local anesthesia dosage for single shot techniques and epidural test dose
  Titration of local anesthesia dosage for continuous techniques
  Pre-existing neurologic damage
  ? More prone to neurologic injury

TABLE 13–7. EPIDURAL ANESTHESIA FOR ACHONDROPLASTIC PATIENTS FOR CESAREAN SECTION

Patient Height and Weight	Epidural Level	Local Anesthetic	Volume	Sensory Level	Author	Complication
122 cm 57 kg	L2–3	3% 2-chloroprocaine	9 ml +9 ml later	T4	Cohen,[14] 1980	Difficulty threading catheter. Inadvertent dural puncture at L3–4
120 cm 48 kg	L2–3	0.75% plain bupivacaine	21 ml	T3–4	Waugaman,[64] 1986	Transient paresthesia with catheter placement
121 cm 73 kg	L2–3 ? L3–4	0.5% plain bupivacaine	12 ml +11 ml saline	C5	Brimacombe,[15] 1990	Difficulty threading catheter: intravenous. Difficulty with second attempt, but successful
111 cm 46 kg	L2–3	0.5% plain bupivacaine	5 ml	T4 on left T6 on right	Wardall,[22] 1990	
119 cm 61 kg	T11–12	2% lidocaine +1:200,000 epinephrine	8 ml	T5	Carstoniu,[19] 1992	

Modified from Carstoniu J, Yee I, Halpern S. Epidural anaesthesia for caesarean section in an achondroplastic dwarf. Can J Anaesth 1992;397:708.

in heart rate expected with the more accepted test dose of 15 μg.[16] Unlike the proportionate short-statured patient, a dosage based on weight may not be appropriate, especially because the spinal cord of achondroplastic patients is larger in relation to the spinal canal.

One brief report describes a successful continuous spinal anesthetic in a pregnant achondroplastic dwarf.[24] A 32-gauge microspinal catheter was used. (This catheter is now withdrawn by the Food and Drug Administration in the US because of concerns over associated neurologic deficits.[65, 66]) A continuous spinal technique using a 20-gauge epidural catheter may be a good alternative if inadvertent dural puncture occurs while attempting epidural catheterization.

Postoperative pain management with neuraxial opioids was mentioned in only one report, wherein epidural diamorphine in 2.5-mg doses was administered every 12 hours.[15] No mention was made of postoperative monitoring in this report. Although a single dose of epidural morphine is the usual practice in our institution, a reduced dosage with increased respiratory monitoring (frequent vital signs and continuous pulse oximetry) in the postoperative period seems appropriate.

TABLE 13–8. EPIDURAL TEST DOSES IN PATIENTS WITH ACHONDROPLASIA

Author	Test Dose
Cohen,[14] 1980	3 ml 3% 2-chloroprocaine
Brimacombe,[15] 1990	2 ml 0.5% plain bupivacaine
Wardall,[22] 1990	3 ml 0.5% plain bupivacaine
Carstoniu,[19] 1992	1 ml 2% carbonated lidocaine with 1:200,000 epinephrine

Anesthesia for Nonachondroplastic Parturients

The general considerations in these patients are similar to those in the achondroplasia patients. Most require a cesarean section for obstetric reasons. Craniofacial deformities may be present, and thus the anesthesiologist should anticipate airway difficulties. Cardiac or pulmonary compromise may be present, depending on the presence of pre-existing thoracic spinal deformities and the degree of uterine impingement on the intrathoracic structures. Cardiac anomalies may be present in some forms of dwarfism; thus, any suggestive cardiac symptoms should be investigated before delivery. As in achondroplasia, other spinal deformities can exist, making regional anesthesia more difficult.

Only two case reports describing anesthetic management in parturients with nonachondroplastic disproportionate dwarfism have been published.[17, 25] One describes a dwarf with spondyloepiphyseal dysplasia congenita who underwent cesarean section with epidural anesthesia. This patient had cervical spine abnormalities and marked thoracic kyphoscoliosis and lumbar lordosis. (Figure 13–3 shows a nonpregnant patient with spondyloepiphyseal dysplasia.) After inadvertent intravenous placement of an epidural catheter, repeat placement was uneventful; 8 ml of 2% lidocaine with 1:200,000 epinephrine was administered to establish a surgical block to T4.[25]

The other case involved an emergency cesarean section performed for vaginal bleeding in a patient with a marginal placenta previa and spondylometepiphyseal dysplasia (Fig. 13–4).[17] This patient had limited neck and jaw mobility and was thought to have "a very high anterior larynx." She underwent awake direct laryngoscopy, which revealed the epiglottis and posterior arytenoids. A rapid-sequence induction with easy intubation was performed. The case was complicated not only by blood loss but also by the presence of pulmonary edema, probably as a consequence of ritodrine administration.[17] No anesthetic complications occurred.

NEONATAL CONSIDERATIONS

Many types of dwarfism can be diagnosed immediately after birth. The incidence of newborn dwarfism in this population greatly depends on the parents' type of dwarfism and the accuracy of the parents' diagnosis.[1] The prognosis for each infant is also dependent on the type of dwarfism exhibited. For example, infants who are homozygous for the achondroplasia gene die either in utero or in the early neonatal period. Infants with other types of dwarfism may have thoracic cage

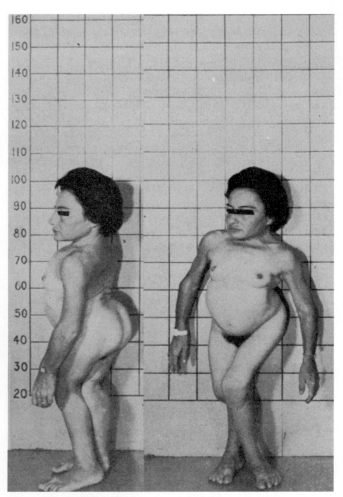

Figure 13–3. Spondyloepiphyseal dysplasia (patient F.L.). Deformities of the spine and limbs with contracture of the pelvis and kyphoscoliosis. (From Tyson JE, Barnes AC, McKusick VA, et al. Obstetric and gynecologic considerations of dwarfism. Am J Obstet Gynecol 1970;108:688.)

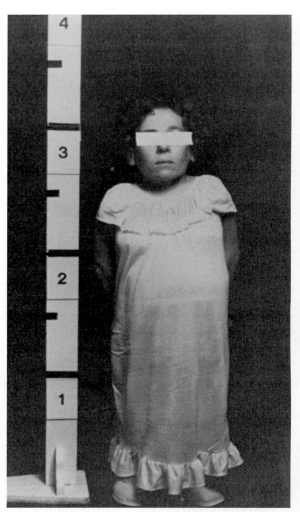

Figure 13–4. Patient with spondylometepiphyseal dysplasia (SMED) 2 days postpartum. Note the short stature and short neck. (From Benson KT, Dozier NJ, Goto J, et al. Anesthesia for cesarean section in patient with spondylometepiphyseal dysplasia. Anesthesiology 1985;63:548.)

abnormalities with respiratory compromise that necessitates ventilatory support. The team responsible for neonatal resuscitation should be notified in advance so that appropriate preparation can be made for delivery of a baby in a potentially compromised condition.

CONCLUSIONS

Currently, very few reports are available in the literature to guide the anesthetic management of parturients of short stature. All pregnant dwarfs have a high incidence of cesarean section, for which they need some type of anesthesia. The physiologic changes of pregnancy often exacerbate the pre-existing mechanical and physiologic abnormalities present in dwarfs. Anesthesia often poses greater risk to these patients. Because numerous forms of dwarfism exist, it is critical that each parturient be evaluated early in pregnancy and her individual needs assessed before anesthetic intervention is undertaken.

References

1. Tyson JE, Barnes AC, McKusick VA, et al. Obstetric and gynecologic considerations of dwarfism. Am J Obstet Gynecol 1970;108:688.
2. Berkowitz ID, Raja SN, Bender KS, et al. Dwarfs: Pathophysiology and anesthetic implications. Anesthesiology 1990;73:739.
3. Orioli IM, Castilla EE, Barbosa-Neto JG. The birth prevalence rates for the skeletal dysplasias. J Med Genet 1986;23:328.
4. Bailey JA. Disproportionate Short Stature: Diagnosis and Management. Philadelphia, WB Saunders, 1973, p 4.
5. Phillips JA. Inherited defects in growth hormone synthesis and action. In Scriver CR, Beaudet AL, Sly WS, Valle D (eds): The Metabolic and Molecular Basis of Inherited Disease, 7th ed. New York, McGraw-Hill, 1995, p 3029.
6. Rimoin DL, Holzman GB, Merimee TJ, et al. Lactation in the absence of human growth hormone. J Clin Endocrinol 1968; 28:1183.
7. Rimoin DL, Merimee TJ, McKusick VA. Growth-hormone deficiency in man: An isolated, recessively inherited defect. Science 1966;152:1635.
8. Amselem S, Duquesnoy P, Attree O, et al. Laron dwarfism and mutations of the growth hormone-receptor gene. N Engl J Med 1989;321:989.
9. Dorland's Illustrated Medical Dictionary, 26th ed. Philadelphia, WB Saunders, 1981.
10. Menashe Y, Sack J, Mashiach S: Spontaneous pregnancies in two women with Laron-type dwarfism: Are growth hormone and circulating insulin-like growth factor mandatory for induction of ovulation? Hum Reprod 1991;6:670.
11. Cheek TG, Gutsche BB. Maternal physiologic alterations during pregnancy. In Shnider SM, Levinson G (eds): Anesthesia for Obstetrics, 3rd ed. Baltimore, Williams & Wilkins, 1993, p 3.
12. Allanson JE, Hall JG. Obstetric and gynecologic problems in women with chondrodystrophies. Obstet Gynecol 1986;67:74.
13. Muller J, Starup J, Christiansen JS, et al. Growth hormone treatment during pregnancy in a growth hormone-deficient woman. Eur J Endocrinol 1995;132:727.
14. Cohen SE. Anesthesia for cesarean section in achondroplastic dwarfs. Anesthesiology 1980;52:264.
15. Brimacombe JR, Caunt JA. Anaesthesia in a gravid achondroplastic dwarf. Anaesthesia 1990;45:132.
16. Moore DC, Batra MS. The components of an effective test dose prior to epidural block. Anesthesiology 1981;55:693.
17. Benson KT, Dozier NJ, Goto H, Arakawa K. Anesthesia for cesarean section in a patient with spondylometepiphyseal dysplasia. Anesthesiology 1985;63:548.
18. Maroteaux P. International nomenclature of constitutional diseases of bones with bibliography. Birth Defects 1986;22:1.
19. Carstoniu J, Yee I, Halpern S. Epidural anaesthesia for caesarean section in an achondroplastic dwarf. Can J Anaesth 1992;39:708.
20. McArthur RDA. Obstetric anaesthesia in an achondroplastic dwarf at a regional hospital. Anaesth Intensive Care 1992; 20:376.
21. Bancroft GH, Lauria JI. Ketamine induction for cesarean section in a patient with acute intermittent porphyria and achondroplastic dwarfism. Anesthesiology 1983;59:143.
22. Wardall GJ, Frame WT. Extradural anaesthesia for caesarean section in achondroplasia. Br J Anaesth 1990;64:367.
23. Kalla GN, Fening E, Obiaya MO. Anaesthetic management of achondroplasia. Br J Anaesth 1986;58:117.
24. Crawford M, Dutton DA: Spinal anaesthesia for caesarean section in an achondroplastic dwarf (letter). Anaesthesia 1992;47:1007.
25. Rodney GE, Callander CC, Harmer M. Spondyloepiphyseal dysplasia congenita: Caesarean section under epidural anaesthesia. Anaesthesia 1991;46:648.
26. Spranger J: Spondyloepiphyseal dysplasia congenita. In Bergsma D (ed): Birth Defects Compendium. London, Macmillan Press, 1979, p 969.
27. Walts LF, Finerman G, Wyatt GM. Anaesthesia for dwarfs and other patients of pathological small stature. Can Anaesth Soc J 1975;22:703.
28. Mayhew JF, Katz J, Miner M, et al. Anaesthesia for the achondroplastic dwarf. Can Anaesth Soc J 1986;33:216.
29. Mather JS. Impossible laryngoscopy in achondroplasia: A case report. Anaesthesia 1966;21:244.
30. Nelson MA: Spinal stenosis in achondroplasia. Proc R Soc Med 1972;65:1028.
31. Yang SS, Corbett DP, Brough AJ, et al. Upper cervical myelopathy in achondroplasia. Am J Clin Pathol 1977;68:68.
32. Morgan DF, Young RF. Spinal neurological complications of achondroplasia. J Neurosurg 1980;52:463.
33. Schreiber F, Rosenthal H: Paraplegia from ruptured lumbar discs in achondroplastic dwarfs. J Neurosurg 1952;9:648.
34. Wynne-Davies R, Walsh WK, Gormley J. Achondroplasia and hypochondroplasia: Clinical variation and spinal stenosis. J Bone Joint Surg 1981;63B:508.
35. Bergstrom K, Laurent U, Lundberg PO. Neurological symptoms in achondroplasia. Acta Neurol Scand 1971;47:59.
36. Alexander E. Significance of the small lumbar spinal canal: Cauda equina compression syndromes due to spondylosis: Part 5. Achondroplasia. J Neurosurg 1969;31:513.
37. Lutter LD, Lonstein JE, Winter RB, Langer LO, et al. Anatomy of the achondroplastic lumbar canal. Clin Orthop 1977;126:139.
38. Schreiber F, Rosenthal H. Paraplegia from ruptured lumbar discs in achondroplastic dwarfs. J Neurosurg 1952;9:648.
39. Cohen ME, Rosenthal AD, Matson DD. Neurological abnormalities in achondroplastic children. J Pediatr 1967;71:367.
40. Ozer FL. Achondroplasia with spinal neurologic complications in mother and son: Case report. Birth Defects 1974;10:351.
41. Lutter LD, Langer LO. Neurological symptoms in achondroplastic dwarfs: Surgical treatment. J Bone Joint Surg 1977;59A:87.
42. Vogl A, Osborne RL. Lesions of the spinal cord (transverse myelopathy) in achondroplasia. Arch Neurol Psychiatr 1949;61:644.
43. Fremoin AS, Garg BP, Kalsbeck J. Apnea as the sole manifestation of cord compression in achondroplasia. J Pediatr 1984;104:398.
44. Reid CS, Pyeritz RE, Kopits SE, et al. Cervicomedullary compression in young patients with achondroplasia. Value of comprehensive neurologic and respiratory evaluation. J Pediatr 1987; 110:522.
45. Kopits SE. Orthopedic complications of dwarfism. Clin Orthop 1976;114:153.
46. Bethem D, Winter RB, Lutter L, et al. Spinal disorders of dwarfism. J Bone Joint Surg 1981;63A:1412.
47. Steinbok, P, Hall J, Flodmark O. Hydrocephalus in achondroplasia. The possible role of intracranial venous hypertension. J Neurosurg 1989;71:42.
48. Thomas IT, Frias JL, Williams JL, Friedman WA. Magnetic resonance imaging in the assessment of medullary compression in achondroplasia. Am J Dis Child 1988;142:989.
49. Freidman WA, Mickle JP. Hydrocephalus in achondroplasia: A possible mechanism. Neurosurg 1980;7:150.
50. Stokes DC, Phillips JA, Leonard CO, et al. Respiratory complications of achondroplasia. J Pediatr 1983;102:534.
51. McKusick VA. Heritable Disorders of Connective Tissue. St. Louis, CV Mosby, 1972, p 750.
52. Hull D, Barnes ND. Children with small chests. Arch Dis Child 1972;47:12.
53. Guilleminault C, Kurland G, Winkle R, et al. Severe kyphoscoliosis, breathing and sleep. Chest 1981;79:626.
54. Stokes DC, Pyeritz RE, Wisa RA, et al. Spirometry and chest wall dimensions in achondroplasia. Chest 1988;93:364.
55. Mueller SM, Bell W, Cornell S, et al. Achondroplasia and hydrocephalus. Neurology 1977;27:430.
56. Smith TH, Baska RE, Francisco CB, et al. Sleep apnea syndrome: Diagnosis of upper airway obstruction by fluoroscopy. J Pediatr 1978;93:891.
57. Levin DL, Muster AJ, Pachman LM, et al. Cor pulmonale secondary to upper airway obstruction. Chest 1975;68:166.
58. Myer CM, Cotton RT. Laryngotracheal stenosis in spondyloepiphyseal dysplasia. Laryngoscope 1985;95:3.
59. Wynne-Davis R, Hall CM, Apley AG. Skeletal dysplasia group: Instability of the upper cervical spine. Arch Dis Child 1989;64:283.
60. Anderson CE, Sillence DO, Lachman RS, et al. Spondylometaphyseal dysplasia, Strudwick type. Am J Med Genet 1982;13:243.

61. Perovic MN, Kopits SE, Thompson RC. Radiological evaluation of the spinal cord in congenital atlanto-axial dislocation. Radiology 1973;109:713.

62. Davison JJ, Davison MC, Hay DM. Gastric emptying time in late pregnancy and labour. J Obstet Gynaecol Brit Commonw 1970;77:37.

63. Cohen SE. The aspiration syndrome. Clin Obstet Gynaecol 1982;9:235.

64. Waugaman WR, Kryc JJ, Andrews MJ. Epidural anesthesia for cesarean section and tubal ligation in an achondroplastic dwarf. J Am Assoc Nurs Anesth 1986;54:436.

65. Rigler ML, Drasner K, Krejcie TC, et al. Cauda equina syndrome after continuous spinal anesthesia. Anesth Analg 1991;72:275.

66. Rigler ML, Drasner K. Distribution of catheter-injected local anesthetic in a model of the subarachnoid space. Anesthesiology 1991;75:684.

SCOLIOSIS AND MAJOR SPINAL SURGERY

∎ ∎ ∎ ∎ ∎ ∎ ∎

Edward T. Crosby, M.D.

Moderate to severe scoliotic curves are not common in women of childbearing age. Most likely, scoliosis is uncommon in this group because screening programs have identified many at-risk patients early in the disease process, resulting in timely intervention and curve correction. Additionally, primary neuromuscular diseases that result in scoliosis are uncommon and may themselves limit the woman's reproductive potential. Despite the fact that women with moderate to severe scoliosis constitute a small population of patients, pregnancy within that population is common. Pregnancy, labor, and delivery are often similar in women with scoliosis with respect to both process and outcome compared with the general population. If the disease process is advanced, however, pregnancy may not only be complicated but also may be life-threatening. In this small subpopulation, a detailed understanding of the pathophysiology of advanced scoliosis and the interaction with pregnancy is necessary to provide effective maternal care.

SCOLIOSIS

Definition and Description

Scoliosis is defined as an appreciable lateral deviation in the normally straight vertical axis of the spine. Scoliosis can be classified according to its cause and a description of the curve, including its magnitude, location, and direction.[1] Scoliosis is divided into structural and nonstructural types, on the basis of spinal flexibility. Nonstructural curves are those seen in postural scoliosis or those related to sciatica or leg length discrepancies. Nonstructural curves are occasionally seen in parturients, developing with progression of the gestation and resolving after delivery. They do not affect the mobility of the spine; they are nonprogressive and resolve with attention to the underlying cause. Structural curves are those of idiopathic scoliosis or resulting from the conditions outlined in Table 14–1. Equal lateral flexibility is lacking which is best appreciated on left and right bending films. Structural curves

are associated with the presence of a fixed prominence, the rib hump, on the convex side of the curve. This prominence is usually best demonstrated in the forward-bend position. Reduced spinal mobility is characteristic of the structural curves. Kyphoscoliosis, which is a combination of kyphosis and scoliosis, is uncommon in parturients. It is usually a congenital disorder, although it may be related to progressive infantile scoliosis or paralytic forms of scoliosis.

The curve of scoliosis is typically described by its angle, location, and direction. The curve angle is determined by the Cobb method, in which the upper and lower end vertebrae of the curves are determined. Lines are drawn through the end points of these vertebrae and the Cobb angle is formed by the intersection of perpendiculars to these lines (Figs. 14–1 and 14–2). The anatomic area of the spine in which the apex of the curve is situated determines the location of the curve. Thoracolumbar curves are most commonly seen, followed in frequency by those affecting only the thoracic or lumbar spines.[2] The lower limit of curves involving the lumbar spine is usually L3 or L4, although relatively few curves extend this far caudad. The direc-

TABLE 14–1. **CONDITIONS ASSOCIATED WITH SCOLIOSIS**

Congenital (vertebral) anomalies
Hemivertebra
Spina bifida
Neurologic disorders
Cerebral palsy
Polio
Neurofibromatosis
Myopathic disorders
Myotonic dystrophy
Muscular dystrophy
Connective tissue disorders
Marfan syndrome
Rheumatoid disease
Osteochondrystrophies
Achondroplasia/hypochondroplasia
Osteogenesis imperfecta
Infection
Tuberculosis
Post-traumatic

tion assigned to the curve is determined by the convexity. Right thoracic curves are the most common curves described in idiopathic scoliosis.

Etiologic Considerations

Scoliosis results from a disruption of the balance achieved in the spine between the static and dynamic structural components, the neuromuscular elements, and the balance and symmetry of the body as a whole. The cause of the majority (85–90%) of cases of scoliosis is unknown (idiopathic). Idiopathic scoliosis is divided into three types: infantile, juvenile, and adolescent.[1] The two types of infantile scoliosis are resolving and progressive. The majority do not progress beyond 30° and resolve spontaneously. Less commonly, and usually in males, the curves are progressive and result in severe deformity early in life. Juvenile scoliosis has its onset in the 4- to 9-year age group, is less common than the adolescent form, and is not as well defined. Adolescent idiopathic scoliosis (AIS), which has its onset between age 10 and the age at skeletal maturity, represents the most common form of idiopathic scoliosis. It usually occurs in an otherwise healthy child, often in association with a family history of the disease.

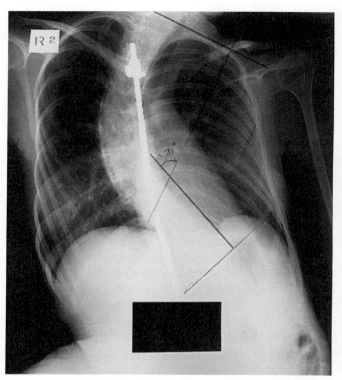

Figure 14–2. Cobb angle—chest radiograph. Cobb angles are represented on this radiograph of a young woman with a progressive spinal muscular atrophy (Kugelberg-Welander syndrome) and a 70° thoracic curve. Note should also be made of the rib separation on the right hemithorax compared with the left. This patient's pelvic film is detailed in Figure 14–6.

The inheritance pattern is consistent with a dominant inheritance with reduced penetrance.[3]

Less common causes of scoliosis are listed in Table 14–1. Of these rarer forms, the most common in parturients are deformities caused by neurologic and myopathic conditions that result in paralytic scoliosis as well as curves resulting from osteochondystrophies. Infectious causes of scoliosis, predominantly tuberculosis-related, are primarily reported from underdeveloped countries.[4]

Incidence and Prevalence

As a result of the prevention of poliomyelitis, surveys reflect largely the incidence of AIS.[3] The incidence of minor curves in the US population, assessed radiographically, is 4 in 1000.[5] The incidence of deformities that reach angles of 35° is 1 in 1000, and of deformities greater than 70° approximately 0.1 in 1000.[6] These larger curves occur predominantly in females. The prevalence of scoliosis is wide, reportedly ranging from 0.3 to 15.3%.[7] Although the prevalence in the American population is 1.8% if minor curvatures (5–10°) are included, the rate in adult females is 10.7%.[8, 9] Over the past 25 years, scoliosis screening programs and early interventions (orthotic braces for curves of 25–40° and

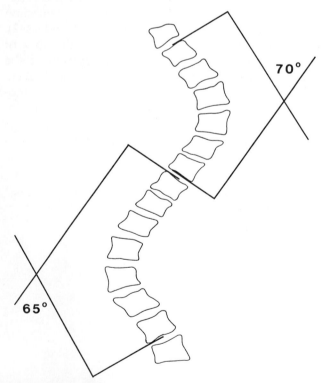

Figure 14–1. Cobb angle—schematic representation. A line is drawn parallel to the superior cortical plate of the proximal end vertebrae and to the inferior cortical plate of the distal end vertebrae. A perpendicular line is erected to each of these lines. The angle of intersection is the (Cobb) angle of the curve. (From Crosby ET: Musculoskeletal disorders. In Chestnut DH (ed): Obstetric Anesthesia: Principles and Practice. St. Louis, Mosby–Year Book, 1994, p 907.)

spinal fusion for curves greater than 40°) have been used to prevent the natural progression of the disease. Evidence suggests a reduced incidence of uncorrected major curves in adults, which is likely due to early diagnosis and intervention.[10]

Severe scoliosis is rare in parturients. The reported incidence varies from 1 in 1500 to 1 in 12,000 pregnancies. This variability may reflect geographic differences in the occurrence rate of etiologic factors.[11] Most of the surveys involved women with severe scoliosis. The rarity of the combination of severe scoliosis and pregnancy is probably a result of the relatively low prevalence of moderate to severe curves in the population, because pregnancy is common in women who have scoliosis. In a postal survey of women diagnosed with scoliosis in Minnesota, 72% of responders had been pregnant, an average of 2.8 times each.[12] More than half of these women (68%) had been diagnosed with idiopathic scoliosis, the majority having adolescent-onset disease. Their mean curve size was 37°, and most of the spinal curves (61%) were thoracic or thoracolumbar, although a significant proportion were lumbar. Fifty-eight percent of the patients had undergone spinal surgery for scoliosis, which may account for the relatively small Cobb angles in the group.

Risk Factors for Curve Progression

Progression of a curve is defined as an increase of 5° or more, as measured by the Cobb method, over subsequent assessments. Progression is most likely to occur in the rapid adolescent growth phase in immature patients; in patients with larger curves (>20°) at the time of original diagnosis; and in patients with double curves at presentation.[13] There is a threefold increase in the risk of progression if the initial curve is measured at greater than 20° than if the curve is less than 20°. In adults, thoracic curves are more likely to progress if the Cobb angle is large (>50°). Although it was once thought that there was little progression after skeletal maturity, observation over decades has shown that moderate curves (60–80°) increase an average of 30°.[15] The natural history of the untreated severe curve is progression of the deformity over time, resulting in early death from cardiopulmonary failure.[3, 14, 15] Long-term follow-up of patients with major uncorrected curves demonstrated that their mortality rate was twice that of the general population, and the average age at death was 46.6 years.[16]

Skeletal Changes in Idiopathic Scoliosis

The skeletal anatomic pathology that results from AIS is complex. Deformation of vertebrae is present, as are abnormal relationships between vertebrae, excess curvature in the frontal plane, loss of normal sagittal plane curves, and rotation in the vertical axis. The vertebral bodies have shorter, thinner pedicles and laminae on the concave side and a narrower vertebral canal (Fig. 14–3). The transverse processes are anatomically abnormal and asymmetric in their spatial orientation. The spinous processes are deformed and skewed from the midline. Vertebral deformation does not occur in curves with Cobb angles of less than 40°.[17] The rotatory component associated with the scoliotic curve is such that the axial rotation of the vertebral body is into the convexity of the lateral curve, and the spinous process is rotated back into the concavity.[18] (Fig. 14–4A) As a result of the rotation of the vertebrae, the ribs on the side of the convexity are pulled backward, producing a prominent posterior angle—the rib hump (Fig. 14–4B) The interlaminar space is shifted more toward the curve convexity than is the spinal process, and the usual anatomic relationship between these structures is altered. This change is important if major neuraxial block is considered, because the underlying structures no longer maintain the same relationships to surface landmarks.

Indications for Intervention and Principles of Corrective Surgery

Curves of less than 20° are considered benign and need not be treated.[13] Nonoperative therapy with

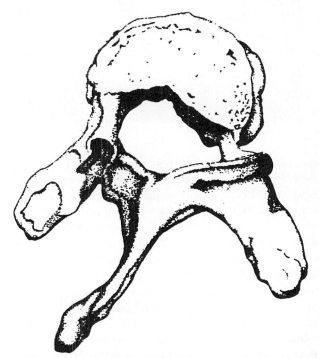

Figure 14–3. Scoliotic deformation of the vertebral body. The vertebra diagrammed is from a spine with a moderate to severe right-sided curve. The body has shorter, thinner pedicles on the concave (left) side and a narrower vertebral canal. The transverse processes are abnormal and asymmetric in their spatial orientation. The spinous process is deformed and skewed from the midline. (See also Figure 14–7.)

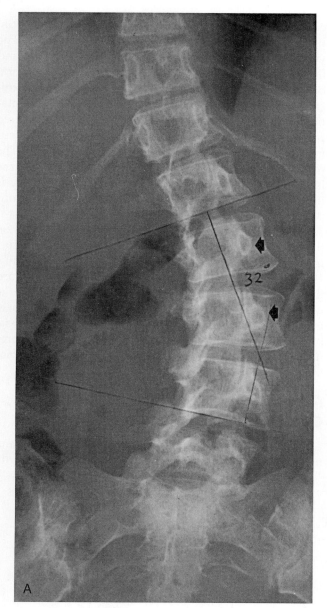

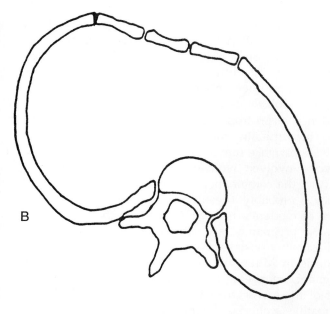

Figure 14–4. Idiopathic scoliosis—lumbar spine. *(A)* X-ray study of the lumbar spine in a 26-year-old woman with idiopathic scoliosis. The spinous process and pedicles *(arrows)* are rotated away from the curve convexity and into the concavity. The epidural space was entered easily by directing the needle about 15° off the perpendicular at the skin level toward the convexity of the curve. (From Crosby ET: Musculoskeletal disorders. In Chestnut DH (ed): Obstetric Anesthesia: Principles and Practice. St. Louis, Mosby–Year Book, 1994, p 908.) *(B)* Rib hump—schematic. As a result of the rotation of the vertebrae, the ribs on the side of the convexity are pulled backward, producing the prominent posterior angle, the rib hump. The intercostal gap is increased in the hemithorax with the hump. (See Figure 14–2.)

braces is utilized for progressive curves in the 20 to 40° range. Fifteen to 20% of the curves in this range do not respond to bracing and require surgery to halt curve progression.[8] Curves less than 40° are not usually fused unless there is documented curve progression, pain related to the curve, or neurologic deficits. The goal of surgery is to fuse the spinal curve and prevent progression of the deformity. Modern surgical techniques consistently yield a 50% reduction of the deformity, without excessive risk. The area fused should be kept as short as possible to maintain the greatest number of mobile articulations, but enough of the spine must be fused to stabilize the deformity. Fusion of the thoracic spine rarely causes any long-term disability, whereas fusion in the lumbar spine often leads to loss of motion and increased stress in the few unfused lower segments. An attempt is usually made to limit the extent of the caudal fusions in the lumbar spine and to avoid

the lumbosacral junction if at all possible. The most common stabilization technique remains the posterior fusion and instrumentation. Anterior spinal surgery is used in more severe curvatures, which are less flexible, or in congenital spinal deformities, which may require combined anterior and posterior procedures.

Harrington reported his first series of patients with structural scoliosis treated by curve correction and internal fixation by spinal instrumentation more than three decades ago.[19] During Harrington instrumentation, hooks are attached at the upper and lower extremes of the curve. The Harrington rod is inserted into the hooks and maximally extended. Bone graft material is obtained from the ilium and placed over the decorticated vertebrae. Following the correction, the patient undergoes a variable period of casting and immobilization to allow for maturation of the bone graft. Additional techniques of spine instrumentation have since been developed. In the Luque technique, rods were secured in place with sublaminar wires.[20] The risks associated with the placement and removal of the sublaminar wires within the spinal canal very much limited the application of this technique.[18] Newer segmental techniques involve a rod system that combines the distraction-compression forces of the Harrington technique with the strength of the Luque segmental fixation technique. The advantage of these newer techniques compared with Harrington fusion is that there is rarely a requirement for postoperative external support (casting) or prolonged immobilization. All techniques described, however, involve spinal instrumentation and extensive bone grafting in the axial spine (Fig. 14–5).

Follow-up studies of patients who underwent early operative corrections of severe scoliotic curves demonstrated improvements in both lung volumes and function postoperatively in some.[21, 22] In others, increases in lung volumes are not always obtained, although lung function is improved or the progression of the restrictive lung disease arrested.[23] Improved function was demonstrated when significant reductions in moderate to severe curves were achieved with Harrington instrumentation or when thoracic kyphosis was normalized.[24, 25] Delaying correction until adulthood appears to reduce the gains made in lung function, when compared with results of earlier correction.[26] Patients who undergo early instrumentation generally do not develop the cardiopulmonary complications that afflict patients with severe and uncorrected disease.[21, 22, 26–28]

Cardiopulmonary Pathophysiology in Idiopathic Scoliosis

Respiratory Pathophysiology

Scoliosis interferes with the formation, growth, and development of the lungs.[29] Because the number of alveoli increase greatly between birth and age 8, the occurrence of scoliosis before lung maturity reduces the number of alveoli formed. The pulmonary vasculature forms in parallel with the alveoli and is likewise affected, resulting in increased pulmonary resistance, pulmonary hypertension, and, in severe cases, right heart failure. The pulmonary pathophysiology of scoliosis also includes the effects of the vertebral and ribcage deformity on the mechanical function of the lung. The key findings that correlate with respiratory compromise are (1) a thoracic curve; (2) thoracic lordosis; and (3) a ribcage deformity. The most common abnormality is a *restrictive* pattern of pulmonary dysfunction with a reduction in lung volume and compliance. This pattern is seen in all patients with thoracic curves greater than 65°. Limitation of ventilatory reserve is present, which is initially manifested as dyspnea on

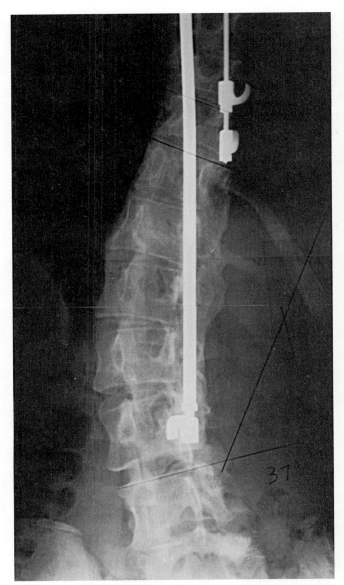

Figure 14–5. Harrington rod instrumentation. Radiograph of the lumbar spine in a 31-year-old woman with thoracolumbar scoliosis corrected with spinal instrumentation. There is rotation of the vertebrae into the curve (toward the rod), and extensive bone grafting is evident adjacent to the rod. Two lumbar interspaces are not involved in the fusion, L4-L5 and L5-S1. (From Crosby ET: Musculoskeletal disorders. In Chestnut DH (ed): Obstetric Anesthesia: Principles and Practice. St. Louis, Mosby–Year Book, 1994, p 909.)

exertion and reduced exercise capacity in the early stages. Progression of the curve results in greater severity of the respiratory compromise.

Although the residual volume (RV) is generally not affected in most patients with restrictive lung disease, functional residual capacity (FRC) is decreased. If the FRC is sufficiently reduced, airways may close during normal tidal breathing, resulting in physiologic shunt and arterial hypoxemia. Total lung capacity (TLC—the volume of the lung at end-maximal inspiration) and vital capacity (VC—the volume that can be exhaled from the lungs starting from maximal inspiration) are both reduced. Normal VC in adults is 70 to 80 ml/kg.

When values are reduced to less than 15 to 18 ml/kg, expiratory airflow may become inadequate to produce an effective cough. Flow rates, as measured against lung volumes, provide a measure of the presence or absence of airway obstruction. These ratios tend to be unaffected in restrictive lung disease, implying that intrinsic airways disease is not typically associated with scoliosis.

The amount of work performed during breathing depends on many factors, the most important of which are the stiffness of the lungs and chest wall and the resistance to flow through the airways. In patients with thoracic scoliosis, the chest wall is stiff, and larger transpulmonary gradients must be generated to achieve airflow. More work is necessary to expand the lungs to any volume than if the chest wall were normal. The actual work done is reduced if patients with scoliosis breathe more rapidly at smaller volumes. A normal dead space in conjunction with small-tidal-volume breathing, however, results in increased dead space (wasted) ventilation. Increased ventilatory requirements may result in a large increment in respiratory work. As the respiratory work increases the potential for respiratory failure also increases. If the respiratory muscles are forced to work at a sustained intensity of greater than 40% of maximum, muscle fatigue and respiratory failure result.[30]

Dyspnea on exertion occurs before the onset of alveolar hypoventilation. The degree of spinal deformity usually correlates with symptom severity. Cardiorespiratory symptoms are not common with curves of less than 70°. Dyspnea is more common as the deformity exceeds 100°, and alveolar hypoventilation occurs when angles exceed 120°. In younger patients with moderate thoracic scoliosis (25–70%), impaired exercise capacity is usually due to deconditioning and lack of regular aerobic exercise and not intrinsic ventilatory impairment.[31] Patients with severe scoliosis (curve >90°) are more likely to experience sleep-breathing abnormalities, night time hypoxemia, and daytime hypercapnia.[32]

Cardiovascular Pathophysiology

Scoliosis and cardiac anomalies may have a common embryologic etiology.[33] In AIS, the incidence of mitral valve prolapse exceeds 25%, and children with congenital heart disease have an increased incidence of scoliosis.[34] Most patients with AIS, however, do not have congenitally abnormal hearts. The cardiovascular abnormality most commonly associated with scoliosis results from the restrictive pulmonary defect. The consequences of impaired lung development and alveolar hypoxemia are increased pulmonary vascular resistance and right ventricular hypertrophy. Permanent changes of the pulmonary vasculature are common with curvatures greater than 65°. Pulmonary hyperten-

sion exists when the mean pulmonary artery pressure (PAP) exceeds 25 mm Hg. Pulmonary hypertension at rest or with exercise occurs in many patients with a moderately advanced deformity long before the onset of detectable right heart failure.[6] The greater the deformity, as measured by the Cobb angle, the greater the PAP. Pulmonary hypertension is mainly attributable to increases in pulmonary vascular resistance (PVR) resulting from hypoxic pulmonary vasoconstriction and anatomic vascular alteration. Persistent hypertension leads to pulmonary arterial wall thickening and fibrosis, and eventually the elevated pressures become irreversible. Administration of enriched oxygen mixtures may decrease PAPs but does not return them to normal.[6] Fixed pulmonary hypertension, unresponsive to supplemental oxygen therapy, carries a grave maternal prognosis during pregnancy and is an indication for termination of pregnancy.[35]

Patients with pulmonary hypertension have a limited ability to increase cardiac output with activity.[36] Because of the limited cardiac output, tachyarrhythmias are not well tolerated and may produce marked systemic hypotension. An increased heart rate can reduce cardiac output, and stroke volume is relatively fixed in the setting of pulmonary hypertension. If the right ventricle fails in the presence of pulmonary hypertension, left ventricular filling decreases and low-output failure and sudden death may occur. Death may be caused by sudden changes in venous return to the right ventricle, with acute left ventricular failure, ischemia, and dysrhythmias. Hypoxia, due to the increased oxygen consumption associated with labor as well as the underlying pulmonary dysfunction, further compromises cardiovascular function.[37] Minute pulmonary emboli may be fatal in established pulmonary hypertension because cardiac reserve may be so marginal that even a small decrease in vascular compliance may fatally compromise ventricular function.

In patients with altered pulmonary vascular pressures, arterial blood gas values often demonstrate a widened alveolar-arterial gradient. Electrocardiographic abnormalities indicative of pulmonary hypertension occur at a late stage and include signs of right atrial dilatation and right ventricular hypertrophy and strain. Electrocardiographic changes do not necessarily parallel the severity of the underlying pulmonary hypertension.[38] Echocardiography may be used to demonstrate changes in right ventricular wall thickness, chamber size, and ventricular function. The typical echocardiographic appearance shows right ventricular and right atrial enlargement with a normal to reduced left ventricular cavity.[39] Midsystolic closure of the pulmonic valve is commonly seen. Closure is demonstrated in Doppler studies to be caused by a reflected pressure wave that is produced by the high PVR, which results in transient retrograde blood flow. Reversal of the normal septal curvature, which is associated with right ventricular pressure overload states, is seen with two-dimensional echocardiography. This septal shift results in impaired left ventricular diastolic compliance.

Scoliosis Associated with Neuromuscular Disease—Cardiopulmonary Manifestations

The pathophysiologic sequelae of neuromuscular scoliosis, when scoliosis develops consequent to a primary neurologic or myopathic disorder, differ from those of idiopathic scoliosis. Abnormal respiratory function results not only because of the skeletal deformity of scoliosis but also because of abnormalities in the central control of respiration and in the supraspinal innervation of muscles. Abnormal respiratory function results also from the loss of muscle function due to lesions of the motor neurons and peripheral nerves or myopathy. Respiratory function may be further compromised by impairment of the airway defense mechanisms caused by loss of control of the pharynx and the larynx, by ineffective cough mechanism, and by infrequent or reduced large breaths. Recurrent aspiration pneumonitis results from compromised airway protective reflexes. The prognosis for the patient with scoliosis caused by neuromuscular disease is worse than that for one with idiopathic scoliosis. Prognosis is determined predominantly by progression of the primary disorder. Scoliosis caused by neuromuscular disease results in irreversible respiratory failure at a young age.

The neuromuscular disorders usually involve both the inspiratory and expiratory muscles, resulting in moderate to severe decreases in inspiratory capacity and expiratory reserve volume. Until the diseases are well advanced or until a significant degree of thoracic scoliosis is superimposed, FRC remains normal. Hypoventilation is a prominent feature of the neuromuscular disorders associated with scoliosis. Diaphragmatic weakness or paralysis attributable to the underlying disorder can further compromise vital capacity. If rib-cage expansion is limited by neuromuscular involvement, respiratory function is severely compromised. Hypoxemia may be present for prolonged periods before the onset of hypercapnia. Pulmonary vasoconstriction, hypertension, and right heart failure occur owing to the same etiologic considerations as for idiopathic scoliosis. A primary myocardial impairment may be superimposed on the acquired cardiovascular derangements in conditions such as muscular dystrophy and Marfan disease.[40]

INTERACTION OF PREGNANCY WITH SCOLIOSIS

Cardiopulmonary Signs and Symptoms of Normal Pregnancy

When evaluating the parturient with significant cardiopulmonary disease, an attempt has to be made to distinguish the signs and symptoms that are consistent with normal pregnancy from those that may herald a deterioration in maternal condition. Although most women complain of dyspnea by the middle of the third trimester, dyspnea begins in many during the first or second trimester. Dyspnea probably results from the woman's subjective awareness of hyperventilation that is universally present in pregnancy. Fatigue and reduced exercise tolerance are common complaints during pregnancy and are probably due to increased body weight. Despite these symptoms, exercise testing shows no deterioration in exercise response during moderate activity. Two features help distinguish physiologic from pathologic dyspnea.[41, 42] Physiologic dyspnea tends to begin earlier in pregnancy and often reaches a plateau or improves as term approaches. It is rarely extreme, and patients can usually maintain daily activities. The dyspnea of cardiopulmonary disorders is progressive, becoming more severe as gestation advances and physiologic demands are increasing. If dyspnea is extreme, has a limiting impact on normal activity, occurs at rest or with minimal exertion, or is associated with a cough, maternal cardiorespiratory decompensation should be ruled out.[41] Dyspnea that is acute in onset or progressive and intractable, especially if coupled with other signs and symptoms (orthopnea, paroxysmal nocturnal dyspnea), is more likely to represent cardiopulmonary disease.

Peripheral edema is common and may be misinterpreted as a sign of right ventricular decompensation. Peripheral edema occurs late in pregnancy, and the incidence increases with maternal age. Jugular venous distension is also seen in late pregnancy as a result of the increase in circulating blood volume.[41] Right-sided pressures are not increased, however. Persistently or significantly elevated jugular venous pressure is a sign of elevated right atrial pressure. Precordial palpation commonly reveals a brisk, diffuse, and laterally displaced left ventricular apical impulse. Prominence of the right ventricle is evident, even to the point of mimicking pulmonary or tricuspid valvular incompetence and atrial septal defect.[41] Pulmonary bibasilar crackles are occasionally present.[41] These crackles result from the atelectasis that occurs as the diaphragm moves cephalad, compressing the lung bases. The crackles typically clear or are very much reduced following a deep inspiration.

Effect of Normal Pregnancy on the Diagnostic Tests of Cardiopulmonary Function

Most studies report an increase in left ventricular end-diastolic dimensions of approximately 6 to 10% with a small increase in end-systolic dimensions near term. Evidence of left ventricular hypertrophy appears by 12 weeks' gestation, with a 50% increase in mass by term.[43] Atrial size is commonly increased, reflecting greater maternal blood volume. The electrocardiogram may show changes in rate, rhythm, interval, and axis. The PR and QT intervals are shortened as a result of the higher resting heart rate. Small Q waves and T-wave inversions are common in lead III and often normalize or decrease with deep inspiration. ST-segment depression and T-wave inversions occur in the limb leads and left precordial leads. They may mimic the electrocardiographic changes of myocardial ischemia.

Increased vascular markings may be evident on chest radiographs. The markings result from both the increased blood volume and the increased anteroposterior chest diameter. Forced vital capacity (FVC) and forced expiratory volume in one second (FEV_1) are unchanged, as is the ratio of FEV_1:FVC, which is used to assess patients for obstructive airways disease. Flow volume loops are also unaffected by pregnancy. Although maximal breathing capacity is not changed, minute ventilation is increased by up to 50% at term. Assessment of arterial blood gas levels reveals an increase in PaO_2 of about 10 mm Hg, a decrease in $PaCO_2$ of a similar magnitude, and a decrease in both serum bicarbonate concentrations and pH of a smaller magnitude.

Impact of Pregnancy on the Spinal Deformity

Pregnancy may exacerbate both the severity of spinal curvature and the cardiorespiratory abnormalities in patients with uncorrected scoliosis. The factors that predict curve progression are the same in parturients as they are in nonpregnant women. Thus, a young skeletally immature woman with scoliosis seems to be at particular risk for curve progression during pregnancy. Curves that are less than 25° or curves that have been stable before the pregnancy do not, as a rule, progress during the pregnancy.[44–46] More severe curves and those that have not yet stabilized may progress. Although maternal morbidity and mortality have been linked by some to the severity of the curve, the true correlation appears to be with the degree of functional impairment present before pregnancy.[4, 47] Patients with severe curves (Cobb angle ≥90°) but good cardiopulmonary function tolerate pregnancy well.[48] The incidence of gestational back pain is higher than expected in patients with uncorrected scoliosis, but not in those who have undergone spinal fusion.[46]

Effect of Pregnancy on the Cardiopulmonary Pathophysiology of Scoliosis

The thoracic cage normally expands in circumference during pregnancy as a result of increases in both an-teroposterior and transverse diameters. Little potential exists for further thoracic cage expansion during inspiration. Inspired volumes in the term pregnant woman are largely attributable to diaphragmatic excursion. If the chest cage is fixed by scoliosis, the diaphragm is entirely responsible for all increments in minute ventilation. As the enlarging uterus enters the abdominal cavity in midgestation, diaphragmatic activity is constrained. FRC decreases to 70 (supine) to 80% (upright) of nonpregnant volume by term gestation. Closing capacity (CC) is also reduced. Even greater than anticipated decreases in FRC and CC may be seen in patients with scoliosis, resulting in ventilation/perfusion mismatch and reduced arterial oxygen content.

Minute ventilation increases by 40 to 50% during pregnancy. In the normal parturient, the rise is primarily a result of increased tidal volume (V_T), whereas respiratory rate is relatively unchanged. In the scoliotic patient with restrictive lung disease, such rises in V_T may not be possible, and the increased minute ventilation is achieved via increased respiratory rate. Increased respiratory rate elevates the work of breathing, and respiratory failure may result. The greater demands on the pulmonary system peak by mid-third trimester. Because the uterus continues to grow, however, it may encroach further on the noncompliant thorax and cause deterioration despite the fact that respiratory demand has stabilized. The onset of new respiratory symptoms or the exacerbation of pre-existent symptomatology during the antepartum period is associated with an increased rate of maternal morbidity as well as a requirement for assisted ventilation around the time of delivery.[47] During labor, minute ventilation of the unmedicated parturient increases by a further 75 to 150% in the first stage and by 150 to 300% in the second stage. Oxygen consumption increases above prelabor values by 40% in the first stage and 70% in the second stage. These levels may be either unattainable or unsustainable by the scoliotic parturient with restrictive lung disease, and respiratory failure may result.

In parturients with neuromuscular scoliosis, decreased lung volumes with advancing pregnancy result in increased ventilation/perfusion mismatching, decreased arterial oxygen content, and carbon dioxide retention. These effects may be especially marked during sleep because of a further reduction in lung volumes due to loss of muscle tone during sleep and enhanced cephalad shift of the diaphragm during supine positioning. The upper airway resistance rises during pregnancy because of mucosal hyperemia, increasing secretions, and occasional development of nasal polyps. These changes predispose the patient to snoring and obstructive sleep apnea.[49] Weakness of the muscles that stabilize the upper airway is common in diffuse muscle disorders; and the weakness may increase the incidence, severity, and maternal-fetal impli-

Elevated Pa_{CO_2}
Bilateral diaphragmatic impairment
Extensive intercostal muscle weakness
Vital capacity less than 1.0 l
Cobb angle greater than 100°

cations of the sleep apnea that develops. A stage of dyspnea on exertion as a prelude to more severe incapacity is seen only rarely in neuromuscular scoliosis. Neuromuscular dysfunction has possibly long since rendered such exertion untenable. Risk factors for ventilatory failure during pregnancy have been identified (Table 14–2).[50]

Cardiac output increases to about 40% by the end of the first trimester and peaks at 50% above nonpregnant levels by the third trimester. Cardiac output is augmented by an increase in both heart rate and stroke volume. Pulmonary vascular pressures are unchanged in the normal parturient. In scoliotic parturients who already have increased PVR, it may not be possible to achieve these increased outputs without further increments in vascular pressures placing an intolerable load on the right ventricle, precipitating right heart failure. Death at the time of delivery or in the early postpartum period is common in parturients with pulmonary hypertension.[37]

Outcome of Pregnancy in Scoliotic Parturients

Isolated cases of maternal death during pregnancy and the postpartum period in patients with scoliosis have been reported, although pregnancy is usually well tolerated with few medical or obstetric complications.[47] In the two Reports on Confidential Enquiries into Maternal Deaths in the United Kingdom covering the years 1985 to 1987 and 1988 to 1990, there were two cases of maternal mortality associated with scoliosis, one in each report.[51, 52] Both patients were admitted to the hospital with deteriorating respiratory status. Both underwent cesarean section and died postoperatively. One death was attributed to adult respiratory distress syndrome and multi-organ failure, the other to air embolism. These deaths, viewed in light of the comments regarding the usually benign course of pregnancy in the scoliotic parturient, probably reflect the lack of homogeneity in the population of parturients with scoliosis.

The reproductive experiences of women with scoliosis depend not only on the severity of the curve and the resulting cardiopulmonary sequelae but also on the presence of underlying neuromuscular disorders. Kafer suggested that complications are more likely to occur in the older parturient (>35 years) with severe scoliosis, or in a parturient with scoliosis associated with an underlying neuromuscular disease.[3] Others at risk are primipara who develop fatigue during long labors. Premature labor occurs more commonly in scoliotic parturients and is independent of the severity of the curve.[12, 47, 53]

The incidence of low-birth-weight infants and congenital anomalies is not increased compared with population averages in women with moderate uncorrected or corrected curves.[12] The likelihood of intrauterine fetal compromise rises with the frequency and severity of maternal hypoxic episodes.[50] Malposition at delivery is not common; in patients without cephalopelvic disproportion, vaginal delivery occurs uneventfully. When scoliosis or other underlying disease distorts pelvic anatomy, operative or instrumented deliveries, perineal tears, and uterine prolapses occur with greater frequency, leading to a higher rate of fetal and maternal morbidity.

In the second stage of labor, the diaphragm not only acts as a respiratory muscle but also has a nonrespiratory function. With expulsive efforts, maximal isometric diaphragmatic contractions are often sustained for 10 to 20 seconds. Diaphragmatic fatigue has been demonstrated in laboring women.[54] Although Gandevia noted that the incidence of acute respiratory failure during delivery is virtually zero in healthy parturients, in the patient whose diaphragm is weak due to neuromuscular disease, the potential for respiratory difficulties is increased.[55] Expulsive forces are also decreased and may lead to a prolonged second stage or even failure of a trial of labor.[42]

Cesarean delivery is necessary in a significant proportion of scoliotic parturients. The incidence is likely to be related to the degree of skeletal deformity, resulting maternal compromise, and cephalopelvic disproportion. In patients with severe curves, the rates for cesarean delivery range up to 52%.[4, 48, 56, 57] Cesarean section is technically more difficult in patients with severe curves, especially those with lumbar spinal involvement. This difficulty is due to the acute anteflexion of the uterus in the small abdominal cavity resulting from the approximation of the xiphisternum and the symphysis pubis. The lower uterine segment may be inaccessible, making classic cesarean section necessary.[57] Kopenhager, however, reporting on 25 cesarean sections in women with severe kyphoscoliosis, noted that classic cesarean section was required in only one.[4]

Patients with corrected scoliosis tolerate pregnancy, labor, and delivery well, although some studies have demonstrated an increased incidence of operative delivery compared with that in normal parturients.[27, 58] Others have noted no increased requirement for operative delivery in patients with corrected scoliosis. In Betz and coworkers report of 355 patients with scoliosis and prior posterior fusion, a cesarean section was necessary in only 2.5% of deliveries.[46]

MANAGEMENT ISSUES IN THE SCOLIOTIC PARTURIENT

Antepartum Assessment and Medical Management

Prepregnancy planning in women with scoliosis serves two purposes. It allows for counseling regarding the risk of inheritable disease in offspring when there is a significant genetic component, and it allows for evaluation of the maternal risk in carrying a gestation to term. The majority of patients with scoliosis have mild to moderate idiopathic curves, and the expectation is that they will tolerate pregnancy, labor, and delivery with an incidence of complications comparable to that in the normal population. Maternal morbidity is predominantly due to cardiopulmonary failure and is related to the site (thoracic) of the curvature and degree of cardiopulmonary compromise before pregnancy. Morbidity and mortality increase if the vital capacity is less than 1 to 1.25 l, if $PaCO_2$ is elevated, or if pulmonary hypertension with ventricular compromise is present.[47, 50, 59–61] These are considered indications for terminating the pregnancy. Pregnancy is well tolerated if antenatal lung volumes exceed 50% of those predicted.[44, 47] Scoliosis secondary to a primary neuromuscular disorder may be associated with a higher gestational morbidity than idiopathic scoliosis.[50] Young women with curves that are greater than 25° and those that involve a double curve and are not yet stable should be advised that there is some risk of progression of the curve while proceeding with the pregnancy. Conversely, there is little risk of progression if the curve is less than 20° or has been stable. There is virtually no risk if the curve has been surgically stabilized.[62]

Antepartum maternal assessment focuses on the mother's cardiorespiratory status with attention to both the history and current status; presence of coexistent disease; and type, status, and patient prognosis of associated neuromuscular disorders. If respiratory compromise is evident, a formal respiratory evaluation is carried out. An assessment is made of the respiratory reserve, including both inspiratory and expiratory muscle function, and of the integrity of the airway protective reflexes. Special attention is given to the presence of dyspnea, tachypnea, and exercise tolerance; recent pulmonary function assessments are noted. Further evaluation is then made with respect to the possible benefits of supplemental oxygen therapy, nocturnal continuous positive airway pressure (CPAP) or even assisted (negative-pressure) ventilation. Patients with curves greater than 60° or those with known cardiac disease require formal cardiologic evaluation to assess ventricular size and function as well as pulmonary vascular pressures.

If the mother's cardiopulmonary status is so compromised that her survival is jeopardized with continuation of the pregnancy, a recommendation to terminate the pregnancy may be made. Despite the risk posed to them, many patients choose to continue with pregnancy. The value of a team approach to these high-risk patients cannot be overemphasized. The team includes medical, obstetric perinatology, neonatology, and anesthesiology consultants; the team can be complemented by nursing and social services personnel. The team meets, in whole and in part, at regular intervals to monitor both the condition of the mother and progress of the pregnancy. A plan is generated regarding the management of the pregnancy and delivery. The plan is relayed to the patient and is propagated through the departments involved. Such an approach to management may reduce the incidence of morbidity and mortality even in very high-risk parturients.[59]

Patients with underlying neuromuscular disease or cardiopulmonary dysfunction related to scoliosis represent a particularly high-risk group for antepartum maternal decompensation. Admission to the hospital for the last weeks of the pregnancy enhances the likelihood that maternal decompensation will be recognized early and morbidity or mortality prevented. Oxygen therapy (2–4 l/min by nasal prongs) intermittently during the day and continuously overnight may improve the maternal condition and reduce fetal risk. Chronic hypoxemia and polycythemia combined with the hypercoagulable state induced by pregnancy increase the risk for thromboembolic events.[60] The wearing of antiembolism stockings is recommended. Consideration should also be given to subcutaneous heparin therapy, with full anticoagulation being reserved for the patient with more severe disease. If necessary, heparin may be reversed at onset of labor to allow for neuraxial analgesia.

Obstetric Management

In parturients with little or no cardiopulmonary compromise at the outset of pregnancy, the expectation is for an uneventful pregnancy and delivery. As the pregnancy advances, the cardiopulmonary signs and symptoms of a normal course must be differentiated from true deterioration in function. The obstetrician-perinatologist is in a sensitive position to monitor for untoward maternal responses to the advancing gestation by virtue of the frequency of contact with the woman. If there is concern that the maternal condition is deteriorating, a re-evaluation by the medical consultant is in order to quantify the change and to initiate therapy. Although right-sided heart failure may mimic pre-eclampsia, peripheral edema being common in both, respiratory symptoms are usually profound in cor pulmonale and are uncommon in pre-eclampsia. Maternal decompensation early in the pregnancy confers an ominous prognosis. Decompensation in late pregnancy and during the early postpartum period is common in the patient with borderline cardiopulmonary function. Obstetric intervention before the completion of the gestation is reserved for compelling maternal or fetal indications.

At term, if maternal cardiopulmonary function and pelvic size are adequate and the fetal condition is good, a trial of labor is permitted and should be successful. Cesarean section is reserved for obstetric indications. A higher incidence of operative delivery may occur in patients with spinal fusion for scoliosis, but this has not been a consistently reported finding.[12, 51, 59, 62]

In patients without major lumbosacral deformity, there is little alteration of the pelvic cavity, and malpresentation is not more frequent.[4, 12, 46] In patients in whom the lumbar spinal deformity is prominent, however, malpresentation is common.[57, 63] Pelvic abnormalities are also more common when scoliosis is associated with neuromuscular disorders, which predisposes the fetus to malpresentation (Fig. 14–6).[50] Uterine function is typically normal in scoliosis; labor is not prolonged and spontaneous vaginal delivery is to be anticipated. In patients with severe disease and especially those with gestational decompensation, cesarean section may be indicated because of maternal compromise. Patients with significant pulmonary hypertension should avoid bearing down, and a forceps-assisted vaginal extraction facilitates delivery in these patients. Oxytocin is a systemic vasodilator, and bolus doses should be avoided in parturients with pulmonary hypertension.

Anesthetic Management

Antepartum Assessment

Patients who require antepartum anesthetic consultation include those with significant maternal cardiopulmonary compromise; thoracolumbar scoliosis with a Cobb angle greater than 30°; and spinal instrumentation and fusion for scoliosis. Initial anesthesiology contact should occur early in gestation, not later than the second trimester. The more severe the maternal condition, the earlier first contact is advised. Ongoing evaluation is carried out via the team conferences alluded to earlier. A plan for anesthetic management is formulated well before delivery. The plan is conveyed to the patient and the other team members.

The underlying etiology of the scoliosis as well as the severity and stability of the curve should be elucidated. In patients with scoliosis resulting from neuromuscular disorders, anesthetic considerations specific to those disorders should be reviewed.[64] Radiographic studies done before the pregnancy and operative notes related to surgical procedures on the spine should be assessed in any patient with a significant scoliosis or previous major spinal surgery before consideration is given to regional anesthesia. Reviewing films taken in the past, even before pregnancy, is usually sufficient to determine not only the underlying anatomy but also the residua of previous surgical interventions. The spine should be examined and note made of the surface landmarks and the interspaces least involved in the deformity.

Analgesia for Labor

Modes of analgesia and anesthesia for labor and delivery can be discussed at the antepartum consultation. Patients with uncorrected thoracolumbar scoliosis may be offered epidural anesthesia for labor and delivery, even if the deformity is severe. Placement of the epidural catheter is technically more demanding than usual. An increased incidence of complications should be anticipated. The midline of the epidural space is deviated toward the convexity of the curve, relative to the spinous process palpable at the skin level (Fig. 14–7).[18] The degree of lateral deviation is determined by the severity of the deformity. The needle should enter the selected interspace and be directed toward the convexity of the curve. The experienced clinician can track the resistance of both the interspinous ligament and the ligamentum flavum to maintain a true course into the epidural space. Structural curves of 30° or less and minor functional curves, such as those

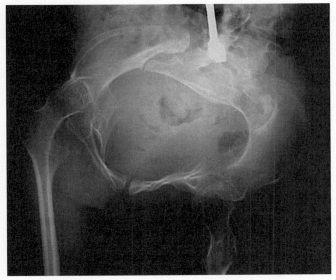

Figure 14–6. Pelvic radiograph. X-ray study of the pelvis in a young woman with a progressive spinal muscular atrophy (Kugelberg-Welander syndrome) demonstrating an inadequate pelvic outlet. She delivered two children by cesarean section under general anesthesia after failed attempts to perform regional anesthesia. Her chest film is detailed in Figure 14–2.

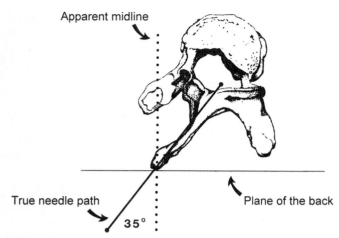

Apparent midline

True needle path

Plane of the back

35°

Figure 14–7. Vertebral displacement and rotation in moderate to severe scoliosis. The vertebral body deviates from the midline and undergoes rotation with the spinous process remaining closer to the true midline (defined as a line drawn from C7 to the sacrum). The interlaminar space is deviated toward the curve convexity. A needle entering the palpated interspinous gap must be directed toward the convexity of the curve to reach the interlaminar gap. The interspinous ligament can be used to determine the angle required. The angle is dependent on the magnitude of the curve.

commonly seen in the term pregnant female, rarely result in much rotatory deviation of the vertebrae. Little accommodation in technique is required for successful needle or catheter placement.

Major spinal surgery in the past is believed by some to represent a relative contraindication to regional anesthesia. This opinion is not shared by me. Regional anesthesia and analgesia may be offered to patients who have experienced previous spinal instrumentations. The incidence of successful block is reduced and complications are more frequent, especially in patients who have had extensive surgeries involving the lumbar spine.[58, 61, 62, 65, 66] Complications include unsuccessful insertions, multiple attempts before successful insertion, false loss of resistance, dural puncture, failed block, or inadequate analgesia. Problems are more frequent in patients with fusions extending to the lower lumbar and lumbosacral interspaces than in those with fusions ending in the upper lumbar spine.[66]

When discussing regional anesthesia with parturients who have previously undergone extensive spinal surgery, consideration should be given to the following:

1. 20% of patients' spines are fused to L4 and L5 levels, leaving few lumbar interspaces uninvolved[58, 67]
2. Reliable surface landmarks are absent following surgery
3. Degenerative changes occur in the spine below the area of fusion at a rate greater than usual, and these changes may increase the likelihood of technical difficulties entering the space or achieving a block[68]
4. Insertion of an epidural needle by either the mid-

line or paramedian approach in the fused area may not be possible because of the presence of instrumentation, scar tissue, and bone graft material[65]
5. A false loss of resistance is common
6. The ligamentum flavum may be injured during surgery, resulting in adhesions in the epidural space or obliteration of the epidural space, which may interfere with spread of local anesthetic injected into the epidural space[69]
7. Obliteration of the epidural space may make accidental dural puncture inevitable
8. It may not be possible to perform an epidural blood patch if a significant postdural puncture headache results
9. Persistent back pain is common in patients with surgically corrected scoliosis (correlates with increasing time since the surgery and extent of fusion)[27, 68]
10. Patients often manifest a high degree of anxiety about their backs and may be reluctant to have a regional block
11. The incidence of malignant hyperthermia may be increased in patients with idiopathic scoliosis or neuromyopathic syndromes that predispose them to scoliosis.[3]

Once the epidural catheter is sited and its position verified, it may be activated with local anesthetic alone or with a local anesthetic-opioid mixture. In parturients with significant cardiovascular compromise, a dilute local anesthetic-opioid mixture (bupivacaine 0.0625%–0.125% with 2–4 µg/ml fentanyl at infusion rates of 8–15 ml/hr) provides excellent first stage and good second stage analgesia with fewer hemodynamic consequences compared with more concentrated local anesthetic solutions.[70, 71] Combined spinal-epidural analgesia is also an option in patients in whom the spinal spaces can be reached. The efficacy and complication profiles of the combined technique are similar to those of epidural analgesia.[72] Intrathecal opioids represent another option for labor analgesia. Although some reports suggest that there is less hemodynamic compromise than with local anesthetics[73–77] others state that the incidence and magnitude of hypotension is similar.[78] Continuous subarachnoid infusions of sufentanil or meperidine for effective labor analgesia has been described in both normal populations and in parturients with severe cardiac disease.[79–81] In the event that the opioid alone provides inadequate pain relief (i.e., perineal pain during second stage), small, hemodynamically innocuous doses of dilute local anesthetic solutions are usually adequate supplements.[79]

The goals in the anesthetic management of parturients with pulmonary hypertension include (1) avoidance of pain, hypertension, hypoxemia, hypercarbia, and acidosis, because these increase PVR; (2) avoidance of myocardial depression because cardiac output will be further decreased; (3) maintenance of intravascular volume and preload; and (4) maintenance of systemic vascular resistance so as to ensure myocardial perfusion and prevent right-to-left shunting. The use of regional block in parturients with pulmonary hypertension is controversial and historically has been avoided.[82] Concerns include reducing venous return with sympatholytic vasodilatation as well as the possibility of creating or augmenting a right-to-left shunt and reducing myocardial perfusion by reducing systemic vascular resistance. Systemic hypotension resulting from regional block may lead to right ventricular ischemia and profound decreases in cardiac output. Because cardiac output may be relatively fixed in patients with pulmonary hypertension, hypotension due to decreased systemic vascular resistance may elicit little effective physiologic compensation and may be difficult to treat pharmacologically.[60] The utilization of small incremental doses of dilute local anesthetic to initiate epidural blockade followed by a continuous infusion, however, should be well tolerated by most parturients.[59]

The introduction of lipid-soluble opioids into the infusing solution reduces both the mass of local anesthetic required and the potential for significant cardiac decompensation with the initiation of regional analgesia. It is a prudent strategy to enhance the safety of regional anesthesia in this subpopulation and is to be highly recommended. Intrathecal administration of lipid-soluble opioids may also be an acceptable strategy to provide labor analgesia in these parturients, although hypotension may result from the administration of intrathecal sufentanil alone.[78]

In patients in whom the lumbar spinal spaces cannot be safely reached, consideration may be given to the performance of a caudal block. Experience with caudal anesthesia is obviously a prerequisite for this option because the potential for harm is considerable.[83] Alternatives to regional block include patient-controlled intravenous analgesia (PCA) with parenteral analgesics (fentanyl, meperidine, nalbuphine) and inhalation of a 50:50 mixture of oxygen and nitrous oxide.[84, 85] If it is concluded at the antepartum assessment that a regional block is not likely to be an option for labor analgesia, referral of the motivated parturient to a trained labor coach for antenatal preparation may be worthwhile. A strategy employing multiple modalities can be designed and implemented and often results in an improved labor experience for the parturient.

Invasive cardiac monitoring is recommended for those patients with significant cardiopulmonary dysfunction. A radial arterial line allows for continuous assessment of maternal blood pressure and serial arterial blood gases. Central venous pressure monitoring is also helpful in parturients with right ventricular dysfunction. Insertion of the central line through the antecubital fossa veins prevents maternal distress resulting from the Trendelenburg position for insertion through the vessels in the neck, particularly in those patients who are experiencing symptomatic cardiopulmonary decompensation. No evidence supports the routine insertion of the pulmonary artery catheter (PAC) in patients with pulmonary hypertension, although current texts in obstetric anesthesia recommend it.[86, 87] The PAC may prove extremely useful in the management of parturients who present in undiagnosed cardiorespiratory distress. PAC may aid in the differentiation of predominant respiratory decompensation from cardiac failure in patients at risk for both. The PAC facilitates intrapartum management, but this is not reflected in improved survival rates.[60, 61] Measurements of baseline cardiac output, right atrial pressure, and PVR may assist in predicting maternal outcome through the intrapartum period. A cardiac output of less than 4 l/min, right atrial pressure greater than 10 mm Hg, and PVR greater than 1000 dynes-sec · cm^{-5}, are all associated with poor maternal outcome.[60]

It may be extremely difficult to pass a catheter into the pulmonary artery in a parturient with pulmonary hypertension due to the dilated right atrium and ventricle, low cardiac output, and tricuspid regurgitation.[36] A special PAC, the Swan-Ganz Guidewire TD Catheter (American Edwards Laboratories, Irvine, CA), facilitates passage in these patients. It has an extra port for the placement of a 0.32-mm guidewire, which serves to stiffen the catheter, preventing both coiling in the dilated chambers and flipping back through the incompetent valve. Tachyarrhythmias, which are commonly precipitated by catheter passage, are likely to be poorly tolerated because cardiac output may decrease significantly. The risk of both pulmonary artery rupture and thrombosis is enhanced when the PAC is used in patients with pulmonary hypertension.[61] Published guidelines regarding PAC support an individual assessment and defend its use when it is determined that the potential benefits are sufficient to overcome the risks associated with PAC in patients with pulmonary hypertension.[88]

Anesthesia for Operative Delivery

Cesarean section may be indicated for maternal or fetal welfare or for obstetric reasons. Parturients with severe scoliosis often are small and frail. During surgery, the rib hump and bony prominences should be padded, with care taken to minimize heat loss. The patient's small size may occasionally necessitate pediatric-sized equipment, such as blood pressure cuffs. Controversy is related to aspects of the anesthetic management of cesarean section in patients with severe scoliosis.[89] Some argue that general anesthesia is preferable because it provides airway and ventilatory control. The alternative is that, unless technical difficulties preclude performance of a regional block or maternal cardiopulmonary decompensation is imminent or present, there is a role for regional anesthesia.[89] A slow incremental extension of an epidural or a subarachnoid block provides ideal conditions for operative delivery and postoperative analgesia. Because local anesthetic dose requirements are variable, an epidural or a subarachnoid catheter is preferable to a single-shot subarachnoid injection. Particular attention should be paid to the dose of local anesthetic because the patient's small size renders usual volumes toxic. In patients with severe curves, there is speculation that subarachnoid hyperbaric local anesthetic solution may pool in dependent portions of the spine, resulting in an inadequate block.[90] Supplementing the block with isobaric formulations of local anesthetic may improve the quality of the block. Supplementation is facilitated with an indwelling subarachnoid catheter, otherwise, it requires multiple dural punctures.

Multiple reports exist about epidural anesthesia in parturients with severe scoliosis, including those with cardiopulmonary compromise and corrective instrumentation. Performance of regional block in these patients is technically demanding and may be complicated by failed or inadequate block. Block quality may be enhanced by supplemental epidural injection of chloroprocaine when dose limits of the other agents have been reached or by subarachnoid injection of small doses of local anesthetic.[91] Reports have been published about extensive spinal blocks associated with profound hemodynamic instability when full-dose subarachnoid injection is made in the setting of pre-existent, albeit inadequate, epidural blockade in parturients.[92–95] If time permits, allowing the epidural block to regress before performing spinal block is recommended.[96] Alternatively, reducing the dose of local anesthetic agent injected into the subarachnoid space by at least 20%, and perhaps as much as 50%, is recommended if partial epidural block is present.[95]

The rate of mortality related to cesarean section in patients with pulmonary hypertension is excessive.[59, 60] The high mortality rate is probably due to the presurgical status of the mother and reflects her poor condition. Few reports exist of survived cesarean delivery with epidural anesthesia in patients with pulmonary hypertension.[61] Prognosis is related to the preoperative maternal condition, with survivors demonstrating good right ventricular function. There is no place for spinal anesthesia for cesarean section in the parturient with significant pulmonary hypertension.

General anesthesia may be indicated because of maternal preference or maternal cardiopulmonary disease or because of technical difficulties related to regional block. A thorough evaluation of the maternal airway is indicated, because a number of conditions associated with scoliosis, including severe scoliosis itself, are associated with difficult laryngoscopy and intubation. Many patients with scoliosis resulting from neuromus-

cular diseases have pre-existing airway obstructions and may have sleep apnea. Because general anesthesia also causes relaxation of the pharyngolaryngeal elements, patients may be at particular risk for airway complications perioperatively.[97] Postoperatively, elements of laryngeal incompetence and impaired swallowing may further decrease the integrity of the airway defense mechanisms.

In normal patients, the FRC falls 18% at induction of anaesthesia, which is attributable to cephalad shift of the diaphragm, ribcage dysfunction or instability, and increased intrathoracic blood volumes.[98–101] Abdominal surgery produces persistent postoperative decreases in FRC that are progressive, becoming evident hours after the end of surgery.[102–106] The decreases in FRC are related to diaphragmatic dysfunction and may persist for up to one week. Atelectasis and ventilation/perfusion abnormalities, which impair gas exchange and result in hypoxemia in normal subjects, may occur. In scoliotic parturients with underlying pulmonary pathology, these effects are augmented and may result in significant postoperative morbidity. Other causes of postoperative hypoxemia that are of particular importance to patients with scoliosis are included in Table 14–3.

Anesthesia, tracheal intubation, and surgery result in mucociliary dysfunction and abnormal or retrograde mucous flow.[107] Reduced competence of the larynx increases the potential for postextubation aspiration in patients already at risk because of both the pregnancy and underlying airway disorders. Coughing and bucking at the end of surgery may transiently and significantly reduce FRC, resulting in further ventilation/perfusion mismatch and hypoxemia.[108] Tracheal extubation after cesarean section in the parturient with gestational hypertension may result in significant increases in both systemic arterial and pulmonary artery pressures.[109] These pressure rises take on added significance in the setting of pre-existing pulmonary hypertension. Criteria for postoperative extubation must include assessment of preoperative respiratory function. An assessment of respiratory muscle strength and ability to support the airway should be made in all patients, but it is particularly important in patients with pre-existing compromise.

Potential hazards of general anesthesia in parturients with pulmonary hypertension include the increased pulmonary artery pressures during laryngoscopy and intubation; adverse effects of positive-pressure ventila-

TABLE 14–3. **FACTORS CONTRIBUTING TO POSTOPERATIVE HYPOXEMIA IN SCOLIOTIC PARTURIENTS**

Increased ventilation/perfusion mismatch
Increased alveolar-to-arterial oxygen gradient
Inhibition of hypoxic pulmonary vasoconstriction
Decreased cardiac output
Underlying pre-existent pulmonary disease
Restriction of chest wall movement

tion on venous return; and negative inotropism of some anesthetic agents. These adverse effects can be largely attenuated by an opioid-supplemented induction and maintenance technique.[61] An obvious potential exists for neonatal respiratory depression with this technique, but the depression is not difficult to manage. Nitrous oxide should be avoided because it increases PVR.[61] The patients should be in an intensive care setting for up to a week following delivery because major cardiopulmonary complications are common during this period.[61]

Management of Acute Maternal Cardiac Decompensation

Parturients with pulmonary hypertension and right ventricular compromise may present in right heart failure and cardiogenic shock during gestation. Mortality attributable to such a presentation is high. Urgent cesarean section is likely to be necessary to achieve maternal and fetal salvage. The immediate goal of therapy in this setting should be to increase cardiac output to maintain systemic blood pressure and prevent right ventricular ischemia.[110] Inotropic support with dopamine may be of value because it improves contractility and increases both cardiac output and blood pressure, while having lesser effects on pulmonary vasoconstriction than adrenaline or noradrenaline.[111] The combination of dopamine and a pulmonary vasodilator may further improve right ventricular function. Although sodium nitroprusside has been provided in this setting, nitroglycerin is also an effective pulmonary vasodilator with fewer effects on the systemic vasculature and on both fetal and uterine activity.[60] If the mother survives the acute event, it is advisable to maintain inotropic support to allow right ventricular afterload and volumes to decrease.[112]

CONCLUSIONS

It should be anticipated that most scoliotic patients will experience pregnancy, labor, and delivery with a similar incidence of complications as the general population. Within the population of scoliotic parturients, however, there is a subpopulation at high risk for morbidity and mortality. These patients are best served by a multidisciplinary team approach. Evidence exists that such an approach results in an improved outcome for both mother and child. Involvement of anesthesiology consultants in these multidisciplinary units is both medically advisable and personally rewarding.

References

1. Goldstein LA, Waugh TR. Classification and terminology of scoliosis. Clin Orthop 1973;93:10.
2. Winter RB. Posterior spinal fusion in scoliosis: Indication, technique and results. Orthop Clin North Am 1979;10:787.
3. Kafer ER. Respiratory and cardiovascular functions in scoliosis and the principles of anesthetic management. Anesthesiology 1980;52:339.
4. Kopenhager T. A review of 50 pregnant patients with kyphoscoliosis. Br J Obstet Gynaecol 1977;84:585.
5. Shands AR, Eisberg HB. The incidence of scoliosis in the state of Delaware J Bone Joint Surg 1955;37A:1243.
6. Bergofsky EH. Respiratory failure in disorders of the thoracic cage. Am Rev Resp Dis 1979;119:643.
7. Chow D. Scoliosis: A surgical perspective. Probl Anesth 1991; 5:40.
8. Winter RB. Adolescent idiopathic scoliosis. N Engl J Med 1986;314:1379.
9. Carter OD, Haynes SG. Prevalence rates for scoliosis in US adults; results from the first National Health and Nutrition Examination Survey. Int J Epidemiol 1987;16:537.
10. Torell G, Nordwall A, Nachemson A. The changing pattern of scoliosis treatment due to screening. J Bone Joint Surg 1981;63A:337.
11. Hung CT, Pelosi M, Langer A, Harrigan JT. Blood gas measurements in the kyphoscoliotic gravida and her fetus: Report of a case. Am J Obstet Gynecol 1975;121:287.
12. Visscher W, Lonstein JE, Hoffman DA, et al. Reproductive outcomes in scoliosis patients. Spine 1988;13:1096.
13. Lonstein JE, Carlson JM. The prediction of curve progression in untreated idiopathic scoliosis during growth. J Bone Joint Surg 1984;66A:1061.
14. Collis DK, Ponseti IV. Long-term follow-up patients with idiopathic scoliosis not treated surgically. J Bone Joint Surg 1969;51A:425.
15. Pehrsson K, Larsson S, Oden A, Nachemson A. Long-term follow-up of patients with untreated scoliosis. A study of mortality, causes of death, and symptoms. Spine 1992;17:1091.
16. Freychuss U, Nilsonne U, Lundgren KD. Idiopathic scoliosis in old age. I. Respiratory function. Acta Med Scand 1968;184:365.
17. Sevastik JA, Aaro S, Normelli H. Scoliosis: Experimental and clinical studies. Clin Orthop 1984;191:27.
18. White AA III, Panjabi MM. Practical biomechanics of scoliosis and kyphosis. In Clinical Biomechanics of the Spine, 2nd ed. Philadelphia, JB Lippincott, 1990, p 127.
19. Harrington PR. Treatment of scoliosis. J Bone Joint Surg 1962;44A:591.
20. Wengner DR, Carollo JJ, Wilkerson JA. Biomechanics of scoliotic correction by segmental spinal instrumentation. Spine 1982;7:260.
21. Gazioglu K, Goldstein LA, Femi-Pearse D, Yu PN. Pulmonary function in idiopathic scoliosis. Comparative evaluation before and after orthopaedic correction. J Bone Joint Surg 1968;50A:1391.
22. Lindh M, Bjure J. Lung volumes in scoliosis before and after correction by the Harrington instrumentation method. Acta Orthop Scand 1975;46:934.
23. Zorab PA, Prime FJ, Harrison A. Lung function in young persons after spine fusion for scoliosis. Spine 1979;4:22.
24. Kumano K, Tsoyoma N. Pulmonary function before and after surgical correction with scoliosis. J Bone Joint Surg 1982; 64A:242.
25. Ogilvie JW, Schendel MJ. Calculated thoracic volume as related to parameters of scoliosis correction. Spine 1988;13:39.
26. Sponseller PD, Cohen MS, Nachemson AL, et al. Results of surgical treatment of adults with idiopathic scoliosis. J Bone Joint Surg 1987;69A:667.
27. Cochran T, Irstam L, Nachemson A. Long term anatomic and functional changes in patients with adolescent idiopathic scoliosis treated by Harrington rod fusion. Spine 1983;8:576.
28. Moskowitz A, Moe JH, Winter RB, Binner H. Long-term followup of scoliosis fusion. J Bone Joint Surg 1980;62A:364.
29. Hamilton PP, Byford LJ. Respiratory pathophysiology in musculoskeletal disorders. Probl Anesth 1991;5:91.
30. Roussos CS, Macklem PT. Diaphragmatic fatigue in man. J Appl Physiol 1977;43:189.
31. Kesten S, Garfinkel SK, Wright T, Rebuck AS. Impaired exercise capacity in adults with moderate scoliosis. Chest 1991;99:663.

32. Mezon BL, West P, Israels J, Kryger M. Sleep breathing abnormalities in scoliosis. Am Rev Respir Dis 1980;122:617.

33. Roth A, Rosenthal A, Hall JE, et al. Scoliosis and congenital heart disease. Clin Orthop 1973;93:95.

34. Hirschfeld SS, Ruder C, Nasch CL, et al. The incidence of mitral valve prolapse in adolescent scoliosis and thoracic hypokyphosis. Pediatrics 1982;70:451.

35. Spinnato JA, Kraynack BJ, Cooper MW. Eisenmenger's syndrome in pregnancy: Epidural anesthesia for elective cesarean section. N Engl J Med 1981;304:1215.

36. Rich S. Primary pulmonary hypertension. Prog Cardiovasc Dis 1998;31:205.

37. Gummerus M, Laasonen H. Eisenmenger complex and pregnancy. Ann Chir Gynaecol 1981;70:339.

38. Kanemoto N. Electrocardiogram in primary pulmonary hypertension. Eur J Cardiol 1980;12:181.

39. Goodman J, Harrison DC, Popp RL. Echocardiographic features of primary pulmonary hypertension. Am J Cardiol 1974;33:438.

40. Sullivan PJ, Miller DR, Wynands JE. Cardiovascular manifestations of musculoskeletal diseases. Probl Anesth 1991;5:107.

41. Zeldis SM. Dyspnea during pregnancy. Distinguishing cardiac from pulmonary causes. Clin Chest Med 1992;13:567.

42. Gilbert R, Auchincloss J. Dyspnea of pregnancy: Clinical and physiological observations. Am J Med Sci 1966;252:270.

43. Robson SC, Hunter S, Moore M, Dunlop W. Serial study of factors influencing changes in cardiac output during human pregnancy. Am J Physiol 1989;256:H1060.

44. Berman AT, Cohen DL, Schwentker EP. The effects of pregnancy on idiopathic scoliosis. A preliminary report on eight cases and a review of the literature. Spine 1982;7:76.

45. Blount WP, Mellencamp DD. The effect of pregnancy on idiopathic scoliosis. J Bone Joint Surg 1980;62A:1083.

46. Betz RR, Bunnell WP, Lambrecht-Mulier E, MacEwan GD. Scoliosis and pregnancy. J Bone Joint Surg 1987;69A:90.

47. Sawicka EH, Spencer GT, Branthwaite MA. Management of respiratory failure complicating pregnancy in severe kyphoscoliosis: A new use for an old technique? Br J Dis Chest 1986;80:191.

48. Siegler D, Zorab PA. Pregnancy in thoracic scoliosis. Br J Dis Chest 1981;75:367.

49. Charbonneau M, Falcone T, Cosio MG, Levy RD. Obstructive sleep apnea during pregnancy: Therapy and implications for fetal health. Am Rev Respir Dis 1991;144:461.

50. Schneerson JM. Pregnancy in neuromuscular and skeletal disorders. Monaldi Arch Chest Dis 1994;49:227.

51. Report on Confidential Enquiries into Maternal Deaths in the United Kingdom 1985–87. London, Her Majesty's Stationery Office, 1991.

52. Report on Confidential Enquiries into Maternal Deaths in the United Kingdom 1988–90. London, Her Majesty's Stationery Office, 1994.

53. Manning CW, Prime FJ, Zorab PA. Pregnancy and scoliosis. Lancet 1967;2:792.

54. Nava S, Zanotti E, Ambrosino N, et al. Evidence of acute diaphragmatic fatigue in a "natural" condition. Am Rev Respir Dis 1992;146:1226.

55. Gandevia SC. Muscle fatigue. Does the diaphragm fatigue during parturition? Lancet 1993;341:347.

56. Jones DH. Kyphoscoliosis complicating pregnancy. Lancet 1964;1:517.

57. Phelan JP, Dainer MJ, Cowherd DW. Pregnancy complicated by thoracolumbar scoliosis. South Med J 1978;71:76.

58. Crosby ET, Halpern SH. Obstetric epidural anaesthesia in patients with Harrington instrumentation. Can J Anaesth 1989;36:693.

59. Smedstead KG, Cramb R, Morison DH. Pulmonary hypertension and pregnancy: A series of eight cases. Can J Anaesth 1994;41:502.

60. Roberts NV, Keast PJ. Pulmonary hypertension and pregnancy—a lethal combination. Anaesth Intensive Care 1990;18:366.

61. Weeks SK, Smith JB. Obstetric anaesthesia in patients with primary pulmonary hypertension. Can J Anaesth 1991;38:814.

62. Daley MD, Morningstar BA, Rolbin SH, et al. Epidural anesthesia for obstetrics after spinal surgery. Reg Anesth 1990;15:280.

63. Chau W, Lee KH. Kyphosis complicating pregnancy. J Obstet Gynaecol Br Commw 1970;77:1098.

64. Bader AM. Neurologic and neuromuscular disease. In Chestnut DH (ed): Obstetric Anesthesia: Principles and Practice. St. Louis, CV Mosby, 1994, p 920.

65. Feldstein G, Ramanathan S. Obstetrical lumbar epidural anesthesia in patients with previous posterior spinal fusion for kyphoscoliosis. Anesth Analg 1985;64:83.

66. Hubbert CH. Epidural anesthesia in patients with spinal fusion. Anesth Analg 1985;64:843.

67. Aaro S, Ohlen G. The effect of Harrington instrumentation on the sagittal mobility of the spine in scoliosis. Spine 1983;8:570.

68. Sponseller PD, Cohen MS, Nachemson AL, et al. Results of surgical treatment of adults with idiopathic scoliosis. J Bone Joint Surg 1987;69A:667.

69. LaRocca H, MacNab I. The laminectomy membrane. Studies in its evolution, effects and prophylaxis in dogs. J Bone Joint Surg 1974;56:545.

70. Chestnut DH, Owen CL, Bates JN, et al. Continuous infusion epidural analgesia during labor: A randomized, double-blind comparison of 0.0625% bupivacaine/0.0002% fentanyl versus 0.125% bupivacaine. Anesthesiology 1988;68:754.

71. Elliott RD. Continuous infusion epidural analgesia for obstetrics: Bupivacaine versus bupivacaine-fentanyl mixture. Can J Anaesth 1991;38:303.

72. Norris MC, Grieco WM, Borkowski M, et al. Complications of labor analgesia: Epidural versus combined spinal epidural techniques. Anesth Analg 1994;79:529.

73. Cohen SE, Cherry SM, Holbrook RH Jr, et al. Intrathecal sufentanil for labor analgesia—sensory changes, side effects and fetal heart rate changes. Anesth Analg 1993;77:1155.

74. Ducey JP, Knape KG, Talbot J, et al. Intrathecal narcotics for labor cause hypotension (abstract). Anesthesiology 1992;77:A997.

75. Camann WR, Mintzer BH, Denney RA, Datta S. Intrathecal sufentanil for labor analgesia: Effects of added epinephrine. Anesthesiology 1993;78:870.

76. Camann WR, Denney RA, Holby ED, Datta S. A comparison of intrathecal, epidural, and intravenous sufentanil for labor analgesia. Anesthesiology 1993;77:884.

77. Honet JE, Arkoosh VA, Norris MC, et al. Comparison among intrathecal fentanyl, meperidine and sufentanil for labor analgesia. Anesth Analg 1991;75:734.

78. D'Angelo R, Anderson MT, Philip J, Eisenach JC. Intrathecal sufentanil compared to epidural bupivacaine for labor analgesia. Anesthesiology 1994;80:1209.

79. Ransom DM, Leicht CH. Continuous spinal analgesia with sufentanil for labor and delivery in a parturient with severe pulmonary stenosis. Anesth Analg 1995;80:418.

80. Leicht CH, Evans DE, Durkan WJ. Intrathecal sufentanil for labor analgesia: Results of a pilot study (abstract). Anesthesiology 1990;73:A980.

81. Johnson MD, Hurley RJ, Gilbertson LI, Datta S. Continuous microcatheter spinal anesthesia with subarachnoid meperidine for labor and delivery. Anesth Analg 1990;70:658.

82. Thornhill MA, Camann WR. Cardiovascular disease. In Chestnut DH (ed): Obstetric Anesthesia: Principles and Practice. St. Louis, CV Mosby, 1994, p 746.

83. Finster M, Poppers PJ, Sinclair JC, et al. Accidental intoxication of the fetus with local anesthetic drug during caudal anesthesia. Am J Obstet Gynecol 1965;92:922.

84. Rayburn W, Leuschen P, Earl R, et al. Intravenous meperidine during labor: A randomized comparison between nursing- and patient-controlled administration. Obstet Gynecol 1989;74:702.

85. Rayburn WF, Smith CV, Leuschen P, et al. Comparison of patient-controlled and nurse-administered analgesia using intravenous fentanyl during labor. Anesth Rev 1991;18:31.

86. Mangano DT. Anesthesia for the pregnant cardiac patient. In Shnider SM, Levinson G (eds): Anesthesia for Obstetrics, 3rd ed. Baltimore, Williams & Wilkins, 1993, p 485.

87. Rocke DA, Rout CC, Orlikowski CEP. Anesthesia and coexisting maternal disease. In Norris MC (ed): Obstetric Anesthesia. Philadelphia, JB Lippincott, 1993, p 451.

88. Practice guidelines for pulmonary artery catheterization. A report by the American Society of Anesthesiologists Task Force on Pulmonary Artery Catheterization. Anesthesiology 1993;78:380.

89. Cheek TG, Banner RN. Orthopedic/neurologic disease. Probl Anesth 1989;3:112.

90. Moran DH, Johnson MD. Continuous spinal anesthesia with combined hyperbaric and isobaric bupivacaine in a patient with scoliosis. Anesth Analg 1990;70:445.

91. Crosby E, Read D. Salvaging inadequate epidural anaesthetics: The chloroprocaine save (letter). Can J Anaesth 1991;38:136.

92. Beck GN, Griffiths AG. Failed extradural anaesthesia for Caesarean section. Complication of subsequent spinal block. Anaesthesia 1992;47:690.

93. Mets B, Broccoli E, Brown AR. Is spinal anesthesia after failed epidural anesthesia contraindicated for Cesarean section? Anesth Analg 1993;77:629.

94. Stone PA, Thorburn J, Lamb KSR. Complications of spinal anaesthesia following extradural block for Caesarean section. Br J Anaesth 1989;62:335.

95. Waters JH, Leivers D, Hullander M. Response to spinal anesthesia after inadequate epidural anesthesia. Anesth Analg 1994;78:1033.

96. Pascoe HF, Jennings GS, Marx GF. Successful spinal anesthesia after inadequate epidural block in a parturient with prior surgical correction of scoliosis. Reg Anesth 1993;18:191.

97. Miller KA, Harkin CP, Bailey PL. Postoperative tracheal extubation. Anesth Analg 1995;80:149.

98. Bergman NA. Distribution of inspired gas during anesthesia and artificial ventilation. J Appl Physiol 1963;18:1085.

99. Brismar B, Hedenstierna GG, Lundquist H, et al. Pulmonary densities during anesthesia with muscular relaxation—a proposal of atelectasis. Anesthesiology 1985;62:422.

100. Muller N, Volgyesi G, Becker L, et al. Diaphragmatic muscle tone. J Appl Physiol 1979;47:279.

101. Westbrook PR, Stubbs SE, Sessler AD, et al. Effects of anesthesia and muscle paralysis on respiratory mechanics in normal man. J Appl Physiol 1973;34:81.

102. Ali J, Weisel RD, Layug AB, et al. Consequences of postoperative alterations in respiratory mechanics. Am J Surg 1974;128:376.

103. Colgan FJ, Whang TB. Anesthesia and atelectasis. Anesthesiology 1968;29:917.

104. Strandberg A, Tokics L, Brismar B, et al. Atelectasis during anaesthesia and in the postoperative period. Acta Anaesthesiol Scand 1986;30:154.

105. Simmoneau G, Vivien A, Sartene R, et al. Diaphragm dysfunction induced by upper abdominal surgery. Am Rev Respir Dis 1983;128:899.

106. Wahba WM, Don HF, Craig DB. Postoperative epidural analgesia: Effects on lung volumes. Can Anaesth Soc J 1975;22:519.

107. Gamsu G, Singer MM, Vincent H, et al. Postoperative impairment of mucous transport in the lung. Am Rev Respir Dis 1976;114:673.

108. Bickler PE, Dueck R, Prutow RJ. Effects of barbiturate anesthesia on functional residual capacity and ribcage/diaphragm contributions to ventilation. Anesthesiology 1987;66:147.

109. Hodgkinson R, Farkhanda J, Hayashi H, Hayashi R. Systemic and pulmonary blood pressure during Caesarean section in parturients with gestational hypertension. Can Anaesth Soc J 1980;27:389.

110. Prewitt RM, Ghigone M. Treatment of right ventricular dysfunction in acute respiratory failure. Crit Care Med 1983;11:346.

111. Holloway EL, Polumbo RA, Harrison DC. Acute circulatory effects of dopamine in patients with pulmonary hypertension. Br Heart J 1975;37:482.

112. Pietkau D, Kettner JD, Slykerman L, et al. Volume versus dopamine to maintain cardiac output as right ventricular afterload increases. Can Anaesth Soc J 1983;30:S69.

First described in 1678, osteogenesis imperfecta comprises a diverse group of genetic disorders of collagen synthesis characterized by bone fragility and fracture propensity.[1-3] Initially referred to as *brittle bone disease*, the severity and clinical presentations are quite varied. At one extreme is a disease incompatible with life, with death occurring either in utero or in the early perinatal period. At another extreme are patients whose disease allows for fairly normal growth and normal fertility. These women can carry a fetus, which may also be affected by osteogenesis imperfecta, to term. Affected women who are pregnant present unique obstetric and anesthetic issues.

DEFINITION

Osteogenesis imperfecta is caused by a mutation in one of the two genes that encode the chains of type 1 collagen, which is the major protein in bone.[1] Expression of the disease is highly variable because the mutations (over 70 have been characterized) occur at different places in the genes. The mutations result in decreased synthesis of collagen, production of defective collagen, or both.[4] Bone fragility is a hallmark of the disease. The frequency of all forms of osteogenesis imperfecta is estimated to be 1 in 5000 to 1 in 10,000 individuals.[1]

CLINICAL CHARACTERISTICS

Osteogenesis imperfecta causes skeletal fragility, with the severity ranging from that resulting in perinatal death to that resulting in only a minimal increase in the incidence of fractures in people who would otherwise be viewed as normal (Table 15–1). All affected patients have osteopenia—bones deficient in mineral and matrix content.[1-3] Fractures occur after minimal or no apparent trauma, and poor healing may lead to limb angulation and asymmetry. Ligamentous laxity is also observed.

CLASSIFICATION

In the past, the disease was classified into two types—*congenita*, referring to the cases resulting in early neonatal death, and *tarda*, referring to those who develop fractures later in life. In 1979, Sillence introduced an expanded classification scheme describing four types of osteogenesis imperfecta, attempting to correlate genetic, morphologic, and biochemical characteristics of affected patients (Table 15–2).[6, 7] This classification is somewhat arbitrary, because varied disease expression results in a continuum of severity and clinical characteristics even within each group. Ongoing studies that correlate genetic with phenotypic information at the molecular level will likely provide the information necessary to further distinguish the variants.

Type I is the common mild form. It results from *abnormally low production* of normal type 1 collagen by fibroblasts,[1] distinguishing it from the other forms. This mechanism explains why patients with type I disease may live essentially normal lives. Although some patients (about 10%) have fractures at birth, most have normal birth weight and length. Bone fragility from osteoporosis is characteristic of type I disease, but bone deformity is not as severe as in other types, and it usually results from fractures or joint laxity rather than from abnormal bone development. Bone fragility may increase with age. Patients with type I disease are the least deformed by osteogenesis imperfecta, and they may become pregnant.

Types II, III, and IV differ from type I in that genetic mutations result in production of *abnormal collagen*. As

TABLE 15–1. **POSSIBLE CLINICAL CHARACTERISTICS OF OSTEOGENESIS IMPERFECTA**

Bone fractures with minimal trauma
Vertebral body collapse—kyphosis and scoliosis
Cervical spine instability from odontoid hypoplasia
Deformed chest cavity
Fragile teeth (dentinogenesis imperfecta)
Blue sclera
Easy bruisability, subcutaneous hemorrhages
Hearing loss

TABLE 15–2. **CLASSIFICATION OF OSTEOGENESIS IMPERFECTA**

Type	Notable Clinical Features
I	Normal stature, mild disease
	Blue sclera
	Conductive hearing loss
	Dentinogenesis imperfecta variable
	Fractures may occur during infancy and childhood
	Normal fertility, pregnancy possible
	Transmitted as an autosomal dominant trait
II	Always lethal in the perinatal period
	Short, deformed limbs; beaded ribs
	Diagnosis by ultrasound
III	Rare, similar to type II, but not as severe
	Severe bone fragility and postnatal growth failure
	Dentinogenesis imperfecta common
IV	Normal sclera
	Moderate bone deformity
	Generalized osteopenia, fractures
	Dentinogenesis imperfecta variable
	Hearing loss variable

From Sillence DO, Senn A, Danks DM. Genetic heterogeneity in osteogenesis imperfecta. J Med Genet 1979;16:101; and Sillence D. Osteogenesis imperfecta: An expanding panorama of variants. Clin Orthop 1981;159:11.

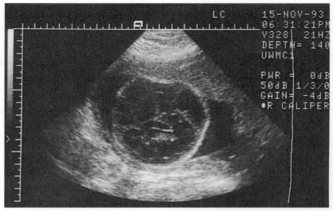

Figure 15–2. Ultrasound image of the head of a fetus with osteogenesis imperfecta type II at 30 weeks' gestational age showing a hypomineralized calvarium, which is easily deformed by the pressure of the ultrasound transducer (coming from the top of the image). (Courtesy of Dr. Edith Cheng, Assistant Professor, Departments of Obstetrics and Gynecology and Medical Genetics, University of Washington.)

such, these forms of the disease are more severe than type I.[4]

Type II (perinatal lethal osteogenesis imperfecta) is incompatible with life. It can be diagnosed with ultrasound as early as about 15 weeks' gestation.[8] Characteristics include extreme bone fragility, short and deformed limbs (Fig. 15–1), minimal calvarial mineralization (Fig. 15–2), and beaded ribs (Fig. 15–3). Death may occur in utero, from abnormalities in development stemming from the bone fragility, or in the early postnatal period, from respiratory failure.

Type III is a rare form of the disease. Because fractures can occur before birth, this form may resemble type II disease. Type III disease generally is less severe than type II and is characterized by severe bone fragil-

ity, progressive bone deformity, and postnatal growth failure. The sclerae may be blue at birth and then lighten to normal. Hearing problems are uncommon. Abnormalities in dentition are common.

Osteogenesis imperfecta *type IV* is probably the most commonly recognized form with a severity intermediate between type I and type III disease. More skeletal deformity is present than in type I disease, with resulting short stature and kyphoscoliosis. Many affected children require intramedullary rods.[3] The sclerae are either normal or grayish. Some patients may have hearing loss. Dentinogenesis imperfecta is common.

TREATMENT

No reliable, successful treatment or cure exists. Drug therapy is aimed at increasing bone density to minimize fractures. Calcitonin (which blocks osteoclastic bone resorption) and sodium fluoride have been tried, but success is difficult to assess given the varied nature of the disease.[1, 2, 5]

Orthopedic management aims to preserve mobility, bone straightness, and bone strength. Standard treatment of fractures employs lightweight casts to maximize mobility. Surgical treatment includes intramedullary rods to straighten bones and support bones with recurrent fractures. Physical therapy is an important part of management, with swimming the safest exercise for these patients.[1, 5]

DIAGNOSIS

The diagnosis is made from clinical information and is considered in patients presenting with osteopenia,

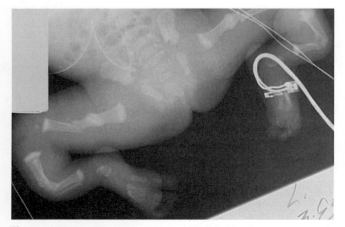

Figure 15–1. Postmortem radiograph of the lower extremities of a term fetus with osteogenesis imperfecta type II or III demonstrating severe bone deformity and evidence of multiple fractures. (Courtesy of Dr. Corinne L. Fligner, Associate Professor, Department of Pathology, University of Washington.)

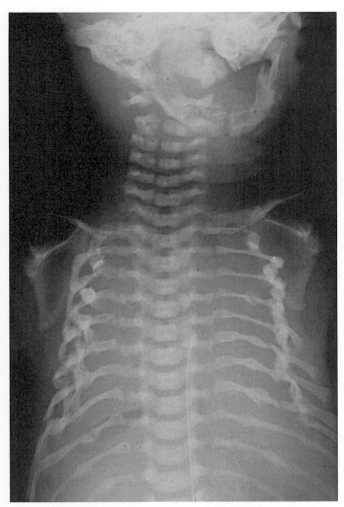

Figure 15–3. Postmortem radiograph of the ribcage of a term fetus with osteogenesis imperfecta type II or III demonstrating multiple rib fractures, which create a "beaded" appearance. (Courtesy of Dr. Corinne L. Fligner, Associate Professor, Department of Pathology, University of Washington.)

short stature, recurrent fractures, and associated symptoms (presenile hearing loss, blue sclerae, dentinogenesis imperfecta). Although mild cases of type I osteogenesis imperfecta remain undetected, advances in prenatal diagnosis of the severe type II and III forms allow the diagnosis to be made early in gestation.

Most cases of type II or III osteogenesis imperfecta are not suspected but are identified on routine ultrasound examinations. Otherwise, the gestation may be carried until there is delivery of a stillborn infant or one that dies soon after birth. Typically, deformed long bones and skull and thoracic abnormalities can be identified by ultrasonography as early as 15 weeks' gestation (see Figs. 15–1 to 15–3). [8, 9]

Munoz and coworkers described three diagnostic criteria for osteogenesis imperfecta with ultrasonography: (1) the femora are more than three standard deviations below the mean length for gestational age; (2) there is marked demineralization of the fetal bones; and (3) there is evidence of multiple fractures. [10] These features

distinguish osteogenesis imperfecta from other short limb skeletal dysplasias (such as thanatophoric dysplasia, achondroplasia, achondrogenesis, hypophosphatasia). Using these criteria, these investigators identified most of the cases in a series of fetuses at risk for the disease. [10] At some centers, if a mother has previously delivered a fetus affected by type II or III osteogenesis imperfecta, a diagnosis can be made by culturing cells from chorionic villus sampling at 10 to 12 weeks. Unlike amniocytes obtained from amniocentesis, these cells produce type 1 collagen, and a defect in the type of collagen produced can be detected. The results are available at about 16 weeks' gestation, allowing the parents the option for pregnancy termination if the fetus is affected.

Transmission of osteogenesis imperfecta type I follows an autosomal dominant pattern. [1] Therefore, a mother with known osteogenesis imperfecta (type I) has a 50% chance of transmitting the disease to her offspring. Ultrasonography can identify prenatal fractures in the fetus (Fig. 15–4). The other types also follow an autosomal dominant pattern of inheritance; however, the recurrence rate of type II (and probably type III) is only about 7% of pregnancies because of gonadal mosaicism. [1]

PARTURIENTS WITH OSTEOGENESIS IMPERFECTA

Women with osteogenesis imperfecta who survive to childbearing age (usually type I) are normally fertile, and the pregnancies can be carried to term. [11] The obstetrician must recognize the diagnosis of osteogenesis

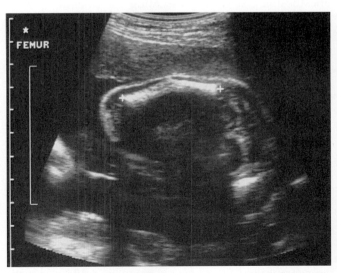

Figure 15–4. Ultrasound image of the femur of a third trimester fetus with osteogenesis type I demonstrating a femur fracture. The diagnosis of osteogenesis type I was suspected in this fetus because the mother gave a history of fractures and had blue sclerae. (Courtesy of Dr. Edith Cheng, Assistant Professor, Departments of Obstetrics and Gynecology and Medical Genetics, University of Washington.)

imperfecta in the pregnant woman and carry out appropriate tests to evaluate the fetus for the presence of the disease. The patients should be referred for anesthetic evaluation early in gestation to allow for suitable preparation.

Delivery mode is influenced by the maternal condition and the status of the fetus. Avoiding labor and vaginal delivery may contribute to an atraumatic delivery in a fetus affected by osteogenesis imperfecta, but this strategy is controversial.[11] The effort and pressure of labor and vaginal delivery may place the mother at risk for fractures. In a review of 15 cases of pregnant women with osteogenesis imperfecta, one of the nine who delivered vaginally suffered fractures of the pubic rami during labor.[12] Previous pelvic fractures and pelvic malformations increase the risk of cephalopelvic disproportion and the need for cesarean delivery. Six of the 15 patients described by Key and Horger underwent cesarean delivery; the indications included cephalopelvic disproportion, fetus with known osteogenesis imperfecta, prior or recent pelvic fracture, and twins.[12]

Delivery mode should be individualized in these women.[13] Carlson and Harlass[11] suggest that the indication for cesarean delivery be no different for these patients than that for healthy patients. The need to assess the maternal pelvic anatomy and the fetus for fractures or deformations and to proceed with cesarean delivery is underscored, if clinical judgment suggests that vaginal delivery increases the risk of either maternal or fetal fractures.

ANESTHETIC CONCERNS

The following issues must be recognized by the anesthesiologist when evaluating the patient with osteogenesis imperfecta: patient fragility, airway abnormality, vertebral column abnormality, bleeding abnormality, and risk of hyperthermia (Table 15–3).[14]

Critical to managing these patients is recognizing the risk of fractures with minimal trauma. The operating room table must be generously padded. Automatic blood pressure cuffs must be avoided; the vigorous inflation (especially with the initial blood pressure measurement) can fracture the humerus.[15] An arterial line for blood pressure monitoring is a reasonable option. Overly vigorous tourniquet application may similarly fracture the bones of the arm. Gentle local pressure and gravity are employed to promote venous distension for intravenous catheter placement or obtaining blood samples. Rough head, neck, and jaw manipulation during laryngoscopy and intubation may cause fractures of the cervical spine, mandible, or teeth. Either gentle laryngoscopy with minimal head, neck, and jaw manipulation or awake fiberoptic intubation is indicated to secure the airway when general anesthesia is administered. It is recommended that the clini-

TABLE 15–3. ANESTHETIC CONCERNS IN THE PARTURIENT WITH OSTEOGENESIS IMPERFECTA

Bone fragility and fractures
  Blood pressure cuff
  Tourniquet for blood draws
  Succinylcholine-induced fasciculations
  Airway positioning for intubation (cervical vertebrae and mandible)
Airway abnormalities
  Large head, large tongue, short neck
  Poor dentition vulnerable to fracture
Kyphoscolioisis
  Restrictive lung disease
  Pre-existing neurologic disease from nerve compression
  Epidural or spinal anesthesia technically difficult
Predisposition to bleeding
  Connective tissue problem
  Platelet dysfunction
Hyperthermia during general anesthesia
  Not malignant hyperthermia per se
  Reflects abnormalities in metabolism
  Responds to cooling measures (skin surface cooling, cold intravenous fluids)

cian avoid succinylcholine-induced fasciculations by using a nondepolarizing muscle relaxant.[14]

A careful airway evaluation is performed because the patient may have a relatively large tongue, short neck, and minimal neck flexion/extension, all of which can complicate laryngoscopy and intubation. Abnormal dentition may complicate osteogenesis imperfecta, resulting in easy fracture of existing teeth during airway manipulation.

Kyphosis and scoliosis resulting from prior vertebral fractures may produce restrictive lung disease from decreased chest wall compliance (Chapter 14). Restrictive lung disease may be aggravated by pectus excavatum. A decreased vital capacity and ventilation/perfusion mismatch can lead to hypoxemia, which, if severe, may progress to cor pulmonale.[16]

Abnormalities of the lumbar spine may contribute to difficulties with regional anesthesia. Although there are reports of successful epidural anesthesia for cesarean delivery, access to the epidural space can be difficult.[17, 18] The paramedian approach to the epidural or subarachnoid space may enhance the success of regional anesthesia in patients with scoliosis. Because prior vertebral fractures may result in nerve compression, a preanesthetic neurologic examination should be performed to document the presence of neurologic deficits. Odontoid hypoplasia has been noted in patients with severe osteogenesis imperfecta, underscoring the need to avoid neck hyperextension during laryngoscopy and intubation.[5]

Some patients with osteogenesis imperfecta report easy bruising. Not only is the etiology of this bruising unclear, but so is the actual risk for bleeding. In a series of patients with osteogenesis imperfecta, about 35% (7/20) of patients had capillary fragility, but more than 90% of patients had a normal bleeding time (an incidence similar to that in the normal population).[19] One proposed mechanism is that abnormal perivascular collagen does not allow normal vessel retraction and constriction after injury. In addition, platelet function studies reveal abnormal aggregation to adenosine phosphate and collagen, and impaired platelet factor 3 release.[20] These abnormalities were found in patients with otherwise normal blood coagulation test results (including platelet count, bleeding time, partial thromboplastin time, and prothrombin time), who did not have clinical evidence of a bleeding tendency. The significance of these abnormalities remains unclear. Furthermore, it is unknown whether there is a relationship between capillary fragility and epidural hematoma formation if blood vessel puncture occurs during epidural catheter placement. It is important to inform the patient with osteogenesis imperfecta and easy bruising of this uncertainty. A coagulogram should be done before anesthesia or surgery in those parturients with a history of easy bruising.

Parturients with osteogenesis imperfecta are also prone to excessive uterine bleeding. In a series reported by Key and Horger, three patients had significant postpartum hemorrhage, one from a uterine rupture, which led to her death, one from retained placenta, and one from a vaginal sulcus tear.[12] Young and Gorstein,[21] in a report of uterine rupture requiring obstetric hysterectomy, suggest that abnormal connective tissue in the uterus may predispose these patients to uterine bleeding. Pathologic examination of the uterus, in their case, revealed decreased collagen content. It is important to recognize the risk of obstetric hemorrhage in such patients. An appropriate approach is to have good intravenous access before delivery and cross-matched blood readily available.

Patients with osteogenesis imperfecta are at risk for developing hyperthermia during general anesthesia. Although malignant hyperthermia has been reported in these patients,[22] the elevated temperature is not currently considered malignant hyperthermia but rather another hypermetabolic state.[23] No muscle rigidity occurs, but there is an increase in oxygen consumption, heart rate, respiratory rate, and cardiac output as well as diaphoresis. A related finding is that up to 50% of patients with osteogenesis imperfecta have elevated serum thyroxine levels.[14] The hyperthermia can usually be controlled with skin surface cooling (Fig. 15–5).[24]

Core temperature must be monitored carefully during surgery, with oxygen administered and skin surface cooling instituted with circulating water or air blankets if core temperature rises. Giving atropine should be avoided because atropine can worsen the hyperthermia by preventing sweating. The problem of hyperthermia may be lessened with regional anesthesia.

Other issues to consider in the patient with osteogenesis imperfecta presenting for surgery are the

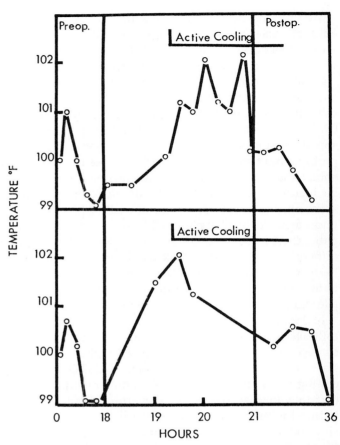

Figure 15–5. Oral temperature measured in a 4-year-old child undergoing orthopedic surgery on two different occasions. Temperature increased from a preoperative level of 99 to 100° F to about 102° F after an hour of anesthesia (oxygen, nitrous oxide, and halothane administered with assisted ventilation) and surgery. Institution of skin surface cooling helped stop the hyperthermia, which resolved after surgery. The hyperthermia was not accompanied by muscle rigidity. (From Solomons CC, Myers DN. Hyperthermia of osteogenesis imperfecta and its relationship to malignant hyperthermia. In Gordon R, Britt B, Kalow W (eds): International Symposium on Malignant Hyperthermia. Springfield, IL, Charles C Thomas, 1973, p 319.)

possible presence of hyperthyroidism, congenital heart disease, and premature arteriosclerosis.

Epidural analgesia is the best option in the patient with osteogenesis imperfecta who presents for vaginal delivery. I suggest placing an epidural catheter relatively early in labor, because placement may be technically difficult owing to abnormal anatomy. Other principles of regional analgesia for labor are similar to those for healthy parturients.

Choosing anesthesia for cesarean delivery in a patient with osteogenesis imperfecta depends upon the degree of urgency and the relevant problems of each patient. Because there are risks associated with both regional anesthesia (block placement difficulty resulting from spine abnormalities) and general anesthesia (airway difficulties) in these parturients, the obstetrician must be aware that rapid induction of any form of anesthesia is unsafe. The scenario of a "crash" cesarean delivery should be avoided.

Two reports describe in detail the successful use of epidural anesthesia for cesarean section in patients with osteogenesis imperfecta.[17, 18] In one, identification of the epidural space was accomplished utilizing the "lateral approach."[18] The response to epidural local anesthetics was variable with 31 ml of 3% 2-chloroprocaine used in one,[18] whereas in the other, only 12 ml of 0.5% bupivacaine was required.[17] No reports exist of spinal anesthesia in parturients with osteogenesis imperfecta, but osteogenesis imperfecta does not preclude spinal anesthesia. In fact, the subarachnoid space may be identified with more certainty than the epidural space in patients with kyphoscoliosis. The relatively unpredictable block height with spinal anesthesia in patients with short stature and the potential for airway difficulties if a total spinal occurred, however, leads me to favor epidural anesthesia over spinal anesthesia, if technically feasible. Continuous spinal anesthesia, allowing titration of anesthetic level, is another option.

In 1992, Cho and coworkers described general anesthesia for cesarean delivery in a parturient with osteogenesis imperfecta who refused regional anesthesia.[25] The investigators described padding the operating room table and using a manual blood pressure cuff to minimize trauma to the arm. Anesthesia was induced with thiopental and vecuronium to avoid succinylcholine-induced fasciculations. Neck manipulation was minimized while the airway was secured with direct laryngoscopy. The patient's esophageal temperature increased to 38.7° C during the case but returned to normal after administration of cool intravenous fluids and skin surface cooling with a circulating water mattress. The patient tolerated the anesthetic and surgery well.

CONCLUSIONS

Osteogenesis imperfecta presents unique obstetric and anesthetic challenges. A viable fetus with type I or IV disease may be delivered vaginally or by cesarean section, depending upon the perceived risk of fetal injury during vaginal delivery. In the parturient with osteogenesis imperfecta (usually type I), the risks of bone fragility, vertebral anatomy abnormality, and airway difficulty must be considered. Regional anesthesia for labor and vaginal delivery or cesarean delivery is the best option, but it may prove technically difficult. The risks of obstetric hemorrhage and hyperthermia are additional considerations.

References

1. Byers PH, Steiner RD. Osteogenesis imperfecta. Annu Rev Med 1992;43:269.
2. Gertner JM, Root L. Osteogenesis imperfecta. Orthop Clin North Am 1990;21:151.
3. Cole WG. Etiology and pathogenesis of heritable connective tissue diseases. J Pediatr Orthop 1993;13:392.
4. Byers PH, Wallis GA, Willing MC. Osteogenesis imperfecta: Translation of mutation to phenotype. J Med Genet 1991;28:433.
5. Marini JC. Osteogenesis imperfecta: Comprehensive management. Adv Pediatr 1988;35:391.
6. Sillence DO, Senn A, Danks DM. Genetic heterogeneity in osteogenesis imperfecta. J Med Genet 1979;16:101.
7. Sillence D. Osteogenesis imperfecta: An expanding panorama of variants. Clin Orthop 1981;159:11.
8. Constantine G, McCormack J, McHugo J, et al. Prenatal diagnosis of severe osteogenesis imperfecta. Prenat Diagn 1991;11:103.
9. Thompson EM. Non-invasive prenatal diagnosis of osteogenesis imperfecta. Am J Med Genet 1993;45:201.
10. Munoz C, Filly RA, Golbus MS. Osteogenesis imperfecta type II: Prenatal sonographic diagnosis. Radiology 1990;174:181.
11. Carlson JW, Harlass FE. Management of osteogenesis imperfecta in pregnancy. J Reprod Med 1993;38:228.
12. Key TC, Horger EO. Osteogenesis imperfecta as a complication of pregnancy. Obstet Gynecol 1978;51:67.
13. Kuller J, Bellantoni J, Dorst J, et al. Obstetric management of a fetus with nonlethal osteogenesis imperfecta. Obstet Gynecol 1988;72:477.
14. Libman RH. Anesthetic considerations for the patient with osteogenesis imperfecta. Clin Orthop 1981;159:123.
15. Oliverio RM. Anesthetic management of intramedullary nailing in osteogenesis imperfecta: Report of a case. Anesth Analg 1973;52:232.
16. Falvo KA, Klain DB, Krauss AN, et al. Pulmonary function studies in osteogenesis imperfecta. Am Rev Resp Dis 1973;108:1258.
17. Cunningham AJ, Donnelly M, Comerford J. Osteogenesis imperfecta: Anesthetic management of a patient for cesarean section: A case report. Anesthesiology 1984;61:91.
18. Bullard JR, Alpert CC, James WF. Anesthetic management of a patient with osteogenesis imperfecta undergoing cesarean section. J S Carolina Med Assoc 1977;73:417.
19. Evensen SA, Myhre L, Stormorken H. Haemostatic studies in osteogenesis imperfecta. Scand J Haematol 1984;33:177.
20. Hathaway WE, Solomons CC, Ott JE. Platelet function and pyrophosphates in osteogenesis imperfecta. Blood 1972;39:500.
21. Young BK, Gorstein F. Maternal osteogenesis imperfecta. Obstet Gynecol 1968;31:461.
22. Rampton AJ, Kelly DA, Shanahan EC, et al. Occurrence of malignant hyperpyrexia in a patient with osteogenesis imperfecta. Br J Anaesth 1984;56:1443.
23. Weglinski MR, Wedel DJ. Differential diagnosis of hyperthermia during anesthesia and clinical import. In Levitt, RC (ed): Anesthesiology Clinics of North America, vol 12. Philadelphia, WB Saunders, 1994, p 475.
24. Solomons CC, Myers DN. Hyperthermia of osteogenesis imperfecta and its relationship to malignant hyperthermia. In Gordon RA, Britt BA, Kalow W (eds): International Symposium on Malignant Hyperthermia. Springfield, IL, Charles C Thomas, 1973, p 319.
25. Cho E, Dayan SS, Marx GF. Anaesthesia in a parturient with osteogenesis imperfecta. Br J Anaesth 1992;68:422.

Acknowledgment

The helpful comments provided by Dr. Edith Cheng, Assistant Professor, Departments of Obstetrics and Gynecology and Medical Genetics, University of Washington, are appreciated.

INTRACRANIAL AND SPINAL CORD LESIONS

■ ■ ■ ■ ■ ■ ■

Mark D. Johnson, M.D., and Frank G. Zavisca, M.D.

Primary and secondary tumors, mass lesions, cerebral trauma and strokes can all occur in the parturient. A stroke is defined as a syndrome of acute neurologic injury following rupture or occlusion of vessels in the central nervous system (CNS). Cerebral vessels can rupture from trauma or inherent weakness. Cerebral vessels can be occluded from within by thrombosis or embolism and can be occluded by a mass lesion.[1-9] The incidence of maternal stroke resulting from bleeding cerebral aneurysm is present in 1 in 6000 to 1 in 30,000 pregnancies, with a 20% mortality and a 50% incidence of permanent neurologic sequelae (Table 16–1).[3, 5] A report indicates that the risk of stroke from cerebral infarction and intracerebral hemorrhage is increased in the 6 weeks after delivery but not during pregnancy.[10]

Few centers have extensive experience treating these disorders, and thus management is based on isolated case reports, basic principles, and common sense. This chapter describes special diagnostic techniques, preoperative care, and surgical and obstetric management. Anesthetic management for neurosurgery, and for labor and delivery, are detailed at the end of the chapter. Specific anesthetic concerns pertinent to each lesion are mentioned in that section. Issues important to the care of the parturient with a CNS disorder include

- The pathophysiology of the lesion
- The impact of pregnancy on the lesion
- The developmental status of the fetus
- The impact of medical management, monitoring, and surgery on the fetus
- The susceptibility to aortocaval compression and gastric aspiration during pregnancy
- The potential for aortocaval compression from lead shielding during diagnostic radiologic procedures
- The maternal versus fetal priority with respect to surgical plan, timing, and route of delivery
- The communication and coordination among the patient, her family, and the medical team (neurologist, neurosurgeon, obstetrician, anesthesiologist, medical consultants, and nurses).

DIAGNOSIS AND SPECIAL TECHNIQUES

A number of intracranial conditions can produce similar symptoms and signs in the parturient (Table 16–2).[1, 3, 4, 6–12] *A high index of suspicion for unusual conditions is important*, because aggressive treatment greatly affects outcome.

In a 1995 case report,[12a] the importance of a reasonable level of clinical suspicion in parturients with symptomatology indicative of raised intracranial pressure was emphasized. These workers described the administration of epidural analgesia to a parturient with an overlooked, large, cerebropontine angle tumor and obstructive hydrocephalus. The epidural administration was associated with a clear exacerbation of CNS symptoms, which in this case were dizziness, paresthesia in both hands, and transient rigid immobility.

A multidisciplinary team approach in a specialized center is critical to ensure that the management of the mother and fetus is planned in a cohesive, structured manner. Clinical symptoms and signs of neurologic disease in pregnancy lead to the performance of more specialized investigations to make or confirm a diagnosis.

Special Diagnostic Tests

A number of special imaging techniques are used for neurologic diagnosis[2, 11, 12] to differentiate the most

TABLE 16–1. TYPES OF STROKES DURING PREGNANCY OR PUERPERIUM*

Hemorrhagic Strokes (6)		Ischemic Strokes (9)	
Saccular aneurysm	1	Arterial thrombosis	2
Arteriovenous malformation	1	Arterial embolism	3
Hypertensive	3	Venous thrombosis	2
Unknown	1	Vasculitis	1
		Moyamoya disease	1

*In 15 women at Parkland Memorial Hospital, Dallas, TX, 1984 to 1990[3]

TABLE 16–2. **SYMPTOMS AND SIGNS RESULTING FROM INTRACRANIAL LESIONS**

Symptoms	Signs
Headaches (if mild may be a warning leak from aneurysm)	Signs of increased intracranial pressure (e.g., hypertension and bradycardia)
Nausea, vomiting	Nuchal rigidity
Blurred vision or diplopia	Altered consciousness
Photophobia	Seizures
Orbital pain	Focal neurologic signs
Loss of vision	Ataxia
Dizziness	Bruits
Respiratory distress	Proteinuria
Epigastric pain	Disseminated intravascular coagulation
Mental changes	

common cause of pregnancy-related neurologic dysfunction, which is eclampsia, from less common, surgically treatable conditions. These techniques include magnetic resonance imaging (MRI) and those that require shielding of the fetus, such as computed tomography (CT) and angiography.

Immobility is required for imaging. Although anesthesia is seldom needed, it may be requested for uncooperative or unstable patients. Technical problems can occur, such as difficulty in positioning the pregnant patient in the scanning apparatus, shielding of the patient and anesthesiologist, and remote access to the patient.

MRI does not emit ionizing radiation, rather it uses powerful magnets to alter temporarily the energy state of hydrogen protons in water. This information is analyzed by computer to create detailed images useful for neurologic diagnosis. Special anesthetic equipment resistant to the intense magnetic field of MRI is needed because the circuit boards of anesthesia machines and monitors may be affected. The magnetic field can also produce hazardous movement of metal clips used for prior surgery. The use of ferromagnetic clips may constitute a contraindication for MRI. Most vascular clips are now made of titanium, which is not ferromagnetic, and thus these are compatible with MRI. MRI is thought to be safe for the fetus, after limited experience with its use in pregnancy.[13]

CT scanning emits ionizing radiation in multiple planes with computer analysis producing images. The images are not as detailed as those from MRI, but CT scanning is more readily available and less expensive.

Angiography utilizes sequential x-rays following injection of contrast media into a blood vessel to obtain a definitive image of lesions. It is invasive and can alter neurologic function, and thus it is performed ideally in an awake patient. Complications that can occur include vessel occlusion from subintimal vascular dissection of dye or hematoma formation and problems directly related to contrast media. Hyperosmolar contrast media can irritate cerebral vessels and produce arterial necrosis, cerebral embolism, sepsis, and temporary va-

sodilatation with intense pain. These complications are treated with steroids, low-molecular-weight dextran, and vasopressors. Hyperosmolar solutions produce an osmotic diuresis, which can lead to dehydration, reduced fetal perfusion, and fluid shifts in the fetal brain.[12, 14] Hypocarbia is used to constrict cerebral vessels, slowing the cerebral circulation and resulting in a greater concentration of dye in the vessels and greater clarity of the angiograms. This brief period of hypocarbia is probably safe for the fetus. Spinal myelograms can produce headache, confusion, and coma from the irritative effects of hyperosmolar dyes and from cerebrospinal fluid leak following lumbar puncture. The small volume of dye needed for a myelogram is unlikely to produce significant osmotic effects in the fetus.

Allergic reactions occur in 2 to 5% of patients undergoing angiography or myelography. In patients with a history of allergy to contrast media, prophylaxis with steroids and antihistamines should be considered. To treat mild allergic reactions, diphenhydramine in 25- to 50-mg doses, has little effect on the fetus. If anaphylaxis occurs, epinephrine, fluids, and cardiopulmonary resuscitation (CPR) may be needed. Hypotension resulting from anaphylaxis can decrease uteroplacental perfusion. Modern contrast media, with a lower ionic content, produce fewer complications.

LESIONS OF THE CNS

The following conditions are discussed: Intracranial hemorrhage, spinal cord hematoma, head trauma, cerebral and spinal cord ischemia, brain tumor, benign intracranial hypertension, hydrocephalus, and CNS infection.

Intracranial Hemorrhage

The pathophysiologic effects of intracranial hemorrhage result from a compressive mass effect and irritative effects of blood and the breakdown products of blood and clots in the CNS. Because the skull is a fixed vault and most intracerebral structures are relatively noncompressible, even a small hemorrhage can result in significant anatomic distortion producing large increases in intracranial pressure (ICP) and reduction in cerebral perfusion. Intracranial hemorrhage has an incidence of 1 to 5 per 10,000 pregnancies and can be categorized as follows:

1. *Subarachnoid hemorrhage* (SAH), which results from bleeding into the subarachnoid space, usually from lesions near the surface of the brain
2. *Intracerebral hemorrhage* (ICH), which results from bleeding into the brain parenchyma. Bleeding can also occur into both areas, regardless of the etiology of the hemorrhage.[2]

Subarachnoid Hemorrhage

Epidemiology and Pathophysiology

Subarachnoid hemorrhage is associated with saccular aneurysms or arteriovenous malformations (AVMs) and occurs in 0.01 to 0.05% of pregnancies.[2, 5, 6, 11, 12, 14–19] In a clinical series of subarachnoid hemorrhage in parturients, 77% resulted from intracranial saccular (Berry) aneurysms and 23% from AVMs. Mortality ranged from 40 to 50%.[5]

Intracranial aneurysms result from a weakening of the internal elastic lamina of large arteries at the base of the brain, usually at a bifurcation. As an aneurysm develops, it often forms a neck with a dome. The vessel wall thins at the site of rupture (most often the dome), and rupture occurs into the subarachnoid space of the basal cisterns, the subdural space, or directly into the underlying brain parenchyma. Aneurysms can leak spontaneously. Precipitating factors for rupture include bleeding disorders, hypertension, and cocaine abuse.[20]

Arteriovenous malformations consist of abnormal, thin-walled communications between the arterial and venous system that can occur in most parts of the brain and spinal cord.[21] A large malformation can produce an arteriovenous shunt sufficient to raise the cardiac output. The vessels are thin and prone to rupture.

Clinical Presentation and Diagnosis

Unruptured aneurysms are usually asymptomatic. Large aneurysms can produce symptoms (including headache and focal neurologic signs) depending on where they are located. A small hemorrhage may produce a severe headache resulting from the irritating effect of blood in the subarachnoid space.[22] Periorbital pain, nausea, and vomiting can occur. Throbbing headache, seizures, and hemorrhage into the brain parenchyma are more characteristic of an AVM. When a major hemorrhage occurs, the following symptoms can ensue:

- Intracranial pressure (ICP) approaches mean arterial pressure, decreasing cerebral perfusion and resulting in a transient loss of consciousness.
- An excruciating headache occurs either before loss of consciousness or upon awakening.
- Bleeding into the underlying brain can produce a localized mass effect.
- Rarely, acute vascular spasm leads to additional focal neurologic signs with stupor, but impaired autoregulation is unlikely.
- The electrocardiogram (ECG) often shows ST and T wave changes similar to those seen following myocardial ischemia, along with a prolonged QRS complex, increased QT interval, and prominent peaked or inverted T waves. The cause of these ECG changes has been debated, but there is evidence that structural myocardial lesions may occur, possibly as a consequence of intense sympathetic activity.[2, 17] These lesions are usually not associated with an elevated creatine phosphokinase (CPK) level. The ECG changes generally do not correlate with the extent of cardiac injury. The grade of SAH may correlate with wall motion abnormalities on echocardiography.

The following complications can result:

- Rebleeding occurs in 10 to 30% of patients in the first 3 weeks following aneurysm rupture, with a mortality of 50 to 60% with each rebleeding episode. Thereafter, the rebleeding rate is 3% per year (less with an AVM).
- Vasospasm occurs in 35% of patients 4 to 11 days following SAH, leading to further neurologic deterioration. Vasospasm may result from irritation by the breakdown products of clot.
- Hydrocephalus occurs in 15 to 20% of patients following aneurysmal SAH, which is the result of blood and cellular exudate blocking efflux of cerebrospinal fluid (CSF). This obstruction is manifested by a gradual decrease in the level of consciousness.
- Cerebral edema may result from irritation of the brain around a subarachnoid clot or from an intracerebral hematoma.
- Hyponatremia can be seen with the syndrome of inappropriate antidiuretic hormone (SIADH).

Subarachnoid hemorrhage is life-threatening, and surgery can be lifesaving; therefore, a CT scan, MRI, and possibly lumbar puncture should be carried out promptly. Angiography is performed to define the lesion for surgical intervention.

Neurosurgical Management

Controversy has existed over the optimal time to operate on parturients suffering from subarachnoid hemorrhage.[1, 5, 11, 12] Early operation to clip an aneurysm reduces the incidence of vasospasm and rebleeding. The patient's condition may be unstable (worsening neurologic status, poorly controlled hypertension), however, and surgery itself may induce vasospasm. One report indicated that surgical management of aneurysms, but not arteriovenous malformations, was associated with lower maternal and fetal mortality,[5] but another report stated that surgical management of both lesions resulted in better outcomes.[23] Current practice favors early clipping of aneurysms to prevent rebleeding, to maintain normotension and normovolemia, and to improve treatment of vasospasm.[17–19] Therefore, the decision to operate is based primarily on neurosurgical considerations.

Effect of Pregnancy and Obstetric Management

In the past it was thought that aneurysms, but not AVMs, had an increased tendency to bleed with advancing gestational age.[22] A further report, however, indicates that both aneurysms and AVMs bleed more frequently with advancing gestational age, which is thought to be due to progressively greater hemodynamic and hormonal changes.[5] This report does not explain the rarity of intracranial hemorrhage during labor and delivery, when hemodynamic changes are maximal. Another report found that hemorrhage resulting from AVMs does not occur in clusters during any particular trimester, but that the incidence in subsequent pregnancies is increased.[21] Further evidence suggests that the incidence and mortality from intracranial hemorrhage in parturients are similar to the general population.[5, 21]

If an aneurysm has been clipped, there is no increased risk to allowing vaginal delivery.[24] If the aneurysm is untreated, the risk of intrapartum rebleeding is greatest if the initial bleeding occurred during the third trimester. An uncorrected AVM is more likely to bleed during labor and delivery than an aneurysm. In both cases, some clinicians recommend elective cesarean delivery at 38 weeks' gestation,[23–25] but others have observed no advantage from operative delivery.[5] With unclipped and previously ruptured aneurysms, we recommend operative delivery.

A combined cesarean section-neurosurgical procedure can be undertaken when indicated.[1, 12, 26–29] If urgent, the neurosurgical procedure is carried out before delivery.[30–32] In patients with obstetric reasons for expeditious delivery, the neurosurgical procedure may be performed at a time remote from delivery.

Anesthetic Management

Aneurysm clipping may be delayed in patients whose condition is unstable.[17, 33] An important preoperative and intraoperative goal is to minimize transmural pressure (mean arterial pressure − intracranial pressure) across the aneurysm wall, to minimize the risk of rebleeding. In the past, minimizing transmural pressure was achieved by sedation, dehydration, and hypotension. Hypovolemia and hypotension in the presence of vasospasm may result in reduced cerebral blood flow and thereby increased ischemia.[33, 34] Although induced hypotension has been used successfully during pregnancy,[30–32] reports have described improved success with normotension before clipping.[17, 33, 34] Specific therapy for cardiac dysrhythmias, neurogenic pulmonary edema, and elevated ICP may require treatment perioperatively.

After surgery, early awakening is desirable in some cases to allow a timely neurologic examination. Urgent CT scan and/or angiography is sometimes needed to rule out intracranial hematoma or vascular injury when acute neurologic defects are found upon the patient's awakening.

General anesthetic considerations for cesarean section are the same as those for neurosurgical procedures. Epidural anesthesia has been given for cesarean section[35, 36] and for vaginal delivery[37–39] in patients with a medically managed intracranial aneurysm. A report described the use of either epidural or general anesthesia for cesarean section in three women with AVMs.[40]

Intracerebral Hemorrhage

Epidemiology and Pathophysiology

Hemorrhage into the brain parenchyma of pregnant patients is often the result of hypertensive disorders.[6, 12, 41] Pregnancy-induced hypertension occurs in 5% of this population and may lead to cerebral hemorrhagic complications. One report described three women with strokes of hypertensive etiology in 90,000 patients studied. Two of these patients had underlying chronic hypertension, and all three patients had residual neurologic deficits.[3] The incidence due to less common etiologies is unknown.

Severe pre-eclampsia causes arterial vasospasm and multifocal petechial hemorrhages; it may be accompanied by SAH.[42] Fibrinoid necrosis of small penetrating arteries has been described following eclampsia and chronic hypertension. Hypertensive ICH typically occurs in the basal ganglia, thalamus, cerebellum, or pons. Intracerebral hemorrhage can also accompany SAH caused by aneurysms or AVMs. Primary ischemic strokes may be associated with hemorrhagic transformation. As with SAH, the risk of ICH in pregnancy is increased with metastatic choriocarcinoma, moyamoya disease, Kaposi's sarcoma, occult carotid-cavernous fistula, bleeding diatheses, and cocaine abuse.[6]

Clinical Presentation and Diagnosis

Pregnant patients with ICH present with an abrupt onset of a neurologic deficit referable to the site of the hemorrhage, commonly accompanied by headache, nausea, and vomiting. In addition to clinical observation and laboratory studies to rule out bleeding disorders, noncontrast CT scan is the most sensitive test to diagnose acute ICH. Contrast CT scan, MRI scan, or angiography may be needed to exclude a structural etiology. It is important to differentiate ICH from SAH, because treatment differs greatly.

Neurosurgical Management

Intracerebral hemorrhage is often not amenable to surgical correction, and it carries a poor prognosis. Treatment is supportive, with control of blood pressure (BP) and ICP. Surgery is reserved for life-threatening elevations of ICP, brainstem herniation, and evacuation of an expanding hematoma that is well defined.

Effect of Pregnancy and Obstetric Management

Pre-eclampsia can elevate ICP. In addition, the cardiovascular effects of labor and delivery can significantly elevate BP, increasing the risk of ICH. Circulating estrogens may dilate abnormal blood vessels, increasing the risk of rupture.

Cesarean section offers no advantage over modified vaginal delivery in limiting hemodynamic stress. Obstetric considerations should determine the mode of delivery. For pre-eclampsia, early delivery may be needed. If a hematoma is present, surgical evacuation may be required early in pregnancy (e.g., ICH resulting from chronic hypertension) with delivery at a later date.

Anesthetic Management

Blood pressure and ICP must be controlled before surgery. The hypertensive or eclamptic patient is particularly difficult to manage in this regard because she has a low intravascular volume, which predisposes her to severe hypotension and decreased fetal perfusion following anesthetic induction.[12] In these cases, optimal fluid replacement is guided by the use of central venous pressure (CVP) and Swan-Ganz catheters (Table 16–3).

In patients with subarachnoid hemorrhage, the ICP is usually not elevated, unless there is an intracranial hematoma. Even in these patients, the ICP usually has normalized by the time they are brought to the operating room. It is imperative that the ICP not be lowered until the dura is opened. By decreasing the ICP, the transmural pressure gradient across the aneurysm can be increased, which heightens the risk of rupture. Diuretics such an mannitol and furosemide (Lasix) may be administered intraoperatively to reduce brain bulk within the skull and facilitate surface exposure. The osmotic effects of mannitol may precipitate cerebral

TABLE 16–3. MANAGEMENT OF ANEURYSMAL CLIPPING: ANESTHETIC GOALS

Prevent hypertension
Maintain normal mean arterial pressure
Maintain normal intracranial pressure*
Maintain normocarbia†
Maintain normal O₂ saturation
Maintain appropriate analgesia, muscle relaxation, amnesia
Monitor intravascular volume status
Mild hypothermia (34–35° C) may be considered to reduce metabolic rate—brain protection (prevent shivering with muscle relaxation)
Head elevation
Left uterine displacement to minimize aortocaval compression

*ICP must not be lowered until the dura is opened to minimize changes in the transmural pressure gradient across the aneurysm
† Hypocarbia potentially reduces placental perfusion

bleeding in the fetus and should be given with caution before delivery.

Mild hypothermia affords some degree of brain protection, but controlled studies regarding the use of hypothermia in patients undergoing cerebral aneurysmal clipping have not been performed to date.

Although global cerebral blood flow tends to be on the lower side of normal in SAH patients, there may be regions of the brain that are susceptible to ischemia primarily because of reduced perfusion in these regions. Maintenance of normal BP is therefore absolutely essential. More and more, the data indicate that controlled hypotension may be detrimental in that it can reduce flow to regions of the brain that are already ischemic.

The value of intravenous antioxidant-free radical scavenger agents, such as barbiturates, calcium channel blockers, lidocaine, and mannitol, has not been established. Steroids may be useful to reduce swelling and inflammatory responses.

Regional anesthesia is generally preferred for hypertensive patients. It avoids the hypertensive response to intubation and reduces the risk of vomiting and aspiration. If general anesthesia is chosen, BP is controlled with labetalol or a titratable drug, such as sodium nitroprusside, using an indwelling arterial line to assess the response to therapy on a beat-to-beat basis.

Postoperatively, the patient is observed for potential pulmonary complications resulting from excess fluid loading. After delivery, administration of a diuretic may minimize this risk. Pre-eclamptic patients are observed for postpartum convulsions; they are managed with magnesium sulfate and/or benzodiazepine therapy.

Spinal Hematoma

Bleeding into the spinal area can occur spontaneously, or rarely an iatrogenic lesion can occur following regional anesthesia.[43–48] Painful, progressive paraplegia results. The only effective treatment is emergency decompression.[48] Spontaneous partial recovery occurs rarely.[49, 50] Symptoms and signs of a spinal hematoma must be differentiated from the pain and motor dysfunction associated with prolapsed intervertebral disc and other neurologic complications of pregnancy.[51]

The physiologic changes of pregnancy can exacerbate a maternal spinal disc problem—spondylolisthesis resulting in nerve root compression and sciatica. Spondylolisthesis is thought to be a consequence of hormonal changes, increased weight, and altered posture. Other peripheral nerve entrapment syndromes such as facial nerve palsy and carpal tunnel syndrome increase in frequency as the gestation progresses. The lateral femoral cutaneous nerve, which provides sensory innervation to the upper anterior thigh, may be injured as the abdomen expands or during pushing when it is stretched under the inguinal ligament. Neurologic examination usually differentiates these lesions based on their single nerve or nerve root distribution.

An iatrogenic epidural or spinal cord hematoma may occur with regional anesthesia in the pregnant patient. Patients who are treated with anticoagulants (even after the spinal, epidural, or delivery) may, rarely, develop bleeding. Pre-eclampsia can also result in impaired coagulation after an epidural has been placed. Considering the vascularity of the epidural space, it is surprising that clinically detectable hematomas are not seen more often.

A spinal hematoma can develop rapidly or insidiously. The hematoma is usually related to arterial bleeding. The patient may complain of severe burning back pain that progresses to motor dysfunction (usually bilaterally) and the loss of bowel and bladder function. Such a scenario is a medical emergency because nerve compression and ischemia result in permanent damage, often in less than 6 hours from the onset of symptoms. An MRI is used for diagnosis followed by immediate surgical decompression by laminectomy, if a hematoma is found. With the onset of symptoms during evaluation, the patient should be treated with narcotic analgesics and sedatives. Normotension, normal oxygen saturation, and normocarbia should be maintained. Mild, generalized hypothermia and local back cooling may be helpful. Free-radical scavengers such as barbiturates, calcium channel blockers, and steroids may be protective. The patient's ventilation must be ensured, and endotracheal intubation with sedation (especially during the MRI) should be considered.

Cerebral Trauma

Various traumatic head injuries have been reported in the parturient.[7, 52] Prompt diagnosis and management can be lifesaving.

Epidemiology and Pathophysiology

The incidence of traumatic brain injury in the US is in the range of 152–430 per 100,000/year in the general population. The mortality rate is 30 per 100,000/year with a large number suffering permanent disabilities. Approximately 7% of pregnant women will suffer a bodily injury, with motor vehicle accidents[53] and alcohol ingestion as major contributory factors.

Head injury may be classified as closed or open (penetrating). Closed injuries may be diffuse or focal. Diffuse injury, often caused by acceleration-deceleration forces, ranges from simple concussion (transient loss of consciousness) to severe axonal disruption. Focal injuries include subdural hematoma, epidural he-

matoma, and cerebral contusion. Subdural hematoma occurs when the bridging veins between the brain and the dural venous sinuses are disrupted as a result of an acceleration injury. Epidural hematomas are caused by rupture of the meningeal arteries, which are embedded in the grooves of the skull, by direct skull trauma. Cerebral contusions are heterogeneous areas of necrosis, infarction, hemorrhage, or edema. Coup contusions result from deformation of the skull at the point of impact, and contrecoup contusions result from deceleration of the brain against the skull. Intracerebral hematomas result from depressed skull fractures, penetrating wounds, or acceleration-deceleration injuries. Missiles produce various injuries. In addition to neurologic damage, major long-term complications of cerebral trauma include epilepsy and hydrocephalus.

Clinical Presentation and Diagnosis

A patient with a concussion injury may present with temporary unconsciousness, disorientation, amnesia, dizziness, disequilibrium, coma, or progress to death. Acute subdural hematomas appear as rapidly expanding mass lesions, with hemiparesis or pupillary abnormalities, or both. Epidural hematomas can appear with immediate loss of consciousness, followed by a lucid interval, later followed by neurologic symptoms such as headache and increased lethargy. Some patients may not experience unconsciousness until after the injury. Symptoms of subarachnoid hemorrhage can also occur. Contusions, hematomas, and missile-related injuries produce various localized and diffuse signs and symptoms.

On admission, history, physical examination, laboratory tests (including coagulation studies and determination of blood gases), and imaging studies are useful to establish the extent of injury to the brain and other systems. If neuroradiologic examination is needed, it should be performed promptly. The fetus can usually be shielded. Radiation of the fetus should be considered a minor risk in lifesaving situations.

Neurosurgical Management

Management includes control of BP, ICP, lung ventilation, maternal cerebral perfusion, and fetal perfusion. Surgical intervention is indicated for subdural and epidural hematomas; for intracerebral hematomas associated with a mass effect and/or neurologic deterioration; for symptomatic ICP greater than 25 mm Hg that is not responding to treatment; for depressed skull fractures and hydrocephalus; and to place ICP monitors.

Effect of Pregnancy and Obstetric Management

The incidence and morbidity of cerebral trauma in pregnant women are similar to those in a nonpregnant population of similar age.[7] In the presence of severe head trauma, injury to other organ systems must be ruled out, especially the vulnerable gravid uterus, with the potential for uterine rupture, placental separation, and fetal trauma. A discussion of fetal injury is beyond the scope of this chapter.

Method of delivery is based on obstetric considerations. Injury may precipitate premature labor, and because the patient, who is in an obtunded condition, cannot indicate that she is in labor, fetal monitoring should be initiated and early delivery anticipated.

Anesthetic Management

Anesthetic management for neurosurgery is similar to that in the nonpregnant patient, with consideration for those factors important in dealing with nonobstetric surgery during pregnancy.[54] Exposure to teratogens is of concern, but judicious use of common agents is safe in the absence of hypoxemia, acidemia, and hypercarbia. Anesthetic management for delivery is similar to that for pregnant patients suffering from ICH (see earlier).

Central Nervous System Ischemia

Cerebral Ischemia

Epidemiology and Pathophysiology

Ischemic strokes result from occlusion of the cerebral circulation (venous or arterial) due to various causes. In one report, ischemic strokes were observed in 9 of 90,000 pregnancies (see Table 16–1).[3] In another report, cerebral thrombosis was present in 1 of 29,000 pregnancies.[55] In India, the incidence of cerebral venous thrombosis was found to be 1 in 250 pregnancies.[56] In a study by Kittner and coworkers,[10] the relative risk for cerebral infarction during pregnancy was 0.7 (adjusted for age and race) compared with a relative risk of 8.7 in the first 6 weeks after delivery.

The hypercoagulable state of pregnancy may, in some situations, contribute to arterial and venous occlusion. For arterial occlusion, specific etiologies in parturients are similar to those in other young adults[8] and include the following categories:

■ Arteriopathies, which include premature atherosclerosis, usually associated with additional risk factors, such as smoking, hypertension, diabetes, hypercholesterolemia, homocystinuria, radiation to the neck, and a family history of arteriosclerosis. Included in this category are arterial dissection and various disorders producing inflammation of the cerebral arteries.
■ Hematologic disorders, which include sickle cell crises, that cause ischemic injury to the vessel wall

with subsequent intimal and medial proliferation; systemic lupus erythematosus (SLE); thrombotic thrombocytopenic purpura (TTP); and a number of less common disorders.
■ Cardioembolism, which includes emboli from artificial valves, mitral valve prolapse, atrial fibrillation, subacute bacterial endocarditis, and other cardiac diseases.[5, 57]
■ Other emboli, which include fat, amniotic fluid, and air, as well as paradoxical emboli from veins in the presence of a patent foramen ovale.
■ A miscellaneous category includes Sheehan syndrome (pituitary infarction following hypotension), migraine-related stroke, and drug-induced stroke. Use of cocaine, heroin, and amphetamines may cause arteritis, vasospasm, embolization of foreign material, and endocarditis.
■ Idiopathic or cause unknown, despite extensive investigation.

Cerebral venous thrombosis is associated with pregnancy, especially in the early postpartum period due to blood loss during delivery and dehydration.[58] Underlying precipitating factors include infection, dehydration, hyperviscosity syndromes (sickle cell disease, malignancy, polycythemia rubra vera, paroxysmal nocturnal hemoglobinuria),[59] procoagulation syndromes (antiphospholipid antibody syndrome, deficiency of protein C and S),[60] and AVM. Thrombosis of the sagittal sinus with extension to the cortical veins is not uncommon. Sagittal sinus thrombosis blocks reuptake of spinal fluid and produces intracranial hypertension. Cortical vein thrombosis produces focal cerebral ischemia and edema, and, when extensive, bland or hemorrhagic infarction.

Clinical Presentation

Cerebral arterial thrombosis is characterized by a gradual onset of focal deficits, whereas arterial emboli produce a more sudden onset of symptoms. Detailed discussion of the focal lesions produced is beyond the scope of this chapter. Cerebral venous thrombosis produces a progressive headache, nausea and vomiting, blurred or double vision, and altered mentation as a consequence of increased ICP. Cortical vein occlusion produces focal or generalized seizures and lateralizing signs that affect the proximal extremities.

Diagnosis

Ischemic strokes must be differentiated from hemorrhagic or structural lesions, which may be surgically treatable. Recurrence of stroke is common; thus aggressive diagnosis and treatment for the underlying medical condition should be pursued. Diagnostic measures include clinical information, extensive laboratory investigation (including coagulation studies), CT, MRI, and angiography when indicated.

Effect of Pregnancy and Obstetric Management

Wiebers and Wishnant[55] found that the incidence of cerebral infarction was increased 13-fold during pregnancy. The hypercoagulable state of pregnancy and hormonal influences play a role in this predisposition.[60] BP should be maintained in the normal range, and hyperventilation should be avoided. Otherwise, obstetric considerations should determine the mode of delivery. Regional anesthesia has been used successfully for operative vaginal and abdominal delivery.

Neurosurgical Management

Management is usually supportive, including therapeutic heparin to minimize recurrence. Only in the case of hemorrhagic transformation of the infarction, with mass effects and increased ICP, should surgery be needed. Surgery may also be required for ventriculoperitoneal shunting and placement of ICP monitors.

Anesthetic Management

Increases of ICP and BP are avoided by the careful induction of epidural analgesia and anesthesia and by the avoidance of pushing in the second stage with assisted vaginal delivery. Reversal of therapeutic anticoagulation is required if a regional anesthetic technique is selected. The risk of creating a dural puncture from epidural insertion must be weighed against the risk of exacerbating hypertension with intubation of the trachea in those parturients with an elevated ICP. Postoperatively, the patient must be observed for extension of the lesion, increased intracranial pressure, and recurrence of emboli.

Spinal Cord Ischemia

The anterior spinal artery syndrome has been reported rarely in parturients suffering severe and/or prolonged hypotension. Patients present with painless paraplegia resulting from spinal cord ischemia.[61] The condition must be differentiated, using imaging studies, from epidural abscess and hematoma. Epidural abscess and hematoma are rarely caused by regional anesthesia, but hematoma is treatable with timely decompression of the mass lesion. Spinal cord ischemia, however, is rarely reversible.

Central Nervous System Neoplasm

Epidemiology and Pathophysiology

Brain tumors, although rare in young patients, may occur during pregnancy.[9, 62] In the US, approximately 90 women per year develop brain tumors while pregnant. The types of tumor are identical to those seen in nonpregnant women of the same age [62, 63] and may be benign or malignant, primary or metastatic. The majority are gliomas, followed by meningiomas, acoustic neuromas, and less common tumors such as choriocarcinomas, which are unique to pregnancy. Spinal tumors represent 12% of CNS neoplasms during pregnancy. Prognosis varies according to the type of tumor.

Gliomas arise from astrocytes and oligodendrocytes, varying in degree of malignancy from slow-growing to highly anaplastic, producing tissue damage and mass effect. Meningiomas are benign tumors that grow slowly from the membranes covering brain and spinal cord, ultimately producing a mass effect. Acoustic neuromas are slow-growing, benign tumors arising from the vestibular portion of the eighth nerve; they are often seen in patients with neurofibromatosis. Pituitary tumors are benign and slow-growing, producing a variety of hormones (growth hormone, adrenocorticotropic hormone [ACTH], prolactin), and visual field defects from compression of the optic chiasm. Choriocarcinoma, an invasive, malignant tumor of trophoblastic origin, is prone to metastasis and may develop after molar pregnancy, abortion, ectopic gestation, or term pregnancy. Metastatic brain lesions are found in 3 to 20% at the time of initial diagnosis of choriocarcinoma.[64, 65] In the spinal cord, hemangiomas and meningiomas are the most common tumors, producing symptoms related to compression of surrounding structures.

Clinical Presentation

Nonspecific symptoms from brain tumors include constant headache and persistent nausea and vomiting resulting from increased intracranial pressure. These symptoms must be differentiated from common headache and morning sickness. Most affected patients demonstrate lateralizing signs, including hemiparesis, sensory loss, visual field defects, and aphasia. Seizures are also common with low-grade gliomas and meningiomas. Seizures may be focal or generalized (with or without a focal onset) and must be differentiated from those resulting from eclampsia. Patients with spinal cord tumors causing compression can present with painless weakness and numbness of the legs, followed by paralysis and loss of sphincter function.

Diagnosis

MRI scanning is best for defining mass lesions, and it does not emit ionizing radiation. CT scanning, although less sensitive, may also be used with proper shielding.

Neurosurgical Management

Low-grade gliomas are slow-growing and are often resected electively after delivery. High-grade gliomas are resected without delay with concomitant radiotherapy and chemotherapy. Because these treatments pose a significant risk to the fetus, decisions about treatment must be individualized. In the case of a slow-growing meningioma, 30% can be completely resected. The remainder require subtotal resection or radiation. Pituitary tumors are treated by transsphenoidal resection, or bromocriptine therapy in the case of prolactinomas. For choriocarcinoma, radiation and chemotherapy are used, and surgery is reserved for those with a single metastatic lesion to the brain or those requiring decompression. Anticonvulsants and corticosteroids are given when indicated. Spinal hemangiomas and meningiomas with rapidly progressing symptoms are treated with decompression laminectomy, but vertebral resection and intradural surgery may be needed.

Effect of Pregnancy and Obstetric Management

Although pregnancy does not influence the presence or type of tumor, it may have profound effects on symptoms. Meningiomas and acoustic neuromas may enlarge during pregnancy, possibly from fluid retention, increased blood volume, and generalized engorgement of blood vessels.[12] Pregnancy hormones may facilitate tumor growth, because 90% of meningiomas and some gliomas have progesterone receptors. Maternal BP, ICP, and seizure activity (if present) must be controlled throughout pregnancy and especially during labor. If there is increased intracranial pressure, many obstetricians prefer to deliver by cesarean section. Similar maternal and fetal outcomes can be achieved, however, with pain-free labor and assisted vaginal delivery.

Anesthetic Management

The anesthetic management is guided by signs and symptoms associated with the tumor.[66] Major considerations are avoidance of extremes in BP and ICP. Labor can be permitted in the absence of elevated ICP with pain control provided by epidural analgesia. If the ICP is elevated, brainstem herniation may follow an inadvertent dural puncture. For cesarean section in a parturient with raised ICP, preinduction measurement and control of ICP and BP are mandatory. An arterial line and ventriculostomy with ICP pressure transducer assist in controlling the response to tracheal intubation so that therapy (antihypertensive drugs, hyperventilation, mannitol) can be titrated to maintain homeostasis.

Central Nervous System Infection

Infection of the brain and spinal cord can become organized into abscesses that produce symptoms similar to those of other mass lesions.[67–72] Anesthetic considerations are the same as those for brain tumors and other space-occupying lesions.

Other Conditions

Benign Intracranial Hypertension

Benign intracranial hypertension or "pseudotumor cerebri"[73] is defined as an increase in ICP without a demonstrable etiology and is a diagnosis of exclusion. The various CNS and systemic causes of elevated ICP are shown in Figure 16–1.

Epidemiology and Pathophysiology

Benign intracranial hypertension is thought to occur in 1 in 1000 pregnancies, with a 30% recurrence rate in subsequent pregnancies.[74, 75] It is reported most often in obese women of childbearing age, suggesting a hormonal etiology.[73] It may occur after chronic use of specific medications (such as tetracycline), but evidence suggests that it is not more common in pregnancy.[1] Overproduction and/or underabsorption of cerebrospi-

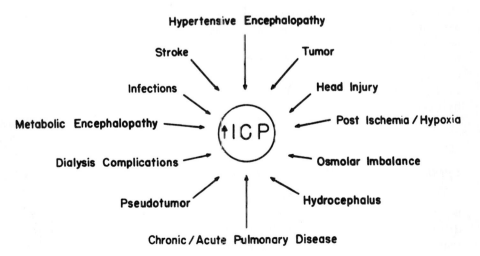

Figure 16–1. Intracranial and systemic causes of intracranial hypertension. (From Shapiro H, Drummond JC. Neurosurgical anesthesia and intracranial hypertension. In Miller RD (ed): Anesthesia, 3rd ed. New York, Churchill Livingstone, 1990, p 1749.)

nal fluid (CSF) are proposed mechanisms. The disease is usually benign, but increased ICP can lead to optic atrophy and blindness.[76]

Clinical Presentation and Diagnosis

Headache, stiff neck, papilledema, and visual disturbances occur from increased ICP. The diagnosis is one of exclusion. CSF pressure is elevated; CSF composition is normal; and results of imaging studies are normal.

Neurosurgical Management

Treatment consists of serial lumbar punctures to drain CSF. Brainstem herniation usually does not occur, because the increase in ICP is uniformly distributed throughout the CNS. Two cases of cerebellar tonsillar herniation have been reported, however, after diagnostic lumbar puncture in patients with this syndrome.[77] These patients presented with severe headache, neck pain, and focal neurologic signs. A shunting procedure (commonly a lumboperitoneal shunt) or optic nerve decompression is required, if the patient experiences progressive loss of vision or optic nerve compression.[74, 76, 78]

Effect of Pregnancy and Obstetric Management

Symptoms worsen during pregnancy,[75] suggesting a hormonal etiology. The condition usually resolves post partum. Obstetric management should not be significantly altered by this disorder.

Anesthetic Management

General anesthesia may be required for placement of a lumboperitoneal shunt, and the usual precautions for nonobstetric surgery during pregnancy apply.[54] Regional analgesia for labor and delivery has been described and was deemed to be safe.[74, 79] If a lumboperitoneal shunt is in place, general anesthesia may be preferable for cesarean section in that the impact of the shunt on extension of regional anesthesia is unknown. Parturients with benign intracranial hypertension and associated headache often undergo a diagnostic spinal tap. Following this procedure, they have the potential to develop a postdural puncture headache, and an epidural blood patch may be considered. Blood placed in the epidural space may increase ICP as a result of hydraulic compression of the dura.[80]

Hydrocephalus

Epidemiology and Pathophysiology

The incidence of pregnant patients with CSF shunts is unknown, but successful treatment of congenital hydrocephalus in childhood has translated into more females with ventricular shunts reaching childbearing

TABLE 16–4. CAUSES OF HYDROCEPHALUS

Congenital aqueductal stenosis
Noninherited, Dandy-Walker anomaly
Acquired, secondary to
Subarachnoid hemorrhage
Infection
Tumor
Inherited neural tube defect

age.[81–83] The causes of hydrocephalus are shown in Table 16–4, all of which may require ventricular shunts to relieve raised ICP.

Clinical Presentation and Diagnosis

The symptoms of raised ICP are headache, nausea and vomiting, ataxia, papilledema, and sixth nerve paresis. In patients with shunts, hydrocephalus may recur when the shunt malfunctions, which is commonly the result of infection or mechanical damage. A physical examination and a CT or an MRI scan should be performed to rule out other causes. If results of the scan are normal, a lumbar puncture can exclude other processes, such as benign intracranial hypertension.

Neurosurgical Management

Shunts are placed or replaced when the patient develops a decreased level of consciousness, worsening headache, vomiting, and/or visual disturbances. Ventriculoperitoneal shunts are the most resistant to infection and are used commonly. Prophylactic antibiotics are recommended to prevent infection of the shunt during revision.

Effect of Pregnancy and Obstetric Management

Pregnancy may precipitate hydrocephalus or may aggravate symptoms in a patient with a previously well-functioning shunt. In the presence of reduced brain compliance, the increased blood volume of pregnancy may lead to increased ICP, which must be controlled. If ICP is normal there are no specific obstetric considerations. Prophylactic antibiotics should be administered, however, especially if the peritoneum is entered for cesarean section or tubal ligation.

Anesthetic Considerations

General anesthesia is used for shunt placement, with emphasis on controlling ICP, by ensuring an adequate anesthetic depth and a beta-blocker such as labetalol. Induction with thiopental is preferred. Regional anesthesia has been given for vaginal delivery in these patients.[83] If ICP is elevated, caution must be advised when epidural anesthesia is induced.

PREOPERATIVE CONSIDERATIONS FOR NEUROSURGERY DURING PREGNANCY

Monitors

It is important to monitor oxygen saturation, electrocardiogram, end-tidal carbon dioxide (CO_2) level, fetal heart rate, direct arterial and central venous pressures, ICP, and occasionally electroencephalographic status and sensory evoked potentials (Table 16–5).

It is essential to monitor ICP in neurosurgical patients.[11] When the brain is injured, swelling often results. Initially, ICP often remains normal because the brain has room to expand within the intracranial cavity, displacing CSF and soft tissue. When the reserves for this expansion are exhausted, however, ICP rises dramatically, and cerebral perfusion is reduced. Increases in ICP produce headache, nausea, and papilledema. Unilateral pupillary dilation, oculomotor or abducens nerve palsy, decreased levels of consciousness, irregular respiration, and cardiovascular changes indicate cerebellar herniation. With an acute increase in ICP, loss of consciousness may occur before signs of herniation are seen. Uterine contractions and pressure on the uterus, both during labor and post partum, can increase ICP. This increase in ICP is a result of fluid shifts and increases in arterial and venous pressure from pain and the Valsalva maneuver. During a uterine contraction, 200 to 300 ml of blood are forced back into the systemic circulation. Shifting of the brain and cerebral edema can raise ICP, but clinical and radiologic signs alone are not always accurate indicators of ICP. Direct measurement may be required to evaluate the effects of therapy. ICP monitoring is employed rarely and is most common for patients with head trauma. Several methods have been used to monitor ICP (Table 16–6).[11, 84]

Electroencephalography (EEG) measures the spontaneous electrical activity of the cerebral cortex, as recorded from the scalp or surface electrodes. Computer analysis of EEG data may be graphically displayed, simplifying interpretation. Focal cerebral ischemia may not be reflected in the EEG, which is a record of overall electrical activity measured remotely from the site of

TABLE 16–5. MONITORS USED FOR NEUROSURGICAL PROCEDURES IN PREGNANCY

Monitor	Considerations
Pulse oximeter	Provides a noninvasive indicator of the patient's oxygenation and may provide an early warning of overhydration and other pulmonary complications
Electrocardiogram	Used to evaluate cardiac status, electrolyte balance, and oxygenation. Following subarachnoid hemorrhage, the ECG often shows characteristic changes.[17] Increased intracranial pressure can also lead to ECG changes,[51] and retraction during posterior fossa surgery may cause dysrhythmias
Fetal heart rate	Evaluates alterations in uteroplacental and fetal perfusion; noninvasive and presently the only available method of monitoring the fetus on an ongoing basis. Changes in FHR pattern may indicate suboptimal uteroplacental perfusion and need for altered fluid management, obstetric intervention, or adjusting maternal hemodynamic status (e.g., during controlled hypotension for neurosurgical procedures)
Indwelling arterial line	Direct arterial pressure measurement is useful for rapidly evaluating and controlling BP and for measuring arterial blood gases
Central venous catheter	Brachial approach for catheterization advantageous, since it avoids cerebral circulation and does not interfere with surgical field. Catheter location should be verified by chest x-ray and pressure trace. Provides accurate assessment of fluid balance. For surgery in sitting position, multiport CVP catheter, with tip at the junction of superior vena cava and right atrium, is used to withdraw air in event of air embolism.[11] A pulmonary artery catheter can detect cardiac and pulmonary complications, air embolism. Useful for fluid balance in patients with elevated ICP; cerebral aneurysms requiring controlled hypotension; severe pregnancy-induced hypertension
Intracranial pressure	Cerebral perfusion pressure (CPP) = mean arterial pressure − ICP; if CPP is inadequate, tissue damage results
Electroencephalogram	Deep anesthesia, cerebral ischemia, and other abnormal states can decrease the amplitude and frequency of the EEG. However, many physiologic factors affect the EEG in the anesthetized patient, so interpretation remains controversial
Evoked potentials	Small electrical signals generated in various nerve pathways following periodic electrical stimulation. These signals are weak, so computerized filtering and averaging of multiple signals are needed. The averaged response is plotted as voltage over time. Latency from stimulation to the evoked response, and amplitude of the response, are altered by anesthetics, ischemia, and other factors.[11] Acute changes intraoperatively may alert anesthesiologist to important alterations in patient's condition
Precordial Doppler	Useful for neurosurgical procedures in sitting position to detect air entrainment (will detect as little as 0.1 ml air in RV). Will also pick up venous air embolus at cesarean delivery
End-tidal carbon dioxide	End-tidal CO_2 monitoring and direct arterial CO_2 measurement allow calculation of arterial-alveolar CO_2 gradient, important in diagnosing pulmonary embolic events

TABLE 16–6. **DEVICES TO MEASURE INTRACRANIAL PRESSURE**

Device	Advantages	Disadvantages
Intraventricular catheter	Accurate Vary fluid to control ICP	Fluid filled—blockage Penetrates brain tissue Infection
Subarachnoid (Richmond) bolt	Technically easy No penetration of brain	Less accurate Fluid filled—blockage Infection
Epidural bolt	Technically easy Less infection	Less accurate Fluid filled—blockage
Fiberoptic bolt	Technically easy Less infection Not fluid filled	Less accurate

injury. Many factors affect the EEG in the anesthetized patient; thus, expert interpretation is required. The EEG may be employed preoperatively for diagnosis, and it may be continued perioperatively.[11]

Control of Intracranial Pressure

Acute increases in ICP and expanding intracranial lesions can result in herniation. Signs and symptoms of herniation include loss of consciousness, lateralizing neurologic signs ("blown pupil"), sudden changes in blood pressure, vomiting, respiratory collapse, and seizures. Acute obstetric disasters (such as amniotic fluid embolism) need to be ruled out. The rapid progression of this life-threatening emergency makes immediate surgical intervention the first priority and diagnostic CT or MRI scan secondary. Immediate treatment may involve cardiopulmonary resuscitation, tracheal intubation, and hyperventilation. The normal intracranial pressure is less than 15 mm Hg and should remain below 20 mm Hg.[85] If the ICP exceeds 25 mm Hg, it may adversely affect cerebral perfusion pressure (CPP). Events associated with an increase in ICP during pregnancy include laryngoscopy, endotracheal intubation, extubation, straining during labor and delivery, and uterine autotransfusion.

A number of methods may be used to control ICP during the perioperative period:

- *Diuretics* decrease brain water, volume of the brain, and ICP (Table 16–7). Osmotic diuretics, such as mannitol, draw water out of the cell when the blood brain barrier (BBB) is intact, but they should be used cautiously. Maternally administered mannitol has the potential to induce intracranial bleeding in the fetal brain. In rabbits, maternal infusion of mannitol draws free water from the fetus, increasing plasma sodium and osmolality, decreasing fetal plasma volume, and leading to fetal dehydration.[15] Similar effects may occur in humans,[16] but moderate doses are usually safe with close monitoring of the fetus and

mother. Tumors, intracranial hemorrhage, infarction, and infection may damage the BBB, allowing mannitol to draw water into these areas, with a resultant increase in ICP. Mannitol can also cause a transient dilation of vascular smooth muscle, leading to a transient increase of ICP. In patients at risk of heart failure (for example, those with eclampsia and severe hypertension) mannitol may precipitate pulmonary edema. Diuretics such as furosemide reduce ICP by inducing a systemic diuresis and decreasing CSF production. Unlike mannitol, they do not produce an increase in cerebral blood volume or osmolality.

- *Corticosteroids* are thought to reduce elevated ICP associated with brain tumors by decreasing swelling and inflammation. It may take hours to days for the steroids to have a significant effect, however. Long-term dexamethasone therapy may cause hyperglycemia, gastrointestinal bleeding, electrolyte disturbances, infection, and fetal adrenal suppression.[5] Short-term corticosteroid therapy is thought to have a minimal effect on the fetus.[16]

- *Acute hyperventilation*, and the resultant hypocarbia, produce transient cerebral vasoconstriction if CO_2 reactivity is intact. This cerebral vasoconstriction reduces cerebral blood volume, and ICP falls by 4% for each 1 mm Hg reduction in Pa_{CO_2}. Maternal hypocarbia, in excess of the normal physiologic pregnancy level of p_{CO_2} 34 mm Hg, shifts the maternal oxyhemoglobin dissociation curve to the left, reducing release of oxygen to the fetus. Excessive maternal hyperventilation also causes a reduction in fetal perfusion secondary to uterine vasoconstriction. (A normal pregnant arterial pH is 7.44, resulting from a physiologic increase in maternal ventilation.) When buffering compensation in CSF lowers bicarbonate levels and returns pH toward normal, hyperventilation becomes ineffective in altering intracranial pH and reducing intracranial pressure. Other methods of managing intracranial pressure are thereby usually

TABLE 16–7. **EFFECTS OF THERAPY FOR INTRACRANIAL LESIONS**

Treatment	Effect on Mother	Effect on Fetus
↑ Fluid intake	↑ Cerebral perfusion	↑ Perfusion
↓ Fluid intake	↔ CPP	↓ Perfusion
Diuretics	↓ ICP IC bleeding	↓ Perfusion IC bleeding
Corticosteroids	↓ ICP	Minimal effect
Hyperventilation	↓ ICP	↓ Perfusion and oxygen delivery
CSF drainage	↓ ICP	↔
Hypothermia	↓ $CMRO_2$ ↓ ICP	?
Barbiturate coma	↓ $CMRO_2$ ↓ ICP ↓ BP	? ↓ Perfusion
Calcium blockers	? ↓ Brain damage?	Probably safe
Free-radical scavengers	? ↓ Brain damage?	?
Angiography	Vessel damage, osmotic diuresis, allergy, sepsis	↓ Perfusion

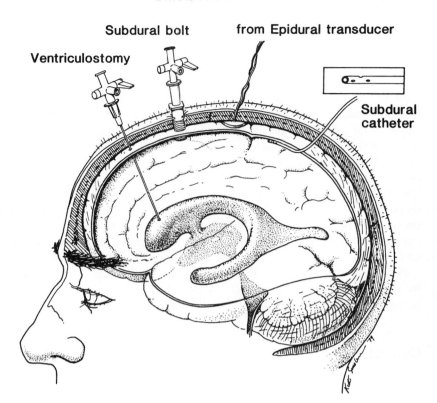

Ventriculostomy   **Subdural bolt**   **from Epidural transducer**

Subdural catheter

Figure 16–2. Commonly employed techniques and sites for intracranial pressure (ICP) measurement. (From Shapiro H, Drummond JC. Neurosurgical anesthesia and intracranial hypertension. In Miller RD (ed): Anesthesia, 3rd ed. New York, Churchill Livingstone, 1990, p 1749.)

instituted while hyperventilation is reduced. Subsequently, hyperventilation can be used again for management of acute exacerbations of ICP. With adequate hydration and monitoring of pCO_2, BP, and fetal heart rate (FHR), moderate degrees of hyperventilation of the parturient (maintaining $PaCO_2$ in the 25–30 mm Hg range) are not harmful to the fetus.

- *Head position* should be neutral, if possible, because neck rotation may decrease venous return, thereby increasing ICP. Head-up tilt improves venous drainage and reduces ICP. Raising the operative site above the level of the heart increases the probability of entraining air emboli into the pulmonary circulation. Arterial pressure and ICP should be measured at brain level and precordial Doppler utilized for early detection of air entrainment.
- *Ventriculostomy* (Figure 16–2) is helpful in monitoring ICP and draining CSF for ICP control. When epidural anesthesia is considered in a patient with increased ICP, CSF can be withdrawn from the ventriculostomy to reduce the risk of brainstem herniation if an inadvertent lumbar puncture occurs.

Intravenous Fluid Management and Blood Pressure Control

In unconscious patients and those with intracranial lesions, fluid and electrolyte balance can be problematic as a result of decreased fluid intake, vomiting, and the use of hyperosmolar dyes for angiography. Severe fluid restriction produces minimal reduction in ICP because fluid loss is isotonic, but it can cause a reduction in uteroplacental perfusion. Intravenous fluid loading is sometimes employed to maintain BP, cerebral perfusion, and fetal perfusion. Hypotension and hypovolemia in the presence of vasospasm can reduce cerebral perfusion,[33, 34] and thus judicious overhydration, while measuring BP and FHR, is appropriate. Glucose-free isotonic solution should be given just before delivery, because hyperglycemia can exacerbate cerebral injury and has neonatal consequences (e.g., hypoglycemia).[86] Before induction of anesthesia, a fluid load of 500 to 1000 ml is useful if the patient is dehydrated. Intraoperatively, 50% of the urinary losses and two to three times estimated blood loss should be replaced with Ringer's lactate solution to avoid the risks associated with hypotension and hypovolemia.

Control of BP throughout the perioperative period is important for maintenance of ICP, CPP, and fetal perfusion. If autoregulation is intact, cerebral blood flow (CBF) is maintained over a wide range of CPP. Autoregulation is altered by ischemia, edema, hemorrhage, infection, and herniation of brain tissue. Cerebral perfusion then becomes passively dependent on BP. Avoidance of hypertension, which may cause cerebral edema and hemorrhage, and hypotension, which may induce cerebral ischemia, is necessary.

Vasopressors and antihypertensives should be selected with the fetus in mind. Ephedrine constricts both capacitance and resistance vessels and increases myocardial contractility, which benefits fetal perfusion but may increase shear stress on sensitive intracranial vessels. Ephedrine must, therefore, be used cautiously. Evidence suggests that phenylephrine, which increases afterload, is safe for the fetus in 20- to 40-μg increments.[87] In large doses, however, phenylephrine has the potential to reduce uteroplacental perfusion because of its alpha-adrenergic effect on uterine vasculature. Antihypertensive agents such as labetalol, hydralazine, trimethaphan, nitroglycerin, and brief infusions of nitroprusside are safe for the fetus in normal dosages.[12] The lack of placental autoregulation means that its perfusion is directly related to maternal mean blood pressure. The effect of volume expanders, diuretics, vasopressors, or vasodilators must be considered in terms of their impact on cerebral perfusion, maternal end-organ perfusion, and placental perfusion. Clearly, in some situations, that which is best for maternal homeostasis may be detrimental to the fetus.

Control of Seizures

Parturients with intracranial lesions may present initially with seizures. Diagnosis can be delayed while the more common causes of seizures in pregnancy (e.g., eclampsia) are ruled out. Definitive treatment for the seizure depends on its etiology (see Chapter 17). Initial control of seizure activity is important, regardless of etiology, to avoid physical injury, pulmonary aspiration, increased systemic and intracranial hypertension, increased cerebral metabolism, and maternofetal hypoxemia. The benefits of controlling a seizure outweigh the risks from potential teratogenicity associated with the use of some anticonvulsants.[5] Midazolam, given in doses up to 5 mg, or a small dose of thiopentone (25–50 mg), produces minimal depression of the fetus. These medications are readily available to the anesthesiologist to treat maternal seizures promptly with minimal fetal respiratory depression in the aforementioned doses. If seizures occur near delivery, respiratory depressant effects of higher doses of benzodiazepines can be treated by ventilatory support of the neonate.

Brain Protection

Various methods may be employed to minimize further neurologic damage in the perioperative period by reducing ongoing damage to surrounding tissues. Many of these methods are experimental, and the effects on the fetus are unknown.

- Hypothermia reduces cerebral metabolic rate for oxygen ($CMRO_2$) by 7 to 8% per 1° C fall in maternal temperature, causing cerebral vasoconstriction. Moderate hypothermia down to 34° C can be produced by surface cooling, which is helpful for reducing

intracranial pressure and protecting the brain against transient ischemic events during neurosurgery.[17] Profound hypothermia may produce dysrhythmias in the mother and fetus, postoperative shivering, increased blood viscosity, altered coagulation, altered drug clearance, and increased infection.[17] Cardiopulmonary bypass may be utilized for acute induction of deep hypothermia and to arrest circulation during resection of giant aneurysms or AVMs for periods up to 1 hour.
- Deep barbiturate coma with pentobarbital may cause cerebral vasoconstriction and reduced ICP and cerebral oxygen consumption during surgery. Hypotension associated with its use, however, may have an adverse impact on fetal perfusion.[17]
- Calcium channel blockers such as nimodipine have shown some efficacy in reducing neurologic damage after ischemic strokes and rupture of cerebral aneurysms.[88] Experience in parturients having neurosurgery is limited, but moderate doses that do not produce severe hypotension are likely to be safe, because nimodipine has been given in the treatment of preeclampsia.[89]
- Midazolam, propofol, and etomidate reduce cerebral oxygen consumption in animals and, in the usual clinical doses, do not appear to harm the fetus.[12]

Anesthetic Management for Neurosurgery during Pregnancy

Emphasis has been placed on selection of surgical procedures with the welfare of the parturient in mind, because the well-being of the mother determines fetal outcome. Likewise, the method of delivery is more often selected based on obstetric considerations, because modern anesthetic management allows stress-free vaginal and cesarean delivery. Anesthetic management for a neurosurgical procedure during pregnancy is similar to that for a nonpregnant patient, with the following exceptions:

- Surgery is best deferred until the second trimester
- The well-being of the fetus is assessed throughout surgery by monitoring fetal heart rate
- Left uterine displacement is ensured to avoid aortocaval compression.

Most anesthetic drugs are safe for the fetus,[54] and second trimester surgery negates concern about teratogenesis. Premature labor can occur following any nonobstetric surgery, and thus early detection with fetal monitoring and prompt treatment is important, although the risk for premature labor is much greater following abdominal or pelvic surgery.

Preoperative Assessment

The impact of preoperative therapy and anesthetic intervention on the mother and fetus should be considered when formulating an anesthetic plan (Tables 16–7 & 16–8). Only in the most severe cases (massive trauma, epidural hematoma, brainstem herniation) is immediate surgery required. Major considerations include the neurologic status of the woman (including level of consciousness and evidence of raised ICP), working diagnosis, cardiorespiratory status, and fetal status. Maternal condition should be as stable as possible before proceeding to surgery, and appropriate monitors should be in place (see earlier).

Preanesthetic and anesthetic goals include controlling BP, CBF, and ICP; avoiding aspiration; and maintaining fetal perfusion. Antacids, metoclopramide, and histamine-2 blockers reduce acidity and volume of gastric fluid. Premedication with sedatives should be avoided in patients whose condition is obtunded out of concern for hypoventilation, possible aspiration, and accurate neurologic evaluation. For an awake, anxious patient, intravenous sedation and analgesia with drugs safe for the fetus (midazolam 1–2 mg and fentanyl 50–100 μg) are useful supplements to anesthetic induction. When indicated, a precordial Doppler ultrasonic transducer is placed over the right sternal border, between the third and sixth intercostal spaces, to detect small amounts (0.25 ml) of venous air entrained during sitting craniotomies,[11] and a multiport CVP catheter is placed to aspirate air if needed.

Induction of Anesthesia

Every parturient is assumed to have a full stomach. The patient should receive preoxygenation. If a nasogastric tube is present, it should be suctioned and removed before induction of anesthesia. After induction of anesthesia, cricoid pressure is applied until the endotracheal tube is secured. The same precautions exist when intubating the trachea of a comatose, unstable non-surgical patient.[4] If the status of the cervical spine is uncertain, rapid intubation with stabilization of the neck by axial traction is done if there is inadequate time to do fiberoptic intubation in an awake patient.

Sodium thiopental (STP) is an anticonvulsant and a cerebral vasoconstrictor. It reduces cerebral blood volume, ICP, and cerebral oxygen consumption. If the patient is adequately hydrated, STP has minimal impact on blood pressure, and thus fetal perfusion and CPP are maintained. Propofol has effects similar to STP and, similar to other cerebral vasoconstrictors, it preserves autoregulation and response to changes in pCO$_2$.[90] Benzodiazepines produce effects qualitatively similar to those of STP, but quantitatively less; because of their slow onset they are seldom used in neuroanesthesia. Etomidate has effects similar to STP, but with less cardiovascular depression, and hence it offers some advantages in the presence of hemodynamic instability. Methohexital is similar to STP but may induce seizures in large doses. Ketamine produces hypertension, increased uterine tone, and increased ICP, and thus it is not recommended in neuroanesthesia. An opioid, such as fentanyl or sufentanil, combined with droperidol, minimally reduces ICP and cerebral oxygen consumption while maintaining cerebral perfusion. Remifentanil and alfentanil have no effect on ICP with a background of isoflurane/nitrous oxide anesthesia in patients undergoing supratentorial craniotomy.[91]

During induction of general anesthesia ICP must be controlled, in some cases necessitating ICP monitoring. Treatment with lidocaine (100 mg), labetalol (5–10 mg increments at 3-minute intervals), an opioid (fentanyl, 50–100 μg), and an induction with sodium thiopental help to minimize hypertension associated with laryngoscopy and intubation and blunt increases in ICP.[11] Prolonged infusions of sodium nitroprusside may induce fetal cyanide toxicity and should be avoided. An adequate depth of anesthesia and complete neuromuscular blockade should be achieved before laryngoscopy and intubation, minimizing the possibility of aspiration, hypertension, and increased ICP. Acute increases in ICP can be treated with hyperventilation, boluses

TABLE 16–8. **EFFECTS OF ANESTHETICS ON MOTHER AND FETUS**

Anesthetic	Effect on Mother	Effect on Fetus
Midazolam	↓ Ventilation/sedation	↓ Ventilation
Opioids	↓ Ventilation/sedation	↓ Ventilation
Thiopental	↓ ICP, ↓ BP	↓ Ventilation ↓ Placental perfusion
Muscle relaxants	Apnea, possible histamine release	Negligible
Tracheal intubation	↑ BP, ↑ ICP; possible intracranial bleed	Negligible
Antihypertensive agents	Stabilizes BP, prevention of intracranial bleed, ± ↑ ICP	Negligible if uterine artery perfusion pressure is adequate
Volatile agents	↑ CBF ↔ ICP ↓ CMR	Negligible if uterine artery perfusion pressure is adequate
Nitrous oxide	↑ CBF ↔ ICP	Negligible
Extubation	↑ BP ∴ potential for intracranial bleeding Hypoxemia	Negligible if mother's condition is stable
Spinal	↓ BP/high spinal block; possible brainstem herniation in presence of raised ICP	Negligible if mother's condition is stable
Epidural	↓ BP; allows for continuous postop pain control; possibility of brainstem herniation after inadvertent dural puncture Possibility of high spinal or local anesthetic toxicity	Negligible if mother's condition is stable

of STP and/or labetalol, or greater concentrations of inhaled anesthetic. After delivery of the fetus, mannitol and furosemide (Lasix) can be administered.

Neuromuscular Blockers

Neuromuscular blockade facilitates adequate endotracheal intubation and operative conditions. Reducing muscle tone also prevents an increase in venous pressure and ICP, which can result from straining or coughing. Succinylcholine (100–120 mg) remains the most reliable neuromuscular blocker in this situation, although the resulting fasciculations may temporarily increase ICP and BP, but this is of little consequence. Precurarization with a small dose of a non-depolarizing blocker (3–6 mg d-tubocurare) reduces, but does not eliminate, fasciculations. This practice, however, can decrease the effectiveness of succinylcholine. If succinylcholine is contraindicated, non-depolarizing neuromuscular agents, such as rocuronium, may be given in a dose 1.5 to 1.75 times the ED_{95}. Rocuronium 0.6 mg/kg produces good to excellent intubating conditions at 60 to 90 seconds. The practice of giving a priming dose (10–20% of total dose) can cause profound muscle weakness in some patients, especially those receiving magnesium sulfate, hence it should be used with caution in pregnancy. Large doses of atracurium may produce hypotension, presumably by releasing histamine. The newer agent, cis-atracurium, is more suitable in this regard. Neuromuscular blockade should be maintained throughout the procedure to avoid increases of ICP resulting from increases of muscle tone.

For a prolonged procedure, a longer acting drug is appropriate. Pancuronium (0.5 mg increments to avoid tachycardia), or doxacurium (0.1 mg/kg) may be administered. If extubation with neurologic evaluation of the patient is planned immediately postoperatively, shorter acting agents are more readily reversed. The choice of neuromuscular blocker is ultimately dependent on the anesthesiologist's experience and the case's requirements.

Maintenance of Anesthesia

The maintenance of anesthesia may be accomplished with a combination of opioid and volatile agents. Intravenous agents are selected for their cerebral and pharmacokinetic effects.[11, 92] Propofol decreases CBF and CMR and preserves autoregulation and reactivity to CO_2. Propofol has a high lipophilicity, fast metabolic rate, and short redistribution half-life. Its adverse hemodynamic effects can be prevented by slow administration. The impact of synthetic opioids on ICP and CBF is insignificant if hyperventilation is ensured.[92]

The commonly used volatile anesthetics halothane, enflurane, and isoflurane produce vasodilation that increases CBF,[92] and they decrease the cerebral metabolic rate. Clinical and laboratory studies have failed to demonstrate a beneficial effect of these agents in terms of neurologic outcome, however. At approximately 1.5 maximal allowable concentration, halothane and enflurane increase CBF more than isoflurane (although these concentrations are seldom needed clinically). Evidence indicates that the newer agent desflurane may elevate ICP more than sevoflurane. Sevoflurane 1% is safe for the fetus when administered during cesarean section.[93] Nitrous oxide increases CBF and ICP, and may attenuate cerebral protection by barbiturates.

Induced hypotension is done occasionally to control bleeding during clipping of intracerebral aneurysms.[30-32, 92] Hypotension may have adverse effects on the fetus, however.[12] If induced hypotension is used, it should be limited in depth and duration, adjusting the mean BP upwards if the FHR pattern becomes unfavorable (e.g., loss of beat-to-beat variability, fetal tachycardia, sudden decelerations). Improvements in FHR pattern have been described after correcting hypoxemia[94] or by increasing flow during cardiopulmonary bypass.[95]

Emergence and Extubation

In many cases, patients are awakened at the end of the procedure, so that neurologic status can be evaluated. Metoclopramide and ranitidine given before extubation reduce the risk of vomiting and aspiration. To avoid increased ICP and hypertension at extubation, lidocaine and antihypertensive agents such as labetalol are useful. The trachea is extubated when protective airway reflexes have returned and the patient is hemodynamically and neurologically stable. ICP and other parameters are monitored in the immediate postoperative period. Patients in severely obtunded or unstable condition, those with pulmonary complications, or those requiring hyperventilation to control ICP require prolonged intubation. Coughing, as a result of tracheal irritation from an endotracheal tube, raises ICP significantly; hence, adequate sedation and analgesia must be maintained in those requiring protracted periods of intubation and ventilation, and neuromuscular paralysis may be required. Superior laryngeal nerve block and instillation of lidocaine into the endotracheal tube are other ways of obtunding the ICP response to laryngeal stimulation.

ANESTHESIA FOR DELIVERY IN A PARTURIENT WITH RAISED ICP

Vaginal Delivery

If vaginal delivery is selected, monitors to measure BP and ICP, if indicated, should be placed before delivery. The labor should be as pain-free as possible, and the second stage should be shortened with oxytocin and forceps delivery to reduce straining. The net effect of these changes on the transmural pressure of aneurysms is unknown.

The decision concerning pain relief must be made in the context of other available methods. Systemic analgesics may depress respiration and increase ICP. Paracervical blockade can provide adequate anesthesia for the second stage for some patients, but it can produce fetal compromise. Pudendal block with local infiltration may be given for delivery, but it is not useful for labor analgesia.

Segmental lumbar or caudal epidural anesthesia reduces the pain of labor and limits straining. If epidural anesthesia is administered when ICP is increased, a "wet-tap" with an epidural needle can cause a sudden leakage of CSF and theoretically can lead to a brain herniation. In addition, a rapid reduction in CSF pressure can increase the transmural pressure in an aneurysm, leading to rupture. The anesthetic technique should therefore be selected with these serious complications in mind. In selected patients, regional anesthesia may be given safely with the proper precautions. If there is concern about increased ICP, a ventriculostomy can be used to measure ICP and to withdraw CSF if needed. Immediately before the catheter is placed, the ventriculostomy should be checked to ensure that fluid can be readily withdrawn.

An epidural bolt measures ICP but cannot be utilized to withdraw CSF. Placement of a lumbar epidural catheter by the most experienced person available reduces the chance of a wet tap. A caudal approach may reduce, but not eliminate, the possibility of a wet-tap, but it is rarely done. If the patient is anxious, some sedation, such as intravenous midazolam 1 to 2 mg, may minimize movement during catheter placement. Spinal anesthesia should not be used if ICP is elevated. In the event of a wet-tap in a patient with elevated ICP, the injection of saline through the catheter while the ventriculostomy is vented has been suggested. A study of a porcine model showed an increase in ICP with epidural injections, with a concomitant reduction in cerebral and spinal cord blood flow.[96] If the epidural route is employed, the injections should be made slowly to minimize such changes.

Cesarean Delivery

Cesarean delivery may be required for obstetric indications. General anesthesia allows a simultaneous neurosurgical procedure.[26, 27] For the patient with a possible difficult airway, the adverse hemodynamic effects of respiratory obstruction and straining, during fiberoptic intubation, must be considered.[97, 98] If lumbar epidural anesthesia is selected, the same considerations apply as for vaginal delivery. Some have employed epidural[36]

and spinal[99] anesthesia for cesarean section in patients with intracranial lesions. It can be argued that spinal anesthesia with a small, pencil-point spinal needle is unlikely to cause a significant CSF leak in patients with raised ICP[99]; this is highly controversial, because few clinicians would use spinal anesthesia in the presence of intracranial hypertension from a space-occupying lesion. If labor occurs when neurosurgery is planned, an emergency cesarean section, followed immediately by an intracranial procedure, may be performed using general anesthesia.

CONCLUSIONS AND FUTURE DIRECTIONS

Many of the lesions discussed in this chapter are uncommon, and thus it is unlikely that a meaningful, controlled study can be done to compare management techniques. Prompt reporting of individual cases and appropriate laboratory research are important, however, because improved management is facilitated by a greater total experience and improved knowledge of related physiology. Advances in neurosurgical, obstetric, and anesthetic management have resulted in a trend to treat the parturient aggressively for her neurologic condition, because the welfare of the fetus ultimately depends on the health of the mother. Appropriate monitoring; rational, pre-emptive control of physiologic variables; communication; coordinated team approach; and timely intervention based on predetermined triage priorities are essential to optimal management.

References

1. Cunningham FG, Mac Donald PC, Gant NF, et al. Neurological and psychiatric disorders. In Cunningham FG, MacDonald PC, Gant NF, et al (eds): Williams Obstetrics, 19th ed. Norwalk, CT, Appleton & Lange, 1993, pp 1243–1258.
2. Kistler JP, Popper AH, Martin JB. Cerebrovascular diseases. In Isselbacher KJ, Braunwald E, Wilson JD, et al (eds): Harrison's Principles of Internal Medicine, 13th ed. New York, McGraw-Hill, 1994, pp 2233–2256.
3. Simolke GA, Cox SM, Cunningham FG. Cerebrovascular accidents complicating pregnancy and the puerperium. Obstet Gynecol 1991;78:37.
4. Biller J, Adams HP Jr. Cerebrovascular disorders associated with pregnancy. Am Fam Phys 1986;33:125.
5. Dias MS, Sekhar LN. Intracranial hemorrhage from aneurysms and arteriovenous malformations during pregnancy and the puerperium. Neurosurgery 1990;27:855.
6. Wilterdink JL, Feldmann E. Cerebral hemorrhage. Adv Neurol 1994;64:13.
7. Jordan BD. Maternal head trauma during pregnancy. Adv Neurol 1994;64:131.
8. Wilterdink JL, Easton JD. Cerebral ischemia. Adv Neurol 1994;64:1.
9. DeAngelis LM. Central nervous system neoplasms in pregnancy. Adv Neurol 1994;64:139.
10. Kittner SJ, Stern BJ, Feeser BR, et al. Pregnancy and the risk of stroke. N Engl J Med 1996;335:768.
11. Bendo AA, Hartung J, Cotrell JE. Neurophysiology and neu-

roanesthesia. In Barash P, Cullen BF, Stoelting RK (eds): Clinical Anesthesia, 2nd ed. Philadelphia, JB Lippincott, 1992, pp 871–918.

12. Rosen MA. Anesthesia for neurosurgery during pregnancy. In Shnider S, Levinson G (eds): Anesthesia for Obstetrics. Baltimore, Williams & Wilkins, 1993, pp 551–62.

12a. Wakeling HG, Creagh Barry P. Undiagnosed raised intracranial pressure complicating labour. Int J Obstet Anesth 1995;4:117.

13. Powell MC. Magnetic resonance imaging in obstetrics. Fetal Maternal Med Rev 1993;5:57.

14. Cunningham FG, MacDonald PC, Gant NF, et al. Imaging modalities in pregnancy. In Cunningham FG, MacDonald PC, Gant NF, et al (eds): Williams Obstetrics, 19th ed. Norwalk, CT, Appleton & Lange, 1993, pp 981–989.

15. Bruns PD, Linder RO, Drose VE, et al. The placental transfer of water from fetus to mother following intravenous infusion of hypertonic mannitol to the maternal rabbit. Am J Obstet Gynecol 1963;86:160.

16. Biggs JSG, Allen JA. Medication and pregnancy. Drugs 1981;21:69.

17. Bekker AY, Baker KZ, Baker CJ, et al. Anesthetic considerations for cerebral aneurysm surgery. Am J Anesthesiol 1995;22:248.

18. Guy J, McGrath BJ, Borel CO, et al. Perioperative management of aneurysmal subarachnoid hemorrhage: Part 1. Operative management. Anesth Analg 1995;81:1060.

19. McGrath BJ, Guy J, Borel CO. Perioperative management of aneurysmal subarachnoid hemorrhage: Part 2. Postoperative management. Anesth Analg 1995;81:1295.

20. Lichtenfeld PJ, Fubin DB, Feldman RS. Subarachnoid hemorrhage precipitated by cocaine snorting. Arch Neurol 1984;41:223.

21. Horton JC, Chambers WA, Lyons SL, et al. Pregnancy and the risk of hemorrhage from cerebral arteriovenous malformations. Neurosurgery 1990;27:867.

22. Robinson JL, Hall CJ, Sedzimir CB. Subarachnoid hemorrhage in pregnancy. J Neurosurg 1972;36:27.

23. Weibers D. Subarachnoid hemorrhage in pregnancy. Semin Neurol 1988;8:226.

24. Holcomb WL, Petrie RH. Cerebrovascular emergencies in pregnancy. Clin Obstet Gynecol 1990;33:467.

25. Robinson JL, Hall CJ, Sedzimir CB. Arteriovenous malformations, aneurysms and pregnancy. J Neurosurg 1974;41:63.

26. Conklin KA, Herr G. Anaesthesia for Caesarean section and cerebral aneurysm clipping. Can Anaesth Soc J 1984;31:451.

27. Lennon RL, Sundt TM, Gronert GA. Combined cesarean section and clipping of intracerebral aneurysm. Anesthesiology 1984;60:240.

28. Kofke WA, Wuest HP, McGinnis LA. Cesarean section following ruptured cerebral aneurysm and neuroresuscitation. Anesthesiology 1984;60:242.

29. Whitburn RH, Laishley RS, Jewkes DA. Anaesthesia for simultaneous cesarean section and clipping of intracerebral aneurysm. Br J Anaesth 1990;64:642.

30. Donchin Y, Amirav B, Sahar A, et al. Sodium nitroprusside for aneurysm surgery in pregnancy. Br J Anaesth 1978;50:849.

31. Dhamee MS, Goh M. Deliberate hypotension for clipping of cerebral aneurysm during pregnancy. Anesthesiol Rev 1985;12:20.

32. Newman B, Lam AM. Induced hypotension for clipping of a cerebral aneurysm during pregnancy: A case report and brief review. Anesth Analg 1986;65:675.

33. Mayberg M, Batjer H, Dacey R, et al. Guidelines for management of aneurysmal subarachnoid hemorrhage. Special report. Stroke 1994;25:2315.

34. Rosenwasser RH, Deljado TE, Buchheit WA, et al. Control of hypertension and prophylaxis against vasospasm in cases of subarachnoid hemorrhage. A preliminary report. Neurosurgery 1983;12:658.

35. Laidler JA, Jackson IJ, Redfern N. The management of Caesarean section in a patient with an intracranial arteriovenous malformation. Anaesthesia 1989;44:490.

36. Gupta A, Hesselvik F, Eriksson L, et al. Epidural anesthesia for cesarean section in a patient with a cerebral artery aneurysm. Int J Obstet Anesth 1993;2:49.

37. Hunt HB, Schifrin BS, Suzuki K. Ruptured berry aneurysms and pregnancy. Obstet Gynecol 1974;43:827.

38. McCausland AM, Holmes F. Spinal fluid pressures during labor: Preliminary report. West J Surg Obstet Gynecol 1957;65:221.

39. Marx GF, Zemaitis MT, Orkin LR. Cerebrospinal fluid pressures during labor and obstetric anesthesia. Anesthesiology 1961;22:348.

40. Hudspith MJ, Popham PA. The anaesthetic management of intracranial haemorrhage from arteriovenous malformations during pregnancy: Three cases. Int J Obstet Anesth 1996;5:189.

41. Sibai BM. Treatment of hypertension in pregnant women. N Engl J Med 1996;335:257.

42. Mercado A, Johnson G, Calver D, et al. Cocaine, pregnancy and postpartum intracerebral hemorrhage. Obstet Gynecol 1989;73:467.

43. Bromage PR. Neurologic complications of regional anesthesia in obstetrics. In Shnider S, Levinson G (eds): Anesthesia for Obstetrics. Baltimore, Williams & Wilkins, 1993, pp 433–453.

44. Packer NP, Cummins BH. Spontaneous epidural hemorrhage. A surgical emergency. Lancet 1978;1:356.

45. Mayumi T, Dohi S. Spinal subarachnoid hematoma after lumbar puncture in a patient receiving antiplatelet therapy. Anesth Analg 1983;62:777.

46. Guy MJ, Zahra M, Sengupta RP. Spontaneous spinal hematoma during general anesthesia. Surg Neurol 1979;11:199.

47. Greensite FS, Katz J. Spinal hematoma associated with attempted epidural anesthesia and subsequent continuous spinal anesthesia. Anesth Analg 1980;59:72.

48. Lao TT, Halpern SH, MacDonald D. Spinal subdural haematoma in a parturient after attempted epidural anaesthesia. Can J Anaesth 1993;40:340.

49. Harik SI, Raichle ME, Reis DJ. Spontaneous remitting spinal hematoma in a patient on anticoagulants. N Engl J Med 1971;284;1355.

50. Messer HD, Forshan VR, Brust JCM, et al. Transient paraplegia from hematoma after lumbar puncture: A consequence of anticoagulation therapy. JAMA 1976;235:529.

51. Holdcroft A, Gibberd FB, Hargrove RL, et al. Neurological complications associated with pregnancy. Br J Anaesth 1995;75:522.

52. Ropper AH. Trauma of the head and spine. In Isselbacher KJ, Braunwald E, Wilson JD, et al (eds). Harrison's Principles of Internal Medicine, 13th ed. New York, McGraw-Hill, 1994, pp 2320–2328.

53. Sims CJ, Boardman CH, Fuller SJ. Airbag deployment following a motor vehicle accident in pregnancy. Obstet Gynecol 1996;88:726.

54. Cohen SE. Nonobstetric surgery during pregnancy. In Chestnut DH (ed): Obstetric Anesthesia, Principles and Practice. St Louis, CV Mosby, 1994, pp 273–293.

55. Wiebers DO, Wishnant JP. The incidence of stroke among pregnant women in Rochester, Minn. 1955–1979. JAMA 1985;254:3055.

56. Srinivasan K. Ischemic cerebral vascular disease in the young. Two common causes in India. Stroke 1984;15:733.

57. Cox SM, Hankins GDV, Leveno KJ, et al. Bacterial endocarditis: A serious pregnancy complication. J Reprod Med 1988;33:671.

58. Wiebers DO. Ischemic cerebrovascular complications of pregnancy. Arch Neurol 1985;42:1106.

59. Roos KL, Pascuzzi RM, Kuharik MA, et al. Postpartum intracranial venous thrombosis associated with dysfunctional protein C and deficiency of protein S. Obstet Gynecol 1990;326:1130.

60. Branch DW. Antiphospholipid antibodies and pregnancy: Maternal implications. Semin Perinat 1990;14:139.

61. Ackerman SE, Mushtaque M, Juneja M, et al. Maternal paraparesis after anesthesia and cesarean section. South Med J 1990;83:695.

62. Hochberg F, Priutt A. Neoplastic disorders of the central nervous system. In Isselbacher KJ, Braunwald E, Wilson JD, et al (eds): Harrison's Principles of Internal Medicine, 13th ed. New York, McGraw-Hill, 1994, pp 2256–2269.

63. Aminoff MJ. Neurological disorders and pregnancy. Am J Obstet Gynecol 1978;132:325.

64. Jones WB. Gestational trophoblastic neoplasms: The role of chemotherapy and surgery. Surg Clin North Am 1978;58:167.

65. Weed JC, Woodward KT, Hammond CB. Choriocarcinoma metastatic to the brain: Therapy and prognosis. Semin Oncol 1982;9:208.

66. Finfer SR. Management of labour and delivery in patients with intracranial neoplasma. Br J Anaesth 1991;67:784.

67. Scheld WM. Bacterial meningitis and brain abscess. In Isselbecher KJ, Braunwald E, Wilson JD, et al (eds): Harrison's Principles of

Internal Medicine, 13th ed. New York, McGraw-Hill, 1994, pp 2296–2309.

68. Usubiaga JE. Neurological complications following epidural analgesia. Int Anesth Clin 1975;13:19.

69. Baker AS, Ojemann RG, Swartz MN, et al. Spinal epidural abscess. N Engl J Med 1975;293:463.

70. Male CG, Martin R. Puerperal spinal epidural abscess. Lancet 1973;1:608.

71. Schreiner EJ, Lipson SF, Bromage PR. Neurological complications following general anaesthesia: Three cases of major paralysis. Anaesthesia 1983;38:226.

72. Ready LB, Helfer D. Bacterial meningitis in parturients after epidural anesthesia. Anesthesiology 1989;71:988.

73. Weisberg LA. Benign intracranial hypertension. Medicine 1975;54:197.

74. Shekleton P, Fidler J, Grimwade J. A case of benign intracranial hypertension in pregnancy. Br J Obstet Gynaecol 1908;87:345.

75. Koontz WL, Herbert WNP, Cefalo RC. Pseudotumor cerebri in pregnancy. Obstet Gynecol 1983;62:324.

76. Abouleish E, Ali V, Tang RA. Benign intracranial hypertension and anesthesia for cesarean section. Anesthesiology 1985;63:705.

77. Parchuri SRA, Lawlor M, Kleinhomer K, et al. Risk of cerebellar tonsillar herniation after diagnostic lumbar puncture in pseudotumor cerebri (abstract). Reg Anesth 1993;18:S99.

78. Douglas MJ, Flanagan ML, McMorland GH. Anaesthetic management of a complex morbidly obese parturient. Can J Anaesth 1991;38:900.

79. Palop R, Choed-Amphai E, Miller R. Epidural anesthesia for delivery complicated by benign intracranial hypertension. Anesthesiology 1979;17:10.

80. Hilt H, Gramm HJ, Link J. Changes in intracranial pressure associated with extradural anaesthesia. Br J Anaesth 1986;58:676.

81. Cusimano MD, Miffe FM, Gentili F, et al. Management of pregnant women with cerebrospinal fluid shunts. Pediatr Neurosurg 1991;17:10.

82. Wisoff JH, Kratzert KJ, Handwerker SM, et al. Pregnancy in patients with cerebrospinal fluid shunts: Report of a series and review of the literature. Neurosurgery 1991;29:827.

83. Gast MJ, Grubb RL, Strickler RC. Maternal hydrocephalus and pregnancy. Obstet Gynecol 1983;62:295.

84. Gilbert HC, Vender JS. Monitoring the anesthetized patient. In Barash P, Cullen BF, Stoelting RK (eds): Clinical Anesthesia, 2nd ed. Philadelphia, JB Lippincott, 1992, pp 737–770.

85. Brown M. Critical care. In Barash P, Cullen BF, Stoelting RK (eds): Clinical Anesthesia, 2nd ed. Philadelphia, JB Lippincott, 1992, pp 1609–1633.

86. Kenepp NB, Shelley WC, Kumar S, et al. Effects on newborn of hydration with glucose in patients undergoing Caesarean section with regional anaesthesia. Lancet 1980;1:645.

87. Thomas DG, Robson SC, Redfern N, et al. Randomized trial of bolus phenylephrine or ephedrine for maintenance of arterial pressure during spinal anaesthesia for Caesarean section. Br J Anaesth 1996;76:61.

88. Popovic EA, Danks RA, Siu KH. Experience with nimodipine in aneurysmal subarachnoid hemorrhage. Med J Aust 1993;158:91.

89. Belfort MA, Saade GR, Moise KJ Jr, et al. Nimodipine in the management of pre-eclampsia: Maternal and fetal effects. Am J Obstet Gynecol 1994;171:417.

90. Fox J, Gelb AW, Enns J, et al. The responsiveness of cerebral blood flow to changes in arterial carbon dioxide is maintained during propofol-nitrous oxide anesthesia in humans. Anesthesiology 1992;77:453.

91. Warner DS, Hindman BJ, Todd MM, et al. Intracranial pressure and hemodynamic effects of remifentanil versus alfentanil in patients undergoing supratentorial craniotomy. Anesth Analg 1996;83:348.

92. Shapiro HM, Drummond JC. Neurosurgical anesthesia. In Miller RD (ed): Anesthesia, 4th ed. New York, Churchill Livingstone, 1994, pp 1897–1946.

93. Gambling DR, Sharma SK, White PF, et al. Use of sevoflurane during elective cesarean birth: A comparison with isoflurane and spinal anesthesia. Anesth Analg 1995;81:90.

94. Katz JD, Hook R, Barash PG. Fetal heart rate monitoring in pregnant patients undergoing surgery. Am J Obstet Gynecol 1976;125:267.

95. Bernal MJ, Miralles JP. Cardiac surgery with cardiopulmonary bypass during pregnancy. Obstet Gynecol Surv 1986;41:1.

96. Grocott HP, Mutch WAC. Epidural anesthesia and acutely increased intracranial pressure: Lumbar epidural space hydrodynamics in a porcine model. Anesthesiology 1996;85:1086.

97. Burns AM, Dorje P, Lawes EG, Nielsen MS. Anaesthetic management of caesarean section for a mother with pre-eclampsia, the Klippel-Feil syndrome and congenital hydrocephalus. Br J Anaesth 1988;61:350.

98. Semple DA, McClure JH, Wallace EM. Arnold-Chiari malformation in pregnancy. Anaesthesia 1996;51:580.

99. Atanassoff PG, Alon E, Weiss BM, et al. Spinal anaesthesia for Caesarean section in a patient with brain neoplasma (letter). Can J Anaesth 1994;41:163.

SEIZURES AND COMA

· · · · · · ·

Ann E. Newton, M.B.

Consideration of central nervous system (CNS) disorders in pregnancy presents a plethora of problematic and sensitive management issues for the medical team. Seizure disorders affect pregnancy, and pregnancy affects seizure disorders. A well-known twofold increase in congenital malformations is associated with epilepsy and antiepileptic drugs (AEDs). Medicolegal and social dilemmas affect the management of maternal vegetative and brain death situations.

SEIZURE DISORDERS

A seizure or convulsion is defined as an abrupt alteration in cortical activity evidenced by a change in consciousness or by a motor, sensory, or behavioral symptom. Epilepsy is the term used for recurrent seizures occurring over months or years, often with a stereotypical clinical pattern.[1]

The neurologic manifestations of epileptic seizures are varied, ranging from a brief lapse of attention to a prolonged loss of consciousness with abnormal motor activity (Table 17–1). Many patients who present following a "fit" have only had an episode of unconsciousness. It is important to consider and exclude other conditions that are commonly confused with epilepsy such as syncope, migraine, and metabolic and cerebral disorders.[2]

Epilepsy is the most common neurologic disorder

TABLE 17–1. CLASSIFICATION OF EPILEPTIC SEIZURES

Generalized Seizures
    Absences (petit mal)
    Bilateral myoclonus
    Infantile spasms
    Clonic seizures
    Tonic seizures
    Tonic-clonic seizures (grand mal)
    Akinetic seizures
Partial Seizures
    With elementary symptoms
    With complex symptoms (temporal lobe)
    Partial seizures becoming generalized
Status Epilepticus

in pregnant women, with seizures usually starting in childhood or early adulthood. Seizures occurring in the peripartum period may be caused by eclampsia. The differential diagnosis of eclamptic seizures includes idiopathic epilepsy, cerebrovascular pathology, mass lesion, infectious disease, drug intoxication or withdrawal, and metabolic disorder.[3]

Management of Seizures

The principles of seizure management are to stop the seizure, maintain an unobstructed protected airway, ensure oxygenation of both mother and fetus, and prevent aspiration. The need for endotracheal intubation must be assessed, and the maintenance of left uterine displacement must be ensured to help preserve fetal oxygenation. Clinical presentation may indicate a need for further investigation and computed tomography (CT) scan or magnetic resonance imaging (MRI) to delineate intracerebral pathology. Early neurosurgical intervention can then be instituted if required. Fetal assessment should be performed using ultrasound and cardiotocography to determine the need for obstetric intervention and operative delivery.

Seizure control may be achieved rapidly, using intravenous benzodiazepines, without deleterious fetal effects. Neonatal problems following intravenous diazepam include hypotension, hypothermia, lethargy, and apnea. Short-acting benzodiazepines are recommended for seizure treatment in labor. Phenytoin may be given with a loading dose of 15 to 18 mg/kg by slow intravenous infusion (12.5–25 mg/min) and maintained by 300 mg/day, starting 12 hours later. Further dosing must be based on serum phenytoin levels (therapeutic range is 10–15 μg/ml) (Table 17–2).[3]

Eclamptic seizures may be single or multiple, potentially leading to status epilepticus. The definitive treatment of eclampsia is to deliver the baby after medical control of the seizure. A report from the Eclampsia Trial Collaborative Group[4] details evidence in favor of the use of magnesium sulfate for routine anticonvulsant management of mothers with eclampsia (Table

TABLE 17-2. MANAGEMENT OF SEIZURES IN PREGNANCY

Airway
Relieve obstruction
Administer oxygen
Assess need for intubation
Circulation
Intravenous access
Ensure left lateral tilt
Drugs
Benzodiazepine initially for control
Diazepam
Midazolam
Phenytoin
    Load 15–18 mg/kg at 12–25 mg/min
    Maintain 300 mg/day (with levels)
Fetal Assessment
Determine obstetric management when mother's condition
    stabilized

17–3). The intravenous regimen consists of a 4-g loading dose over 5 minutes, followed by an infusion of 1–2 g/hour for 24 hours, with a further 2 to 4 g given intravenously (IV) for recurrent convulsions. Magnesium sulfate may cause hypotonia, hyporeflexia, and lethargy in the newborn. Maternal magnesium sulfate serum levels of more than 6 mEq/l may cause loss of patellar reflexes, whereas lethargy and respiratory depression are seen at levels above 8 to 10 mEq/l.[3]

Status epilepticus is defined as recurrent seizures without a return to consciousness or prolonged seizure activity beyond a 30-minute period.[3] The management principles include seizure cessation and prevention, airway management, and identification of a precipitating cause. Maternal and fetal risks are high, with the potential consequences of irreversible maternal brain injury and fetal hypoxia, ischemia, bradycardia, and death. Teramo and Hiilesmaa reported 29 cases of status epilepticus in labor with the death of nine mothers and 14 infants.[5] A case report has been published, detailing generalized tonic-clonic maternal seizures associated with a reassuring fetal heart rate pattern and normal fetal acid-base status and oxygenation.[6]

Adequate initial treatment with a benzodiazepine is essential to stop and prevent seizures, because phenytoin and phenobarbitone have a longer latency. Tracheal intubation, assisted ventilation, and phenobarbital titration to electroencephalographic (EEG) burst suppression may be required.

Effect of Pregnancy on Epilepsy

Hormonal effects on seizure frequency have been recognized since the late nineteenth century. Estrogen

TABLE 17-3. COLLABORATIVE ECLAMPSIA TRIAL: INTRAVENOUS MAGNESIUM SULFATE THERAPY

Intravenous loading	4 g over 5 min
Intravenous maintenance	1–2 g/hour
If recurring convulsions	2–4 g IV over 5 min

level peaks are related to an increase in seizure frequency, and progesterone is related to anticonvulsant effects. Seizure susceptibility may correlate best with the estrogen/progesterone ratio.[7] Other factors implicated in the interplay between epilepsy and pregnancy are those of increased weight (water and sodium), mild respiratory alkalosis, and psychological stress.[8]

The influence of pregnancy on the frequency of epileptic seizures has been examined by retrospective and prospective studies with varying results. In one prospective study, seizure frequency did not change in 50% of pregnancies, decreased in 13%, and increased in 37%.[9] Therapeutic drug noncompliance, sleep deprivation (68%), and inadequate medication (47%) were postulated as the determinants of the course of epilepsy in pregnancy. Another prospective report of 154 pregnancies showed a 14% decrease, 32% increase, and 23% unchanged seizure frequency, with 31% being seizure free during pregnancy and 3 months post partum.[10] Gjerde showed no statistical difference between seizure frequency before and during pregnancy.[11] Reasons cited for these other differences are potential interpretive problems in previous prospective studies of accurate evaluation of seizure severity and frequency; lack of nonpregnant controls; and variations in AED treatment before and during pregnancy in some patients.

Plasma concentrations of AEDs fall during pregnancy. Reasons for this decrease include less patient compliance (due to possible anxiety and missed doses in labor); absorption and protein binding; and an increase in volume of distribution, hepatic and renal clearance, and body weight.[12] Folic acid supplementation may also result in lowered AED levels. Maternal folate deficiency has been linked to spontaneous abortion, placental abruption, and fetal malformations, and folate should be prescribed at the first antenatal visit.

The unbound (free) portion of the AED is biologically active, and it is the unbound level of drug, rather than its total level, that is related to seizure control and toxicity development. Ideally, the unbound level should be established before conception and the medication regimen modified to achieve monotherapy. Free drug levels should be measured monthly during the first and second trimesters and then every 2 weeks in the third trimester. Close monitoring of serum levels, with dose adjustment after delivery, identifies the rebound increases that can occur despite no change in drug dosing.[8]

Effect of Epilepsy on Pregnancy

People who suffer from epilepsy may have a lower fertility rate. Anovulatory cycles have been reported, and there is evidence that tonic-clonic and partial seizures can cause a raised prolactin level. AEDs also affect the hypothalamic-pituitary axis.[7]

Several studies suggest that pregnancies of epileptic mothers display an increase in complications and adverse outcomes. These problems include hyperemesis, vaginal bleeding, pre-eclampsia, premature labor, postpartum hemorrhage, and higher obstetric intervention rates.[12] Other studies show no difference in outcomes as compared with those in nonepileptic patients.[13] Reasons proposed for nonconcordance of study results include difficulty in assessing spontaneous miscarriage rates, bias in the reporting of vaginal bleeding, difficulty in differentiating between an epileptic and eclamptic seizure, and higher induction rate resulting in preterm deliveries (<37-week gestation).

Loss of fetal heart rate variability due to AEDs may lead to a diagnosis of fetal compromise and an alteration of delivery management. AEDs, which are membrane stabilizers, may increase the duration of labor and the incidence of vaginal bleeding by decreasing the strength of uterine contractions and decreasing the coagulation factors and platelet number and function.[8]

Effect of Epilepsy on the Fetus and Neonate

The effects of maternal epilepsy on the fetus and neonate may be due to the condition itself, AED use, or a combination of both. Seizures during pregnancy expose the fetus to the risk of blunt trauma, hypoxia, and acidosis with the potential sequelae of neurologic damage and intrauterine death. Status epilepticus requires rapid intervention and carries the risk of maternal and fetal death.

Phenobarbitone may increase the incidence of nonreactive, nonstress test results. Intravenous diazepam causes loss of baseline variability within 2 minutes of administration (lasting 1 hour without acidosis, as determined with fetal vein pH). Long-term anticonvulsant therapy is associated with an increase in breech presentation, possibly from a lowering of the frequency or strength of fetal limb movements and hence an inhibition of spontaneous version.[8]

The application of a fetal scalp electrode carries a potential risk of bleeding by an effect of AEDs on fetal blood coagulation. Hemorrhagic disease of the newborn is a potentially life-threatening vitamin K–deficiency disorder in infants born to mothers taking AEDs. Vitamin K supplements are recommended in the last month of pregnancy.

All AEDs are found in breast milk, with the amount related to the degree of plasma protein binding. Barbiturates, primidone, ethosuccimide, and benzodiazepines have the highest concentrations in breast milk, whereas phenytoin and valproate are lower. Lethargy and poor breast-feeding in the neonate indicate the need to change to bottle feeding to prevent toxicity, especially in the preterm infant or the infant in the

early neonatal period.[13] Clonazepam and diazepam are associated with lethargy, hypotonia, and apnea in neonates because the half-life is two to four times longer than in adults.[14] Apnea monitoring and observing the infants for signs of drug withdrawal are recommended.[13, 15]

A twofold increase (to 6%) is seen in the incidence of congenital malformations. Reported malformations include orofacial cleft, congenital heart defect, microcephaly, mental retardation, distal limb hypoplasia, and nail dysplasia. AEDs are implicated in teratogenesis, but the contribution from a genetic component related to epilepsy is also postulated. Children of epileptic fathers have increases in malformations similar to those of children born to epileptic mothers. The term *fetal hydantoin syndrome* has been coined, but the abnormalities are also linked to barbiturates. Abnormalities due to trimethadione are more serious, with high rates of malformation and stillbirth.[17] Valproic acid therapy in pregnancy carries a 1% risk of neural tube defects.[17]

Obstetric Management

Pregnancies in epileptic mothers are regarded as high-risk. The obstetrician and neurologist ideally should begin management of the patient before she conceives. If the mother fulfills the criteria, anticonvulsant drug withdrawal or monotherapy is the goal. This adjustment has the advantages of minimal drug exposure for the fetus and the least-possible medication to control seizures in the mother. Phenytoin, barbiturate, or carbamazepine are recommended. Obstetric management goals include the abolition of seizures during pregnancy and delivery and the birth of a healthy infant (Table 17–4).

The consequences of seizures are fetomaternal hyp-

TABLE 17–4. **MANAGEMENT OF THE EPILEPTIC IN PREGNANCY**

Preconception

Counseling
Withdraw AEDs, if appropriate
    If seizure-free
    If normal EEG
Or try to achieve monotherapy (avoid trimethadione and valproic acid)
Establish and maintain therapeutic drug levels

Postconception

Counseling
Maintain AED regimen
Monitor free drug levels regularly
Vitamin supplements
    Folic acid 1 mg daily
    Vitamin K 5–10 mg/day (from 36 wks)

Peripartum

Parenteral anticonvulsants

oxia and acidosis, whereas status epilepticus is a life-threatening event for both mother and fetus.

Counseling the epileptic mother is necessary to ensure compliance with medication and provide information on fetal malformation rates. Breast-feeding is not contraindicated unless the infant shows signs of lethargy. Possible infant withdrawal symptoms should be discussed.

Anticonvulsant drug levels must be maintained throughout labor. Intravenous administration may be necessary owing to decreased gastrointestinal absorption. Loss of fetal heart rate variability with AEDs, fetal bradycardia with prolonged recovery following a grand mal seizure in labor, maternal postictal drowsiness, and CNS depression with rapid intravenous control of seizures make the epileptic mother a potential candidate for obstetric intervention. Maternal epilepsy, however, is not synonymous with operative delivery.

Suggested criteria for emergency cesarean section specific for the epileptic parturient include generalized seizures during labor, threat of fetal asphyxia, and lack of active participation in labor due to drowsiness. Elective cesarean section may be indicated if there is a neurologic deficit with inability to cooperate, deterioration in seizure control late in the third trimester, or history of seizures during heavy physical exercise or mental stress (Table 17–5).

Anesthetic Management

When considering the anesthetic implications of maternal epilepsy, clinicians must be aware of the many potential drug interactions that may occur. Clinicians must also consider how the antiepileptic medication modifies standard anesthetic techniques and how anesthetic drugs and techniques interact with the epileptic condition. Phenobarbitone and phenytoin are probably the most commonly prescribed anticonvulsants, and both are active inducers of microsomal enzymes. Enzyme induction affects AED metabolism and enhances breakdown of other substances such as narcotics, neuromuscular blocking drugs, and volatile anesthetic agents. Hence, hepatic enzyme induction by AEDs has the potential to affect drug dosing and production of toxic metabolites (e.g., fluoride ions from enflurane and sevoflurane).

TABLE 17–5. **CRITERIA FOR CESAREAN SECTION IN THE EPILEPTIC PARTURIENT**

Elective	Emergency
Neurologic deficit	Generalized seizure in labor
Deterioration in third-trimester seizure control	Threat of fetal asphyxia
Occurrence of seizures with exercise and stress	Maternal somnolence and lack of cooperation in labor

Phenobarbitone, a CNS depressant, decreases the dose requirements for induction and maintenance of anesthesia and increases the susceptibility to the respiratory depressant effects of opioids. Some anesthetic agents, such as enflurane, are epileptogenic, particularly in the presence of hypocapnia. Methohexital, ketamine, etomidate, and aliphatic phenothiazines are also epileptogenic. Tricyclic antidepressants lower the seizure threshold. Opioids cause neuroexcitatory phenomena in animals but not in humans. Meperidine, but more so its metabolite normeperidine, with its long half-life, can cause CNS excitability. Laudanosine, a metabolite of atracurium, can be epileptogenic, but this is unlikely to occur in humans. Propofol (not yet approved for obstetric use) has been implicated in epileptogenesis, with myoclonic activity and opisthotonos during clinical use. The amide local anesthetics, in low concentrations, are anticonvulsant, but in high concentrations (plasma lidocaine level $\geq$ 10 μg/ml) cause convulsions. The action of nondepolarizing neuromuscular blockers may be enhanced by concomitant AEDs. Yet, with long-term phenytoin, there may be resistance to pancuronium, vecuronium, and perhaps, d-tubocurarine, but not to atracurium.

The anesthesiologist must consider the side effects of AEDs. Phenytoin may cause gingival hyperplasia, osteomalacia, gastrointestinal symptoms, lupus-like reactions, and hepatocellular sensitivity reactions. Depletion and altered metabolism of folate can cause megaloblastic anemia or peripheral neuropathy. Other hematologic reactions include leukopenia, anemia, and, rarely, agranulocytosis and aplastic anemia. Barbiturates may cause rash, osteomalacia (vitamin D responsive), hypoprothrombinemia, megaloblastic anemia, and peripheral neuropathy related to folate deficiency. Carbamazepine side effects include rash, lymphadenopathy, and splenomegaly. An antidiuretic hormone (ADH) effect may induce water retention, producing emesis and mental confusion. Carbamazepine can also cause transient and sometimes persistent leukopenia, and, rarely, agranulocytosis and aplastic anemia may be life-threatening.[19, 20]

Anesthesia and Analgesia During Labor

Cooperation of obstetrician, neurologist, and anesthesiologist is emphasized. The prevention and prompt treatment of intrapartum seizures and the provision of effective labor analgesia to reduce potentially seizure-provoking anxiety and hyperventilation are the goals of anesthesia care. Evaluation should be carried out with emphasis on the adequacy of control, the side effects of therapy, the patient's mental and physical ability to cooperate, and the proposed obstetric management.

Inhalational and parenteral opioid analgesia can be used. The dose may require modification to prevent augmentation of CNS depression in the parturient already partially sedated from anticonvulsants such as diazepam. Epidural analgesia instituted within the accepted guidelines provides superior pain relief. In my opinion, coagulation assessment is indicated before instituting an epidural block. *[The editors are of the opinion that in the absence of clinical evidence of a coagulopathy, or other risk factors, a full coagulation evaluation is unwarranted.]* Epidural analgesia should be established incrementally to avoid high plasma concentrations of local anesthetic, and an infusion of dilute local anesthetic should be titrated to maintain a T8–10 block throughout labor. Early detection of intravascular migration of the epidural catheter is especially pertinent in these patients to avoid high local anesthetic plasma levels, which can induce seizures.

Anesthesia for Cesarean Section

Cesarean section may be elective or emergent. The choice of general or regional anesthesia is determined by the combination of maternal, fetal, and obstetric factors. Postictal and drug-induced somnolence and status epilepticus mandate general anesthesia, recognizing the potential interaction between anesthetic agents and AEDs and the need to protect the airway.

Regional anesthesia is appropriate for elective cesarean section in a patient who is medically stable. Epidural anesthesia may be the preferred technique, however, because there is a questionable association between spinal anesthesia and potentiation of seizure activity.[21] Despite the many potential problems facing the pregnant epileptic woman, most have a stable gestational course and deliver a healthy infant.

THE COMATOSE PARTURIENT

Coma is the term used to describe a state of unconsciousness from which a person cannot be aroused. A multitude of etiologies exist, all of which may complicate pregnancy and pose great threat to the mother and fetus (Table 17–6). Further along the continuum of CNS deficits are the entities of chronic vegetative state and brain death, which pose many dilemmas, especially when considered in the context of a viable pregnancy.

Principles of Management of Coma in Pregnancy

The immediate goal is prevention of further nervous system damage. Hypotension, hypoglycemia, hypoxia, hypercapnia, and hypothermia should be rapidly corrected, and seizures should be controlled. The unconscious parturient is at risk from gastric regurgitation

TABLE 17–6. DIFFERENTIAL DIAGNOSIS OF COMA

Intracranial	Extracranial
Vascular	*Hypotension*
Hemorrhage	Hemorrhage
Subarachnoid	Myocardial infarct
Intracerebral	Septic shock
Infarction	*Hypertension*
Thrombus	Encephalopathy
Embolus	Eclampsia
Vasculitis	*Metabolic*
Tumor	Endocrine
Hemorrhage	Hepatic
Edema	Renal
Abscess	Hypoxia
Hemorrhage	Hypercarbia
Edema	*Drugs/Toxins*
Infection	*Physical*
Meningitis	Hypothermia
Encephalitis	Electrocution
Trauma	
Edema	
Hemorrhage	
Subdural	
Extradural	
Intracerebral	
Epilepsy	
Postictal	
Status epilepticus	

and aspiration pneumonitis and requires endotracheal intubation as a matter of urgency, if cyanosis and hypoventilation are not corrected with supplemental oxygen. The maternal condition may allow rapid neurologic assessment before administration of anesthetic agents to facilitate endotracheal intubation. Left uterine displacement must be provided. Fetal viability should be assessed as soon as possible after maternal stabilization.

Results of patient history and a thorough clinical examination with neurologic and laboratory evaluation indicate the possible need for neuroimaging techniques such as CT scanning, MRI, MR angiography, and conventional angiography. Appropriate maternal abdominal shielding is required. An accurate diagnosis allows for development of an individualized, definitive management plan, utilizing a multidisciplinary approach. Input from the indicated medical and paramedical specialties is necessary to provide multifaceted care.

In general, neurosurgical considerations dictate management in the case of life-threatening intracranial hemorrhage. Obstetric decisions, however, are based on fetal viability. In mothers with Hunt and Hess grades IV and V post-subarachnoid hemorrhage, supportive intensive care is preferred to early repair.[22] Brain tumors, especially meningiomas, may increase in size during pregnancy. Symptomatology and time of presentation depend on tumor location. Subsequently, the outcome for the fetus is determined by the individual circumstances. If the fetus is viable and neurosurgical intervention mandatory, cesarean section before craniotomy may be indicated (Chapter 16).[23] Steroids may be administered to enhance fetal lung maturity.

Cortical venous thrombosis (CVT) may occur during pregnancy or puerperium in the setting of venous stasis, hypercoagulability, and/or endothelial injury. CVT may be mistaken for eclampsia (or may be associated with it) or aneurysmal rupture. Increased intracranial pressure (ICP) is present as a result of impaired cerebral spinal fluid absorption related to venous obstruction. Treatment with anticoagulants may cause intracranial bleeding (if cerebral infarction is present) or uterine bleeding in the puerperal period. Management of patients with CVT involves supportive therapy and anti-seizure medications. The patients usually recover rapidly and spontaneously without neurologic sequelae.[24, 25]

Hypoglycemic coma, not associated with insulin therapy, is rare in pregnancy, chiefly because pregnancy confers insulin resistance. Insulinoma may be diagnosed with simultaneous determination of plasma glucose, insulin, and C-peptide levels in the fasting state. In one case report, treatment consisted of 50% glucose infusion and supportive care until a pancreatic tumor was excised post partum.[26]

Another rare cause of hypoglycemia in pregnancy is lymphocytic hypophysitis, causing anterior pituitary deficiency in the absence of a radiographically identifiable pituitary tumor or neurofibroma. In one report, treatment consisted of an initial 50% glucose infusion with good response followed by thyroxine and cortisol replacement—once the diagnosis of panhypopituitarism was established.[27]

Prolonged maternal hypoglycemia may cause precipitous fetal compromise. During short-lived maternal hypoglycemia the fetal heart rate pattern changes, displaying acceleration-deceleration patterns and nonreactive tachycardia with return to a fully reactive tracing and normal baseline reading with treatment.[28]

Anesthetic Management

The anesthetic care of the parturient with raised ICP follows the same general guidelines as those of the nonpregnant patient. The hypertensive response to laryngoscopy and intubation should be obtunded, cerebral perfusion pressure maintained, and ICP reduced by the usual well-accepted pharmacologic and physical methods. Direct blood pressure monitoring is recommended.

Additional factors to consider include avoidance of supine hypotension and relative contraindication to succinylcholine. The normal arterial Pco_2 at term is already 28 to 32 mm Hg, and further reduction may decrease placental blood flow. Control of brain edema with mannitol may produce fetal and amniotic dehy-

dration. Dexamethasone and furosemide can be given. Fetal heart rate should be monitored throughout the perianesthetic period.

Management of Maternal Vegetative State and Brain Death

A chronic vegetative state is defined as a subacute or chronic condition that sometimes occurs after brain injury and consists of a return of wakefulness accompanied by an apparent total lack of cognitive function. The vital functions of respiration, blood pressure, and thermal regulation are retained and may be subject to periods of overactivity.

Brain death results from total cessation of cerebral blood flow at a time when cardiorespiratory function remains preserved by artificial life support. It is a diagnosis made according to strict criteria. Brainstem and hypothalamic centers do not function, resulting in a lack of spontaneous respiration, hypotension, hypothermia, and panhypopituitarism, including diabetes insipidus with concomitant treatment problems.

Somatic survival can be maintained for a long period (usually much shorter in the case of brain death). If the maternal condition is stable, intrauterine fetal maturation and development can proceed. Fetal growth assessment by serial ultrasound examinations and sequential biophysical profile scores are used as indices of fetal well-being. Such examinations also aid detection of major congenital malformations.

Supportive intensive care includes respiratory support, ranging from tracheobronchial toilet to mechanical ventilation (mandatory in brain death); hemodynamic monitoring and cardiovascular support; nutritional support (enterally or parenterally) appropriate to the caloric requirements of pregnancy; maintenance of body temperature; treatment of infection; physiotherapy; and thromboembolism prophylaxis. The timing of delivery, often by classic cesarean section, is determined by maternal condition and fetal maturity. Betamethasone may be administered to stimulate lung maturation, if indicated.

Case reports in the literature outline scenarios and management issues. Fulminant subacute sclerosing panencephalitis (SSPE) is a rare cause of rapid neurologic deterioration culminating in a vegetative state. Pregnancy as a state of natural immunosuppression was suggested as the trigger for the delayed onset and fulminant course of this measles-virus–associated, progressive, fatal disease in two pregnant women. One mother developed the disease post partum, whereas the other became ill at week 14 and stuporous 2 weeks later. Supportive and intensive obstetric care was provided, and cesarean section was performed after the onset of spontaneous labor at 33 weeks' gestation.[29]

The management of a pregnant patient with irreversible anoxic brain damage who is in a persistent vegetative state from 14 weeks' gestation until delivery at 34 weeks by cesarean section is described by Hill and coworkers.[30] Management issues in this case included seizure control, respiratory support, enteral feeding, antidysrhythmic therapy, hyperthermia control, and fetal monitoring with biophysical profile scoring and lung maturity assessment. They stressed a team approach to decision-making with each case being assessed individually with regard to the likelihood of maternal survival and fetal prognosis with continued life support.[30]

CONCLUSIONS

Advances in intensive care, life-support systems, and neonatology make possible the continuation of pregnancy in the vegetative-state or brain-dead parturient. Moral and ethical problems abound regarding withdrawal of support from the vegetative-state mother post partum. No rules can be made. Each case must be assessed individually and with liaison among family members, legal advisors, ethicists, and members of the multidisciplinary care team.

Questions regarding consent and cessation of treatment, planned cesarean section, and perimortem cesarean section are complex and require medicolegal solutions.

References

1. Martin JB, Ruskin J. Faintness, syncope and seizures. In Isselbacher KJ, Braunwald E, Wilson JD, Martin JB, Fauci AS, Kasper DL (eds): Harrison's Principles of Internal Medicine, 13th ed. New York, McGraw-Hill, 1994, p 90.
2. Rubenstein D, Wayne D. Neurology. In Lecture Notes on Clinical Medicine, 4th ed. Oxford, Blackwell Scientific Publications, 1990, p 113.
3. Kaplan PW, Repke JT. Eclampsia. Neurol Clin 1994;12:565.
4. Eclampsia Trial Collaborative Group. Which anticonvulsant for women with eclampsia? Evidence from the Collaborative Eclampsia Trial. Lancet 1995;345:1455.
5. Teramo K, Hiilesmaa VK. Pregnancy and fetal complications in epileptic pregnancies: A review of the literature. In Janz D, Bossi L, Dam M, et al (eds): Epilepsy, Pregnancy and the Child. New York, Raven Press, 1982, p 53.
6. Goetting MG, Davidson BN. Status epilepticus during labor. A case report. J Reprod Med 1987;32:313.
7. Mattson RH, Cramer JA. Epilepsy, sex hormones and antiepileptic drugs. Epilepsia 1985;26:S40.
8. Robertson IG. Prescribing in pregnancy. Epilepsy in pregnancy. Clin Obstet Gynecol 1986;13:365.
9. Schmidt D, Canger R, Avanzini G, et al. Change of seizure frequency in pregnant epileptic women. J Neurol Neurosurg Psychiatry 1983;46:751.
10. Bardy AH. Incidence of seizures during pregnancy, labor and puerperium in epileptic women: A prospective study. Acta Neurol Scand 1937;75:356.
11. Gjerde IO, Strandjord RE, Ulstein M. The course of epilepsy during pregnancy: A study of 78 cases. Acta Neurol Scand 1988;78:198.
12. Yerby MS. Problems and management of the pregnant woman with epilepsy. Epilepsia 1987;28:S29.
13. Rayburn WF, Lavin JP Jr. Drug prescribing for chronic medical disorders during pregnancy: An overview. Am J Obstet Gynecol 1986;155:565.
14. Shelton RC, Ebert MH. Drugs and the Central Nervous System. In Wood M, Wood AJJ (eds): Drugs and Anesthesia. Pharmacology for Anesthesiologists, 2nd ed. Baltimore, Williams & Wilkins, 1990, p 586.
15. Fisher JB, Edgren BE, Mammel MC, et al. Neonatal apnea associated with maternal clonazepam therapy. A case report. Obstet Gynecol 1985;66:S34.
16. Clifford DB. Seizures and pregnancy. Am Fam Physician 1984;29:271.
17. Garden AS, Benzie RJ, Hutton EM, et al. Valproic acid therapy and neural tube defects. Case reports. Can Med Assoc J 1985;132:933.
18. Hiilesmaa VK, Bardy A, Teramo K. Obstetric outcome in women with epilepsy. Am J Obstet Gynecol 1985;152:499.
19. Shelton RC, Ebert MH. Drugs and the Central Nervous System. In Wood M, Wood AJJ (eds). Drugs and Anesthesia. Pharmacology for Anesthesiologists, 2nd ed. Baltimore, Williams & Wilkins, 1990, p 592.
20. Drummond JC, Shapiro HM. Cerebral Physiology. In Miller RD (ed). Anesthesia, 3rd ed, vol 1. New York, Churchill Livingstone, 1990, p 638.
21. Aravapalli R, Abouleish E, Aldrete JA. Anesthetic implications in the parturient epileptic patient. Anesth Analg 1988;67:S3.
22. Raps EC, Galetta SL, Flamm ES. Neurointensive care of the pregnant woman. Neurol Clin 1994;12:601.
23. DeGrood RM, Beemer WH, Fenner DE, et al. A large meningioma presenting as a neurologic emergency in late pregnancy. Obstet Gynecol 1987;69:439.
24. Ravindran RS, Zandstra GC, Viegas J. Postpartum headache following regional analgesia; a symptom of cerebral venous thrombosis. Can J Anaesth 1989;36:705.
25. Younker D, Jones MM, Adenwala J, et al. Maternal cortical vein thrombosis and the obstetric anesthesiologist. Anesth Analg 1986;65:1007.
26. Galun E, Ben-Yehuda A, Berlatzki J, et al. Insulinoma complicating pregnancy: Case report and review of the literature. Am J Obstet Gynecol 1986;155:64.
27. Notterman RB, Jovanovic L, Peterson R, et al. Spontaneous hypoglycemic seizures in pregnancy. A manifestation of panhypopituitarism. Arch Intern Med 1984;144:189.
28. Confino E, Ismajovich B, Menachem PD. Fetal heart rate in maternal hypoglycemic coma. Int J Gynaecol Obstet 1985;23:59.
29. Wirguin I, Steiner I, Kidron D, et al. Fulminant subacute sclerosing panencephalitis in association with pregnancy. Arch Neurol 1988;45:1324.
30. Hill LM, Parker D, O'Neill BP. Management of maternal vegetative state during pregnancy. Mayo Clin Proc 1985;60:469.

SPINAL CORD INJURY, SPINA BIFIDA, TETHERED CORD SYNDROME, AND ANTERIOR SPINAL ARTERY SYNDROME

. . . .

Roanne Preston, M.D., and Edward T. Crosby, M.D.

Patients with diseases of the spinal cord may present in obstetric units, although not commonly. Patients with spinal cord injuries and spina bifida present more frequently in obstetric practice as a result of the improved surgical techniques and rehabilitation therapy in recent decades. Tethered cord syndrome in adults is now a well-recognized entity. Although rare, it may be seen in an obstetric patient. Anterior spinal artery syndrome remains mainly a disease of older patients, although the use of neuraxial epinephrine has been implicated in some cases in younger patients.

SPINAL CORD INJURY

The incidence of spinal cord injury (SCI) is 25 to 30 in 1 million population in North America. The majority of the victims are young, and in Canada 20% of them are female.[1, 2] Advances in acute and rehabilitation care have led to improvements in outcomes, with victims able to attain higher levels of independent function after SCI than was previously possible. Rehabilitation emphasizes integration back into society. Cord-injured patients are encouraged to work, establish relationships, and begin or continue families.

Pregnancy in patients with spinal cord injury is therefore no longer as rare. Following the injury there is a period of amenorrhea of 3 to 9 months.[3] The average time to pregnancy following SCI is 4 to 13 years, but the average age at pregnancy and time interval since injury have been decreasing.[3–5] Since the first published case report of successful pregnancy in a quadriplegic in 1953, there have been numerous articles on care of the pregnant SCI patient.[6] The majority of the literature involves chronic spinal cord injury, although there are some reports on management of the patient with acute spinal injury during pregnancy.[7–12] Appropriate management decisions in providing care to parturients with SCI are dependent on knowledge of (1) the pathophysiology of spinal cord injury and (2) the impact of pregnancy on the medical complications of spinal injury.

Acute Spinal Injury

Pregnant women constitute less than 1% of the total admissions for acute injury to trauma centers.[7] Acute spinal injuries incurred during pregnancy are uncommon. The injuries often lead to fetal loss, however, with a high incidence of miscarriages, stillbirths, and fetal abnormalities (14/45 cases in a review from the 1970s).[8, 9] Patients in the second trimester have the worst outcomes, in part because of the uterine trauma resulting in placental abruption or direct fetal trauma.[8–12] If the fetus remains viable, two approaches to the management of the mother with spinal cord injury have been advocated. Enforced bed rest with spinal immobilization until the fetus reaches a viable age and then combined cesarean section and spinal stabilization at one surgery have constituted one approach. The risks of prolonged bed rest including thromboembolic phenomenon and acquired secondary neurologic injury may favor early surgical intervention. With early intervention, there are concerns about the impact on the fetus of prolonged surgery in the prone position and about the potential hemodynamic instability occurring from spinal shock. Because of the small number of cases reported, the actual risk of preterm labor is unknown.[3, 13, 14] Unstable thoracolumbar fractures invariably require early surgical stabilization, and body braces may compromise the growing fetus.

The initial phase of acute spinal cord injury, lasting 3 to 6 weeks, is known as *spinal shock*. This period of spinal shock is due to the sudden interruption of suprasegmental descending neurons, which normally keep spinal motor neurons in a continuous state of readiness.[15] Spinal shock is characterized by flaccid paralysis below the level of the lesion and loss of all sensory modalities, temperature regulation, and spinal reflexes (tendon and autonomic). Cardiovascular effects include hypotension (possibly severe), bradycardia with high thoracic lesions, and dysrhythmias. Because of absent vasomotor tone, the extremities lose heat rapidly if left exposed, and they develop dependent edema. A prolonged period of paralytic ileus may be observed. Cervical lesions at C2 to C4 usually mandate ventilatory support for a prolonged period or permanently whereas lower cervical lesions may require ventilation initially until the thoracic cage muscles recover function. During the acute-injury phase, patients with high thoracic lesions may have significant impairment of the ability to cough or clear the airway of secretions. Patients are thereby highly susceptible to aspiration and pneumonia.

Treatment of spinal shock includes high-dose steroids, surgical stabilization of fractures, and supportive care in intensive care units. Following the stage of flaccid paralysis, SCI patients usually develop exaggerated reflexes with muscle spasms, upper motor neuron–injury pattern tendon reflexes, and autonomic hyperreflexia.

Medical Complications in Chronic Cord Injury

Following the initial period of spinal shock (3–6 weeks), the situation stabilizes as chronic spinal cord injury. Most neurologic improvement is made early, usually in the first year after injury, although some patients continue to make slow progress over the subsequent few years.[15, 16] Patients with cervical and high thoracic levels of injury typically have impaired pulmonary function with decreased respiratory reserve. Pulmonary sequelae result in poor cough and recurrent infections. Chronic or recurrent urinary tract infection with calculi formation may lead to deterioration in renal function. Deep vein thrombosis and decubitus ulcers remain persistent concerns in the wheelchair-bound patient. Anemia of chronic disease is common, but the use of iron supplements may cause deterioration in bowel function. Many SCI patients have low blood pressure on the basis of low blood volume as well as impaired capacitance vessel function.[17]

Pregnancy may aggravate many of these conditions (Table 18–1). Anemia is worsened, and the risk of deep vein thrombosis is enhanced. The respiratory changes of pregnancy include further loss of functional residual capacity and expiratory reserve volume that compromises cough mechanics. The expanding uterus limits diaphragm excursion; this is particularly important in the patient with cervical cord injury who may be entirely dependent on the diaphragm for respiratory function. Labor normally puts an enormous demand

TABLE 18–1. MEDICAL COMPLICATIONS OF SPINAL CORD INJURY AGGRAVATED BY PREGNANCY

Pulmonary
  Decreased respiratory reserve
  Atelectasis and pneumonia
  Impaired cough
Hematologic
  Anemia
  Thromboembolic phenomenon
Urogenital
  Chronic urinary tract infections
  Proteinuria
  Renal insufficiency
  Urinary tract calculi
Dermatologic
  Decubitus ulcers
Cardiovascular
  Hypotension
  Autonomic hyperreflexia

From Crosby ET, St. Jean B, Reid D, et al. Obstetrical anaesthesia and analgesia in chronic spinal cord-injured women. Can J Anaesth 1992;39:489.

on ventilation, and it may actually cause acute diaphragmatic fatigue.[18–21] Although this fatigue is not reflected in a clinical deterioration in the normal parturient, labor may not be tolerated in the respiratory-compromised SCI parturient. Much of the increased minute ventilation in labor is precipitated by the pain of parturition. Patients with high cord injuries may be spared both the pain and the resultant increased ventilatory demands.

As weight increases and ligaments become more lax, transfers may become more difficult. Decubitus ulcers may result as the parturient becomes less mobile with advancing gestation. Pregnancy predisposes her to more urinary stasis, which results in increased urinary tract infection (UTI) rates.[4, 22] Intermittent catheterizations result in less morbidity than indwelling bladder catheters, but the frequency may have to be increased as gestation advances. Orthostatic changes in blood pressure may be augmented by the decreased systemic vascular resistance that results from the hormonal changes of pregnancy, and such changes may produce symptoms.

Management of the Parturient with Chronic Spinal Cord Injury

Antepartum and Medical Management

Patients with chronic spinal cord injuries should have a medical assessment before conception to determine their ability to tolerate the pregnancy medically. Many SCI patients take medications for spasticity such as baclofen and diazepam. The safety of baclofen in pregnancy has not been established. Withdrawal of these drugs should be over several days to prevent increased spasticity. Diazepam has been associated with an increased incidence of lip and palate malformations,[23] although further studies dispute this.[24] Fetal benzodiazepine syndrome, however, has been described, which includes growth retardation, dysmorphism, and CNS dysfunction.[25] In view of this finding, benzodiazepines should be stopped before conception. Pulmonary function needs to be evaluated early in pregnancy to identify those at risk of respiratory deterioration.[26] Pulmonary function tests are recommended, and respiratory consultation should be sought if there is evidence of significant compromise in pulmonary function.[1] Some patients may actually require ventilator assistance during late pregnancy. Negative-pressure ventilators are ideally suited to this task. Smoking does much to enhance the morbid potential of pregnancy in SCI parturients, and every effort to dissuade the patient from smoking should be made.

Obstetric Management

The most common problems encountered during pregnancy in SCI patients are UTIs (80%), anemia (30–60%), and pressure sores (26%).[1] Preterm labor may be more common in SCI parturients, and unattended delivery may occur because of the difficulty of ascertaining when labor has begun in the absence of painful contractions. An increased need arises for second-stage instrumentation and assisted delivery.[3, 4, 22, 27–30] Earlier reports of a high incidence of fetal malformations[30, 31] and prematurity have not been confirmed in subsequent literature.[27–29]

Obstetric management begins with the assessment of pelvic adequacy. Patients who suffered the injury before puberty should have this assessment early in the pregnancy.[1, 26] If the pelvis is deemed to be adequate, vaginal delivery should be anticipated, although there is an increased requirement for assisted delivery because of the loss of abdominal musculature needed for expulsive efforts.[5, 32] Preterm labor is treated with β_2 agonists and magnesium sulfate.[1, 29, 30] A risk of precipitating respiratory failure arises with magnesium sulfate in the susceptible patient because of its muscle relaxation effects.[33] Because of the risk of painless labor in patients with high injury levels, weekly cervical examinations are performed after 28 weeks, with hospitalization if cervical dilation occurs.[1] Some centers have routine admission at 36 to 37 weeks to prevent unattended delivery.[27] Consensus exists that cesarean section be reserved for obstetric indications. During labor, specific nursing care for SCI should continue, such as frequent turning to prevent pressure sores and providing optimal bladder care. Education from nurses about pregnancy and SCI is very important for the patient's physical and mental well-being during labor.

The most dangerous complication during labor and delivery is autonomic hyperreflexia (AH). Failure to identify patients at risk and provide appropriate prophylaxis and treatment for episodes of AH remains an important medical and legal issue.[1, 3, 22] The American College of Obstetricians and Gynecologists (ACOG) guidelines published in 1993 recommend early initiation of epidural block to prevent AH in those patients at high risk.[1] If epidural block is not available immediately, the guidelines recommend that vasodilator treatment be initiated. If induction of labor is planned, patients at high risk for AH should have epidural block initiated before induction commences.[1, 2, 30] Ergotamine in the third stage should be avoided because of the potential of precipitating autonomic hyperreflexia.[27]

No evidence of an increased incidence of pre-eclampsia exists in this patient population.[1, 26, 34]

Anesthetic Management

Problems in SCI patients of relevance to the anesthesiologist include (1) an increased incidence of premature labor and painless, precipitous labor; (2) a need for pain relief in labor; (3) an occurrence of muscle spasms in labor; and (4) a frequent requirement for assisted delivery. Prophylaxis must be given for autonomic hyperreflexia. Hyperkalemia with succinylcholine use in patients with subacute injury is an additional concern. Antepartum anesthesia consultation is encouraged and should be routine for parturients with SCI.[28] During this visit, the likely requirements and options for analgesia, including the risks and benefits, may be discussed. Patients with an injury level below T10 are likely to experience normal labor pain. Patients with incomplete levels between T6 and T10 may not experience typical labor pain, but they may be subject to extreme leg and abdominal spasms with contractions. Patients with complete injury levels above T5 have painless labor but are at high risk for autonomic hyperreflexia, whereas those with complete level between T5 and T10 are at low risk.

Autonomic hyperreflexia, or the mass autonomic response, was first reported in 1890, but was not well described until 1954.[35] AH is a life-threatening reflex caused by a mass sympathetic response to noxious stimuli that is not modulated by the supraspinal influences of the central nuclei.[27, 36] AH is commonly seen in patients with spinal cord injuries whose level of injury is T5 or above (85–90% incidence). AH is less common in patients with lesions between T5 and T8 (50–65%) and is rare with lesions below T8.[37, 38] Most patients have complete lesions.[3] Incomplete lesions allow for craniocaudad neural traffic and the potential for supraspinal modulation of spinal reflexes. This syndrome requires an intact sympathetic system below the level of the lesion, and hence it is not seen in cases of cord infarction.

The reflex is initiated by a noxious stimulus entering the dorsal horn of the spinal cord, passing into sympathetic neurons in the intermediolateral columns of the lateral horns. These sympathetic neurons travel to the paraspinal sympathetic chain and allow for propagation of these impulses cephalad, caudad, and peripherally. A large sympathetic outpouring causes vasoconstriction and visceral spasm. In those spinal levels above the lesion, which are influenced by supraspinal modulation, reflex and compensatory vasodilation occurs. If the lesion is above the midthoracic level, however, there is insufficient vasodilator reserve to counteract the vasoconstriction; therefore, severe systemic hypertension occurs. Baroreceptor response to the hypertension results in centrally mediated bradycardia and vasodilation above the lesion level.[37, 39, 40] Clinical signs and symptoms include severe hypertension, bradycardia, sweating, blurred vision, increased skin temperature, facial flushing, and nasal congestion.[2] Reported morbidity resulting from the hypertension has included retinal hemorrhage, intracranial hemorrhage,[33, 40] hypertensive encephalopathy,[40] seizure,[3] atrioventricular (AV) conduction abnormalities including sinus arrest,[39, 41] fetal arrhythmia, and uteroplacental insufficiency leading to fetal hypoxemia.[1]

Many patients at risk for autonomic hyperreflexia give a history of AH episodes with visceral (bladder or rectal) overdistension. Labor is a potent stimulus, however, and AH may be precipitated for the first time with parturition.[3, 42, 43] Maximal noxious stimulation occurs in the perineal region innervated by S2 to S4, and AH may not be present until perineal stretching occurs in the late first stage or early second stage of labor.[27, 39] Other stimuli associated with labor include vaginal examination, instrumentation, amniotomy, and oxytocin infusion.[2] The differential diagnosis is pre-eclampsia. The two are usually simple to distinguish clinically because of the sudden onset of AH. Hypertension is often episodic in AH, coinciding with contractions. In addition, the lack of nondependent edema and proteinuria characteristic of pre-eclampsia helps support the diagnosis.

Several options are available for treating AH during labor. Early reports recommended the combined use of anxiolytics with antihypertensives.[22] Blood pressure control was not optimal, but there was no morbidity attributable to the AH. Labor analgesia was not thought to be necessary in most SCI patients. Direct arterial vasodilators such as sodium nitroprusside and hydralazine have been used with varying success, as have calcium channel, ganglionic (trimethaphan), and adrenergic (guanethidine) blocking agents.[1, 44, 45] Hypertension may be episodic in labor-induced AH. Maternal blood pressure may initially be very high during contractions, despite antihypertensive therapy, then very low in the intervening period before onset of the next contraction. Pure β-blocking drugs are not recommended because of potential uterine vessel vasoconstriction. The combined α- and β-blocker labetalol, however, has been given successfully.[27, 41] In-

creasingly, epidural analgesia has become the method of choice for both prophylaxis and treatment of AH in labor.[1, 2, 4, 26, 27, 38, 46–48]

The issue remains as to when to initiate epidural analgesia. Some have proposed that epidural block be initiated when signs of AH are detected. The contrary view is that all patients considered at risk for AH should have prophylactic epidural block initiated at onset of labor or during induction of labor.[1, 2, 27, 38, 44] Given the seriousness of the syndrome and the potential for morbidity resulting from an episode of AH, prevention is the best option. It is prudent to begin with dilute local anesthetic solutions to minimize the hypotensive effects while still providing AH prophylaxis. Bupivacaine has been administered extensively in various concentrations for prevention of AH and provision of labor analgesia. A solution of 0.1 to 0.125% at 8 to 10 ml/hr probably represents a reasonable initial concentration and infusion rate. The concentration or the infusion rate can be increased as needed to control pain or AH. Epidural fentanyl as the sole agent has been ineffective in one case report by Abouleish and coworkers.[49] The role of lipid-soluble opioids has not been determined, but if fentanyl is employed, it should be as an adjunct to a local anesthetic. Intraspinal and epidural meperidine have been given successfully to treat autonomic hyperreflexia.[2, 50] Meperidine has local anesthetic properties and can be employed as a bolus of 1 mg/kg epidurally or 0.25 mg/kg intrathecally.

Careful assessment of the upper level of block is mandatory, as is frequent blood pressure measurement. Invasive monitors are not required routinely but may be in specific situations. Pulse oximetry is recommended in patients with high cord lesions who are receiving neuraxial opioids.

Regional Anesthesia

Neither stable neurologic disease nor major spinal surgery represents absolute contraindication to regional anesthesia. Technical difficulties may be experienced in performing the block in parturients with abnormal anatomy, and there is an increased risk of accidental dural puncture and inadequate and failed blocks.[51] Regional anesthesia may cause significant hypotension in patients who already have low blood pressure because of the combined effects of spinal injury and pregnancy.[50] Patients with SCI are often near-maximally vasodilated as a baseline state. Provided that adequate prehydration (20 ml/kg) is administered before initiation of regional block, blood pressure should remain stable.[2, 17, 38]

Spinal anesthesia can be employed for SCI parturients, with the awareness that it is harder to control anesthesia levels, and hypotension may be more problematic. Some recommend against its use for these reasons.[38] Spinal block does provide consistently better sacral anesthesia than epidural block, however, and this may represent an advantage when good sacral anesthesia is needed.[52]

No consensus exists as to the most appropriate monitors for an SCI patient in labor. Presence of a low baseline blood pressure and the possibility of AH can be used to justify routine invasive hemodynamic monitors (arterial line, central venous pressure).[26, 38] We believe that noninvasive monitoring techniques are adequate in the majority of cases.

Anesthesia for Cesarean Section

The choice of anesthetic technique for cesarean section is influenced not only by maternal condition but also by whether the requirement is for AH prophylaxis alone or with surgical anesthesia. Regional block is primarily required to provide AH prophylaxis through visceral anesthesia in high cord injury (above T5). The relevant somatic nerves no longer function in these cases. A gentle surgical technique should be encouraged to minimize visceral stimulation and reduce the risk of precipitating an AH crisis. Uterine exteriorization should be avoided.

Regional anesthesia is of benefit in the postpartum period by providing good pain relief with neuraxial opioids via epidural catheters that can be left in place. Spinal anesthesia may be technically simpler to perform than epidural anesthesia, but the potential for more severe hypotension and the concern for further impairing respiratory mechanics by a high block are acknowledged.

General anesthesia prevents AH when it is deep enough to prevent response to noxious genitourinary stimuli. Tracheal intubation does not initiate AH. Rapidly acting antihypertensive agents such as sodium nitroprusside and labetalol should be available. There are implications of SCI on neuromuscular relaxant use. Succinylcholine has been associated with massive hyperkalemia when administered between 72 hours after injury and up until 6 months or more after injury. This effect is likely to result from the proliferation of extrajunctional neuromuscular receptors on muscle that has been denervated by the neurologic injury.[32] Nondepolarizing muscle relaxants are recommended for tracheal intubation and maintenance during general anesthesia in all SCI patients during the first year after injury.

Anesthesiologists will see more pregnant patients with spinal cord injuries in the future. These patients have a multitude of chronic problems related to the injury that may affect pregnancy. Preterm labor is not uncommon, and patients may present in advanced stages of labor. Labor analgesia may not be required in many, but those with high-level lesions are at risk of developing autonomic hyperreflexia despite painless labor. Anesthesia personnel must be involved in the care of these parturients. Epidural block is the treatment of choice for avoiding AH.

The patients should be seen in anesthesia consultation ante partum. At that time, a determination of autonomic hyperreflexia risk is made. Arrangements can be made for evaluation of pulmonary function to identify those at risk of respiratory deterioration in pregnancy or labor. A discussion of the requirement for analgesia during labor and the options available can take place at this visit. Patients with high cord lesions may require intensive management and should be cared for in centers capable of offering such treatment. Staff must be educated about the issues related to the care of SCI patients, in particular those with AH. Vaginal delivery should be anticipated in most patients.

Induction of labor in patients at high risk of developing AH should probably not be initiated until a functioning epidural catheter is in situ. Regional anesthesia can be used in SCI patients and is the treatment of choice for AH.

SPINA BIFIDA

Spina bifida describes a variety of congenital abnormalities that arise as a result of failed closure of the neural tube. Spina bifida is categorized as spina bifida cystica (or aperta), which encompasses meningocele, myelomeningocele, rachischisis, and anencephaly; and spina bifida occulta, which encompasses a wide range of minor defects of mesodermal, neural, or ectodermal origin (Fig. 18–1 and Table 18–2). The solitary finding of defective laminar arches, which may itself be a variant of normal, is not usually described as spina bifida occulta.[53] The incidence of spina bifida cystica varies from 0.5 to 2.5 in 1000 births in North America and the United Kingdom, respectively. The incidence of spina bifida occulta ranges from 10 to 50% of the adult population based on the presence of defects seen radiologically in the vertebral spinous processes and lamina.[54, 55]

TABLE 18–2. **FORMS OF SPINA BIFIDA OCCULTA ACCORDING TO TISSUE OF ORIGIN**

Mesodermal	Neural	Ectodermal
Defective laminar arch	Distal hydromyelia	Nevi
Diastematomyelia	Spinal cord adhesions (without obvious cause)	Hairy patches
Intra/extradural bands		Dermal sinuses
Lipomas	Meningocele manque (aborted herniation of nerve roots)	Cutaneous dimples
Dermoid cyst		

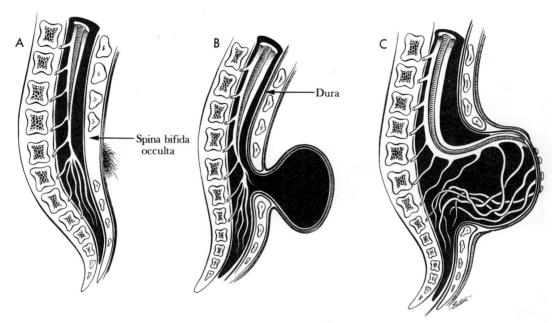

Figure 18–1. Grades of spina bifida. *(A)* Spina bifida occulta. *(B)* Meningocele. *(C)* Myelomeningocele. (From Warkany J. Congenital Malformations: Notes and Comments. Chicago, YearBook Medical Publisher, 1971, p 273.)

Early repair of meningoceles and myelomeningoceles as well as advances in the treatment of the complications, such as infection and hydrocephalus, have resulted in an increasing number of spina bifida cystica patients reaching childbearing age.[54] Numerous case reports have appeared describing issues in the management of labor and delivery in these patients.

Spina Bifida Occulta

A computed tomography (CT) scan study of patients with low back pain or sciatica found spina bifida occulta at S1 in 207 of 1200 patients ages 18 to 72. A decreased incidence of the finding occurred in the older patients. Of patients with occulta lesions, 82% had posterior disc herniation at L4–L5 or L5–S1.[55] Another study found a high incidence of lumbar disc degeneration in young patients with spina bifida occulta. These patients were all less than 20 years old, and 54% had lumbar disc disease at L3–L4, L4–L5, L5–S1.[56] Sixty percent of spina bifida occulta occurs between L4 and S2 levels.[57] The clinical significance of isolated bony arch abnormalities is not yet established, but spina bifida occulta has been associated with chronic back problems, enuresis, and neurologic problems, which reflect its many variants.[55]

Magnetic resonance imaging (MRI) has improved the diagnosis of occult spinal dysraphism, defining lesions that are missed on plain radiographs.[58, 60] Anomalies detected by MRI include tethered cord, diastematomyelia, syringocele, and diplomyelia. Patients with cord abnormalities have cutaneous stigmata in 50 to 70% of cases. Only 30% of these patients have symptoms due to the cord anomalies.[59–61] Patients with isolated vertebral arch anomalies usually have neither cutaneous stigmata nor underlying cord anomalies.[57]

Anesthetic Management of Patients with Spina Bifida Occulta

The implications for obstetric anesthesia management of the patient with spina bifida occulta are few. Most cases consist of an asymptomatic, isolated bony defect at a low spinal level. Regional anesthesia is not contraindicated, and the only recommendation is to perform the block at a site remote from the level of the anomaly. Supporting ligaments, specifically the interspinous ligament and the ligamentum flavum, may be abnormal at the level of the lesion, resulting in an increased potential for accidental dural puncture.[62] The epidural space may also be discontinuous across the lesion, and inadequate or failed block may result. Patients with occulta lesions who have underlying cord anomalies often have cutaneous signs and may have neurologic signs and symptoms. These patients should be assessed antenatally by an anesthesiologist so that relevant neurologic data and consultations can be obtained. Issues related to regional anesthesia, such as direct trauma to the low-lying tethered cord and increased potential for inadequate blocks or dural puncture, can then be discussed fully. Because the majority of spina bifida occulta lesions are at low lumbar or sacral levels and represent fairly trivial anatomic anomalies, they have little impact on regional anesthesia.

Spina Bifida Cystica

The long-term outlook for patients with spinal bifida cystica has improved over the past 50 years.[63, 64] The majority of spina bifida patients are now operated on in the first 24 hours of life. Improved surgical techniques allow closure of large defects. Improved treatment of infection and hydrocephalus has reduced early mortality to 3 to 8%. Most patients develop hydrocephalus (a Chiari II malformation is usually associated with significant cystica lesions), but not all require shunts to be placed. A lower incidence of tethered cord syndrome (4%) also occurs because of improved closure techniques. A study of patients from 1976 to 1986 found that 84% were functional ambulators.[63] Patients with repaired lumbar meningoceles usually have only mild neurologic deficits confined to the lower limbs.[62, 64]

Associated anomalies of the gastrointestinal, skeletal, cardiac, and renal systems may affect development.[65, 66] Myelomeningocele is a dynamic neurologic lesion that eventually produces orthopedic, neurologic, and genitourinary complications. Progressive spinal deformities are seen in up to 90% of patients, with findings of scoliosis, kyphosis, and lordosis.[67] Developmental paralytic scoliosis is the most common type; it results from an imbalance of the paravertebral muscles. This form of scoliosis usually undergoes rapid progression with growth.[68, 69] Congenital scoliosis also occurs, owing to bony abnormalities such as hemivertebrae and multiple rib fusions. The progression is slower, and often significant kyphosis is present. Tethered cord syndrome may also cause scoliosis.[70] The surgical treatment consists of releasing the tethered cord and affixing spinal instrumentation. The release of a symptomatic tethered conus often arrests progression of the curvature in patients with lumbosacral but not thoracic lesions.[67] Progressive lordosis and kyphosis are also significantly reduced. Deterioration in function may also occur in spina bifida because of the development of syringomyelia or shunt dysfunction.[70] Many patients have poor hand control and other manipulative difficulties despite the distance of the lesion from the cervical cord.[71]

Impact of Pregnancy on Spina Bifida Cystica

Several features of spina bifida cystica may affect the course of pregnancy and delivery, as shown in Table 18–3. The management of patients with significant kyphoscoliosis is discussed in Chapter 14. Spina bifida patients may find that they are less mobile during pregnancy as their weight increases, and they may be more susceptible to deep vein thrombosis and decubitus ulcers. The changes in the lumbosacral spine resulting from both hormonal relaxation and expanding abdominal girth may adversely affect both wheelchair fitting and mobility.[72] Impaired renal function may worsen because of the increased incidence of urinary tract infection. The higher abdominal pressure created by the expanding uterus may impair diaphragm func-

TABLE 18–3. NEUROLOGIC AND STRUCTURAL RESIDUA IN ADULTS WITH SPINA BIFIDA

Abnormality	Implications for Pregnancy and Delivery
Sacral agenesis	May permit vaginal delivery despite small pelvis
Pelvic abnormalities (contracted, misshapen)	Abnormal lies and presentations that may preclude vaginal delivery
Short stature	Respiratory problems as uterus expands More likely to have cesarean section
Scoliosis (may be severe)	Cardiorespiratory Mobility problems Technical difficulties with regional anesthesia
Tethered cord syndrome	Neurologic deterioration Cord trauma with regional anesthesia
Shunts	Raised ICP Infection
Chronic bladder problems	Worsened during pregnancy Renal impairment
Motor and sensory deficits	No labor pain Autonomic hyperreflexia Precipitous labor

tion in spina bifida patients, especially those who have short stature or scoliosis. Diaphragmatic fatigue during labor may occur, resulting in the need for ventilatory support and operative delivery.[73]

Medical and Obstetric Management

Patients with spina bifida should consult with medical and obstetric personnel before conception to ensure that medical complications of their disease are minimized. No clear evidence exists of an increased risk of fetal abnormalities in women with spina bifida, but there are case reports documenting fetal malformations.[74, 75] Genetic counseling before conception is also recommended. Respiratory function should be assessed and followed in patients with compromise and in those at risk for decompensation during the pregnancy. Patients with shunt-controlled hydrocephalus require assessment of shunt function. The sites of peritoneal drainage should be noted. Many spina bifida patients have short stature and contracted pelvis that may preclude vaginal delivery. Pelvic assessment should therefore be made early in the pregnancy. Patients have often had prior radiographic assessment of the pelvic area, usually for orthopedic evaluations. A review of these films may be sufficient to generate an opinion on pelvic adequacy.[76]

Numerous case reports have appeared dealing with management of pregnancy and parturition in spina bifida patients. Some frequent complications include preterm labor, UTIs, difficult pelvic examinations due to leg contractures, and damage to ureteroileostomies during cesarean sections.[74, 76–79] Cesarean section should be performed only for obstetric reasons; spina bifida is not an indication for operative delivery.[76]

Anterior sacral meningocele is an extremely rare form of spina bifida that may not be diagnosed until puberty or even during pregnancy, when compression of the neural sac by the growing uterus occurs. Implications for pregnancy include associated sacral and coccygeal malformations, and the effects of the sacral mass on delivery.[62, 78]

Anesthetic Management

Regional anesthesia is not contraindicated in patients with fixed neurologic deficits or previous spinal surgery, although technically it may be more difficult to perform. A high success rate for epidural analgesia in patients with spinal instrumentation can be achieved with prudent persistence.[51, 79] Concern is warranted about an increased potential for accidental dural punctures and incomplete blocks.[72, 79] Vaagenes and coworkers recommend performing the epidural above the level of the lesion if possible, to decrease the likelihood of finding an abnormal epidural space and causing a dural puncture. The hanging drop or air balloon technique to identify the epidural space may be more effective if abnormal ligaments are present, although relatively few anesthesiologists have experience with these techniques.[79] Local anesthetic dose requirements may be decreased in spina bifida patients. Theories advanced to explain this finding include altered dural permeability and abnormally small volume epidural spaces surrounding the lesion.[62, 79]

Spinal anesthesia is thought to be contraindicated because of the unpredictability of local anesthetic dose requirements.[62, 72] In contrast, spinal anesthesia has been used successfully for cesarean section in two case reports by Nuyten and Broome.[80, 81] Spinal anesthesia was said to be technically simpler and provided a more predictable block. Nuyten used a spinal catheter to manipulate the level of block. The risk of cord damage by needle insertion is believed to be minimal if the clinician chooses a site below the anatomic lesion level. If the patient has a shunt, appropriate function of the shunt with no evidence of raised intracranial pressure (ICP) should be confirmed before performing spinal anesthesia. In spina bifida patients with lesion levels above T5–T7, potential exists for autonomic hyperreflexia during labor. Such lesions, however, usually coexist with central nervous system malformations that are incompatible with life and rarely, if ever, are seen.

An increasing number of patients with spina bifida will have children in the future, and the management issues specific to this syndrome must be recognized. The patients require antepartum anesthetic assessment so that all options are analyzed and discussed. Obstetric anesthetic care of the patient with spina bifida provides many challenges. In its mildest form, spina bifida occulta, there may be an increased risk of accidental dural puncture while performing epidural blocks. The more severely affected patients with spina bifida cystica may present with significant scoliosis, surgically scarred backs, respiratory compromise, and obstetric problems such as preterm labor and pelvic abnormalities that preclude vaginal delivery. In the past, most patients did not receive regional anesthesia for labor, and cesarean section was often performed using general anesthesia. An increasing number of reports document successful epidural and spinal anesthesia in these patients.

TETHERED CORD SYNDROME

Tethered cord syndrome (TCS), also known as *tight filum terminale, cord traction syndrome, filum terminale syndrome*, and *tethered conus*, was first described in 1953 by Garceau, although it was probably reported as early as 1918.[82, 83] It is a neurologic syndrome caused by longitudinal traction on the conus medullaris. Initially recognized in pediatric patients after meningomyelocele repair, it has now become an accepted, albeit rare, entity in adults, with more than 120 case reports in the literature. Patients present between the ages of 17 and 76 with a mean age of symptom onset of 33 years and a mean age of diagnosis of 39 years.[84–98]

Tethered cord syndrome is commonly associated with spinal dysraphism, and there are varying degrees of incomplete fusion of the neural arch. Associated anomalies include spina bifida occulta (the most frequent finding in adults),[85, 91] diastematomyelia, syringomyelia, lipoma, dermoid cyst, intra- and extradural bands, and meningocele manque.[85, 86, 99] The underlying pathology causing cord tethering includes thickened filum terminale, intradural lipoma, spinal adhesion, and postsurgical fibrous band. A thickened filum terminale is the most common finding in adults, but there may be more than one pathologic finding. Almost all children who have had a meningocele repair have evidence of a thickened filum and/or low-placed conus medullaris, yet only 15% develop TCS.[82, 100, 101]

The onset of symptoms is related to the degree of traction on the conus. The onset of symptoms in adults typically occurs in two patterns. (1) There is direct trauma to the spine or momentary excessive stretching of the tight conus by extreme flexion of the neck or hips; and (2) there are longstanding mild and static neurologic symptoms that suddenly progress, or new symptoms appear.[91] In the largest published series on adult-onset TCS, 44% followed the second pattern.[91] Some patients with postmeningocele repair do not present with TCS until adolescence and do not represent either of the described patterns.[82, 95, 101]

In adults the major complaint is pain (80% in study by Pang and coworkers[91]), usually in the lower limbs and perineal region. Other presenting symptoms include sphincter dysfunction (57%), leg weakness, and sensory deficit (65%), as well as trophic ulceration.[88-91, 96] Cutaneous stigmata of spinal dysraphism such as dorsal midline nevi, lipomas, skin tags, dimples, and hairy patches are found in only 50% of adulthood TCS but are very common in childhood TCS.[85, 86, 102] Foot deformities and progressive scoliosis are unusual in adults and are more common in children. Often, a precipitating event initiates the symptoms of adult-onset TCS. These precipitating events include childbirth (lithotomy position), sexual intercourse, motor vehicle accidents causing hip flexion, exercising and weightlifting,[89] lumbar spondylosis and herniated discs, direct blows to the back, and falls on the buttocks.[91]

The most helpful diagnostic tools are CT and MRI (Fig. 18–2).[88-90, 92] Myelography demonstrates the position of the conus medullaris as well as the classic horizontal or cephalad direction of exiting sacral nerve roots. It does not delineate well the underlying cause. Plain radiographs of the spine reveal vertebral anomalies in more than 95% of adults.[86, 91, 92] About 70% of adult patients have additional elements of spinal dysraphism, other than spina bifida occulta, as detected by CT, MRI, or surgery.[86] Initial descriptions of the syndrome required that the conus be in an abnormally low position, defined as below the body of L2.[83, 91] In adults, however, 15 to 18% of patients with TCS have a normally positioned conus, as shown in Figure 18–3.[86, 92]

Surgical release of the filum terminale relieves tension and results in dramatic improvement in pain symptoms and motor and sensory functions. Unfortunately, sphincter function usually remains impaired.[85, 91]

Although rare, adult-onset tethered cord syndrome does occur during the childbearing years.[88, 90, 91, 94] The presenting symptoms of back pain and urologic problems may delay diagnosis of the syndrome or may result in misdiagnosis.[88] The underlying pathology frequently discloses the presence of spina bifida occulta, and in 85% of cases the conus medullaris ends below the body of L2. Less than 50% of adults have cutaneous stigmata of spinal dysraphism, and most recall some precipitating event to the onset of their symptoms, including childbirth.

Evidence for adult-onset TCS includes the presence of static neurologic deficits from childhood; pain in the perineal, anal, and gluteal regions or the lower limbs, which may worsen with prolonged bed rest; and shock-like sensations up and down the spine on forward bending similar to those of Lhermitte phenomenon; bilateral lumbosacral sensorimotor deficits; cutaneous stigmata; and bladder complaints with spastic symptoms predominating over hypotonic symptoms. Two cases are reported of young female patients presenting with classic lumbar disc symptoms of radicular pain and dermatomal sensory loss.[93] One was found to have spina bifida occulta at L3–L4, and the other had normal plain radiographs. Both had a low-lying conus at L4. Neither patient had cutaneous stigmata. Another case report involved a 24-year-old female with a history of persistent back pain and bladder symptoms since a previous pregnancy.[94] She had no cutaneous stigmata, but had spina bifida occulta at S2, and low-lying conus. The underlying pathology of the TCS was choristoma. One case report appears in the obstetric literature of a patient with a history of giant lumbar hairy nevus who developed new unilateral neurologic symptoms following delivery with epidural analgesia.[103] On MRI views she had a tethered cord and, on clinical examination after the delivery, she was found to have a smaller right foot and an absent ankle jerk. The precipitating factor of the new neurologic symptoms may have been the result of the fetal head compression, the position during childbirth, or the epidural itself.

Anesthetic Management in Parturients With Tethered Cord Syndrome

Clinically, the importance of this syndrome in the practice of obstetric anesthesia lies in the greater potential for direct spinal cord trauma while performing regional anesthesia, due to the low-lying conus medullaris.[100] The syndrome may not become symptomatic until the precipitating event such as childbirth occurs, and regional anesthesia may be implicated. The risks of epidural anesthesia in this group of patients are

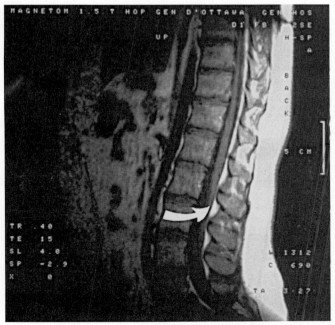

Figure 18–2. MRI scan of a 23-year-old female with a tethered spinal cord. The white arrow indicates conus medullaris, located at the level of the L3 vertebral body.

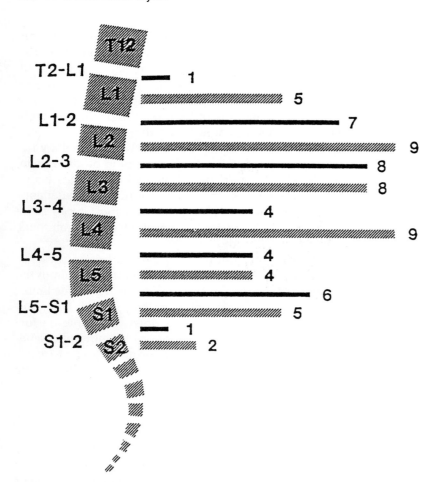

Figure 18–3. Graph shows distribution of the positions of the coni in 73 patients. (From Warder DE, Oakes WJ. Tethered cord syndrome: The low-lying and normally positioned conus. Neurosurgery 1994; 34:598.)

unknown. Such problems emphasize the importance of taking a careful history and performing a neurologic examination in all parturients requesting regional anesthesia who have complaints of significant back pain or neurologic symptoms. In patients with known TCS, regional anesthesia is not contraindicated, but it should be performed below the level of the conus if known, or as low as possible if not. Direct needle trauma to the conus does not necessarily produce typical lancinating pain,[100] but such pain on performing a regional technique mandates immediate removal of the needle or catheter. Epidural anesthesia may be safer than spinal anesthesia because of the low fixed spinal cord. Intrapartum management of patients with known tethered cord syndrome should include avoidance of a prolonged lithotomy position.

ANTERIOR SPINAL ARTERY SYNDROME

Anterior spinal artery syndrome (ASAS) is a rare neurologic syndrome caused by occlusion of the anterior spinal artery, usually in the lower thoracolumbar cord area.[104, 105] First described in 1909 by Spiller in an individual who was found to have thrombosis of the anterior spinal artery at autopsy, the syndrome describes a constellation of neurologic symptoms caused by occlusion of the anterior spinal artery. Symptoms include dissociated sensory function with preservation of proprioception and light touch and loss of motor function. Pathophysiologic events leading to ASAS include vessel occlusion, marked vasoconstriction, and local interference with spinal cord blood flow. It usually is seen in the older population with atherosclerosis and is associated with aortic reconstructive surgery, significant hypotension in the presence of major regional anesthesia, or, in younger patients, underlying vasculitic diseases (Table 18–4).

The spinal cord blood supply is derived from the anterior and posterior spinal arteries. The single anterior spinal artery supplies blood to the anterior two thirds of the spinal cord, areas that subserve motor and coarse sensory function (Fig. 18–4). The anterior spinal artery originates at the foramen magnum from branches of the vertebral arteries. During its course down the spinal cord it receives contributions from seven to ten radicular arteries. It does not have a well-developed continuous course, and the feeder arteries from the descending aorta are variable.[106] The major supply in the lower thoracic and lumbar cord is from the artery of Adamkiewicz, which enters the cord between T5 and L4. If the artery enters high, there are few

TABLE 18–4. REPORTED CAUSES OF ANTERIOR SPINAL ARTERY SYNDROME[*104, 105, 107, 109, 110, 116]

Most frequent (more than 20 cases)
Thoracic aneurysm repair
Abdominal aneurysm repair
Less frequent (10 to 15 cases)
Epidural epinephrine use
Syphilis
Spinal cord angioma
Rare (fewer than 10 cases)
Thrombosis
Postinfectious
Metastatic cancer
Cervical spondylosis
Mitral valve emboli
Hypotension
Post-sympathectomy
Vigorous exercise
Spontaneous epidural bleeding
Intravenous vasoconstrictor use

*Excluding 14 cases of unknown etiology.

thoracic medullary vessels and less vascular supply to the thoracic cord. The paucity of supply and poor anastomoses between the anterior and posterior spinal arteries create watershed areas in the cord where supply to the spinal cord is tenuous, most notably the lower thoracic spinal cord.

ASAS is diagnosed on the basis of a combination of clinical findings and radiographic evaluation. Clinically, there is usually a sudden onset of progressive paraparesis, bladder dysfunction, and sensory loss to pain and temperature. Some patients initially experience pain in the neck or back before the onset of neurologic symptoms.[107] MRI has replaced myelography and angiography of the spinal cord as the diagnostic technique of choice.[104] Treatment to reverse the process is limited to high-dose steroids for vasculitis[108] or to anticoagulants and antiplatelet agents for embolic phenomena.[109] In one report, three patients in the acute phase were given injections of dexamethasone and uro-

kinase directly into the artery of Adamkiewicz with good results.[107] Recovery from the syndrome is limited in those patients with occlusive lesions, aortic disorders, and angiomas. Residual bladder dysfunction often remains, even when there is improvement in motor and sensory function.[107]

A report appears in the literature of anterior spinal artery thrombosis in younger patients with a vascular malformation of the cord.[110] In the obstetric population there is one case report involving a diabetic patient with scleroderma who developed ASAS following epidural anesthesia for cesarean section.[111] No hypotension occurred during anesthesia, and the patient was noted to be paraparetic 12 hours after the epidural analgesia wore off. An epidural hematoma was ruled out, but the epidural venogram revealed a compressed, collagen-filled epidural space with poor venous supply. It was postulated that a sudden marked rise in epidural pressure had occurred, with the addition of local anesthetic volume causing compression of the vascular supply. In addition, two case reports implicate epidural catheter irritation as a cause of vasospasm of the anterior spinal artery or segmental feeder arteries. One report involved an epidural technique for labor analgesia. Shortly after delivery the patient developed sudden onset of paraparesis with preservation of posterior column function. The epidural catheter was removed; complete resolution of the neurologic symptoms occurred over the ensuing 30 minutes.[112] In the other case, postoperative analgesia provided by an epidural technique caused a similar transient ASAS.[113]

The addition of drugs for vasoconstriction, such as epinephrine, to local anesthetic solutions used for major regional anesthesia has been postulated to cause vasoconstriction of the anterior spinal artery, resulting in ASAS.[114, 115] A series of 11 cases of paraplegia following epidural anesthesia is attributed to epinephrine.[116] Dog studies by Usubiaga and Dohi and coworkers,

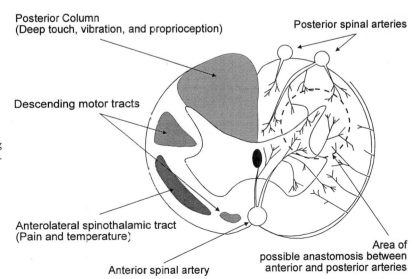

Figure 18–4. Cross-section of the spinal cord showing arterial blood supply and areas of sensorimotor function.

Posterior Column
(Deep touch, vibration, and proprioception)

Posterior spinal arteries

Descending motor tracts

Anterolateral spinothalamic tract
(Pain and temperature)

Anterior spinal artery

Area of possible anastomosis between anterior and posterior arteries however, have demonstrated that clinically relevant concentrations of epinephrine in the epidural space do not cause sufficient impairment of spinal cord blood flow to result in ASAS.[106, 117] Other etiologic factors (resulting in neurologic impairment following epidural anesthesia) include direct needle trauma, chemical myelopathy, symptomatic decompensation of coincidental tumor or vascular malformation, and infection. In the presence of pre-existing disease of the spinal arteries, however, or in periods of significant hypotension, the epinephrine in the epidural space may cause enough vasoconstriction of the anterior spinal artery to impair blood flow and cause ASAS.[106, 116] In the childbearing population, it is rare to find significant arteriosclerosis, but diseases with vasculitic components such as systemic lupus erythematosus, scleroderma, and Takayasu's arteritis may be present and may affect spinal cord blood flow.[108] In these so-affected patients it seems prudent to avoid epinephrine or other vasoconstrictors in the epidural or subarachnoid spaces.

Obstetric Implications of Anesthesia in the Anterior Spinal Artery Syndrome

As above, risk groups in the obstetric population include those with scleroderma, vasculitic diseases such as lupus, Takayasu's giant cell arteritis, Raynaud's syndrome, and atherosclerosis. Avoidance of epinephrine-containing local anesthetic solutions in these patients seems prudent. Any obstetric patient having major regional anesthesia may be at risk from severe hypotension and, when associated with neuraxial epinephrine, the risk of developing ASAS is introduced.[116] The incidence and duration of severe hypotension during major regional blockade can be reduced by vigilance and prompt treatment. The risk of ASAS in this group must be extremely low, however, and available information suggests that pre-existing vascular disease or malformation is a necessary cofactor. Pregnancy may cause increased susceptibility to impairment of spinal cord blood flow due to engorged venous plexi, especially during second-stage pushing. Catheter-induced vasospasm may yield a clinical picture similar to ASAS and should be considered in the differential diagnosis. Appropriate management should include an immediate withdrawal of the catheter and a neurologic evaluation.

CONCLUSIONS

Diseases of the spinal cord in women in the childbearing years range from the rare to the merely uncommon. Medically challenged patients, however, are encouraged to integrate fully into society. One role being adopted that was actively discouraged in an earlier era is that of mother. For this reason, greater

numbers of cord-compromised patients will present for obstetric anesthesia care in the future. Appropriate management decisions are based on an appreciation of the disease processes as well as the interaction between these processes and pregnancy. The challenge is to produce outcomes in these patients comparable to those in the general obstetric population, which is best achieved when care is provided in a cooperative setting. Assisting in the care of these women can be a tremendously gratifying experience.

References

1. Obstetric management of patients with spinal cord injury. ACOG committee opinion. Int J Gynecol Obstet 1993;42:206.
2. Crosby E, St-Jean B, Reid D, et al. Obstetrical anaesthesia and analgesia in chronic spinal cord-injured women. Can J Anaesth 1992;39:487.
3. Cross LL, Meythaler JM, Tuel SM, et al. Pregnancy, labor and delivery post spinal cord injury. Paraplegia 1992;30:890.
4. Baker ER, Cardenas DD, Benedetti TJ. Risks associated with pregnancy in spinal cord-injured women. Obstet Gynecol 1992;80:425.
5. Cross LL, Meythaler JM, Tuel SM, et al. Pregnancy following spinal cord injury. West J Med 1991;154:607.
6. Nilsson DE. The delivery of a quadriplegic patient confined to a respirator. Am J Obstet Gynecol 1953;65:1334.
7. Esposito TJ, Gens DR, Smith LG, et al. Trauma during pregnancy. A review of 79 cases. Arch Surg 1991;126:1073.
8. Goller H, Paeslack V. Pregnancy damage and birth complications in the children of paraplegic women. Paraplegia 1972;10:213.
9. Goller H, Paeslack V. Our experiences about pregnancy and delivery of the paraplegic woman. Paraplegia 1970;8:161.
10. Oppenhimer WM. Pregnancy in paraplegia patients. Two case reports. Am J Obstet Gynecol 1971;110:784.
11. Patterson RM. Trauma in pregnancy. Clin Obstet Gynecol 1984;27:32.
12. Albright J, Sprague B, El-Khoury B, et al. Fractures in pregnancy. In Buchsbaum HJ (ed): Trauma in Pregnancy. Philadelphia, WB Saunders, 1979, p 143.
13. Crosby WM. Traumatic injuries during pregnancy. Clin Obstet Gynecol 1983;26:902.
14. Paonessa K, Fernand R. Spinal cord injury and pregnancy. Spine 1991;16:596.
15. Adams RD, Victor M (eds). Diseases of the spinal cord. In Principles of Neurology, 4th ed. New York, McGraw Hill, 1989, p 720.
16. Piepmeier JM, Jenkins NR. Late neurological changes following traumatic spinal cord injury. J Neurosurg 1988;69:399.
17. Desmond JW, Laws AK. Blood volume and capacitance vessel compliance in the quadriplegic patient. Can Anaesth Soc J 1974;21:421.
18. Contreras G, Gutierrez M, Beroiza T, et al. Ventilatory drive and respiratory muscle function in pregnancy. Am Rev Respir Dis 1991;144:837.
19. Gilroy RJ, Mangura BT, Lavietes MH. Rib cage and abdominal volume displacements during breathing in pregnancy. Am Rev Respir Dis 1988;137:668.
20. Nava S, Zanotti E, Ambrosino N, et al. Evidence of acute diaphragmatic fatigue in a "natural" condition. The diaphragm during pregnancy. Am Rev Respir Dis 1992;146:1226.
21. Gandevia SC. Does the diaphragm fatigue during parturition? (letter). Lancet 1993;341:347.
22. Young BK, Katz M, Klein SA. Pregnancy after spinal cord injury: Altered maternal and fetal response to labor. Obstet Gynecol 1983;62:59.
23. Safra MJ, Oakley GP Jr. Association between cleft lip with or without cleft palate and prenatal exposure to diazepam. Lancet 1975;2:478.

24. Czeizel A. Lack of evidence of teratogenicity of benzodiazepine drugs in Hungary. Reprod Toxicol 1988;3:183.
25. Laegreid L, Olegard R, Wahlstrom J, et al. Abnormalities in children exposed to benzodiazepines in utero. Lancet 1987; 1:108.
26. Greenspoon JS, Paul RH. Paraplegia and quadriplegia: Special considerations during pregnancy and labor and delivery. Am J Obstet Gynecol 1986;155:738.
27. Hughes SJ, Short DJ, Usherwood MM, et al. Management of the pregnant woman with spinal cord injuries. Br J Obstet Gynaecol 1991;98:513.
28. Craig DI. The adaptation to pregnancy of spinal cord injured women. Rehabil Nurs 1990;15:6.
29. Catanzarite VA, Ferguson JE II, Weinstein C, et al. Preterm labor in the quadriplegic patient. Am J Perinatol 1986;3:115.
30. Verduyn WH. Spinal cord injured women, pregnancy and delivery. Paraplegia 1986;24:231.
31. Robertson DN. Pregnancy and labor in the paraplegic. Paraplegia 1972;10:209.
32. Hughes SC. Anesthesia for the pregnant patient with neuromuscular disease. In Shnider SM, Levinson G (eds): Anesthesia for Obstetrics, 2nd ed. Baltimore, Williams & Wilkins, 1987, p 426.
33. Abouleish E. Hypertension in a paraplegic patient (letter). Anesthesiology 1980;53:348.
34. Greenland VC, Young BK. When the mother is paraplegic. Contemporary Ob/Gyn 1984;Aug:201.
35. Ciliberti BJ, Goldfein J, Rovenstine EA. Hypertension during anesthesia in patients with spinal cord injuries. Anesthesiology 1954;15:273.
36. Desmond J. Paraplegia: Problems confronting the anaesthesiologist. Can Anaesth Soc J 1970;17:435.
37. Schonwald G, Fish KJ, Perkash I. Cardiovascular complications during anesthesia in chronic spinal cord injured patients. Anesthesiology 1981;55:550.
38. Boucher M, Santerre L, Menard L, et al. Epidural and labor in paraplegics. Can J Obstet Gynecol 1991;Feb:130.
39. Erickson RP. Autonomic hyperreflexia: Pathophysiology and medical management. Arch Phys Med Rehabil 1980;61:431.
40. McGregor JA, Meeuwsen J. Autonomic hyperreflexia: A mortal danger for spinal cord-damaged women in labor. Am J Obstet Gynecol 1985;151:330.
41. Wanner MB, Rageth CJ, Zach GA. Pregnancy and autonomic hyperreflexia in patients with spinal cord lesions. Paraplegia 1987;25:482.
42. Ellis FR. Neuromuscular disease and anaesthesia. Br J Anaesth 1974;46:603.
43. Cheek TG, Banner RN. Orthopedic/neurologic diseases. Problems in Anesthesia 1989;3:112.
44. Tabsh KMA, Brinkman CR, Reff RA. Autonomic dysreflexia in pregnancy. Obstet Gynecol 1982;60:119.
45. Ravindran RS, Cummins DF, Smith IE. Experience with the use of nitroprusside and subsequent epidural analgesia in a pregnant quadriplegic patient. Anesth Analg 1981;60:61.
46. Speilman FJ. Parturient with spinal cord transection: Complications of autonomic hyperreflexia (letter). Obstet Gynecol 1984;64:147.
47. Stirt JA, Marco A, Conklin KA. Obstetric anesthesia for a quadriplegic patient with autonomic hyperreflexia. Anesthesiology 1979;51:560.
48. Watson DW, Downey GO. Epidural anesthesia for labor and delivery of twins of a paraplegic mother. Anesthesiology 1980;52:259.
49. Abouleish EI, Hanley ES, Palmer SM. Can epidural fentanyl control autonomic hyperreflexia in a quadriplegic parturient? Anesth Analg 1989;68:523.
50. Baraka A. Epidural meperidine for control of autonomic hyperreflexia in a paraplegic parturient. Anesthesiology 1985;62:688.
51. Crosby ET, Halpern SH. Obstetric epidural anaesthesia in patients with Harrington instrumentation. Can J Anaesth 1989; 36:693.
52. Lambert DH, Deane RS, Mazuzan JE. Anesthesia and the control of blood pressure in patients with spinal cord injury. Anesth Analg 1982;61:344.
53. Frank JD, Fixsen JA. Spina bifida. Br J Hosp Med 1980;24:422.
54. Farine D, Jackson U, Portale A, et al. Pregnancy complicated by maternal spina bifida. J Reprod Med 1988;33:323.
55. Avrahami E, Frishman E, Fridman Z, et al. Spina bifida occulta of S1 is not an innocent finding. Spine 1994;19:12.
56. de Bakker HM, Roos RA, Voormolen JH, et al. Lumbar disk degeneration in spinal dysraphism. Am J Neuroradiol 1990;11:415.
57. McAllister VL. Plain Spine X-Rays. In James CCM, Lassman LP (eds): Spina Bifida Occulta. Orthopaedic, Radiological and Neurosurgical Aspects. London, The Whitefriars Press, 1981, p 60.
58. Tripathi RP, Sharma A, Jena A, et al. Magnetic resonance imaging in occult spinal dysraphism. Australas Radiol 1992;36:8.
59. Yamane T, Shinoto A, Kamegaya M, et al. Spinal dysraphism: a study of patients over the age of 10 years. Spine 1991;16:1295.
60. Azimullah PC, Smit LM, Rietveld-Knol E, et al. Malformations of the spinal cord in 53 patients with spina bifida studied by magnetic resonance imaging. Childs Nerv Syst 1991;7:63.
61. Scatliff JH, Kendall BE, Kingsley DP, et al. Closed spinal dysraphism: Analysis of clinical, radiological, and surgical findings in 104 consecutive patients. Am J Neuroradiol 1989;152:1049.
62. Halpern SH. Musculoskeletal disorders and pregnancy: Anesthetic considerations. Problems in Anesthesia 1991;5:163.
63. Reigel DH, McLone DG. Myelomeningocele: Operative treatment and results—1987. Concepts Pediatr Neurosurg 1988;8:41.
64. McCullough DC, Johnson DL. Myelomeningocele repair: Technical considerations and complications. Concepts Pediatr Neurosurg 1988;8:29.
65. Schweitzer ME, Balsam D, Weiss R. Spina bifida occulta. Spine 1993;18:785.
66. Chatkupt S, Ruzicka PO, Lastra CR. Myelomeningocele, spinal arteriovenous malformations and epidermal nevi syndrome: A possible rare association? Dev Med Child Neurol 1993;35:737.
67. Reigel DH, Tchernoukha K, Bazmi B, et al. Change in spinal curvature following release of tethered spinal cord associated with spina bifida. Pediatr Neurosurg 1994;20:30.
68. Muller EB, Norwall A. Prevalence of scoliosis in children with myelomeningocele in Western Sweden. Spine 1992;17:1097.
69. Banta JV, Becker G. The natural history of scoliosis in myelomeningocele. Orthop Trans 1986;10:18.
70. Rekate HL. Neurosurgical management of the child with spina bifida. The tethered spinal cord. In Rekate HL (ed): Comprehensive Management of Spina Bifida. Boston, CRC Press, 1991, p 93.
71. Jansen J, Taudorf K, Pedersen H, et al. Upper extremity function in spina bifida. Childs Nerv Syst 1991;7:67.
72. Eisenach JC. Orthopaedic disease. In James FM, Wheeler AS, Dewan DM (eds): Obstetric Anesthesia: The Complicated Patient, 2nd ed. Philadelphia, FA Davis, 1988, p 238.
73. Shneerson JM. Pregnancy in neuromuscular and skeletal disorders. Monaldi Arch Chest Dis 1994;49:227.
74. Fujimoto A, Ebbin AJ, Wilson MG, et al. Successful pregnancy in woman with myelomeningocele (letter). Lancet 1973;1:104.
75. Opitz JM. Pregnancy in a woman with myelomeningocele. Lancet 1973;1:368.
76. Richmond D, Zaharievski I, Bond A. Management of pregnancy in mothers with spina bifida. Eur J Obstet Gynecol Reprod Biol 1987;25:341.
77. Ellison FE Jr. Term pregnancy in a patient with myelomeningocele, ureteroileostomy, and partial paraparesis. Am J Obstet Gynecol 1975;123:33.
78. Wynn JS, Mellor S, Morewood GA. Pregnancy in patients with spina bifida cystica. Practitioner 1979;222:543.
79. Vaagenes P, Fjaerestad I. Epidural block during labour in a patient with spina bifida cystica. Anaesthesia 1981;36:299.
80. Nuyten F, Gielen M. Spinal catheter anaesthesia for Caesarean section in a patient with spina bifida. Anaesthesia 1990;45:846.
81. Broome IJ. Spinal anaesthesia for Caesarean section in a patient with spina bifida cystica. Anaesth Intensive Care 1989;17:377.
82. Oi S, Yamada H, Matsumoto S. Tethered cord syndrome versus low-placed conus medullaris in an over-distended spinal cord following initial repair for myelodysplasia. Childs Nerv Syst 1990;6:264.
83. James CCM, Lassman LP. Tight filum terminale and tethered cord syndromes. In James CCM, Lassman LP (eds): Spina Bifida Occulta. London, The Whitefriars Press, 1981, p 202.
84. Yamada S, Knierim D, Yonekura M, et al. Tethered cord syndrome. J Am Paraplegia Soc 1983;6:58.

85. Hendrick EB, Hoffman HJ, Humphreys RP. The tethered spinal cord. Clin Neurosurg 1983;30:457.

86. Warder DE, Oakes WJ. Tethered cord syndrome: The low-lying and normally positioned conus. Neurosurgery 1994;34:597.

87. Balagura S. Late neurological dysfunction in adult lumbosacral lipoma with tethered cord. Neurosurgery 1984;15:724.

88. Simon RH, Donaldson JO, Ramsby GR. Tethered spinal cord in adult siblings. Neurosurgery 1981;8:241.

89. Fain B, Vellet D, Hertzanu Y. Adult tethered cord syndrome. S Afr Med J 1985;67:985.

90. Salvati M, Ramundo EO, Artico M, et al. The tethered cord syndrome in the adult. Report of three cases and review of the literature. Zentralbl Neurochir 1990;51:91.

91. Pang D, Wilberger JE. Tethered cord syndrome in adults. J Neurosurg 1982;57:32.

92. Warder DE, Oakes WJ. Tethered cord syndrome and the conus in a normal position. Neurosurgery 1993;33:374.

93. Gokay H, Barlas O, Hepgul KT, et al. Tethered cord in adult mimicking the lumbar disc syndrome: Report of two cases. Surg Neurol 1993;39:440.

94. Molleston MC, Roth KA, Wippold FJ, et al. Tethered cord syndrome from a choristoma of mullerian origin. J Neurosurg 1991;74:497.

95. Barolat G, Schaeffer D, Zeme S. Recurrent spinal cord tethering by sacral nerve root following lipomyelomeningocele surgery. J Neurosurg 1991;75:143.

96. Adamson AS, Gelister J, Hayward R, et al. Tethered cord syndrome: An unusual cause of adult bladder dysfunction. Br J Urol 1993;71:417.

97. Russell NA, Benoit BG, Joaquin AJ, al Fayez N. Adult diastematomyelia. Can J Neurol Sci 1994;21:72.

98. Lesoin F, Petit H, Destee A, et al. Spinal dysraphia and elongated spinal cord in adults. Surg Neurol 1984;21:119.

99. Giles LGF. Review of tethered cord syndrome with a radiological and anatomical study: Case report. Surg Radiol Anat 1991;13:339.

100. Heinz ER, Rosenbaum AE, Scarff TB, et al. Tethered spinal cord following myelomeningocele repair. Neuroradiology 1979;131:153.

101. Tamaki N, Shirataki K, Kojima N, et al. Tethered cord syndrome of delayed onset following repair of myelomeningocele. J Neurosurg 1988;69:393.

102. Hoffman HJ, Hendrick EB, Humphreys RP. The tethered spinal cord: Its protean manifestations, diagnosis and surgical correction. Childs Brain 1976;2:145.

103. Morgenlander JC, Redick LF. Spinal dysraphism and epidural anesthesia. Anesthesiology 1994;81:783.

104. Takahashi S, Yamada T, Ishii K, et al. MRI of anterior spinal artery syndrome of the cervical spinal cord. Neuroradiology 1992;35:25.

105. Kume A, Yoneyama S, Takahashi A, et al. MRI of anterior spinal artery syndrome. J Neurol Neurosurg Psychiatry 1992;55:838.

106. Usubiaga JE. Neurological complications following epidural anesthesia. Int Anesthesiol Clin 1975;13:9.

107. Baba H, Tomita K, Kawagishi T, et al. Anterior spinal artery syndrome. Int Orthop 1993;17:353.

108. Markusse HM, Haan J, Tan WD, et al. Anterior spinal artery syndrome in systemic lupus erythematosus. Br J Rheumatol 1989;28:344.

109. Satran R. Spinal cord infarction. Stroke 1987;22:13.

110. Foo D, Rossier AB. Anterior spinal artery syndrome and its natural history. Paraplegia 1983;21:1.

111. Eastwood DW. Anterior spinal artery syndrome after epidural anesthesia in a pregnant diabetic patient with scleroderma. Anesth Analg 1991;73:90.

112. Ben-David B, Vaida S, Collins G, et al. Transient paraplegia secondary to an epidural catheter. Anesth Analg 1994;79:598.

113. Richardson J, Bedder M. Transient anterior spinal cord syndrome with continuous postoperative epidural analgesia. Anesthesiology 1990;72:764.

114. Kozody R, Pahlaniuk RJ, Wade JG, et al. The effect of subarachnoid epinephrine and phenylephrine on spinal cord blood flow. Can Anaesth Soc J 1984;31:503.

115. Porter SS, Albin MS, Watson WA, et al. Spinal cord and cerebral blood flow responses to subarachnoid injection of local anesthetics with and without epinephrine. Acta Anaesthesiol Scand 1985;29:330.

116. Urquhart-Hay D. Paraplegia following epidural analgesia. Anaesthesia 1969;24:461.

117. Dohi S, Takeshima R, Naito H. Spinal cord blood flow in dogs: The effects of tetracaine, epinephrine, acute blood loss and hypercapnia. Anesth Analg 1987;66:599.

The peripheral nervous system includes all the neural structures outside the pial membrane of the spinal cord and brainstem.[1] Peripheral neuropathy results from a disturbance of function and structure of the peripheral motor, sensory, and autonomic neurons. Because degeneration of the peripheral axon results from primary disorders of the anterior horn cell and sensory neuron in the dorsal root ganglion, these are included in the peripheral neuropathies. By clinical convention, however, disorders such as poliomyelitis and motor neuron disease are not included.[2]

Disease of the peripheral nervous system is of particular importance to the anesthesiologist if, as a consequence of the disease, the patient is likely to be adversely affected by any of the drugs or techniques used. Pregnancy may exacerbate some peripheral neuropathic conditions; it may be an indirect cause of others; or it may impose special management considerations on the immunologically mediated syndromes.

Peripheral neuropathy may occur as a primary disease or as a component of a multitude of diseases with multisystem manifestations. Consequently, the impact of the disease and its treatment on pregnancy (and the impact of pregnancy on the disease) and on fetal development and neonatal well-being depend on the nature, extent, and therapy of the disease.

CLASSIFICATION OF PERIPHERAL NEUROPATHY

The topic of peripheral nerve disease is broad and complex. To help clarify the many different and overlapping presentations it is helpful to consider anatomy, histopathology, symptomatology, neurophysiology, and etiology (Table 19–1). The following section focuses on specific peripheral neuropathies and their interaction with the pregnancy, developing fetus, and anesthesia.

Acquired Demyelinating Polyneuropathies

Guillain-Barré Syndrome or Acute Inflammatory Demyelinating Polyneuropathy

Guillain-Barré syndrome (GBS), an inflammatory, demyelinating disease of peripheral nerves, rarely complicates pregnancy. Its occurrence is similar to that in the general population of 1.7 in 100,000.[3]

The experimental model of GBS, experimental allergic neuritis, gives credence to the theory that the clinical manifestations of this disorder are a result of a cell-mediated immunologic reaction directed at peripheral nerves.[4] A viral etiology is suggested by the occurrence of a similar polyneuritis in patients with acquired immunodeficiency syndrome (AIDS) and with a preceding Epstein-Barr virus (EBV) or cytomegalovirus (CMV) infection.[4–7] The pathology of GBS is characterized by inflammation, demyelination, and axonal degeneration in the peripheral nervous system.[7]

Symptomatology

Clinical features include a symmetrical weakness of proximal as well as distal musculature usually involving the lower extremities before the upper, with the trunk, intercostal, neck, and cranial muscles affected later. The symptoms evolve over several days or weeks and peak at 1 month. The weakness can progress to total motor paralysis within a few days. Dysautonomia is common and is usually short-lived; it may be manifest by sinus tachycardia or bradycardia, facial flushing, profuse or absent diaphoresis, labile blood pressure, and urinary retention. Inappropriate antidiuretic hormone secretion (SIADH)–induced hyponatremia occurs frequently, especially in patients requiring mechanical ventilation. Transient diabetes insipidus is a rare complication. Cerebrospinal fluid (CSF) examination usually reveals an acellular rise in protein by the end of the first week, and electrophysiologic studies reveal conduction block and axonal degeneration.[1]

TABLE 19–1. CLASSIFICATION OF PERIPHERAL NEUROPATHIC CONDITIONS

Anatomy	Symptomatology	Neurophysiology	Etiology
Mononeuropathy		Focal conduction block	Entrapment
			Myxedema
			Acromegaly
			Compression
			Trauma
			Vasculitis/inflammatory
			Periarteritis nodosa (PAN)
			Systemic lupus erythematosus (SLE)
			Sjögren disease
			Sarcoid
			Leprosy
	With subclinical neuropathy		Diabetes
			Alcoholism
			Vasculitis
Multiple mononeuropathy		Axonopathy	Vasculitis
			Diabetes
			Sarcoid
			AIDS
			Leprosy
		Myelinopathy	CIDN
Polyneuropathy	Motor		Acute (GBS, porphyria)
			Chronic
			Hereditary
			Lead
	Sensory		Diabetes
			Vasculitis
			Drugs
			AIDS
			Amyloid
	Autonomic		Diabetes
			Uremia
			Vitamin B_{12} deficiency
			Porphyria
			Drugs
		Axonopathy	Acute (toxins, porphyria)
			Subacute systemic disease
			Chronic hereditary
		Myelinopathy	Acute (GBS, HIV)
			Chronic (CIDN, HIV, inherited)

The course of GBS, concurrent with pregnancy, is similar to that in nonpregnant patients, with weakness peaking within 1 month and remaining on a plateau for a variable period before beginning slow improvement.

Treatment

The essence of therapy is respiratory assistance and careful nursing. The patient's condition may deteriorate unpredictably and rapidly, mandating hospitalization where intensive care facilities are available. Sequential evaluation of respiratory function using clinical assessment, spirometry, and blood gas estimation ensures that endotracheal intubation and mechanical ventilation are instituted appropriately.

Tracheostomy is performed in anticipation of the need for prolonged mechanical ventilation and effective tracheobronchial toilet. Other treatment modalities include cardiovascular support and control with volume expansion and vasoactive drugs, as indicated; maintenance of electrolyte balance; and prevention of deep venous thrombosis and pulmonary embolism.

In severe GBS, early plasmapheresis decreases the duration of mechanical ventilation and the time to independent walking. Plasmapheresis has been employed successfully during pregnancy.[8] Autonomic instability, a particular problem in pregnant women with GBS, may be overcome by fluid loading before the procedure. Pooled human immunoglobulin has been suggested as an alternative to plasmapheresis with as yet unproven efficacy.[9] Steroids are not recommended.[10]

Prognosis

Mechanical ventilation is required by 10 to 23% of patients, and there is a mortality rate of 3 to 7%.[11] Death may occur early from dysautonomia or respiratory arrest, or late from pulmonary embolism and complications of prolonged immobilization.[12]

Interaction of GBS With Pregnancy, Developing Fetus, and Neonate

Pregnant women have mildly restricted respiration determined by the size of the gravid uterus. Thus, when affected by GBS, they may need assisted ventilation earlier and longer than would otherwise be expected. The pregnancy-imposed predisposition to thromboembolism is compounded because of prolonged immobilization. Heparin and low-molecular-weight heparin are the preferred anticoagulants because they do not cross the placenta.[13]

A review by Nelson and McLean[12] indicates the absence of fetal effects attributable to the disease itself or to ventilatory support. This observation suggests that the immunopathogenesis involves factors, such as IgM and immune complexes, that do not cross the placenta. It is reasonable to reassure a pregnant woman with GBS that the fetus will not be affected.[12]

Obstetric Management

Pregnancy, labor, and delivery proceed normally with no evidence to suggest that uterine function is altered in affected parturients. Those requiring respiratory support may go into premature labor.[3] Autonomic instability with unpredictable cardiovascular response precludes tocolytic therapy. Despite strong uterine contractions, the inability to push increases the likelihood of instrumental delivery. Hopkins states that cesarean section in a patient requiring mechanical ventilation may lessen the high mortality rate,[14] but others state that the condition is not affected by pregnancy or pregnancy termination.[12] Quinlan and coworkers[3] believe that unnecessary obstetric intervention must be strongly resisted.

Anesthetic Management

In assessing these patients, clinicians must determine the exact nature of the neurologic deficits. The GBS parturient may have bulbar dysfunction, which increases the risk of aspiration pneumonitis and impinges on her already reduced respiratory reserve. The motor deficit, causing weakness and/or paralysis, interferes with the ability to bear down, whereas a sensory deficit beyond T10 may render uterine contractions painless.[15]

Epidural anesthesia for labor and delivery is described in a case report by McGrady.[16] Bupivacaine 0.25% in small volumes provided excellent labor analgesia, and when cesarean section was required 8 hours later, satisfactory anesthesia was achieved with 7 ml of bupivacaine 0.5%. No apparent ill effects were attributable to the epidural. Successful labor epidural analgesia has also been reported following recovery from GBS.[17] Each case should be assessed individually, keeping in mind that GBS may have a relapsing course.

When general anesthesia is required for cesarean section, acid aspiration prophylaxis is mandatory, utilizing pharmacologic agents (nonparticulate antacid, H_2 receptor blockers, and metoclopramide), cricoid pressure, and rapid-sequence induction with endotracheal intubation. As with many other neuromuscular disorders, depolarizing muscle relaxants are absolutely contraindicated, but nondepolarizing muscle relaxants may be given in reduced doses. Induction can be achieved with thiopentone sodium, but if autonomic instability exists, severe hypotension may result. Adequate preoperative hydration usually prevents severe hypotension.[18] The standard criteria for extubation must be satisfied, and ventilatory assistance may be necessary postoperatively. Keeping in mind the natural history of the disease, patient management is best achieved in the intensive care unit.

Chronic Inflammatory Demyelinating Neuropathy

Chronic inflammatory demyelinating neuropathy and polyradiculoneuropathy (CIDN, CIDPN) appear to be affected by pregnancy.[19–21] Relapse may occur during the latter half of pregnancy, sometimes post partum, and occasionally with the use of oral contraceptives. Treatment may include corticosteroids, plasmapheresis, and human immunoglobulin. Immunosuppressive agents such as azothioprine, cyclophosphamide, and cyclosporin A have been tried but they have unpleasant and serious side effects.

The fetus and neonate are not affected by the disease itself. Obstetric and anesthetic management are similar to those for GBS.

Metabolic Polyneuropathies

This section addresses the peripheral neurologic manifestations of various metabolic disorders. A full description is found in Chapter 20.

Porphyric Polyneuropathy

The porphyrias are disorders associated with an inherited or acquired disturbance in heme biosynthesis. Each is characterized by a unique pattern of overproduction, accumulation, and excretion of intermediates of heme biosynthesis. Each pattern is a metabolic expression of deficiency of heme biosynthetic pathway enzymes. The clinical manifestations are intermittent attacks of nervous system dysfunction and/or sensitivity of skin to sunlight.[22] A neuropsychiatric syndrome occurs with the hepatic porphyrias, which include acute intermittent porphyria (AIP), hereditary coproporphyria (HCP), and variegate porphyria (VP). Photosensitive cutaneous lesions also occur in VP. The incidence of the gene for AIP is 1 in 10,000 to 1 in 30,000 population.

A severe, rapidly advancing, more or less symmetrical polyneuropathy often occurs with abdominal pain, psychosis, and convulsions. It is precipitated by some drugs (Table 19–2). A resultant increase occurs in pro-

TABLE 19–2. PORPHYRINOGENIC DRUGS

Sulfonamides	Succinimide anticonvulsants
Griseofulvin	Alcohol
Estrogens	Ergot preparations
Barbiturates	Benzodiazepines
Phenytoin	

duction of aminolevulinic acid (ALA) and porphobilinogen. Motor neuropathy usually predominates, but sensory and autonomic involvement may be evident. Facial paralysis, dysphagia, and ocular palsies are features of the most severe cases, simulating GBS. The course of the polyneuropathy is variable, with mild cases regressing in a few weeks, severe cases rapidly progressing to respiratory or cardiac paralysis, and slowly progressing cases leaving a severe sensorimotor paralysis that takes months to improve.

Pathologic findings vary from normal-appearing myelin sheaths to degeneration of both axons and myelin sheaths in most peripheral nerves. Diagnosis is confirmed by finding large amounts of porphobilinogen and ALA in the urine. The urine turns dark on standing owing to the oxidation of porphobilinogen to porphobilin.[1]

Treatment consists of respiratory support; beta blockers, if tachycardia and hypertension are severe; intravenous glucose to suppress the heme biosynthetic pathway; and pyridoxine (100 mg bid) on the supposition that vitamin B_6 depletion has occurred. Glucose (20 g/hr IV, 500 g/day) to inhibit ALA production and hematin (4 mg/kg IV daily for 3–14 days) are recommended as the most direct and effective treatment. Complications of hematin treatment are rare but consist of thrombophlebitis, coagulopathy, and hemolysis. A dose of 1 mg·kg^{-1}·day^{-1} of hematin is said to reverse attacks with no clinical anticoagulant effect. Prevention of attacks is of the utmost importance because they can be precipitated by porphyrinogenic drugs (see Table 19–2) and deliberate fasting.[23]

Interaction with Pregnancy and Fetal Effects

Pregnancy may precipitate an acute attack, either during the pregnancy or in the postpartum period, in 50% of patients.[24] In a series of 55 cases, Brodie and coworkers observed one maternal death and a fetal mortality of 15%.[25] If pregnancy continues, it is probable that the newborn will be healthy.[25]

Obstetric Management

The treatment of this disorder is outlined earlier. The potential problem of heme-induced coagulopathy is rare if coagulation is normal beforehand. Conservative glucose therapy is best, but if there is no response, hematin (freshly reconstituted, lyophilized) is administered. Relatively low doses reverse acute attacks and

have no clinically significant effect on coagulation parameters. The complications of hematin therapy in pregnancy are unknown.[23]

Anesthetic Management

As with any patient with a peripheral neuropathy, it is important to determine the extent of existing neurologic deficit and rule out involvement of the autonomic nervous system. Autonomic irritability (sweating, hypertension, tachycardia, salivation, loss of pupillary reflexes, and sphincter control) can be provoked by any drug or anesthetic technique that excites sympathetic activity. The early autonomic end-organ denervation sensitivity gives way to eventual autonomic paralysis with postural hypotension, sensitivity to blood and fluid loss, and reduction in cardiac output with intermittent positive-pressure ventilation (IPPV).

Porphyrinogenic drugs are avoided. Local anesthetic agents, opioids, inhalational agents, and muscle relaxants are all safe. Ketamine has been administered as an induction agent,[24] but comment was made on diagnostic difficulty regarding the cause of postoperative psychosis. Propofol, although not yet recommended for obstetric use, is not porphyrinogenic.[26] In my opinion, an incremental epidural technique with meticulous attention to intravascular volume status is appropriate for labor analgesia and is an alternative to general anesthesia for cesarean section.

Diabetic Neuropathy

The consequences of pregnancy for the chronic complications of diabetes including retinopathy, nephropathy, neuropathy, and hypertension are not clear.[27] Neuropathy is most common in patients older than 50 years, uncommon in those younger than 30 years, and rare in children.[1] A clear relationship exists between the duration of diabetes and development of peripheral neuropathy. Improvement of motor neuron conduction and resistance of ischemic conduction block after therapy are recognized.[28] Several clinical neuropathic syndromes have been delineated (Table 19–3).

Little has been written regarding the effect of pregnancy on diabetic neuropathy, but blood glucose control may determine the development or progression of neuropathy.[29] Other approaches such as aldose-reduc-

TABLE 19–3. DIABETIC PERIPHERAL NEUROPATHY

1. Acute mononeuropathy
2. Painful and predominantly motor mononeuritis multiplex
3. Subacute or chronic symmetrical proximal motor and variable sensory neuropathy
4. Chronic lower limb distal symmetrical sensory neuropathy
5. Autonomic neuropathy involving bowel, bladder, and cardiovascular reflexes
6. Painful thoracoabdominal radiculopathy

tase inhibitors, gangliosides, and symptomatic treatments with amitryptyline, carbamazepine, and phenytoin have been taken.[30]

Management

Close liaison among the obstetrician, endocrinologist, anesthesiologist, and neonatologist is necessary to provide optimal outcome for the diabetic mother and her offspring. The risks of insulin-dependent diabetes mellitus to the fetus and neonate include congenital malformations, macrosomia with shoulder dystocia, hypoglycemia, respiratory distress syndrome, hypocalcemia, hyperbilirubinemia, polycythemia, and death.

If neuropathy is present, the nature of the deficit must be known. Pupillary and lacrimal dysfunction, impaired sweating and vascular reflexes, postural hypotension, and atonicity of bowel and bladder signify autonomic neuropathy. Diabetic gastroparesis may be treated with metoclopramide.[30] The administration of general anesthesia to the pregnant diabetic patient mandates emphasis on the cardiovascular and gastrointestinal implications of autonomic dysfunction and blood glucose control and the potential for difficult intubation. Epidural, spinal, or combined spinal-epidural anesthesia is suitable for labor analgesia with both vaginal delivery and cesarean section. Rapid and aggressive treatment of hypotension using intravenous fluids (nondextrose) and ephedrine is essential to maintain an already compromised uteroplacental blood flow and to prevent fetal hypoxia and acidosis.[31, 32]

Hypothyroid Polyneuropathy

Unless hypothyroidism is mild, pregnancy is unlikely to occur, because affected women are chronically anovulatory. The occurrence of neuropathy in association with hypothyroidism is infrequent and seldom severe.[1] Subjective improvement and complete or near-complete reversibility of neuropathic signs follow treatment with thyroid hormone.[30]

Uremic Polyneuropathy

Uremia refers to the clinical syndrome observed in patients suffering from profound loss of renal function, regardless of etiology. Chronic renal failure ultimately leads to disturbances of every organ system, including the central, peripheral, and autonomic nervous systems. Peripheral neuropathy is a relatively common complication of advanced renal failure. Sensory involvement exceeds motor involvement, lower extremities are affected more than upper, and distal portions of the extremities are affected more than the proximal. Most agree that the neuropathy improves or stabilizes with effective hemodialysis, and in some early cases complete recovery can occur. A few reports suggest that hemodialysis is ineffective and that peritoneal dialysis may be superior. Occasionally, vitamin B_{12} deficiency is the cause. Renal transplantation produces a clearcut improvement in virtually all cases in a period of 6 to 12 months.[1, 30] An accelerated uremic neuropathy that simulates GBS has been identified.[33] Successful pregnancies can occur in parturients on chronic dialysis or with renal transplants. Dialysis may be instituted in a mother with deteriorating renal function to allow fetal viability before delivery.[34]

Anesthetic management is determined not by the presence of uremic neuropathy but by the many other concurrent problems such as fluid and electrolyte imbalance, acidosis, anemia, platelet dysfunction, hypertension, and drug treatment. A detailed discussion of these problems is beyond the scope of this chapter.

Hereditary Polyneuropathies

Charcot-Marie-Tooth Neuropathy or Hereditary Sensorimotor Neuropathy

The hallmarks of this class of polyneuropathy are genetic origin; symmetry of effects; and slow, progressive degeneration of functionally related systems of fibers and axon-myelin fiber loss. The disease is usually inherited as an autosomal dominant trait, and occasionally autosomal recessive. A rare variant with X-linked dominant inheritance has been reported.[35] Onset is usually during late childhood, rarely later. Distal muscle atrophy begins in the feet and legs and later involves the hands. Rarely the sensory loss is severe, which can lead to the development of lower limb perforating ulcers. The main disability is due to a combination of sensory ataxia and weakness with foot drop and instability of the ankles. Usually there is no disturbance of autonomic function.

This neuropathy is divided into types I and II on the basis of conduction velocity in the median nerve, which is slow in type I (<38 m/s) and near normal in type II. Type I cases have a peak onset during the first decade, whereas type II cases have a peak onset in the second decade. Both motor and sensory signs are more severe in type I.

There is no known treatment. Stabilization of the ankles by arthrodesis is indicated if foot drop is severe and the disease is nonprogressive. Light braces and shoes with springs may help to overcome foot drop.[1]

The disease may undergo exacerbation during pregnancy owing to endoneural edema with return to baseline following delivery. There is no effect on the fetus.[36]

Obstetric and Anesthetic Management

Some case reports have indicated the possibility of succinylcholine-induced hyperkalemia[37] and malignant hyperthermia (MH) susceptibility.[38] A review of 86 cases of anesthesia for Charcot-Marie-Tooth disease (CMTD) in nonpregnant patients lends some support to the safe utilization of succinylcholine and MH-triggering agents; although the relatively small sample size does not exclude a potential link.[39] In one patient with unstable exacerbated CMTD, succinylcholine was avoided for fear of an exaggerated hyperkalemic response.[40] General anesthesia for cesarean section was done as this patient was unable to tolerate the supine position because of intercostal muscle weakness. She also required postoperative ventilatory support.[40]

Regional anesthesia has been administered in suitable patients for labor analgesia and cesarean section. The benefits lie in reduction of the work of breathing and complete avoidance of depolarizing muscle relaxants and MH triggering agents.

Dejerine-Sottas Neuropathy

This disorder (also called hereditary sensorimotor neuropathy [HSMN] III) usually has a recessive inheritance pattern, with an earlier onset than CMTD. It is a slowly progressive demyelinating disease. Pain and paresthesias in the feet are early symptoms, which are followed by the development of symmetrical weakness and wasting of the distal portions of the limbs. Sensation is impaired in a distal distribution, and the tendon reflexes are absent. No important changes occur in autonomic function. The ulnar, median, radial, posterior cervical, and peroneal nerves stand out like tendons but are not tender.

I have found no anesthetic or pregnancy case reports, but I do follow the guidelines for CMTD regarding the use of depolarizing relaxants.

Refsum's Disease

Refsum's disease (also called HSMN IV) is a rare, autosomal recessive disorder with onset in late childhood, adolescence, or early adulthood. Diagnosis is based on a combination of clinical manifestations—retinitis pigmentosa, cerebellar ataxia, and chronic polyneuropathy coupled with an increase in blood phytanic acid. Cardiomyopathy and neurogenic deafness are present in most patients. The polyneuropathy is sensorimotor, distal, and symmetrical in distribution, affecting legs more than arms, with all forms of sensation being reduced and tendon reflexes lost. The metabolic defect is in the utilization of dietary phytol.

Anesthetic considerations include avoidance of succinylcholine, assessment of left ventricular function to allow optimal fluid loading, and careful titration of epidural local anesthetic. Epidural blockade is advantageous because it reduces afterload without depressing myocardial contractility. The rapidity of onset and difficulty in control of block height relatively contraindicate spinal anesthesia in parturients with cardiomyopathy.

Dysautonomia

Dysautonomia may be primary or idiopathic, or the condition may be due to systemic disease.[41] The familial (primary) type (Riley-Day syndrome) is a rare autosomal recessive genetic disorder found in the Ashkenazi Jewish population and affects the development of the autonomic and sensory nervous systems.[42] It is characterized by autonomic instability (abnormal sweating, vasomotor control loss, labile hypertension), impaired taste with absence of fungiform papillae, diminished pain and temperature sensation, hyporeflexia, episodic fever, vomiting attacks with frequent episodes of aspiration pneumonia, blunted responses to hypoxia and hypercarbia, alacrima, and corneal anesthesia with ulceration.

Patients are unable to produce a sympathetic response owing to deficient stores or release of norepinephrine. Because of chronic exposure to low levels of catecholamines, there is supersensitivity to exogenous transmitter substances (both adrenergic and cholinergic).

Symptomatic treatment includes elastic extremity garments, mineralocorticoids, and metoclopramide.[30] Some patients do reach adulthood and become pregnant.

Anesthetic Considerations in Labor, Delivery, and Cesarean Section

The parturient with dysautonomia is at greater risk than the healthy parturient because of the already reduced respiratory reserve, together with the tendency to vomiting and aspiration, blunted respiratory response, inability to compensate for intravascular volume depletion, and denervation sensitivity.

Histamine receptor type-2 blockers (e.g., ranitidine) and prokinetics (metoclopramide) should be considered for aspiration prophylaxis. Supplemental oxygen and modified posture may improve respiratory function. Early recognition and treatment of intravascular volume depletion may attenuate hemodynamic instability. Because of the predisposition of the patient to vomiting and respiratory control disturbance, parenteral and inhalational analgesics are hazardous.

Norepinephrine deficiency and an unpredictable response to vasopressors may be a relative contraindication to traditional spinal or epidural anesthesia. Yet, considering that inadequate analgesia can precipitate an autonomic crisis, one alternative is epidural or spinal opioids (with appropriate respiratory monitoring) for first-stage pain relief without sympathetic blockade. Pudendal or saddle block is required for second stage anesthesia. My preference is epidural analgesia, which is carefully titrated utilizing incremental doses of local anesthetic, following optimal intravenous fluid loading.

Anesthesia for cesarean section has been achieved successfully with local infiltration, which avoids the risks of induction of general anesthesia.[42] The principles of general anesthesia for dysautonomia are acid aspiration prophylaxis, meticulous intravascular volume repletion, judicious thiopentone induction, and inhalational and neuromuscular blocker maintenance. Modest narcotic analgesia, augmented by local anesthetic infiltration, should provide effective postoperative pain relief, because patients have a reduced analgesic requirement.

Intermittent positive-pressure ventilation (IPPV) reduces venous return and, hence, systolic blood pressure. For this reason, ventilation pressures should be kept as low as possible. Direct arterial pressure monitoring and postoperative ventilation should be considered. Roizen[43] recommends titration of direct-acting cardiovascular drugs to treat either sympathetic excess or deficiency. These drugs include phenylephrine (vasoconstrictor), isoproterenol (increases heart rate), and esmolol (decreases heart rate) rather than agonists or antagonists that may indirectly release catecholamines.[43] Controversy surrounds the use of esmolol in obstetrics because it crosses the placenta and causes transient hypotension in fetal sheep. It is rapidly eliminated, however, from fetal plasma.[44] Sodium nitroprusside does not alter uterine blood flow or vascular resistance, but concern remains regarding pregnancy owing to the possibility of fetal cyanide toxicity. Careful short-term administration is unlikely to cause fetal compromise.[45]

Vasculitic Neuropathy

Peripheral neuropathy is common in many vasculitic syndromes and may be the only manifestation of the underlying disease (Table 19–4).[1, 46] It may be a true multiple mononeuropathy, an overlapping mononeuropathy, or a distal symmetrical polyneuropathy. Because most of these diseases are multisystem diseases that may be influenced by pregnancy, an interdisciplinary team approach should be employed to manage these parturients.

TABLE 19–4. **SOME ANGIOPATHIC NEUROPATHIES**

Syndrome	Incidence of Peripheral Neuropathy (%)
Polyarteritis nodosa	50–75
Churg-Strauss disease	50
Rheumatoid arthritis	1–5
Systemic lupus erythematosus	10
Wegener's granulomatosis	20

Sarcoidosis

This is a disease of unknown etiology that appears to be a systemic granulomatous reaction involving any tissue. Sarcoidosis is a rare cause of subacute or chronic polyneuropathy of asymmetric type that may be associated with polymyositis. Central nervous system involvement can occur at the stalk of the pituitary, resulting in diabetes insipidus, or in the cerebellum, producing ataxia.[1] Involvement of a single nerve often takes the form of a facial palsy. In other cases, multiple cranial nerves are affected successively.

Pulmonary infiltration results in a restrictive type of lung disease with decreased vital capacity and functional residual capacity. Myocardial involvement may produce heart block, heart failure, paroxysmal dysrhythmia, and cor pulmonale. Uveitis, keratoconjunctivitis sicca, parotitis, hepatosplenomegaly, lupus pernio, and generalized lymphadenopathy also occur. Hypercalcemia develops in 10% of patients. Steroids are given to treat progressive lung disease and threatened vital organs.[47]

Sarcoidosis is not exacerbated by pregnancy, and treatment is the same as that for the nonpregnant patient. Obstetric and anesthetic management is dictated by the cardiopulmonary status of the mother.[48]

Nutritional and Toxic Peripheral Neuropathy

Deficiency States

In the Western world, nutritional polyneuropathy is usually associated with alcoholism. Mothers who have significant systemic disease related to alcohol abuse are usually older than 30 years of age. A distal symmetrical polyneuropathy (DSPN) occurs in alcoholics and is clinically indistinguishable from those due to diabetes mellitus, malnutrition, and human immunodeficiency virus (HIV) infection. Hypotheses as to the cause of DSPN in alcoholics are those of direct toxicity and of poor nutrition with deficiency of thiamine, pyridoxine, pantothenic acid, and folic acid, or a combination of the B vitamins.[49]

The DSPN has no effect on the course of pregnancy, but other alcohol-related organ dysfunction places the mother at increased risk. Alcohol abuse results in myriad acute and chronic complications, such as withdrawal seizures, aspiration pneumonitis, cardiomyopathy, liver dysfunction, peptic ulcer disease, malabsorption, pancreatitis, esophageal varices, coagulopathy, endocrine effects, and immunologic suppression.

The adverse fetal effects of alcohol have long been recognized with the description of the fetal alcohol syndrome.[50] Other teratogenic effects of alcohol exposure are well known, and high rates of infant mortality, adverse perinatal outcomes, and prematurity have been linked to maternal alcohol abuse.

Obstetric and anesthetic considerations are not determined by the neuropathy, although documentation of the deficit is important. It is the identification of other organ dysfunction that determines management. Coagulopathy may preclude regional anesthesia, whereas anxiety and acute intoxication may dictate general anesthesia. Altered pharmacokinetics and pharmacodynamic tolerance in the alcoholic make modification of general anesthesia necessary.

Poisoning With Heavy Metals and Solvents

Heavy metals cannot be metabolized; they persist in the body and exert their toxic effects by combining with one or more of the reactive groups essential to physiologic function (Table 19–5).[1, 51, 52] Exposure may occur as a consequence of high concentrations in soil or water; leaching from utensils and cookware or industry and mining sites; using pesticides and therapeutic agents; and burning fossil fuels containing heavy metals. Another source is the tetraethyl lead added to gasoline.

Lead poisoning produces effects on the gastrointestinal, neuromuscular, central nervous, hematologic, and renal systems. The neuromuscular syndrome ("lead palsy") is now rare. The muscle groups involved are usually the most active (extensors of forearm, wrist, and fingers; and extraocular muscles), often affecting those on the dominant side. Wrist drop and, to a lesser extent, foot drop have been considered pathognomonic for lead poisoning. No sensory involvement occurs. Evidence of permanent neurologic sequelae from levels of lead previously thought safe raised fears of damage to the fetus and newborn with subsequent prohibition of organic lead salt additives to gasoline and consumer products. Treatment of lead poisoning consists of removal from the source of exposure and administration of chelating agents (ethylenediaminetetraacetic acid [EDTA] and penicillamine).

Thallium is used as an insecticide and rodenticide, a catalyst in fireworks, an ingredient in the manufacture of optical lenses, an alloy in industry, and an element in cardiac perfusion imaging. Immediate symptoms of thallium toxicity are gastrointestinal, with nervous system involvement (peripheral sensory, motor and, less frequently, autonomic) beginning within a week of ingestion. Symptoms include paresthesia, myalgia, weakness, tremor, ataxia, and, less commonly, tachycardia, hypertension, and salivation. Treatment includes administration of Prussian blue and mannitol or magnesium sulfate for gut decontamination and potassium chloride (KCl) to enhance renal excretion. Administration of systemic chelating agents is avoided because they may worsen the neurologic symptoms.

Inorganic arsenic does not cross the blood-brain barrier but does cross the placenta. It causes chromosomal breaks in cultured human leukocytes and teratogenetic effects in hamsters. Manifestations of chronic arsenic poisoning include a sensory and peripheral motor neuritis usually affecting the legs more than the arms. Acute treatment includes administration of ipecac or performance of gastric lavage, cardiovascular stabilization, administration of dimercaprol and D-penicillamine, and hemodialysis, as indicated.

Poisoning with mercury may produce a sensorimotor neuropathy similar to that caused by arsenic, although mercury primarily affects the central nervous system. Organic or methyl mercury is highly lipid-soluble and readily crosses the blood-brain barrier and placenta; it is also readily found in breast milk. Elemen-

TABLE 19–5. **POISONING WITH HEAVY METALS**

Substance	Effects Nervous System	Effects Fetal	Effects Other	Treatment
Lead	Neuromuscular syndrome Wrist drop Foot drop Extraocular	Danger assumed	GIT Renal Hematologic	Remove source by chelation (EDTA)
Thallium	Sensorimotor Autonomic		GIT	Prussian blue Mannitol Magnesium } Gut decontamination KCl- ↑ renal excretion Thiocarbamate
Arsenic	Sensorimotor	Chromosomal breaks		Ipecac Gastric lavage CVS support Dimercaprol Penicillamine Hemodialysis
Mercury	CNS mostly Sensorimotor	Cortical/cerebellar atrophy		

GIT = gastrointestinal tract; KCl = potassium chloride; CVS = cardiovascular system; CNS = central nervous system

tal mercury is poorly absorbed by the gastrointestinal (GI) tract but is readily absorbed by the lungs as a vapor. Inorganic mercury salts are absorbed through the GI tract and skin.[52] Prenatal poisoning produces cerebral palsy as a result of cortical and cerebellar atrophy.

A distal symmetrical, predominantly sensory axonopathy may follow exposure to certain hexacarbon industrial solvents such as n-hexane (in contact cement), methyl-*N*-butyl ketone (in plastic-coated and color-printed fabrics), dimethylaminopropionitrile (DMAPN) (in the manufacture of polyurethane foam), methyl bromide (in fumigants), and ethylene oxide (in gas sterilants).

Treatment of the multisystem disturbances, including peripheral neuropathy, associated with heavy metal and solvent poisoning is directed at life-threatening acute complications. Anesthetic management of the parturient is determined by the obstetric situation and degree of organic dysfunction present. Potential fetal effects are noted earlier.

Drug-induced Neuropathies

A large number of drugs are known to produce neuropathy (Table 19–6). The major problem is diagnosis and, once it is established, avoiding further exposure.[1, 2] Drug-induced neuropathy has no specific effect on pregnancy, nor pregnancy on the neuropathy, but the condition necessitating the use of the drug and the treatment regimen itself may have implications for the mother and developing fetus. Once the deficit is accurately documented, anesthetic options are governed by the obstetric situation and maternal medical profile.

Peripheral Neuropathy Due to Infections

GBS commonly follows a viral illness by 1 to 3 weeks. Diseases that have been implicated in GBS include infectious mononucleosis; mycoplasma infection; viral hepatitis; exanthemata; and CMV, *Campylobacter jejuni*, and HIV infections.

Diphtheritic sensorimotor polyneuropathy is now a rare cause of peripheral neuropathy. It occurs 5 to 8 weeks following the exotoxic cranial nerve symptoms of dysphagia, nasal voice, and pupillary accommodation loss. The disease may be confused with GBS, but the obstetric and anesthetic implications are similar.[1]

Leprosy is a major worldwide cause of peripheral neuropathy. Leprous neuritis is a multiple mononeuropathy affecting nerves lying close to the skin, particularly the median, ulnar, peroneal, and facial. The first signs are cutaneous, with the clinical and immunologic manifestations forming a continuum from polar tuber-

TABLE 19–6. DRUG-INDUCED PERIPHERAL NEUROPATHY

Drug	Comment
Isoniazid	SMN
	Pyridoxine prevents
Pyridoxine	Sensory (in large doses)
Nitrofurantoin	SMN
	Uremia also causes SMN
Vincristine	Dose-related SMN
	May develop foot drop
Cisplatin	Sensory
Chloramphenicol	Mild sensory
	Optic neuropathy–associated
Phenytoin	Mild SMN
Dapsone	Motor
Amiodarone	SMN in 5%
Perhexiline	Sensory
Metronidazole	Mild sensory
Lithium	SMN
Flecainide	Sensory

SMN = sensorimotor neuropathy

culoid to polar lepromatous leprosy. Transmission is by direct contact or through respiratory mucosa, with low infectivity and long incubation period of 3 to 5 years. Congenital infection does not occur. Dapsone, a folate antagonist, is the mainstay of therapy. Dapsone is inexpensive and is safe in pregnancy. Dapsone itself may cause a dose-related motor neuropathy (see Table 19–6).

All levels of the neuraxis may be affected in the HIV-infected parturient or one with acquired immunodeficiency syndrome (AIDS). Peripheral neuropathy exists in multiple forms, either associated with the infection itself or as a result of therapy with antiviral or other neurotoxic drugs (Table 19–7).[53] Treatment includes symptomatic relief with medications such as tricyclics, carbamazepine, vitamin B_{12} for DSPN (if deficiency-related), plasmapheresis and steroids for GBS and CIDPN, and ganciclovir for CMV neuropathy. The ob-

TABLE 19–7. PERIPHERAL NERVE SYNDROMES IN HIV INFECTION

Type	Comment
DSPN	Most commonly painful
	Etiology
	CMV
	Neurotoxic
	ddC, ddI
	Vitamin B_{12} deficiency
IDPN	Similar to GBS, CIDPN
Mononeuritis multiplex	Associated with CMV infection
Progressive	Commonly CMV–related, CD4<50
polyradiculopathy	Treatment with ganciclovir
Autonomic	Treatment
	Fluid/electrolyte management
	May require fluorocortisone/ antiarrhythmic medications

DSPN = distal symmetrical polyneuropathy; CMV = cytomegalovirus; ddC = dideoxycytidine; ddI = dideoxyinosine; IDPN = inflammatory demyelinating peripheral neuropathy; GBS = Guillain-Barré syndrome; CIDPN = chronic inflammatory demyelinating polyradiculoneuropathy

stetric and fetal implications of HIV are discussed elsewhere (see Chapter 24).

Anesthetic management of these so-affected patients requires strict attention to safety issues for both patient and anesthesiologist. Because the spectrum of neurologic dysfunction associated with HIV may be progressive, discussion documentation and informed consent are absolute requirements before embarking on regional anesthesia.[54, 55] Thorough assessment of both the symptomatic and asymptomatic patient is essential because of the myriad, possible associated conditions of malignancy and opportunistic infections, which have anesthetic implications.

Nerve Entrapment Syndromes and Miscellaneous Nerve Lesions

Pregnancy, delivery, and puerperium may be associated with a number of nerve and plexus lesions.

Cranial Nerve Lesions

Idiopathic facial nerve palsy, as described by Bell, occurs more frequently in the obstetric population, with most cases arising in the third trimester. Permanent dysfunction is not usual, and most recover gradually within the first 3 months post partum. Treatment with prednisone has been successful with no apparent adverse effect on the parturient or fetus.[56] Temporary isolated cranial nerve lesions (e.g., abducens nerve palsy) can occur after unintentional dural puncture associated with epidural analgesia.

Horner's syndrome is a side effect of lumbar epidural anesthesia and has been described following a dose of a local anesthetic agent insufficient to produce sensory analgesia.[57] A case report exists of Horner's syndrome after epidural anesthesia associated with partial paralysis of the brachial plexus (ulnar nerve) and trigeminal nerve.[58] The patient presented with paresthesia and numbness of the left side of the face in the distribution of the maxillary and mandibular division of the trigeminal nerve. Motor block was manifested by an inability to open the mouth.[58]

Upper Extremity Neuropathies

Carpal Tunnel Syndrome

Median nerve entrapment producing carpal tunnel syndrome may occur during pregnancy (gestational carpal tunnel syndrome), resolving post partum. It may develop post partum (i.e., lactational carpal tunnel syndrome), however, with resolution after weaning.[59]

Neuralgic Amyotrophy (Brachial Plexus Neuropathy)

Neuralgic amyotrophy is a syndrome of sudden onset of upper extremity pain proceeding rapidly to muscle weakness and sensory and reflex impairment. This condition may be spontaneous, heredofamilial, or gestational. Pain usually resolves in a few weeks, whereas motor recovery may take months.

The familial form is inherited in an autosomal dominant fashion. Affected women are prone to attacks during pregnancy or shortly after delivery, and there may or may not be a recurrence with subsequent pregnancies.[60]

Lower Limb Neuropathies

Several pregnancy-related complications have been observed. It is not uncommon for women to develop back pain (usually sacroiliac dysfunction) in late pregnancy. It is unusual, however, for back pain to be due to nerve root compression. Lumbar disc herniation with severe radiculopathy in pregnancy was reviewed in 48,760 consecutive deliveries.[61] Five cases were managed conservatively in the antepartum period, followed by planned cesarean section delivery. There is one report of an L5 radiculopathy due to compression by a uterine leiomyoma.[62] Ipsilateral leg swelling was a feature.

Parturitional lumbosacral plexus injuries occur with a frequency of 1 in 2000 vaginal deliveries.[63] The injuries are usually unilateral. Patients present with pain in the thigh and leg, with symptoms and signs of injury to the superior gluteal and sciatic nerves. If lumbosacral plexus injury occurs with delivery, cesarean section may be considered for subsequent deliveries. Obstetric femoral neuropathy is observed following vaginal delivery (prolonged lithotomy positioning with abduction and external hip rotation) or cesarean section (psoas muscle retractor pressure).

Compression of the lateral cutaneous nerve of the thigh, as it passes between the two prongs of the inguinal ligament attachment to the anterior superior iliac spine, produces meralgia paresthetica. Meralgia paresthetica causes uncomfortable paresthesia and sensory impairment over the anterolateral aspect of the thigh. An increased incidence is found in the third trimester, possibly from the stretching of the nerve by the expanding abdominal wall and the increased lordosis of pregnancy. Spontaneous improvement after delivery is usual. Treatments include bed rest, local anesthetic block, and medial transposition of the nerve.[1, 59]

Peroneal neuropathy may result from compression at the fibular head during labor by palmar pressure, stirrups, squatting, and sustained knee flexion.[59]

Obstetric and Anesthetic Implications

Some of these are addressed in the sections dealing with the individual nerve lesions. Occasionally, elective cesarean section may be advised for maternal reasons. Epidural analgesia and anesthesia in labor and delivery may result in their implication in neurologic injury and, thus, potential for a medicolegal diagnostic dilemma. The list of "obstetric" nerve palsies is quite long, with a number pertaining to the lumbosacral segments of the spinal cord. Thorough assessment with detailed history, examination, investigation, and appropriate multidisciplinary referral (neurologic and/or orthopedic) is mandatory to identify those at risk of obstetric-related neuropathies. The parturient must give informed consent before the institution of epidural or spinal anesthesia. Detailed documentation of the procedure must be done. Epidural analgesia during labor may mask the symptoms of an acute disc prolapse, which can occur de novo, during labor and delivery.[64] If a persistent neurologic deficit appears following delivery, the history, mode of delivery, and detailed anatomic analysis of the lesion must be considered carefully to establish cause. Appropriate treatment can then be initiated. Neuroimaging must be performed early, if indicated, to diagnose such catastrophic events as epidural hematoma or abscess.

CONCLUSIONS

The anesthetic management of the parturient with puerperal neuropathic signs and symptoms requires a well-coordinated team approach with close liaison among the anesthesiologist, obstetrician, other medical specialists, and paramedical personnel. Regardless of whether neuropathy is the predominant symptom or a relatively minor component of a multisystem disorder, the nature and extent of the neurologic deficit must be documented meticulously. Pregnancy may exacerbate the neurologic dysfunction in a few disorders, and knowledge of this possibility is helpful in preoperative patient assessment. Of paramount importance is an unhurried, detailed, antenatal discussion with the mother about the risks and benefits of the anesthetic options, considering the disease, the pregnancy, and the fetus.

References

1. Diseases of the peripheral nerves. In Adams RD, Victor M (eds): Principles of Neurology, 5th ed., p 1117. New York, McGraw-Hill, 1993,
2. Thrush D. Investigation of peripheral neuropathy. Br J Hosp Med 1992;48:13.
3. Quinlan DJ, Moodley J, Lalloo BC, et al. Guillain-Barre syndrome in pregnancy. A case report. S Afr Med J 1988;73:611.
4. Waksman BH, Adams RD. Allergic neuritis: An experimental disease of rabbits induced by the injection of peripheral nerve tissue and adjuvants. J Exp Med 1955;102:213.
5. Hart IK, Kennedy PGE. Guillain-Barre syndrome associated with cytomegalovirus infection. Q J Med 1988;67:425.
6. Cornblath D, McArthur J, Jennedy P, et al. Inflammatory demyelinating peripheral neuropathies associated with HTLV-III infection. Ann Neurol 1987;21:32.
7. Feasby TE. Inflammatory demyelinating polyneuropathies. Neurol Clin 1992;10:651.
8. Hurley TJ, Brunson AD, Archer RL, et al. Landry-Guillain-Barré Strohl Syndrome in pregnancy: Report of three cases treated with plasmapheresis. Obstet Gynecol 1991;78:482.
9. van der Meche FG, Schmitz PI, Dutch Guillain-Barré Study Group. A randomized trial comparing intravenous immune globulin and plasma exchange in Guillain-Barré syndrome. N Engl J Med 1992;326:1123.
10. Guillain-Barré Syndrome Steroid Trial Group. Ineffectiveness of high dose intravenous methylprednisolone in Guillain-Barré syndrome. Lancet 1991;2:1064.
11. Winer JB, Hughes RA, Greenwood RJ, et al. Prognosis in Guillain-Barré syndrome. Lancet 1985;1:1202.
12. Nelson LH, McLean WT Jr. Management of Landry Guillain-Barré syndrome in pregnancy. Obstet Gynecol 1985;65:25S.
13. Flesa HC, Kapstrom AB, Glueck HI, et al. Placental transport of heparin. Am J Obstet Gynecol 1965;93:570.
14. Hopkins A. Neurologic disorders. In De Swiet M (ed): Medical Disorders in Obstetric Practice. London, Blackwell Scientific Publications, 1984, p 1975.
15. Bravo RH, Katz M, Inturrisi M, et al. Obstetric management of Landry-Guillain-Barré Syndrome: A case report. Am J Obstet Gynecol 1982;142:714.
16. McGrady EM. Management of labour and delivery in a patient with Guillain-Barré syndrome (letter). Anaesthesia 1987;42:899
17. Hall JK, Straka PF. Successful epidural analgesia in a primigravida after recovery from Guillain-Barré syndrome. Reg Anesth 1988;13:129.
18. Martz DG, Schreibman DL, Matjasko MJ. Neurological diseases. In Katz J, Benumof J, Kadis LB (eds): Anesthesia and Uncommon Diseases, 3rd ed. Philadelphia, WB Saunders, 1990, p 567.
19. Jones MW, Berry K. Chronic relapsing polyneuritis associated with pregnancy (letter). Ann Neurol 1981;9:413.
20. McCombe PA, McManis PG, Frith JA, et al. Chronic inflammatory demyelinating polyradiculoneuropathy associated with pregnancy. Ann Neurol 1987;21:102.
21. Novak DJ, Johnson KP. Relapsing idiopathic polyneuritis during pregnancy. Immunological aspects and a literature review. Arch Neurol 1973;28:219.
22. Desnick RJ. The porphyrias. In Isselbacher KJ, Braunwald E, Wilson JD, et al (eds): Harrison's Principles of Internal Medicine, 13th ed. New York, McGraw-Hill, 1994, p 2073.
23. Loftin EB III. Hematin therapy in acute porphyria (letter). JAMA 1985;254:613.
24. Bancroft GH, Lauria JI. Ketamine induction for cesarean section in a patient with acute intermittent porphyria and achondroplastic dwarfism. Anesthesiology 1983;59:143.
25. Brodie MJ, Moore MR, Thompson GG, et al. Pregnancy and the acute porphyrias. Br J Obstet Gynaecol 1977;84:726.
26. Parikh RK, Moore MR. A comparison of the porphyrinogenicity of diisopropylphenol (propofol) and phenobarbitone. Biochem Soc Trans 1986;14:726.
27. Berk MA, Miodovnik M, Mimouni F. Impact of pregnancy on complications of insulin-dependent diabetes mellitus. Am J Perinatol 1988;5:359.
28. Ward JD. Barnes CG, Fisher DJ, et al. Improvement in nerve conduction following treatment in newly diagnosed diabetics. Lancet 1971;1:428.
29. Service FJ, Daube JR, O'Brien PC, et al. Effect of blood glucose control on peripheral nerve function in diabetic patients. Mayo Clin Proc 1983;58:283.
30. Hallett M, Tandon D, Berardelli A. Treatment of peripheral neuropathies. J Neurol Neurosurg Psychiatry 1985;48:1193.
31. Datta S, Kitzmiller JL, Naulty JS, et al. Acid-base status of diabetic mothers and their infants following spinal anesthesia for cesarean section. Anesth Analg 1982;61:662.
32. Kenepp NB, Kumar S, Shelley WC, et al. Fetal and neonatal hazards of maternal hydration with 5% dextrose before caesarean section. Lancet 1982;1:1150.
33. Ropper AH, Accelerated neuropathy of renal failure. Arch Neurol 1993;50:536.
34. Hou S. Peritoneal and hemodialysis in pregnancy. Baillieres Clin Obstet Gynaecol 1987;1:1009.
35. Hahn AF, Brown WF, Koopman WJ, et al. X-linked dominant motor and sensory neuropathy. Brain 1990;113:1511.
36. Pollock M, Nukada H, Kritchevsky M. Exacerbation of Charcot-Marie-Tooth disease in pregnancy. Neurology 1982;32:1311.

37. Beach TP, Stone WA, Hamelberg W. Circulatory collapse following succinylcholine: Report of a patient with diffuse lower motor neuron disease. Anesth Analg 1971;50:431.
38. Roelofse JA, Shiipton EA. Anaesthesia for abdominal hysterectomy in Charcot-Marie-Tooth disease. A case report. S Afr Med J 1985;67:605.
39. Antognini JF. Anaesthesia for Charcot-Marie-Tooth disease: A review of 86 cases. Can J Anaesth 1992;39:398.
40. Brian JE Jr, Boyles GD, Quirk JG Jr, et al. Anaesthetic management for cesarean section of a patient with Charcot-Marie-Tooth disease. Anesthesiology 1987;66:410.
41. Sweeney BP, Jones S, Langford RM. Anaesthesia in dysautonomia: Further complications. Anaesthesia 1985;40:783.
42. Lieberman JR, Cohen A, Wiznitzer A, et al. Cesarean section by local anesthesia in patients with familial dysautonomia. Am J Obstet Gynecol 1991;165:110.
43. Roizen MF: Anaesthetic implications of concurrent diseases. In Miller RD (ed): Anesthesia, 3rd ed. New York, Churchill Livingstone, 1990, p 811.
44. Ostman PL, Chestnut DH, Robillard JE, et al. Transplacental passage and hemodynamic effects of esmolol in the gravid ewe. Anesthesiology 1988;69:738.
45. Willoughby JS. Sodium nitroprusside, pregnancy and multiple intracranial aneurysms. Anaesth Intensive Care 1984;12:351.
46. Kissel JT, Mendell JR. Vasculitic neuropathy. Neurol Clin 1992;10:761.
47. Rubenstein D, Wayne D. Respiratory disease. In Lecture Notes on Clinical Medicine, 4th ed. Oxford, Blackwell Scientific Publications, 1990, p 298.
48. de Regt RH. Sarcoidosis and Pregnancy. Obstet Gynecol 1987;70:369.
49. Charness ME, Simon RP, Greenberg DA. Ethanol and the nervous system. N Engl J Med 1989;321:442.
50. Jones KL, Smith DW, Ulleland CN, et al. Pattern of malformation in offspring of chronic alcoholic mothers. Lancet 1973;1:1267.
51. Klaassen D. Heavy metals and heavy-metal antagonists. In Hardman JG, Limbird LE (eds): Goodman and Gilman's The Pharmacological Basis of Therapeutics, 9th ed. New York, McGraw-Hill, 1996, p 1649.
52. Graef JW. Heavy metal poisoning In Isselbacher KJ, Braunwald E, Wilson JD, et al (eds). Harrison's Principles of Internal Medicine, 13th ed. New York, McGraw-Hill, 1994, p 2461.
53. Simpson DM, Olney RK. Peripheral neuropathies associated with human immunodeficiency virus infection. Neurol Clin 1992;10:685.
54. Davies JM, Thistlewood JM, Rolbin SH, et al. Infections and the parturient: Anaesthetic considerations. Can J Anaesth 1988;35:270.
55. Greene ER Jr. Spinal and epidural anaesthesia in patients with the acquired immunodeficiency syndrome (letter). Anesth Analg 1986;65:1090.
56. Dorsey DL, Camann WR. Obstetric anaesthesia in patients with idiopathic facial paralysis (Bell's palsy): A 10-year survey. Anesth Analg 1993;77:81.
57. Mohan J, Potter JM. Pupillary constriction and ptosis following caudal epidural analgesia. Anaesthesia 1975;30:769.
58. Sprung J, Haddox D, Maitra-D'Cruze AM. Horner's syndrome and trigeminal nerve palsy following epidural anaesthesia in obstetrics. Can J Anaesth 1991;38:767.
59. Rosenbaum RB, Donaldson JO. Peripheral nerve and neuromuscular disorders. Neurol Clin 1994;12:461.
60. Lederman RJ, Wilbourn AJ. Postpartum neuralgic amyotrophy (abstract). Neurology 1993;43:A190.
61. LaBan MM, Perrin JC, Latimer FR. Pregnancy and the herniated lumbar disc. Arch Phys Med Rehabil 1983;64:319.
62. Heffernan LPM, Fraser RC, Purdy RA. L-5 radiculopathy secondary to a uterine leiomyoma in a primigravid patient. Am J Obstet Gynecol 1980;138:460.
63. Feasby TE, Burton SR, Hahn AF. Obstetrical lumbosacral plexus injury. Muscle Nerve 1992;15:937.
64. Forster MR, Nimmo GR, Brown AG. Prolapsed intervertebral disc after epidural analgesia in labour. Anaesthesia 1996;51:773.

METABOLIC DISEASE

A large number of inherited disorders of metabolism are known (Table 20–1), not all of which influence perioperative management and anesthesia. Excluded from this review are those in which death is likely to occur before adulthood, those in which subfertility renders pregnancy unlikely, and those in which the disease presents after reproductive age. Disorders highlighted are those that may be seen by an obstetric anesthesiologist (either because of their prevalence or, for some rare conditions, because modern management confers an improved chance of fertility). Malignant hyperthermia; plasma pseudocholinesterase deficiency; and inherited hematologic, endocrine, connective tissue, or bone disorders are considered in detail in other chapters. In all these rare disorders, a basic tenet of management is to refer to a specialist in the relevant field of medicine, to coordinate a multidisciplinary approach, and to make a thorough and early antenatal assessment, with documentation of a plan of management.

Lysosomal Storage Diseases

Lysosomes are cytoplasmic organelles that enclose an acid environment and contain enzymes that hydrolyze macromolecules. The diseases discussed involve mainly single-gene defects affecting one or more lysosomal enzymes. The diseases are of autosomal recessive inheritance. They include the lipid and glycoprotein storage disorders, mucopolysaccharidoses, mucolipidoses, and the hyperphenylalaninemias. Prenatal

TABLE 20–1. **VARIOUS METABOLIC DISORDERS**

Disorder	Key Clinical Features	Obstetric Implications	Anesthetic Implications
McArdle disease	Skeletal muscle myopathy with exercise, rarely myoglobinuric renal failure Adults lead relatively normal life No cardiac involvement	Fertility unaffected Pregnancy and fetus unaffected Disease unaffected by pregnancy	Provide IV dextrose Caution with tourniquets, noninvasive BP cuffs, body temperature changes Use regional techniques For GA, avoid succinylcholine and monitor nondepolarizers
Adult Gaucher disease	Splenomegaly and marrow replacement (secondary pancytopenia) Bone lesions	Fertility unaffected Pregnancy and fetus unaffected Disease usually unaffected	Assess bony deformity Monitor anemia and thrombocytopenia Use regional techniques if possible Prepare for postpartum hemorrhage
Phenylketonuria	Neonatal diagnosis and dietary therapy prevent mental retardation	Fertility unaffected Elevated maternal phenylalanine confers high risk of early pregnancy loss, neonatal retardation, and neonatal cardiac anomalies	Assess antenatally because of high risk of obstetric intervention
Homocystinuria	Neonatal diagnosis and dietary therapy may prevent mental retardation and seizures Thromboembolism, cerebrovascular disease, osteoporosis	High rate of early pregnancy loss and premature labor from placental accidents Anticoagulation often required	Assess antenatally because of high risk of obstetric intervention Plan for regional techniques if possible

diagnosis of both hetero- and homozygotes is often available.[1]

Pompe Disease

Pompe disease, or type II glycogen storage disease, is one of a group of genetic disorders involving pathways for the synthesis, storage, and utilization of glycogen. Those enzyme deficiencies related to liver conversion of glycogen to glucose are classified hepatic-hypoglycemic forms, and those related to muscle conversion of glycogen to lactate form the muscle-energy group. Pompe disease, one of the latter, is a deficiency of α-glucosidase. Weakness, but not cardiac symptoms, is a feature, and the condition may be misdiagnosed as muscular dystrophy. Involvement of respiratory muscles may lead to respiratory failure. Thus, careful preoperative assessment of respiratory function, including arterial blood gas analysis and pulmonary function testing, is necessary before deciding on anesthetic management for surgery during pregnancy.

McArdle Disease

McArdle disease, or glycogen storage disease V, is a rare autosomal recessive hereditary myopathy due to a deficiency of glycogen myophosphorylase, which is required for the conversion of glycogen to lactate during anerobic exercise.[2] Although more prevalent in males, affected individuals are otherwise healthy, and, because fertility is unaffected, pregnancy is likely. The accumulation of glycogen in skeletal muscle produces symptoms of muscle fatigue and cramping during exercise. The diagnosis is usually made in early adulthood. Affected individuals, who may find exercise levels at which they remain asymptomatic, lead a normal existence. Symptoms can be reduced by glucose or fructose ingestion before exercise. A history of myoglobinuria is usually present after severe exercise, but it rarely precipitates acute renal failure. The myocardium and myometrium are usually unaffected, although a case with an abnormal cardiac conduction pathway has been reported.[3] The liver is normal and muscle wasting is uncommon, except in older patients in the upper limbs. Diagnosis is based on assay of serum lactate (with failure to rise), pyruvate, muscle enzyme, and myoglobin levels during ischemic exercise testing.[2] Confirmation is by muscle biopsy and gene studies.

Obstetric and Anesthetic Implications

Pregnancy has been described and appears relatively uneventful.[4, 5] Regional anesthesia confers its usual advantages. Successful, uneventful epidural anesthesia for cesarean section and postoperative analgesia have been reported in the second pregnancy of a woman with McArdle's disease.[6] General anesthesia for cesarean section has been described in the same woman.[5] On theoretical grounds, succinylcholine should be avoided owing to the risk of myoglobinemia, myoglobinuria, and possible renal failure.[7] In both Coleman's case report[5] and in a case after use in a child,[8] the response to nondepolarizing relaxants was normal. A modified rapid-sequence induction using a nondepolarizing drug, with monitoring of neuromuscular block, seems appropriate. Rocuronium (0.6 mg/kg) is probably the preferred agent because of its rapid onset and intermediate duration.[9] Vecuronium 0.1 mg/kg is an alternative, although onset to good intubating conditions is slower and duration of action longer.[10] Another alternative is awake intubation, which is mandatory if difficult intubation is anticipated. No known association exists with malignant hyperthermia. The risk of compromised postoperative respiratory function resulting from myopathy is unlikely in the reproductive age group, but it should be considered.

The use of tourniquets or frequently repeated noninvasive blood pressure recordings is inadvisable, because muscle atrophy is thought to follow repeated episodes of ischemia.[11] Repeated application of an automated blood pressure device has precipitated muscle cramps.[5] Pyrexia, hypothermia, and shivering should all be avoided on the grounds of the poor temperature compensatory mechanisms and the risk of myoglobinemia with severe shivering.

The perioperative administration of intravenous dextrose as a substrate has also been recommended,[7] but the strategy requires titration to maintain normoglycemia, because the fetal and neonatal consequences of maternal hyperglycemia must be considered.[12]

Cori Disease

Cori disease, or debrancher enzyme deficiency, is a rare hepatic-hypoglycemic form of glycogen storage disease, which in mild cases may appear initially in adulthood with a myopathy similar to that of McArdle disease.[2] Important additional anesthetic considerations are the high risk of hypoglycemia with fasting and the presence of cardiac myopathy.

Adult Gaucher Disease

Adult Gaucher disease is one of three forms of Gaucher disease. It is the type I non-neuronopathic form, the most common lysosomal storage disease, and like several others is common in Ashkenazi Jews, in whom the incidence is 1 in 2500. This lipidosis is due to a deficiency of β-glucocerebrosidase, which leads to the accumulation of glucosylceramide, mainly in the reticuloendothelial system. This results in organomegaly, hematologic complications secondary to marrow and splenic involvement, and bony lesions. Enzyme therapy is available but prohibitively expensive. The future, however, holds promise of recombinant enzyme trials and gene replacement therapy.[1, 13]

Obstetric Implications

Fertility is unaffected, and a number of successful pregnancies have been reported.[14, 15] Among the few contraindications to pregnancy are pancytopenia and bleeding as a consequence of marrow infiltration. Splenectomy should be performed (preferably in the second trimester to avoid fetal loss) only on hematologic grounds. Skeletal deformities do not usually affect the pelvis, and thus vaginal delivery can be anticipated. The effect of pregnancy is variable. Some women experience improvement, although more frequently those mildly affected show no change or a deterioration. Neither splenic rupture nor deterioration in liver function has been reported. Mild chronic anemia and thrombocytopenia may occur, and in one series a quarter of the women required blood transfusion for severe anemia or postpartum hemorrhage.[15] The disease otherwise has no effect on obstetric outcome, and fetal growth and development are unaffected.[14, 15]

Anesthetic Implications

Specific antenatal assessment should be directed toward relevant bony deformity, anemia, and thrombocytopenia. The latter warrants regular hematologic monitoring, because it may influence decisions regarding regional techniques and may mandate preparation for postpartum hemorrhage (PPH). Platelet transfusion is not worthwhile because of rapid splenic consumption. It is reassuring that in Goldblatt and Beighton's series[14] of 11 women and 21 pregnancies, only 3 women had thrombocytopenia. Although two of these had a total of seven pregnancies complicated by PPH of undocumented etiology, a transfusion was required only once.

Forbes Disease

Forbes disease (a deficiency of amylo-1,6-glucosidase) has implications similar to adult Gaucher disease, although problems with glucose metabolism may be exaggerated during pregnancy. If insulin is required for the management of gestational diabetes, hypoglycemia is a major risk due to the impaired release of glucose from glycogen.[13, 16]

Mucolipidosis II

Mucolipidosis II is a rare disorder with the patient presenting with progressive skeletal deformities from the first decade and mild mental retardation, but survival to adulthood is common in females.[1] Its specific importance to the anesthesiologist lies in the likelihood of aortic and mitral valvular disease.

Disorders of Amino Acid Metabolism and Storage

Phenylketonuria

Phenylketonuria, or PKU, has an incidence of 1 in 10,000, making it one of the more common disorders of amino acid metabolism, which collectively occur in about 1 in 1000 live births. It is due to reduced activity of liver phenylalanine hydroxylase, which is required to convert phenylalanine to tyrosine. This defect leads to accumulation of phenylalanine and its precursor phenylpyruvic acid in the blood, urine, and tissues, resulting in early mental retardation unless dietary treatment is instituted immediately after birth (elimination of dietary proteins and substitution with an artificial amino acid mixture very low in phenylalanine). With neonatal screening (the Guthrie test) and early detection, plus continued childhood dietary control, many affected women, free of mental handicap, and others with milder forms of the hyperphenylalaninemias, are now reaching reproductive age.[13, 17] It is estimated that there will be 500 fertile women with PKU in the United Kingdom (UK), for example, by the year 2000.[18]

Obstetric and Anesthetic Implications

Although fetal outcome is not affected by the inheritance of PKU, the presence of elevated maternal phenylalanine, and subsequent fetal accumulation, causes serious damage. Abortion is common; more than 75% of infants have microcephaly and are mentally retarded, and the incidence of congenital cardiac anomalies, especially tetralogy of Fallot, is high.[19] If maternal dietary therapy is to improve prognosis, it must be started before conception,[18] because even reintroduction of diet in the first trimester does not guarantee a normal neonate.[20] These issues can create considerable psychological stress in the mother. In the future, transfer of normal genes to liver cells may allow women to maintain normal phenylalanine levels without dietary therapy.[21]

To date, there are no case reports of anesthesia during pregnancy, but the obstetric anesthesiologist should review each case at an early stage of pregnancy because the risk of a maternal operative procedure is high. It seems unlikely that specific modifications to management would become necessary on the basis of mild hyperphenylalaninemia alone.

Homocystinuria

Homocystinuria due to cystathionine β-synthase deficiency is the most common of seven distinct disorders (incidence 1 in 200,000) of homocystine metabolism. Increased plasma levels of homocystine and methionine and decreased cystine levels lead to manifestations such as mental retardation, seizures, dislocated optic lens, osteoporosis, and thromboembolism. Pathophysiology is a consequence of the interference of homocystine in crosslinking of collagen and increased platelet adhesiveness. Early diagnosis and treatment of homocystinuria with pyridoxine, plus methionine restriction, allow a benign clinical course.[17]

Obstetric and Anesthetic Implications

An international review of the condition identified 108 pregnancies among 47 affected women, who were mainly those with response to pyridoxine and higher intelligence.[22] Pregnancy loss was very high in a small number of individuals, but even heterozygotes with modest elevations of homocystine have high perinatal mortality with increased rates of placental infarction and abruption.[23] Thromboembolism is a major concern, and cerebrovascular disease has also been reported.[13] Because pregnancy itself is a hypercoagulable state, these women may require prophylactic anticoagulation antenatally (e.g., with subcutaneous heparin), with continued therapy following delivery.[13] The obstetric anesthesiologist needs to make an antenatal assessment, in conjunction with the obstetric and medical teams, and formulate a management plan that preserves the option of regional analgesia and anesthesia. Our practice is to aim for planned delivery, allowing the effects of heparin to wear off (usually 6 hours after dosing, with confirmatory coagulation tests, if indicated) before using a regional technique or before elective surgery. In some countries, many units do not consider routine cessation of subcutaneous heparin necessary.[23]

Porphyrias

The porphyrias are inherited or acquired disorders of specific enzymes (encoded by a single gene) within the heme biosynthetic pathway (Figure 20–1), characterized by overproduction of porphyrin intermediates in erythroid cells or the liver. Tissue accumulation of porphyrins or decrease in heme production leads to diverse clinical manifestations.

Classifications include *acute* and *nonacute* (presentation) and *erythropoietic* or *hepatic* porphyria. The erythropoietic group cause mainly cutaneous photosensitivity, with anesthesia having no special impact. Patients with the four diseases of the acute hepatic group present with acute crises. Steroids, female hormones, and nutrition influence the production of porphyrins, such that acute intermittent porphyria, for example, often appears in women after puberty or in pregnancy, but rarely after menopause. Diagnosis may be difficult, and the differential diagnosis includes eclampsia, thiamine deficiency, Guillain-Barré syndrome, ruptured aneurysm, and venous thrombosis. Laboratory testing for major metabolites may be confirmatory, but latent carriers may not demonstrate classic excretion patterns. All family members of an affected individual should be treated as being at risk.[24–26]

This review considers only the three acute porphyrias that are relevant to pregnancy and that may be triggered by drugs used in obstetric and anesthetic practice. The principles applying to obstetric anesthesia for acute intermittent porphyria also hold true for *variegate porphyria* (VP) (which is most prevalent in South Africa, affecting 1 in 20,000), and for *hereditary coproporphyria* (HC).

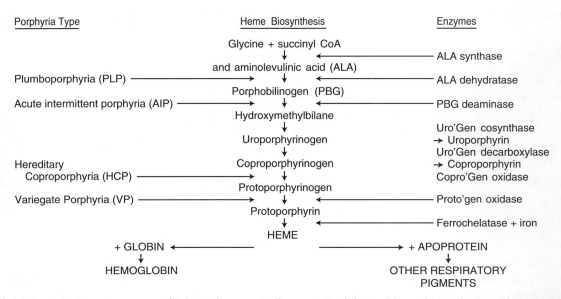

Figure 20–1. The porphyrias are a group of inherited or acquired enzymatic defects of heme biosynthesis, with each type showing a characteristic pattern of overproduction and accumulation of heme precursors based on the location of the enzymatic defect in the heme synthetic pathway. (Modified from Jensen NE, et al. Anesthetic considerations in porphyrias. Anesth Analg 1995;80:591.)

Acute Intermittent Porphyria

Acute intermittent porphyria, or AIP, is an autosomal dominant condition of variable expressivity resulting from a half-normal level of porphobilinogen deaminase (also known as hydroxymethylbilane synthetase). This enzyme is required to convert porphobilinogen formed from δ-aminolevulinic acid, or ALA, to hydroxymethylbilane. The disease is widespread, but it is most common in Northern Europe (incidence 1 in 20,000–25,000).

Most heterozygotes remain asymptomatic until clinical manifestations are precipitated by diet (e.g., starvation resulting from hyperemesis gravidarum or caloric restriction postoperatively), drugs, hormones, infections, alcohol, anesthesia, or surgery. Acute attacks are characterized by severe abdominal pain, vomiting, anxiety, confusion, psychiatric disturbance, and autonomic instability with hypertension and tachycardia (Table 20–2). Dehydration and electrolyte disturbances and new neurologic symptoms typically follow. Prominent also are muscle weakness and polyneuropathy, often asymmetric, with paresis and parasympathetic dysfunction sometimes persisting after resolution of the attack. The neuropathy, which involves axonal degeneration and is primarily a motor deficit (especially of the proximal and cranial nerves), may be due to a deficiency in heme or a neurotoxic effect of elevated ALA levels. Seizures occur in 10 to 20% of cases and may be partly due to hyponatremia resulting from vomiting, diarrhea, and poor oral intake. Persistent hypertension and renal impairment are occasionally seen, but attacks usually resolve over hours to days. ALA and porphobilinogen levels are increased in plasma and urine, and they fall with resolution of attacks.[24]

Porphyric crises are managed supportively by withdrawal of precipitating drugs, reversal of factors increasing ALA synthetase activity (hydration, correction of hyponatremia, glucose administration, treatment of infection), hospitalization, and monitoring. Opioids can be required for pain, antiemetics for nausea, and β-blockers for hypertension and tachycardia. Early intravenous infusion of hematin (a hydroxide of heme) and heme arginate (which is more stable and has fewer side effects) for several days, inhibits ALA synthase in the liver, leading to a response within days and improved outcome.[24–28]

Obstetric Implications

During pregnancy, the activity of erythrocyte porphobilinogen deaminase is not affected.[29] A modest increase occurs in urinary excretion of ALA, porphobilinogen, and porphyrin,[30] although this increase is much smaller than those seen during an acute attack. The incidence of acute attacks tends to rise during pregnancy, however, probably due to higher levels of estrogen and progesterone, both of which are known to precipitate attacks in nonpregnant women. In a review published in 1977 by Brodie and coworkers,[31] 50 cases were evaluated. The maternal mortality was 2% and fetal mortality 13%. Over 50% of affected women had an acute attack during pregnancy, 25% of these commencing after delivery, although many women had been treated with unsafe drugs. The risk of an attack appeared lower in VP (25%) and HC (33%). A later review of the world literature found that 60% of porphyric pregnancies achieved viability, but an exacerbation occurred in 95%.[32] Maternal mortality was over 40%. In AIP, the incidence of spontaneous abortion and hypertension was higher in women who suffered an acute attack of porphyria, and fetal weight was lower than that of asymptomatic women.[31] If no acute attacks occur, fetal outcome is good, and pregnancy is uneventful.

It may be difficult to distinguish an acute porphyric attack from eclampsia. Magnesium sulfate has been recommended as the tocolytic of choice in porphyria and is the anticonvulsant of choice for eclampsia.[28] Pregnancy does not appear to change the natural history of the disease.[33]

Anesthetic Implications

Drug Pharmacology. Great interest lies in drug-induced attacks, because many drugs that are commonly used during pregnancy and in anesthetic practice may be dangerous (Table 20–3). The reader is referred to excellent reviews by Harrison[25] and Jensen[26] and their coworkers. The safety of drugs in porphyria is based on testing in animal models (in which the interspecies variations in response are noted) and clinical reports, such that for many drugs evidence is conflicting or clinical experience insufficient to draw firm conclusions. It is important to recognize precipitants other than drugs and to be aware that known triggers do not consistently induce attacks. Hyperemesis gravidarum has been reported as a possible trigger.[34] The administration of dextrose infusions during labor or following cesarean section has been recommended to prevent hypoglycemia, which is a known trigger, although careful monitoring of maternal blood glucose levels is necessary before delivery to minimize the risk of neonatal hypoglycemia.[12]

When considering prophylaxis against aspiration of gastric contents, metoclopramide is "probably safe" and ranitidine "contentious."[25] Various other drugs encountered in obstetrics should be avoided, including the ergot derivatives, calcium channel antagonists, hydralazine, clonidine, and α-methyldopa. Midazolam, temazepam, lorazepam, droperidol, and phenothiazine antiemetics likely are safe (see Table 20–2).

Regional Analgesia and Anesthesia. Although both lidocaine and bupivacaine are porphyrogenic in some,

TABLE 20–2. **THE ACUTE PORPHYRIAS**

Disorder	Key Clinical Features	Obstetric Implications	Anesthetic Implications
Acute intermittent porphyria	Acute attacks feature abdominal pain, vomiting, behavioral disturbance, autonomic instability, polyneuropathy, weakness, and seizures Triggers include specific drugs and hormones; dehydration and hypoglycemia; infection and stress; and many anesthetic drugs Management is supportive therapy and intravenous infusion of heme arginate	Fertility unaffected Incidence of acute attacks increases and maternal mortality is 2–40% An acute attack confers an increased risk of early pregnancy loss, stillbirth, and fetal growth retardation	Avoid prolonged vomiting or fasting and correct associated abnormalities Avoid drugs that precipitate acute porphyria Give IV dextrose prn Use regional techniques, preferably subarachnoid, if possible (except during acute attack)

but not all, experimental animal models, bupivacaine is considered safe and lidocaine uncertain.[26] Nevertheless, both drugs have been used frequently, and no local anesthetic has been reported to have triggered an attack.[25] Regional blocks, especially spinal techniques that require low doses of local anesthetic, are thus strongly supported.[25, 35] Both epidural analgesia and anesthesia have been employed uneventfully in pregnant patients with porphyria.[36–38] Recommendations to avoid regional anesthetics, published previously, were based on fears of litigation, in the event that neuropathy worsened after delivery. Such recommendations can no longer be supported, provided that the possibility of autonomic dysfunction is considered, preoperative peripheral neuropathy assessed and documented, and appropriate consent obtained. It seems prudent,

TABLE 20–3. **CLASSIFICATION OF DRUGS COMMONLY USED IN ANESTHESIA FOR PATIENTS WITH ACUTE PORPHYRIA**

Drug group	Safe (S) Possibly safe (PS)		Contentious (C) No data (ND)		Unsafe (U) Probably unsafe (PU)	
Intravenous induction agents	Propofol	PS	Ketamine	C	Barbiturates	U
	Midazolam	PS			Etomidate	PU
Inhalation agents	Nitrous oxide	S	Halothane	C	Enflurane	PU
	Cyclopropane	S	Isoflurane	ND		
	Diethyl ether	S				
Muscle relaxants	Curare	S	Atracurium	ND	Alcuronium	PU
	Succinylcholine	S	Pancuronium	C		
	Vecuronium	PS				
Neuromuscular blockade reversal	Atropine		Glycopyrrolate	ND		
	Neostigmine	S				
Local anesthetics	Procaine	S	Lidocaine	C	Mepivacaine	PU
	Amethocaine	PS	Prilocaine	C		
			Bupivacaine	C		
Analgesics	Morphine	S	Alfentanil	ND	Pentazocine	U
	Meperidine	S	Sufentanil	ND	Tilidine	U
	Fentanyl	S				
	Buprenorphine	S				
	Naloxone	PS				
	Acetaminophen	S				
Anxiolytics	Temazepam	S	Diazepam	C	All other benzodiazepines	U
	Lorazepam	PS	Triazolam	C		
	Droperidol	S	Oxazepam	C		
	Phenothiazines	S				
Anti-arrhythmics	Procainamide	S	Lidocaine	C	Verapamil	U
	β-blockers	S	Mexiletine	ND	Nifedipine	U
			Bretylium	ND	Diltiazem	U
			Disopyramide	C		
Other cardiovascular drugs	Epinephrine	S	β-Agonists	ND	Hydralazine	U
	Phentolamine	S	α-Agonists	ND	Phenoxybenzamine	U
			Sodium nitroprusside	ND		
Bronchodilators	Corticosteroids	PS	Hexaprenaline	ND	Aminophylline	U
	Albuterol	S				
Gastric—for cesarean section	Metoclopramide	PS	Ranitidine	C	Cimetidine	PU
	Droperidol	S				

Classification of drugs commonly used in anesthesia for patients with an acute porphyria.
Modified from Harrison GG, Meissner PN, Hift RJ. Anaesthesia for the porphyric patient. Anaesthesia 1993; 48:417.

however, to avoid regional anesthesia during an acute crisis, because mental state changes may result in lack of cooperation, and hemodynamic instability is likely.[26]

General Anesthesia. Women with AIP are at particular risk from conventional general anesthesia (GA) for cesarean section. Thiopentone has accounted for the majority of drug-induced attacks, and thus barbiturates must be avoided. Therefore, it is crucial to make and document a plan, in advance, if urgent cesarean section under GA proves to be necessary. Of the other intravenous induction agents, etomidate is probably unsafe, but ketamine (a suitable drug for normal parturients) has been given uneventfully in porphyria, including for cesarean section.[39] Its classification as "contentious"[25] is based on animal evidence and isolated and somewhat doubtful case reports. There is widespread support for the probable safety of propofol,[25, 26] which is a suitable intravenous drug for cesarean section in healthy parturients.[40–42] Kantor and Rolbin[38] reported on propofol for induction of GA for cesarean section, following an inadequate intraoperative epidural block. The clinical course was uneventful, although the urinary porphobilinogen level was elevated on the first postpartum day. Muscle relaxants and opioids, which are safe or are probably safe, include succinylcholine and vecuronium, morphine, meperidine, and fentanyl. The volatile agents are generally considered safe. Enflurane is classified "probably unsafe" on animal data alone, although both enflurane and isoflurane have been administered to humans and no acute attacks have been ascribed to them. Halothane is considered the agent of choice, and it has been employed extensively in porphyric patients with convincing clinical and biochemical evidence for its safety.[25, 43] Atropine and neostigmine are also safe.

DISEASES INVOLVING THE LIVER

Various congenital and acquired liver diseases may appear during pregnancy, in particular, viral hepatitis. Clinically significant disease is uncommon but is of increasing importance as a cause of maternal mortality. The interested reader is referred to comprehensive reviews of liver disease in pregnancy[44] and pregnancy in patients with chronic liver disease and cirrhosis,[45, 46] and book chapters detailing the viral diseases, acute liver failure, malignancies, and other diseases incidental to pregnancy.[47] No attempt is made to detail in full the anesthetic considerations for the perioperative management of patients with severe hepatic dysfunction, because this information is readily available in standard texts.

Many uncommon conditions involving the liver confer minimal or no risk to maternal and fetal outcome. Examples are the hyperbilirubinemias, which are relatively benign disorders characterized by elevations of unconjugated bilirubin (Gilbert disease) or conjugated bilirubin (Dubin-Johnson and Rotor syndromes). About 50% of affected women experience an increase in jaundice during pregnancy, but fetal outcome is good.

This review concentrates on metabolic liver diseases and liver disorders unique to pregnancy, with the exception of severe pre-eclampsia with liver involvement.

Various changes occur in hepatic physiology, biochemistry, and anatomy during pregnancy.[47] These include unchanged hepatic blood flow (which is thus a smaller proportion of cardiac output); increased splanchnic, portal, and esophageal venous pressure in late pregnancy (with 60% of healthy women having transient esophageal varices); and reduced clearance of drugs that depend on blood flow, owing to a larger volume of distribution. Results of liver function tests are generally unchanged, with the exception of elevated serum lipids, falling serum albumin, rising α_1-, α_2-, and β-globulins, and mildly elevated serum alkaline phosphatase (ALP). These changes persist for several weeks post partum.

Uncommon Diseases Involving the Liver

Wilson Disease

Wilson disease, or hepatolenticular degeneration, is an autosomal recessive condition in which there is an abnormality in the hepatic excretion of copper. This condition probably occurs because hepatic lysosomes lack the normal mechanism to excrete copper into bile for subsequent elimination in the stool. Excess copper then inhibits the formation of the plasma copper protein ceruloplasmin. The worldwide prevalence is 1 in 30,000, and about half of those affected remain asymptomatic until early adulthood. The accumulation of free and tissue copper leads to toxic pathogenic changes in the liver, brain, and other organs, although renal function usually does not change. About 50% of patients present with hepatic involvement (acute and chronic hepatitis, cirrhosis, or occasionally fulminant hepatitis with hemolytic anemia). The remainder display extrahepatic disturbances, usually neurologic (movement disorders including tremor, spasticity, chorea, dysphagia, and dysarthria) or psychiatric and behavioral. Occasionally the diagnosis is made after repeated spontaneous abortion or amenorrhea, or on detection of golden deposits of copper in Descemet's membrane of the cornea (Kayser-Fleischer rings). Unfortunately, the protean manifestations mean misdiagnosis often occurs. Confirmation of the diagnosis is made by detection of low plasma and high urinary copper levels and low blood ceruloplasmin assay, or by liver biopsy with copper assay.[48]

Treatment is based on rapid removal and detoxification of copper deposits. Treatment involves lifelong continual therapy, because relapse results from noncompliance and is fatal within a few years (Table 20–4).

TABLE 20–4. **UNCOMMON LIVER DISEASES**

Disorder	Key Clinical Features	Obstetric Implications	Anesthetic Implications
Wilson's disease	Toxic copper deposition causes hepatic damage, neurologic (usually movement) disorders, and psychiatric disturbance Treatment is to reduce copper levels with chelators (e.g., penicillamine) or zinc	Subfertile unless well-controlled Continuation of treatment is essential to avoid relapse Low risk of teratogenicity with penicillamine	Assess and monitor liver function, coagulation, esophageal varices, bulbar involvement, and drug effects For GA, use drugs appropriate for patients with liver dysfunction Prepare for postpartum hemorrhage
Budd-Chiari syndrome	Patients present with ascites, hepatomegaly, and liver failure Coagulopathy is common The disease may be associated with polycythemia rubra vera or paroxysmal nocturnal hemoglobinuria	Consult a hepatic physician regarding management The fetal prognosis poor	Assess and monitor liver function, coagulation, and hematologic disorders Look for lupus anticoagulant and treat with subcutaneous heparin if present
Primary biliary cirrhosis	Variable presentation from asymptomatic to cirrhosis Diagnosis is based on mitochondrial antibodies and liver biopsy	Pregnancy and the fetus are unaffected in well-compensated disease	Monitor liver function and coagulation Use vitamin K and blood factor replacement as indicated

Four effective therapies are available for both prevention and treatment.[49] Chelating agents have been successfully employed to increase renal copper excretion substantially, with oral penicillamine (plus vitamin B_6 to counteract its antipyridoxine effect) the first therapy of established value. Potential problems with this drug include sensitivity, toxicity (granulocytopenia, thrombocytopenia, nephrotic syndrome, systemic lupus erythematosus, Goodpasture syndrome, and myasthenia gravis), and possible teratogenicity. Birth defects occur in rats and have been described in four newborns of penicillamine-treated mothers.[50] Currently, other drugs utilized include zinc (which blocks intestinal absorption of copper), a chelator trientine,[51] and tetrathiomolybdate (which forms copper complexes to reduce toxicity and blocks gut absorption). Zinc is considered the treatment of choice for asymptomatic and pregnant patients because of its efficacy and lack of toxicity.[49, 52] For those with hepatic or neurologic involvement, additional drugs are required.[49] Liver transplant has been successful for fulminant hepatitis.

Obstetric Implications

In untreated disease, amenorrhea, subfertility, and spontaneous abortion are common, as is maternal morbidity in the unlikely event of pregnancy. When penicillamine or zinc treatment is begun early in the disease, fertility is good. In the absence of severe liver disease, portal hypertension, and esophageal varices, pregnancy is not contraindicated. Pregnancy sometimes has a favorable effect on serum copper levels (attributed to estrogen-induced elevation of plasma ceruloplasmin); however, copper and ceruloplasmin levels usually rise slowly.[53–55] Clinical improvement or remission lasting into the puerperium may also occur.[48, 54, 56] The continu-

ation of treatment, usually at reduced dosage, is important to avoid relapse,[48, 57–59] which may manifest as severe hemolytic crisis (requiring blood transfusion and plasma exchange) and fulminant, fatal liver failure.[59] In addition, the fetus of the untreated woman may show liver damage owing to high copper levels.[55] As mentioned, penicillamine may be teratogenic, although the overall risk is low, with 18 women producing 29 normal infants in one series.[60] Experience with trientine is limited. It is teratogenic in the rat; however, no teratogenetic effects have been reported in small human series.[51] No trials of zinc are available, but on the basis of case reports, zinc appears safe,[49, 52, 61, 62] and it has been recommended.[49] It is possible that it may be protective against some fetal abnormalities.[63]

Anesthetic Implications

Case reports of anesthesia during pregnancy in women with Wilson disease are rare.[64] Patients require careful assessment, particularly of psychological status, liver disease severity, thrombocytopenia, coagulopathy, drug-induced toxicity, and neurologic involvement affecting the bulbar muscles. Renal and liver function tests, blood screening, and coagulation screening are indicated. Liver assessment may include imaging by ultrasonography or magnetic resonance and liver biopsy. Esophagoscopy may be warranted to reveal varices. If varices are detected, epidural analgesia and instrumental delivery are indicated to avoid straining and variceal hemorrhage.[65]

In general, regional techniques are valuable if not contraindicated by an unacceptable cost-benefit analysis because of concern regarding subdural or epidural hematoma. Severe neurologic deficits involving cranial nerves and compromise of upper airway reflexes may mandate GA, but are unlikely. When GA is given to those with significant liver dysfunction, considerations include the use of atracurium and volatile anesthetics with minimal hepatic metabolism (e.g., isoflurane) and the maintenance of hepatic and renal blood flow. Penicillamine has been associated with a myasthenic-type syndrome and possible prolongation of neuromuscular blockade, adding weight to the importance of the cautious administration of muscle relaxants and appropriate monitoring.[64]

Careful attention to asepsis for prevention of infection is necessary if penicillamine-induced bone marrow toxicity has occurred. Extra precautions against intra- and postpartum hemorrhage (e.g. appropriate fasting, additional venous access, crossmatching of blood, rapid infusion devices, consultations with laboratory personnel and a hematologist) may be necessary if a bleeding disorder is present.

Budd-Chiari Syndrome

The Budd-Chiari syndrome is a disease of uncertain etiology characterized by large hepatic vein obstruction leading to centrilobular liver necrosis. It is associated with polycythemia rubra vera, paroxysmal nocturnal hemoglobinuria, and altered coagulation. Clinical features include ascites, liver enlargement, and occasionally acute liver failure. Diagnosis is assisted by ultrasonographic Doppler flow studies and liver biopsy. Management in pregnancy is difficult, because spironolactone is not of established safety,[66] and surgical intervention for shunts is associated with high mortality.[67]

More than 30 cases have been described in pregnancy or the puerperium, although in the past affected women were advised against pregnancy because of the fear of hepatic venous thrombosis.[47] In a series reporting 105 cases, one presented during pregnancy and 15 presented post partum.[67] Patients usually present between the first and third week after delivery and may be resistant to attempts at revascularization. Maternal prognosis is poor.[68] Fetal outcome depends on maternal well-being, but prognosis is usually poor, with only a few successful pregnancies reported.[47]

In addition to assessment of liver function, the anesthesiologist should search for hematologic abnormalities such as antithrombin III deficiency, lupus anticoagulant, and hemolytic anemia.

Primary Biliary Cirrhosis

Primary biliary cirrhosis has a wide clinical spectrum and variable natural history, with affected pregnant woman potentially asymptomatic. The diagnosis is based on detection of mitochondrial antibodies and liver biopsy results. Maternal and fetal outcomes are variable, with good prognosis in well-compensated disease.[47, 69] Attention should be given to preoperative assessment, particularly the need for vitamin K therapy before delivery when cholestyramine has been used.

Uncommon Liver Diseases Unique to Pregnancy

Acute Fatty Liver of Pregnancy

Acute fatty liver of pregnancy, or AFLP, has long been recognized as a clinical entity distinct from hepatitis, but it remains of uncertain etiology (Table 20–5). Although estimates of the occurrence lie between 1 in 10,000 and 1 in 15,000 deliveries,[70, 71] these estimates probably represent underdiagnosis. The diagnosis can be difficult to establish, but early detection is still preferable because mortality is lower if intensive supportive therapy is provided and early delivery achieved.[72] Nevertheless, collective data published since 1980 show a maternal mortality of 18% and fetal mortality of 23%,[47] and AFLP contributed to 6 of 20 direct maternal deaths in the Report on Confidential Enquiries into Maternal Deaths in the United Kingdom 1985 to 1987. This represented a similar number to that ascribed to each of sepsis, ruptured uterus, and anesthesia.[72]

AFLP is characterized histologically by panlobular microvesicular fat vacuolation of hepatocytes, with periportal sparing and minimal inflammation (in contrast to hepatitis). In severe cases, postmortem changes of multi-organ fat infiltration and hemorrhage have been noted. Although the disease is unique to pregnancy, the features are similar to those of Reye's disease in children, and a defect in mitochondrial β-oxidation of fatty acids may be responsible.[73]

Depression of glucose-6-phosphatase activity leads to hypoglycemia, impaired fat transport, and fat accumulation in the liver. Blood abnormalities vary with severity, but abnormalities begin with mildly elevated serum bilirubin and elevated liver enzyme levels. Serum aminospartate transferase (AST) level is often lower than that seen with acute hepatitis, whereas ALP and uric acid levels are greater. Hypoglycemia is common and may be profound. Marked neutrophil leukocytosis with left shift and microangiopathic hemolytic anemia with thrombocytopenia are often present, as is disseminated intravascular coagulation with elevated fibrin degradation products and low antithrombin III. Oliguria is accompanied by electrolyte and renal biochemistry abnormalities, including rising serum creatinine level and, in severe disease, metabolic acidosis.[47, 74]

AFLP typically occurs in the third trimester in both nulliparous and multiparous women, although it may occur as early as 20 weeks' gestation or even post partum.[47] Symptoms develop acutely over no more than 1 week and are nonspecific, commonly including abdominal pain, malaise, nausea and vomiting, fever, and, subsequently, jaundice. Jaundice during preg-

TABLE 20–5. **UNCOMMON LIVER DISEASES UNIQUE TO PREGNANCY**

Disorder	Key Clinical Features	Obstetric Implications	Anesthetic Implications
Acute fatty liver of pregnancy (AFLP)	Patients usually present in late pregnancy with malaise, nausea, abdominal pain, and, later, jaundice Severe features include hypoglycemia, metabolic acidosis, sepsis, liver failure with coagulopathy, and renal dysfunction Manifestations often overlap with pre-eclampsia Management is intensive care (dextrose, antibiotics, vitamin K, etc.), maternal and fetal monitoring. Expedite delivery Natural history is a complete postpartum resolution of disease	Intensive fetal monitoring is required Early delivery may avoid fetal death and prevent maternal mortality	Optimize medical management and monitor maternal and fetal condition Obtain good intravenous access for dextrose and drug administration Probable cesarean section Treat coagulopathy and prepare for peripartum or gastrointestinal hemorrhage Use regional block if not contraindicated Use drugs appropriate for patients with severe hepatic dysfunction
Intrahepatic cholestasis of pregnancy (IHCP)	Patients present in late pregnancy with pruritus and later malaise and mild jaundice Management may include cholestyramine, steroids, and antihistamines All treatments have poor efficacy Rapid postpartum resolution occurs	Monitor maternal and fetal status Preterm delivery is common Increased risk of fetal distress and fetal death in utero Give the neonate vitamin K prophylaxis	Assess and monitor liver function and coagulation Prepare for postpartum hemorrhage If appropriate, consider peripartum steroid coverage
Hyperemesis gravidarum	Severe vomiting and dehydration Minor liver function abnormalities	Increased risk of early fetal loss	Optimize antiemetic therapy Correct fluid and electrolyte imbalance

nancy is, however, more commonly due to viral hepatitis, cholestasis, bile duct obstruction, or pre-eclampsia.[75] Less frequent manifestations of AFLP are headache, backache (pancreatitis), hematemesis, necrotizing enterocolitis, and fulminant acute liver failure, with impaired consciousness, severe hypoglycemia, renal failure, gastrointestinal bleeding, and encephalopathy. Pruritus is uncommon, being present in 5 to 30%.[47]

Pre-eclampsia is frequently present, and the clinical picture overlaps, with hypertension and similar hematologic and histologic features. Indeed, pre-eclampsia may be one of several microvesicular diseases of the liver, with AFLP representing the most severe form.[75, 76] The diagnosis of AFLP is usually based on typical clinical and biochemical findings in the absence of evidence for viral hepatitis (which has a different clinical course and biochemistry and is confirmed by screening for viral markers) or drug-induced hepatitis. Ultrasonographic or computed tomographic imaging of liver fat accumulation may not be positive, and liver biopsy is often not possible due to bleeding risk. Other differential diagnoses include alcoholic hepatitis and autoimmune or other overlapping disorders of a predominantly hematologic nature.

Management is supportive, with emphasis on early diagnosis; intensive treatment of profound hypoglycemia, gastrointestinal hemorrhage, sepsis, and pancreatitis; and correction of coagulopathy. Although neonatal abnormalities are less common than in severe pre-eclampsia, fetal and neonatal complications include prematurity, growth retardation, intrapartum hypoxia,

and hypoglycemia. Widespread fatty infiltration has been described in infants.[77]

Clinical outcome is best determined by clinical assessment. Severe cases mandate early delivery, because striking improvement in liver function invariably follows and prognosis is improved.[78, 79] Immediate delivery is crucial if significant deterioration in maternal or fetal condition occurs, and thus early preparation should be made for obstetric emergencies and planned delivery. Postpartum maternal recovery is rapid, although intensive care facilities are still required because of the risk of maternal hypoglycemia for several days. Hepatic rupture, pancreatitis, and neurologic complications are added risks. A successful liver transplant has been performed in the postpartum period.[80, 81] Subsequent pregnancies are usually normal, although recurrence has been reported.

Anesthetic Assessment

Assessment should be directed toward optimizing medical treatment and monitoring maternal and fetal condition. Blood pressure, blood glucose, fluid and electrolyte status, coagulation status, and acid-base balance must be checked regularly. Good venous access (e.g., central venous catheter, if possible) allows infusion of dextrose, replacement of low serum calcium, correction of hypovolemia, maintenance of adequate urinary output, and treatment of hypertension. Prophylactic administration of an H_2-receptor antagonist, such as ranitidine, is warranted to reduce the risk of gastric erosion, ulceration, and esophagitis.

Vitamin K administration is often necessary, including in the postpartum period when the risk of hemorrhage is high. Administration of fresh frozen plasma and factor concentrates (for clinical bleeding in the presence of coagulopathy or based on laboratory test results after hematologic consultation) may be of value, and platelet transfusion is indicated if the count is less than 20,000 to 30,000 or perioperative bleeding occurs in the presence of thrombocytopenia. Crossmatched blood should be available at all times.

Analgesia and Anesthesia

Only two reports exist on the anesthetic management of AFLP. In one, epidural anesthesia, which preserves liver blood flow, was administered uneventfully.[82] Except for mild cases, delivery is usually by cesarean section, and severe coagulopathy frequently contraindicates regional anesthesia, as in the case report by Corke.[83] If coagulopathy or thrombocytopenia contraindicates regional analgesia because of an increased risk of bleeding, intramuscular injections, acetylsalicylic acid, and nonsteroidal anti-inflammatory drugs should also be avoided. If regional block is feasible, a theoretical argument can be made for spinal anesthesia (because of the smaller needle and reduced risk of vessel puncture) with either subarachnoid morphine or intravenous systemic opioid analgesia postoperatively. If epidural techniques are employed in the presence of thrombocytopenia, it may be advisable to remove the epidural catheter after delivery, because the nadir of platelet count usually occurs 24 to 72 hours later. In addition to the usual obstetric considerations, the aim of general anesthesia should be to maintain liver and renal blood flow. An argument has been proposed for induction with propofol,[83] on the basis that it has normal pharmacokinetics in cirrhosis and no effect on hepatic blood flow[84] whereas studies of thiopentone show conflicting results, including in some a decrease in hepatic flow.[85] Isoflurane may be the volatile agent of choice.[86] Nitrous oxide ideally is avoided.[86] Atracurium has well-recognized advantages in patients with hepatic impairments.[87]

Intrahepatic Cholestasis

Intrahepatic cholestasis of pregnancy, or IHCP, has been reported in up to 2% of pregnancies, half demonstrating a recurrent autosomal dominant form. Reduction in bile flow and in bile and bile salt excretion may be the consequences of a combination of genetically determined and environmental factors, with increased sensitivity to elevated estrogen and progesterone levels. Patients with IHCP usually present in the third trimester, but sometimes they present as early as the sixth gestational week.[88, 89] Pruritus (which is generalized, is worse at night, and responds poorly to treatment) is the classic symptom. In about 50% of cases, jaundice develops after a week or two. In some countries, IHCP accounts for up to 20% of cases of jaundice in pregnancy, a rate second only to viral hepatitis. Malaise, nausea, and abdominal discomfort are common, but pain warrants investigation for viral hepatitis or cholelithiasis. Other differential diagnoses include autoimmune disorders, sclerosing cholangitis, primary biliary cirrhosis, extrahepatic cholestasis, drug toxicity, and Dubin-Johnson syndrome. Laboratory investigations of severe cases show mildly raised liver ALT, AST, and total (mainly conjugated) bilirubin levels.[47] Traditional treatment with phenobarbitone (to induce hepatic enzymes and provide sedation) has generally been abandoned. Cholestyramine, which acts as an anion-exchange resin to bind bile acids, steroids (prednisolone up to 30 mg/day), and antihistamines may be given. Intravenous S-adenosyl-L-methionine has also been tried, but in general, the results of all treatments are disappointing.[89]

Obstetric and Anesthetic Implications

Increased bile salts can be detected within the fetal circulation (although bilirubin does not cross the placenta significantly), and adverse fetal outcomes are common, with preterm labor in up to 60%, stillbirths even in mild cases, and fetal distress and meconium in labor in 11 to 33%.[89, 90] Close fetal monitoring is essential. Induction of labor may be necessary in severe cases, usually on the basis of rising maternal bile acid levels or deterioration of fetal condition.

The neonate requires vitamin K therapy to prevent intracranial bleeding. Maternal symptoms usually resolve within a couple of days of delivery, although occasionally jaundice persists.[47]

The obstetric anesthesiologist should assess the severity of liver dysfunction, in particular checking coagulation status, because derangement may require regular therapy with vitamin K. Vitamin K treatment is particularly likely with cholestyramine, because the latter binds the fat-soluble vitamins (A, D, E, and K). Postpartum hemorrhage occurs in up to 20% of cases,[89] and preparation for the management of peripartum hemorrhage should be made.

Hyperemesis Gravidarum

Hyperemesis gravidarum is associated with elevations of serum AST levels in up to 25% of cases, probably from liver injury resulting from starvation and dehydration in the presence of high estrogen levels and increased susceptibility. Synthetic function remains normal.[91] These abnormalities reverse with treatment. The obstetric anesthesiologist should ensure that fluid and electrolyte abnormalities have been corrected by intravenous hydration and replacement and that pharmacologic antiemetic therapy has been instituted.

References

1. Beaudet AL. Lysosomal storage disease. In Isselbacher KJ, Braunwald E, Wilson JD, et al (eds): Harrison's Principles of Internal Medicine, 13th ed. New York, McGraw-Hill, 1994.
2. Beaudet AL. The glycogen storage disease. In Isselbacher KJ, Braunwald E, Wilson JD, et al (eds): Harrison's Principles of Internal Medicine, 13th ed. New York, McGraw-Hill, 1994.
3. Ratinov G, Baker WP, Swaiman KF. McArdle's syndrome with previously unreported electrocardiographic and serum enzyme abnormalities. Ann Intern Med 1965;62:328.
4. Cochrane P, Alderman B. Normal pregnancy and successful delivery in myophosphorylase deficiency (McArdle's disease). J Neurol Neurosurg Psychiatry 1973;36:225.
5. Coleman P. McArdle's disease. Problems of anaesthetic management for Caesarean section. Anaesthesia 1984;39:784.
6. Samuels TA, Coleman P. McArdle's disease and Caesarean section (letter). Anaesthesia 1988;43:161.
7. Ellis FR. Inherited muscle disease. Br J Anaesth 1980;52:153.
8. Rajah A, Bell CF. Atracurium and McArdle's disease (letter). Anaesthesia 1986;41:93.
9. Abouleish E, Abboud T, Lechevalier T, et al. Rocuronium (Org 9426) for Caesarean section. Br J Anaesth 1994;73:336.
10. Hawkins JL, Johnson TD, Kubicek MA, et al. Vecuronium for rapid-sequence intubation for cesarean section. Anesth Analg 1990;71:185.
11. Field RA. The glycogenoses: von Gierke's disease, acid maltase deficiency and liver glycogen phosphorylase deficiency. Am J Clin Pathol 1968;60:20.
12. Morton KE. Fluid management during labour: a British view. Int J Obstet Anesth 1993;2:147.
13. Walters BNJ, de Swiet M. Bone disease, disease of the parathyroid glands and some other metabolic disorders. In De Swiet M (ed): Medical Disorders in Obstetric Practice, 3rd ed. Oxford, Blackwell Science, 1995.
14. Goldblatt J, Beighton P. Obstetric aspects of Gaucher disease. Br J Obstet Gynaecol 1985;92:145.
15. Zlotogora J, Sagi M, Zeigler M, Bach G. Gaucher disease type I and pregnancy. Am J Med Genet 1989;32:475.
16. Confino E, Pauzner D, Lidor A. Pregnancy associated with amylo-1,6-glucosidase deficiency (Forbes' disease). Case report. Br J Obstet Gynaecol 1984;91:494.
17. Rosenberg LE. Inherited disorders of amino acid metabolism and storage. In Isselbacher KJ, Braunwald E, Wilson JD, et al (eds): Harrison's Principles of Internal Medicine, 13th ed. New York, McGraw-Hill, 1994.
18. Drogani E, Smith I, Beasley M, Lloyd JK. Timing of strict diet in relation to fetal damage in maternal phenylketonuria. Lancet 1987;2:927.
19. Lenke RR, Levy HL. Maternal phenylketonuria and hyperphenylalaninemia. An international survey of the outcome of untreated and treated pregnancies. N Engl J Med 1980;303:1202.
20. Bovier-Lapierre M, Saint-Dizier C, Freycon F, et al. Deux enfants nes de mere phenylcetonurique. Echec d'un regime pauvre en phenylalanine instite pendant la deuxieme grossesse. Pediatrie 1974;29:51.
21. Medical Research Council Working Party on Phenylketonuria. Phenylketonuria due to phenylalanine hydroxylase deficiency: An unfolding story. Br Med J 1993;306:115.
22. Mudd SH, Skovby F, Levy HL, et al. The natural history of homocystinuria due to cystathionine β-synthase deficiency. Am J Hum Genet 1985;37:1.
23. Burke G, Robinson K, Refsum H, et al. Intrauterine growth retardation, perinatal death, and maternal homocysteine levels (letter). N Engl J Med 1992;326:69.
24. Desnick RJ. The porphyrias. In Isselbacher KJ, Braunwald E, Wilson JD, et al (eds): Harrison's Principles of Internal Medicine, 13th ed. New York, McGraw-Hill, 1994.
25. Harrison GG, Meissner PN, Hift RJ. Anaesthesia for the porphyric patient. Anaesthesia 1993;48:417.
26. Jensen NF, Fiddler DS, Striepe V. Anesthetic considerations in porphyrias. Anesth Analg 1995;80:591.
27. Mustajoki P, Nordmann Y. Early administration of heme arginate for acute porphyric attacks. Arch Intern Med 1993;153:2004.
28. Kanaan C, Veille JC, Lakin M. Pregnancy and acute intermittent porphyria. Obstet Gynecol Surv 1989;44:244.
29. Sassa S, Kappas A. Lack of effect of pregnancy or hematin therapy on erythrocyte porphobilinogen deaminase activity in acute intermittent porphyria. N Engl J Med 1989;321:192.
30. DeKlerk M, Weideman A, Malan C, Shanley BC. Urinary porphyrins and porphyrin precursors in normal pregnancy. Relationship to urinary total oestrogen excretion. S Afr Med J 1975;49:581.
31. Brodie MJ, Moore MR, Thompson GG, et al. Pregnancy and the acute porphyrias. Br J Obstet Gynaecol 1977;84:726.
32. Neilsen DR, Neilsen RP. Porphyria complicated by pregnancy. West J Surg Obstet Gynecol 1985;66:134.
33. Zimmerman TS, McMillin JM, Watson CJ. Onset of manifestations of hepatic porphyria in relation to the influence of female sex hormones. Arch Intern Med 1966;118:229.
34. Milo R, Neuman M, Klein C, et al. Acute intermittent porphyria in pregnancy. Obstet Gynecol 1989;73:450.
35. Bohrer H, Schmidt H. Regional anesthesia as anesthetic technique of choice in acute hepatic porphyria. J Clin Anesth 1992;4:259.
36. Brennan L, Halfacre JA, Woods SD. Regional anaesthesia in porphyria (letter). Br J Anaesth 1990;65:594.
37. McNeill MJ, Bennet A. Use of regional anaesthesia in a patient with acute porphyria. Br J Anaesth 1990;64:371.
38. Kantor G, Rolbin SH. Acute intermittent porphyria and Caesarean delivery. Can J Anaesth 1992;39:282.
39. Bancroft GH, Lauria JL. Ketamine induction for cesarean section in acute intermittent porphyria and achondroplastic dwarfism. Anesthesiology 1983;59:143.
40. Dailland P, Cockshott ID, Lirzin JD, et al. Intravenous propofol during cesarean section: Placental transfer, concentrations in breast milk and neonatal effects. A preliminary study. Anesthesiology 1989;71:827.
41. Yau G, Gin T, Ewart MC, et al. Propofol for induction and maintenance of anaesthesia at Caesarean section. A comparison with thiopentone/enflurane. Anaesthesia 1991;46:20.
42. Capogna G, Celleno D, Sebastiani M, et al. Propofol and thiopentone for caesarean section revisited: Maternal effects and neonatal outcome. Int J Obstet Anesth 1991;1:19.
43. Meissner PN, Harrison GG, Hift RJ. Propofol as an I.V. anaesthetic induction agent in variegate porphyria. Br J Anaesth 1991;66:60.
44. Knox TA, Olans LB. Liver disease in pregnancy. New Engl J Med 1996;335:569.
45. Varma RR. Course and prognosis of pregnancy in women with liver disease. Semin Liver Dis 1987;7:59.
46. Lee WM. Pregnancy in patients with chronic liver disease. Gastroenterol Clin North Am 1992;21:889.
47. Fagan EA. Disorders of the liver, biliary system and pancreas. In De Swiet M (ed): Medical Disorders in Obstetric Practice, 3rd ed. Oxford, Blackwell Science, 1995.
48. Scheinberg IH. Wilson's disease. In Isselbacher KJ, Braunwald E, Wilson JD, et al (eds): Harrison's Principles of Internal Medicine, 13th ed. New York, McGraw-Hill, 1994.
49. Brewer GJ. Practical recommendations and new therapies for Wilson's disease. Drugs 1995;50:240.
50. Rosa FW. Teratogen update: Penicillamine. Teratology 1986;33:127.
51. Walshe JM. Trientine and pregnancy in Wilson's disease. Q J Med 1986;58:81.
52. Lao TTH, Chin RKH, Cockram CS, Leung NWY. Pregnancy in a woman with Wilson's disease treated with zinc. Asia-Oceanic J Obstet Gynaecol 1988;14:167.
53. O'Leary JA, Novalis GS, Vosburgh GJ. Maternal serum copper concentration in normal and abnormal gestations. Obstet Gynecol 1966;28:112.
54. Sherwin A. The course of Wilson's disease during pregnancy and after delivery. Can Med Assoc J 1960;83:160.
55. Oga M, Matsui N, Anai T, et al. Copper disposition of the fetus and placenta in a patient with untreated Wilson's disease. Am J Obstet Gynecol 1993;169:196.
56. Dreifuss FE, McKinney WM. Wilson's disease (hepatolenticular degeneration) and pregnancy. JAMA 1966;195:960.
57. Dupont P, Irion O, Beguin F. Pregnancy in a patient with treated Wilson's disease: A case report. Am J Obstet Gynecol 1990;163:1527.
58. Nunns D, Hawthorne B, Goulding P, Maresh M. Wilson's disease in pregnancy. Eur J Obstet Gynecol Rep Biol 1995;62:141.

59. Shimono N, Ishibashi H, Ikematsu H, et al. Fulminant hepatic failure during perinatal period in a pregnant woman with Wilson's disease. Gastroenterol Jpn 1991;26:69.

60. Scheinburg IH, Steinlieb I. Pregnancy in penicillamine-treated patients with Wilson's disease. N Engl J Med 1975;293:1300.

61. Hoogenraad TU, Van Den Hamer CJA, Van Hattum J. Effective treatment of Wilson's disease with oral zinc sulphate. Two case reports. Br Med J 1984;289:273.

62. Hartard C, Kunze K. Pregnancy in a patient with Wilson's disease treated with D-penicillamine and zinc sulfate. A case report and review of the literature. Eur Neurol 1994;34:337.

63. Leonard A, Gerber GB, Leonard F. Mutagenicity, carcinogenicity and teratogencity of zinc. Mutat Res 1986;168:343.

64. el Dawatly AA, Bakhamees H, Seraj MA. Anesthetic management for cesarean section in a patient with Wilson's disease. Middle East J Anesthesiol 1992;11:391.

65. Heriot JA, Steven CM, Sattin RS. Elective forceps delivery and extradural anaesthesia in a primigravida with portal hypertension and oesophageal varices. Br J Anaesth 1996;76:325.

66. Lewis JH, Weingold AB. The use of gastrointestinal drugs during pregnancy and lactation. Am J Gastroenterol 1985;80:912.

67. Khuroo MS, Datta DV. Budd-Chiari syndrome following pregnancy. Report of 16 cases with roentgenologic, hemodynamic and histologic studies of the hepatic outflow tract. Am J Med 1980;8:113.

68. Ilan Y, Oren R, Shouval D. Postpartum Budd-Chiari syndrome with prolonged hypercoagulability state. Am J Obstet Gynecol 1990;162:1164.

69. Nir A, Sorokin Y, Abramovici H, Theodor E. Pregnancy and primary biliary cirrhosis. Int J Gynaecol Obstet 1989;28:279.

70. Kaplan MM. Acute fatty liver of pregnancy. N Engl J Med 1985;313:367.

71. Purdie JM, Walters BN. Acute fatty liver of pregnancy: Clinical features and diagnosis. Aust N Z J Obstet Gynaecol 1988;28:62.

72. Miller D, Romero R. Management of hepatic failure in pregnancy. In Berkowitz RL (ed): Critical Care of the Obstetric Patient. New York, Churchill Livingstone, 1983.

73. Grimbert S, Fromenty B, Fisch C, et al. Decreased mitochondrial oxidation of fatty acids in pregnant mice: Possible relevance to development of acute fatty liver in pregnancy. Hepatology 1993;17:628.

74. Sjögren CMH. Hepatic emergencies in pregnancy. Med Clin North Am 1993;77:1115.

75. Brown MA, Passaris G, Carlton MA. Pregnancy-induced hypertension and acute fatty liver of pregnancy: Atypical presentations. Am J Obstet Gynecol 1990;163:1154.

76. Minakami H, Oka N, Sato T, et al. Preeclampsia: A microvesicular fat disease of the liver? Am J Obstet Gynecol 1988;159:1043.

77. Schoeman MN, Batey RG, Wilcken B. Recurrent acute fatty liver of pregnancy associated with a fatty acid oxidation defect in the offspring. Gastroenterology 1991;100:544.

78. Burroughs AK, Seong NH, Dojcinov DM, et al. Idiopathic acute fatty liver of pregnancy in 12 patients. Q J Med 1982;204:481.

79. Riely CA, Latham PS, Romero R, Duffy TP. Acute fatty liver of pregnancy. A reassessment based on observations in nine patients. Ann Intern Med 1987;106:703.

80. Ockner SA, Brunt EM, Cohn SM, et al. Fulminant hepatic failure caused by acute fatty liver of pregnancy treated by orthoptic liver transplantation. Hepatology 1990;11:59.

81. Amon E, Allen SR, Petrie RH, Belew JE. Acute fatty liver of pregnancy associated with preeclampsia: Management of hepatic failure with postpartum liver transplantation. Am J Perinatol 1991;8:278.

82. Antognini JF, Andrews S. Anaesthesia for caesarean section in a patient with acute fatty liver of pregnancy. Can J Anaesth 1991;38:904.

83. Corke PJ. Anaesthesia for caesarean section in a patient with acute fatty liver of pregnancy. Anaesth Intensive Care 1995;23:215.

84. Servin F, Cockshott ID, Farinotti R, et al. Pharmacokinetics of propofol infusions in patients with cirrhosis. Br J Anaesth 1990;65:177.

85. Gelman S. General anaesthesia and hepatic circulation. Can J Physiol Pharmacol 1987;65:1762.

86. Gelman S, Fowler KC, Smith KR. Liver circulation and function during isoflurane anesthesia in dogs. Anesthesiology 1983;59:A224.

87. Cook DR, Brandon BW, Stiller RL, et al. Pharmacokinetics of atracurium in normal and liver failure patients. Anesthesiology 1984;61:A433.

88. Berg B, Helm G, Petersohn L, Tryding N. Cholestasis of pregnancy. Clinical and laboratory studies. Acta Obstet Gynecol Scand 1986;65 107.

89. Shaw D, Frohlich J, Wittmann BA, Willms M. A prospective study of 18 patients with cholestasis of pregnancy. Am J Obstet Gynecol 1982;142:621.

90. Reid R, Ivey KJ, Rencoret RH, Storey B. Fetal complications of obstetric cholestasis. Br Med J 1976;1:870.

91. Sheehan HL. The pathology of hyperemesis and vomiting of late pregnancy. J Obstet Gynaecol Br Emp 1939;46:685.

CHAPTER

MALIGNANT HYPERTHERMIA

M. Joanne Douglas, M.D.

Malignant hyperthermia (MH) is an inherited disorder of skeletal muscle that produces a hypermetabolic syndrome when susceptible individuals (MHS) are exposed to the triggering anesthetic agents.[1] The known triggering agents are volatile anesthetics (halothane, isoflurane, enflurane, sevoflurane, and desflurane)[1–7] and succinylcholine. They act by causing a sudden rise in intramyoplasmic calcium, which results in increased skeletal muscle metabolism.[8] The diagnostic characteristics of acute MH are acidosis (combined metabolic and respiratory), muscle dysfunction (increased creatine kinase [CK], myloglobinuria, rigidity, hyperkalemia), and evidence of inheritance. Although the disorder is called *malignant hyperthermia*, marked elevation of temperature is often a late sign.[9] The increase in intracellular calcium may be due to a mutation in the ryanodine receptor such that the threshold stimulus for calcium release is lowered or a defect in modulation occurs at the receptor.[9]

In a study of MH in susceptible swine, Ryan and coworkers[8] demonstrated the sequence of events during a reaction. An increase in free myoplasmic calcium precedes an increase in end-tidal CO_2, which is followed by a decrease in SpO_2. These changes are then followed by tachycardia and lastly hyperthermia. Dantrolene reversed these changes in the same order. Hypermetabolism (increased end-tidal CO_2) begins when the intracellular calcium level rises above 0.6 to 0.7 μm, whereas muscle contracture and rigidity occur above 1.0 μm.[8]

MH AND INHERITANCE

MH is inherited in an autosomal dominant fashion with variable penetrance.[10] The RYR1 gene (responsible for the ryanodine receptor in skeletal muscle) appears causal for MH in pigs[11] and some humans.[12–20] Linkage studies attempting to isolate a single responsible gene in humans have demonstrated that human MH is multigenic.[20, 21] Correlation between deoxyribonucleic acid (DNA) testing and results of the caffeine halothane contracture test (CHCT, also known as the in vitro

contracture test, IVCT) has not been conclusive.[13] A possible reason for this uncertainty is the lack of 100% specificity for the CHCT.[22]

CLINICAL PICTURE OF MH

The classic picture of MH is that of an elevation in the end-tidal CO_2, elevation of oxygen consumption (may result in cyanosis or decreased SaO_2), acidosis (metabolic and respiratory), and muscle destruction (increased CK, myoglobinuria, hyperkalemia). These features result in tachycardia, tachypnea, unstable blood pressure (BP), dysrhythmia, and increased temperature. Muscle rigidity (either masseter muscle rigidity [MMR] at the time of intubation or generalized rigidity) is another sign. Approximately 10% of MH cases are fulminant and require rapid diagnosis and aggressive treatment.[23]

Although much debate has focused on the significance of MMR, especially in children, most consider its development a warning sign of impending MH. Although some use the terms *MMR* and *trismus* interchangeably, Hannallah and Kaplan[24] have classified MMR as an inability to open the mouth fully but intubation is possible, whereas trismus is the total inability to open the mouth and to perform intubation.[24] They consider both to be an early sign of MH and recommend discontinuing anesthesia unless it is required urgently. Some cases of incomplete relaxation (increased force is required to open the mouth) may be a normal variant of response to succinylcholine.[25] Under this circumstance, some advocate continuing anesthesia with nontriggering agents and close monitoring.[26] In one series of adult patients with MMR, 25% tested positive for MH using the caffeine halothane contracture test.[27]

In pigs, hyperthermia[28] can trigger MH in the absence of anesthetic triggers, whereas prior hypothermia attenuates MH.[29, 30] Elevated levels of CO_2 and potassium, and therapy with exogenous calcium or adrenergic agents, do not increase the chance of MH.[31–34]

RARE ENDOCRINE DISORDERS
■ ■ ■ ■ ■ ■ ■

Larry C. Gilstrap, III, M.D., and Donald H. Wallace, M.D.

Several different endocrinopathies may complicate pregnancy and may have significant adverse effects on both the mother and the fetus. Diagnosis may prove difficult because of numerous etiologies, and pregnancy can mask or mimic symptoms and signs of endocrine disease. Although thyroid disease and diabetes are relatively common during pregnancy, serious complications of these diseases, such as thyroid storm and diabetic ketoacidosis, are uncommon or rare. These uncommon complications are discussed in this chapter along with some of the other rare endocrinopathies. We emphasize the importance of team management of crises and emergencies.

THYROID STORM

Hyperthyroidism is relatively common in the general population, and hyperthyroidism or thyrotoxicosis occurs in approximately 1 in 2000 pregnant women.[1, 2] The majority of cases of hyperthyroidism in pregnancy are caused by Graves disease, although the condition may also be caused by thyroiditis, toxic adenoma, multinodular goiter, and gestational trophoblastic disease.[1-3] Fortunately, the most serious complication of hyperthyroidism, thyroid storm, is rare even in untreated pregnant women. This exaggerated hypermetabolic state occurs in 2% or less of pregnancies complicated by thyrotoxicosis.[4-6]

Signs, Symptoms, and Laboratory Findings

Pregnant women with thyroid storm have high fever, tachycardia, dysrhythmia, dehydration, and central nervous system signs and symptoms (Table 22–1). Nausea, vomiting, and diarrhea may also occur.

Cardiac function may be significantly affected in women with thyrotoxicosis and thyroid storm.[4, 5, 7] Hyperdynamic cardiac function may progress to significant depression in cardiac function if thyrotoxicosis has been present or untreated for a protracted period of time.[7] Davis and colleagues[4] reported heart failure in

12% of women with thyrotoxicosis during pregnancy. It is important to recognize the potential for cardiac failure when considering β-adrenergic blocker therapy in these women.

Laboratory tests are of little value in distinguishing thyroid storm from untreated thyrotoxicosis. The pregnant woman with thyroid storm has elevated thyroid function test results, including an elevated free thyroxine (T_4), free T_4 index, and free triiodothyronine (T_3) index. Thyroid-stimulating hormone (TSH) level is extremely low or undetectable. Leukocytosis may be present.

Maternal Effects

Thyroid crisis or thyroid storm is a life-threatening condition and should be treated as a medical emergency. Prompt recognition and treatment are essential to survival of both the mother and fetus; maternal mortality has been reported in approximately 15% of cases.[3, 5]

Fetal Effects

Thyroid storm may result in premature labor, premature birth, and intrauterine fetal demise. If the fetus is alive when the mother presents with thyroid crisis, there is often a nonreassuring fetal heart rate (FHR) pattern characterized by FHR tachycardia, decreased or absent beat-to-beat variability, and late deceleration. This abnormal FHR pattern generally improves with correction of the maternal metabolic derangement.

Thyrotoxicosis may develop in about 1% of neonates

TABLE 22–1. SIGNS AND SYMPTOMS OF THYROID CRISIS OR "STORM"[3-5]

Fever (101°F)	Congestive heart failure
Dehydration	Agitation, disorientation
Tachycardia	Coma
Atrial fibrillation	Vomiting and diarrhea

as a consequence of the transplacental passage of thyroid-stimulating immunoglobulin (TSI).[6] Thyrotoxicosis is usually transient (1–3 months).

Management

Pregnant women with thyroid storm should be admitted for intensive monitoring because they are often dehydrated and require vigorous hydration with crystalloids. Electrolyte abnormalities must be corrected and fever treated with a cooling blanket and acetaminophen. Propranolol is useful for the treatment of tachycardia, but cardiac failure should be ruled out and the electrocardiograph (ECG) monitored continuously.

Propylthiouracil (PTU) is started at an initial dose of 1 g, followed by 200 mg every 6 hours. PTU can be given via a nasogastric tube if the woman is comatose or is unable to tolerate oral intake. Potassium iodide (supersaturated potassium iodide solution, SSKI) should be given 1 hour after PTU administration and repeated every 8 hours, as needed. Lithium is a reasonable alternative to potassium iodide.[8] Corticosteroids (dexamethasone 2 mg IV every 6 hours for a total of 8 mg) are recommended by some to further block the conversion of T_4 to T_3. A treatment protocol is summarized in Table 22–2.

It is of paramount importance to not jeopardize the mother's life when her condition is unstable by performing an emergent cesarean section for fetal indications. As previously mentioned, the fetal condition generally improves with correction of the maternal metabolic derangement. Following the diagnosis and institution of therapy, a search should be made for underlying precipitating conditions, such as acute pyelonephritis or chorioamnionitis.

Anesthetic Considerations for Cesarean Delivery

Emergency obstetric and anesthetic management includes careful evaluation of the airway, recognizing

TABLE 22–2. A MANAGEMENT PROTOCOL FOR PREGNANT WOMEN WITH THYROID CRISIS[1,3,5,7]

Hospitalization
Intensive nursing care
Invasive hemodynamic monitoring
Hydration
Evaluate for heart failure
PTU 1000 mg po initially, followed by 200 mg po q6h
Sodium iodide (SSKI)* 5 drops q8h
Lithium carbonate 300 mg q6h if unable to tolerate SSKI
Propranolol 1 mg/min IV or 40 to 80 mg po q4h, if no heart failure
Dexamethasone 2 mg IV q6h for total of 8 mg
Look for precipitating causes (e.g., acute pyelonephritis)

*To be given 1 hour after PTU to block excessive hormone build-up

that significant enlargement of the thyroid gland can obstruct the trachea or a bronchus. Drugs such as ketamine,[9] which stimulate the sympathetic nervous system, must be avoided. Propranolol is contraindicated in the presence of congestive cardiac failure, bronchial asthma, and chronic obstructive pulmonary disease. Excess anxiety and sympathetic nervous system activation are of concern in the awake patient, even in the presence of successful regional anesthesia. Sedation with midazolam may lead to loss of recall of the delivery and increased potential for respiratory depression, pulmonary aspiration, and neonatal sedation. These side effects are unlikely to occur, however, if the dose of midazolam is restricted to 1 to 2 mg IV and is given in 0.5 mg increments. High levels of circulating thyroid hormones increase β-adrenergic receptors,[10] and thus epinephrine should not be added to local anesthetic solutions owing to the risk of an exaggerated circulatory response.

When required, phenylephrine is the pressor of choice in bolus doses of 20 to 40 μg. Adverse fetal effects have not been observed with these doses. With careful management, either general anesthesia or regional anesthesia is acceptable for cesarean delivery that is performed when the maternal condition has been stabilized. Postoperative monitoring also is essential because a crisis can occur in the recovery unit.[7] A diagnosis of a hyperthyroid state during general anesthesia is made on the basis of the history and intraoperative vital signs, which demonstrate a hypercatabolic state. Regional anesthesia can be accomplished safely if there are no signs of high-output cardiac failure.[11] Continuous epidural anesthesia has the advantage of slower onset of sympathetic blockade, with time to position the patient and to administer fluid boluses and small doses of phenylephrine to prevent hypotension.[11]

OTHER THYROID DISORDERS

Hypothyroidism

Most women affected by hypothyroidism experience infertility owing to chronic anovulation. One report described 100 women with untreated hypothyroidism who completed pregnancy.[12] The etiology of subclinical hypothyroidism includes subtotal thyroidectomy (38%), radioiodine therapy (27%), and primary hypothyroidism (27%). Clinical features consist of diminished deep tendon reflexes (69%), fatigue (44%), hair loss (44%), dry skin (38%), and brawny edema (19%). Diagnosis is confirmed by demonstrating a reduced T_4 serum level (mean 2.8 mg/dl, compared with a normal value during pregnancy of 8–16 mg/dl) and a striking elevation of TSH to 88 mIU/dl (normal value <10 mIU/dl).[12]

TABLE 22–3. DRUGS ALTERING THYROID FUNCTION

Drugs That Decrease TSH Secretion	Drugs That Alter T₄ and T₃ Transport in Serum	Drugs That Alter T₄ and T₃ Metabolism

Dopamine
Glucocorticoids
Octreotide
 	
Drugs That Alter Thyroid Hormone Secretion
 	
Decreased thyroid hormone secretion
  Lithium
  Iodide
  Amiodarone
  Aminoglutethimide
Increased thyroid hormone secretion
  Iodide
  Amiodarone
	Increased serum thyroxine-binding globulin (TBG) concentration
	  Estrogens
	  Tamoxifen
	  Heroin
	  Methadone
	  Mitotane
	  Fluorouracil
	Decreased serum TBG concentration
	  Androgens
	  Anabolic steroids (e.g., danazol)
	  Slow-release nicotinic acid
	  Glucocorticoids
	Displacement from protein-binding sites
	  Furosemide
	  Fenclofenac
	  Mefenamic acid
	  Salicylates
		Increased hepatic metabolism
		  Phenobarbital
		  Rifampin
		  Phenytoin
		  Carbamazepine
		Decreased T₄ 5'-deiodinase activity
		  Propylthiouracil
		  Amiodarone
		  β-Adrenergic-antagonist drugs
		  Glucocorticoids
		
		Cytokines
		
		Interferon-α
		Interleukin-2

Adapted from Surks MI, Sievert R: Drugs and thyroid function. N Engl J Med 1995; 333:1688. Copyright 1995 Massachusetts Medical Society. All rights reserved.

Hypothyroidism is associated with a high frequency of spontaneous abortion and early pregnancy loss. An increased risk of pre-eclampsia, placental abruption, anemia, cardiac dysfunction, and postpartum hemorrhage may exist.[12] The role of thyroid hormones in fetal growth and development and brain maturation has yet to be clarified.[13] Low birth weight is a recognized risk in the neonates of affected mothers, and there is increased risk of perinatal morbidity and mortality. Newborn screening programs followed by appropriate treatment of those with congenital hypothyroidism are associated with normal physical and intellectual development.[14–18] It remains unclear whether treatment in utero of the occasional fetus with hypothyroidism is necessary or desirable. Low-normal or occasional low intelligence quotients (IQs) have been observed in some children presenting with congenital hypothyroidism who had very low serum T₄ levels and very high thyrotropin concentrations with delayed bone maturation at birth. These observations have led to the suggestion that hypothyroidism in utero may be associated with irreversible mental retardation.[15–17]

Therapy of hypothyroidism in the pregnant patient with levothyroxin, 0.1 mg/day, is similar to replacement therapy in the nonpregnant patient, and there are no known adverse fetal effects. In considering the placenta a barrier to the maternal-fetal flux of thyroid hormones, it has been established that there are marked maternal to fetal gradients of free T₄ and T₃.[19–22] At delivery, maternal serum free T₄ and T₃ concentrations are twice those in cord serum.[20] Cord serum T₄ concentrations are decreased by 20 to 50% in newborns with thyroid agenesis or with a total defect in thyroid hormonogenesis compared with those in normal newborns.[21] The small amount of T₄ transferred to the fetus contributes to T₃ concentrations in the fetal brain and minimizes the effects of fetal hypothyroidism.[22]

Thyroid Dysfunction and Drugs

Various drugs affect thyroid function through their actions on production, secretion, transport, and metabolism of thyroid hormones (Table 22–3). Iodine-containing medications and radiographic contrast agents can affect thyroid function (Table 22–4). In addition to inorganic iodide, partial deiodination of iodine-containing organic compounds may induce persistent hypothyroidism.[23]

Enzymes that facilitate deiodination, glucuronidation, and sulfation are affected by a variety of drugs.[23] Phenobarbital increases T₄ and T₃ metabolism by stimulating hepatic microsomal drug-metabolizing enzyme activity. Phenytoin and carbamazepine also increase T₄ and T₃ metabolism in this way, and they cause

TABLE 22–4. IODINE CONTENT OF MEDICATIONS AND RADIOGRAPHIC CONTRAST AGENTS

Agent	Iodine Content
Iodides	
Potassium iodide (saturated solution)	≈25 mg/drop
Pima syrup (potassium iodide)	255 mg/ml
Lugol solution (potassium iodide + iodine)	≈7 mg/drop
Iodo-Niacin	115 mg/tablet
Antiasthmatic Drugs	
Mudrane	195 mg/tablet
Elixophyllin-KI (theophylline) elixir	6.6 mg/ml
Iophylline	2 mg/ml
Antiarrhythmic Drugs	
Amiodarone	75 mg/tablet
Radiographic Contrast Agents	
Iopanoic acid	333 mg/tablet
Ipodate sodium	308 mg/tablet
Intravenous preparations	140–380 mg/ml

Adapted from Surks MI, Sievert R: Drugs and thyroid function. N Engl J Med 1995;333:1688. Copyright 1995 Massachusetts Medical Society. All rights reserved.

hypothyroidism in patients treated with T_4. Transient hypothyroidism has been reported in patients with hypersensitivity reactions to phenytoin.[24]

The numerous ways in which the thyroid may be affected by drugs are related to the site of drug interaction.[23] Depending on the site of drug action and the underlying thyroid disorder, either hypothyroidism or hyperthyroidism may result. In patients with thyroid autonomy (e.g., multinodular goiter or hyperfunctioning thyroid adenoma), the drugs may result in hyperthyroidism.[23]

Thyroid Disorder From Treatment With Cytokines

Long-term therapy with cytokines in patients with chronic inflammatory disorders or tumors may result in thyroid dysfunction.[23] An increased risk for thyroid dysfunction occurs if antithyroid antibodies are present before treatment.[23] Interferon-α has been associated with antithyroid microsomal antibodies in 20% of patients, and transient hypothyroidism or hyperthyroidism or both may result.

Anesthetic Management and the Hypothyroid Patient

When replacement therapy has been adequate during the antepartum period, either general anesthesia or regional anesthesia is satisfactory, if operative delivery is required. If the patient is hypothyroid, however, there may be extreme sensitivity to induction agents, opioids, and sedatives. Minimal doses of sodium pentothal or ketamine are given for emergency cesarean delivery using general anesthesia. In some, nitrous oxide alone may cause unconsciousness. Careful titration of neuromuscular blocking agents is critical because of reduced skeletal muscle activity. Abnormal respiratory control mechanisms and physiologic responses to hypoxia and hypercarbia mandate monitoring of oxygen saturation and end-tidal CO_2.

Overall, anesthetic management includes monitoring for critical myocardial and hemodynamic effects of depressant drugs. A peripheral nerve stimulator may not be reliable in the severely hypothyroid patient.[25] The management of the hypothyroid patient population is further complicated by altered metabolism and inactivation of drugs, primary adrenal insufficiency, electrolyte and free-water clearance abnormalities, hypoglycemia, delayed gastric emptying, and skeletal and respiratory muscle dysfunction. Impaired response to hypoxemia, altered consciousness, and coma are potentially life-threatening.

If delivery cannot be delayed until treatment is instituted, the stress of labor or surgery may unmask a reduction in adrenal cortical function. Other serious end-organ effects include anemia, cardiomegaly, cardiomyopathy, conduction abnormality, and heart rate and stroke volume reduction. Invasive hemodynamic monitoring may be indicated in the presence of hypovolemia and abnormal baroreceptor reflexes. Placental abruption and pre-eclampsia are additional serious risks in the hypothyroid pregnant patient.

DIABETIC COMA

Diabetic Ketoacidosis

As with thyroid crisis, diabetic ketoacidosis (DKA) is relatively uncommon during pregnancy, although diabetes itself is relatively common. DKA may occur for the first time during pregnancy in women with previously undiagnosed diabetes. Treatment of premature labor with corticosteroids and/or β sympathomimetics can be a precipitating event.[26] Other associated factors include serious infection and neglect of care.

Signs, Symptoms, and Laboratory Findings

Signs and symptoms vary depending on the degree and stage of metabolic derangement. Women with DKA often present with nausea, vomiting, dehydration, altered mental status, polyuria, polydipsia, rapid respiration, and shortness of breath. They may have a "fruity breath" because of acetone formation.

Laboratory findings include hyperglycemia, ketonuria, ketonemia, and metabolic acidosis (arterial blood pH<7.30, and a decrease in bicarbonate). The major source of ketones is lipolysis (Fig. 22–1). This results from increased catecholamine secretion associated with decreased or no insulin.[27]

Besides dehydration, pregnant women with DKA may have electrolyte abnormalities such as hyponatremia and hyperkalemia. When the serum potassium levels are normal, the total body potassium is very low.

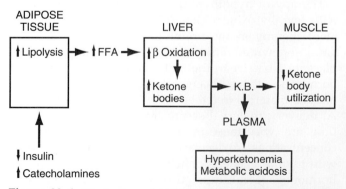

Figure 22–1. Mechanism of ketone body production in diabetic ketoacidosis. (FFA = free fatty acids; KB = ketone bodies. (Redrawn from Hagay ZJ. Diabetic ketoacidosis in pregnancy: Etiology, pathophysiology, and management. Clin Obstet Gynecol 1994;37:39.)

Montoro and coworkers[28] have summarized their experience with 20 consecutive cases of ketoacidosis in pregnancy. These workers divided their patients into two groups—those with a live fetus and those with a dead fetus. The characteristics of the pregnant women in these two groups are summarized in Table 22–5.

Maternal Effects

DKA is a life-threatening condition, and, albeit rare, it may result in maternal mortality. As with thyroid crisis, prompt recognition and treatment are essential to a good outcome for both the mother and fetus.

Fetal Effects

Dehydration, associated with DKA, may affect uteroplacental blood flow and along with acidosis can cause fetal demise. In Montoro's series, the fetal mortality rate was 35%, but there were no fetal deaths following initiation of therapy.[28] Interestingly, 30% of the cases of DKA and more than half of the fetal deaths occurred in women with unrecognized, new-onset diabetes.

The fetus of a woman with DKA often manifests a nonreassuring FHR pattern, with late decelerations and decreased or absent beat-to-beat variability. As with other maternal life-threatening disorders, the condition of these women must be stabilized before delivery is attempted (especially by emergency cesarean delivery). Moreover, once dehydration, acidosis, and electrolyte imbalance are corrected, the FHR often reverts to a normal pattern.

Management

Treatment includes correction of dehydration, electrolyte imbalance, acidosis, and, most importantly, hyperglycemia. Initial hydration consists of 1 to 2 l of isotonic saline over 1 to 2 hours to restore intravascular volume. Following saline hydration, sufficient crystalloid is administered to maintain adequate renal blood flow and uteroplacental blood flow, as evidenced by good urine output and a "normal" FHR pattern. This approach often requires 6 or more liters of fluid in the first 24 hours.

Insulin can be given several different ways, but we prefer a continuous insulin infusion at an initial rate of approximately 5 to 6 IU per hour. Once the blood glucose level falls below 250 mg/dl, the insulin infusion is decreased to 0.5 to 2 IU per hour, and an infusion of 5% dextrose in 1/2 normal saline is started. Potassium is administered if the level is less than 5.0 mEq/l and if the urine output is adequate.[27] Bicarbonate replacement is controversial, but generally it is recommended if the arterial pH is less than 7.10. Obviously, an underlying cause of DKA, such as infection, should be treated.

Hypoglycemic Coma

Pregnant women are particularly susceptible to severe hypoglycemia, especially in the first trimester when hyperemesis is common. Other causes are summarized in Table 22–6.

TABLE 22–5. CHARACTERISTICS OF PATIENTS WITH DIABETIC KETOACIDOSIS*

	Group 1	Group 2	p Value
No. patients	13	7	
Age (year)	25 ± 4.8	25.2 ± 4.6	
Parity	0.8 ± 1.2	0.5 ± 0.8	
Weight (kg)	66.3 ± 16.1	77.2 ± 21.7	
Gestational age (wk)	24.2 ± 7.4	30.9 ± 9.1	<0.05
New-onset diabetes	15%	57%	<0.001
Glucose (mg/dl)	374 ± 100	830 ± 400	<0.005
Na$^+$ (mEq/l)	134.1 ± 4.1	130.3 ± 5.4	
K$^+$ (mEq/l)	4.7 ± 0.8	4.8 ± 0.6	
Cl$^-$ (mEq/l)	106.5 ± 4.8	105.5 ± 7.7	
BUN (mg/dl)	14.2 ± 4.9	22.7 ± 9.8	<0.025
Osmolality (mmol/kg)	295.0 ± 10.9	311.0 ± 21.0	<0.025
Serum acetone (dilutions)	1:8 ± 4	1:9.6 ± 5.5	
Arterial pH	7.23 ± 0.08	7.19 ± 0.12	
Bicarbonate (mEq/l)	7.0 ± 2.3	5.7 ± 3.8	
Anion gap (mEq/l)	24.5 ± 6.0	28.1 ± 7.2	
Fluid requirements (ml)	5551 ± 3372	5087 ± 3493	
Insulin requirements (units)	127 ± 9.7	202 ± 115	<0.05
Length of resolution (hr)	28.6 ± 9.7	38.5 ± 13.5	<0.05

* Group 1: fetus alive; group 2: fetus dead
Na$^+$: sodium; K$^+$: potassium; Cl$^-$: chloride
From Montoro MN, Myers VP, Mestman JH, et al. Outcome in pregnancy in ketoacidosis. Am J Perinatol 1993;10:17.

TABLE 22–6. **CAUSES OF HYPOGLYCEMIA IN DIABETIC PREGNANT PATIENTS**

Hyperinsulinism
Excess activity
Anorexia
Abnormal counterregulatory responses
Anti-insulin antibodies
Antibodies to insulin receptors
Impaired absorption of insulin
Impaired intake (morning sickness, diarrhea, etc.)
Dead fetus
Factitious insulin use
Increased insulin sensitivity (first trimester)

From Reece AE, Homko CH, Wiznitzer A: Hypoglycemia in pregnancy complicated by diabetes mellitus. Clin Obstet Gynecol 1994;37:50.

Signs, Symptoms, and Laboratory Findings

Hypoglycemic coma may be preceded by irritability, tachycardia, nausea, diaphoresis, and mental confusion.[29] It is important to rule out ketoacidosis as a cause of altered consciousness in the pregnant diabetic woman. It is generally not difficult to distinguish hypoglycemia from hyperglycemia by measuring serum glucose and acetone levels. Moreover, hypoglycemia is relatively common during pregnancy whereas DKA is rare.

Maternal Effects

Significant hypoglycemia (i.e., blood glucose levels less than 30 mg/dl) can lead not only to coma but also to seizures and even death.

Fetal Effects

Fortunately, it appears that maternal hypoglycemia has little adverse effect on the fetus. No evidence exists to date to suggest that it is teratogenic.[29–31] Mild to moderate hypoglycemia is not associated with an increase in the frequency of nonreassuring FHR patterns.[29] Severe hypoglycemia resulting in seizures and/or coma, however, can indirectly affect fetal well-being.

Treatment

Treatment is relatively simple and primarily consists of raising the level of maternal plasma glucose. Raising the level can be accomplished by either glucose infusion or glycogen injection.[31]

Anesthetic Considerations

The timing of delivery is determined jointly by the obstetrician and anesthesiologist to ensure that the patient's condition is optimal. The preanesthetic evaluation should be completed as early as possible to allow assessment and correction of acid-base status and fluid and electrolyte abnormalities. If nonpharmacologic methods of pain control do not provide adequate relief in labor, continuous epidural analgesia is beneficial. Pain can lead to stimulation of the hypothalamic-hypophyseal axis, causing excess release of catecholamines, which oppose insulin activity and affect glucose homeostasis. Effective, regional anesthesia decreases circulating levels of catecholamines,[32, 33] reducing the potential for critical decreases in uteroplacental blood flow in patients with chronic uteroplacental insufficiency.

We recommend administration of serial 3-ml test doses of 0.25% bupivacaine to achieve a T10 sensory level with maintenance of analgesia by continuous epidural infusion (CIE) using a dilute bupivacaine solution (e.g., 0.125%) to which 2 μg/ml fentanyl has been added. Supplements of epidural fentanyl (50–100 μg) and additional 3-ml epidural boluses of bupivacaine (0.125–0.5%) may be given as needed. It is important to pay careful attention to positioning of the parturient to avoid aortocaval compression. Positioning can be achieved by left uterine tilt with a wedge under the right hip or with lateral posture. Frequent noninvasive brachial cuff blood pressure recordings for 30 minutes are recommended whenever epidural therapy is initiated or supplemented.

Combined spinal-epidural (CSE) and spinal anesthesia are suitable alternatives to epidural anesthesia, provided that aortocaval compression and hypotension are avoided. Intrathecal injection of lipid-soluble opioids produces rapid-onset analgesia.[34–37] The blood pressure and respiratory rate are monitored for 30 minutes after initiating this technique because there is a report of serious respiratory depression after intrathecal sufentanil during labor.[38] The CSE method is clinically useful if there is insufficient time to achieve adequate epidural pain relief for delivery (e.g., low-dose intrathecal plain bupivacaine 0.25% [2.5 mg] results in rapid pain relief). The epidural catheter is available to prolong or increase anesthesia.[39]

For forceps delivery, sensory blockade is increased with epidural boluses of 3 to 5 ml of bupivacaine 0.5% or lidocaine 2%. Sensory level of the extended segmental block should be T10 to S5. For cesarean delivery the block is extended to the T4 level. Acute fluid loads of crystalloid should be dextrose free,[40–43] and prophylactic ephedrine is administered to avoid hypotension. Local anesthetic solutions containing epinephrine have the potential to reduce uteroplacental blood flow and should be administered cautiously.[44–49]

PHEOCHROMOCYTOMA

Pheochromocytoma is a rare complication of pregnancy but is life-threatening when it does exist. Although most tumors are located in the adrenal medulla, approximately 10% can be found in the sympathetic ganglia.[50]

Multiple Endocrine Adenomas and Sporadic Pheochromocytomas

Pheochromocytomas may be part of various multiple endocrine adenoma (MEA) or neoplasia (MEN) syndromes (Table 22–7).[50–52] A study of 82 nonpregnant patients with pheochromocytoma compared the characteristics of sporadic pheochromocytoma with those of MEN-2 or von Hippel-Lindau (VHL) disease.[53] Of these 82 patients, 23% were familial carriers; 19% had VHL disease; and 4% had MEN-2. Prospectively, in 79 patients at risk for pheochromocytoma, 36 (46%) had a total of 42 unsuspected pheochromocytomas. Out of 130 patients with 185 pheochromocytomas, 43 had VHL disease, 24 had MEN-2, and 63 had sporadic tumors. Patients with familial and sporadic pheochromocytomas were different in mean age at diagnosis (32 versus 46 years), multifocal localization (55 versus 8%), and malignancy (0 versus 11%). Screening of all patients with pheochromocytomas is indicated to avoid further morbidity and mortality in the patients and their families.

Pheochromocytomas are rare during pregnancy.[54, 55] In a series of 139 cases reviewed by Schenker and Granat,[55] there were 56 maternal deaths—14 in the antepartum period, one intrapartum, and 35 within 3 days post partum. The most common causes of death were cardiovascular accident, cardiac arrest, and arrhythmia. Of 162 pregnancies in this report, only 45% of the fetuses survived.[55]

Signs, Symptoms, and Diagnosis

Hypertension is the most common sign of this condition, occurring in 98% of cases.[51, 52] Typically, 95% of pregnant women with pheochromocytoma present with one or more symptoms including headaches, pal-

TABLE 22–7. MULTIPLE ENDOCRINE NEOPLASIA (MEN) SYNDROMES AND PHEOCHROMOCYTOMA[50–53]

MEN-2A (WERMER'S SYNDROME)
Pancreatic β-cell islet adenoma
Pheochromocytoma
Medullary thyroid carcinoma
Hyperparathyroidism
Carcinoid syndrome
Adrenal cortical adenoma

MEN-2B (SIPPLE'S SYNDROME)
Mucocutaneous neuroma
Pheochromocytoma
Medullary thyroid carcinoma
Ganglioneuromas of visceral anatomic plexuses

pitations, and excessive sweating.[55] Normal pregnant women complain of these same symptoms, however. Biochemical tests and radiologic imaging are essential to detect pheochromocytoma.[53] No unanimity exists as to the single best test, although the highest sensitivity appears to be measurement of plasma catecholamines and lowest sensitivity, measurement of urinary vanillylmandelic acid (VMA).[56] Analytic methods for familial or sporadic pheochromocytomas include urinary norepinephrine, epinephrine, and vanillylmandelic acid levels measured by spectrofluorometry. Blood samples for plasma norepinephrine and epinephrine and plasma chromogranin A levels, determined by radioimmunoassay, are obtained after the patients have been supine for 30 minutes.[53] Serum parathyroid hormone level is measured by immunoradiometric assay.[53]

Diagnostic imaging procedures include abdominal ultrasonography, computed tomography (CT), magnetic resonance imaging (MRI), and ^{123}I meta-iodobenzyl guanidine scintigraphy (MIBG).[53] Provocative tests, for example, for phentolamine or histamine, are generally not recommended during pregnancy.[56] The clonidine suppression test, which suppresses catecholamines in patients with essential hypertension but not with pheochromocytoma,[56] has yet to be evaluated in pregnancy and may cause significant hypotension. Prospective evaluation of screening methods,[53] as compared with other studies, revealed the lower sensitivity of ultrasonography of 40% (versus 90–95%). Sensitivity for abdominal CT was 76% (versus 70–98%), MIBG scintigraphy 95% (versus 78–95%), and abdominal MRI 95% (versus 86–100%). Sometimes it is difficult to distinguish between the signs and symptoms of pheochromocytoma and those of pre-eclampsia, especially during the late second and third trimesters.

Maternal Effects

As mentioned, pheochromocytoma in association with pregnancy is life-threatening, and prompt diagnosis and treatment are essential to good outcome. Reported maternal mortality ranges from approximately 3% to nearly 50%.[50–52, 54, 55] Mortality is lower when the diagnosis is made antenatally,[54] treating with α-adrenergic blockers.[55, 57]

Fetal Effects

Fetal loss is reportedly as high as 50%.[52] With treatment using α-adrenergic blockers, however, fetal mortality is decreased to approximately 20%.[57]

Management

Pheochromocytoma during pregnancy may be managed either medically or surgically. Although the definitive treatment for this tumor is surgical, most clinicians utilize medical management during pregnancy with α-adrenergic blocking drugs. Phenoxybenzamine is usually given as an oral dose of 10 mg twice daily and increased by 10 mg/day until symptoms are controlled.[52] Phenoxybenzamine can also be administered intravenously if needed and has no known adverse fetal effects. Prazosin (α-blocker) can also be given, but labetalol (α- and β-blocker) should not be given until α-blockade is achieved.[50, 52]

Treatment

For the pregnant patient at or near term, medical management consists of phenoxybenzamine until the baby is delivered.[55] Maternal mortality is lower with cesarean delivery than vaginal delivery, and it is possible for the tumor to be resected at the time of delivery.[55]

Anesthetic Considerations

The pregnant woman with pheochromocytoma often requires cesarean section. Ten to fourteen days of phenoxybenzamine therapy may be needed to achieve adequate α-blockade, as demonstrated by a blood pressure of about 160–170/90 mm Hg. A tilt test should result in orthostatic hypotension of not less than 80/55 mm Hg.[58, 59] Serial hematocrit measurements decrease as intravascular volume increases from α_1- and α_2-receptor blockade. Before delivery, the electrocardiograph (ECG) should be free of ST-T segment changes and should show infrequent premature ventricular contractions.

Sedation with oral lorazepam the night before surgery and 2 hours preoperatively reduces maternal anxiety and activation of the sympathetic nervous system. Antacid prophylaxis (sodium citrate, metoclopramide, and ranitidine) is administered to reduce the risk of aspiration. The patient is sedated with intravenous fentanyl and small doses of midazolam, if required. In addition to the usual noninvasive monitors (ECG, pulse oximetry), the radial artery is cannulated using local anesthesia to directly measure the blood pressure. A second, large-bore peripheral intravenous cannula (14 or 16 gauge) is established to allow for rapid infusion of warmed crystalloids and colloids intraoperatively. Alfentanil (20–30 μg/kg) or fentanyl (2–3 μg/kg) and lidocaine (1–2 mg/kg) is administered to reduce the incidence of ventricular dysrhythmias and prevent or attenuate the pressor response to tracheal intubation. These drugs are given immediately before induction with 4 mg/kg sodium pentothal and 1.5 mg/kg succinylcholine.

Controlled ventilation with a nitrous oxide and oxygen mixture and isoflurane is acceptable for maintenance of general anesthesia. Normocarbia, oxygen-ation, and adequate depth of general anesthesia are maintained. Sodium nitroprusside (SNP, 50 mg added to 500 ml of 5% dextrose solution) can be infused to control blood pressure intraoperatively (average adult dose 3 μg·kg^{-1}·min^{-1}, maximum dose not to exceed 800 μg/min). If the surgery includes removal of the pheochromocytoma, SNP should be terminated when the adrenal vein is clamped. Typically, recovery from the SNP infusion occurs within 1 to 2 minutes, thus preventing a rapid fall in blood pressure once the tumor is removed.

After the umbilical cord is clamped intraoperative analgesia is maintained with fentanyl or sufentanil by bolus or infusion. Neuromuscular blockade is monitored with a peripheral nerve stimulator and vecuronium is administered, as required. Drugs that release histamine, such as atracurium and morphine, are avoided, because histamine releases catecholamines from chromaffin granules. Preference should be given to drugs like vecuronium, fentanyl, and etomidate, which do not cause histamine release. Other neuromuscular blocking drugs are available[60] (for example, cis-atracurium) that have a lower incidence of side effects, including those related to histamine release.

A randomized, controlled trial compared three general anesthetic techniques and one combined general/regional technique[61] for pheochromocytoma resection in nonobstetric patients. All patients had been treated preoperatively with α-adrenergic blockade, and β blockade was added to suppress dysrhythmia and tachycardia. Intraoperatively, hypertension was controlled with SNP infusion and increased depth of anesthesia. Fluid boluses, decreased depth of anesthesia, and phenylephrine infusion were effective in the management of hypotension. Dysrhythmias were treated with 0.1- to 0.5-mg boluses of propranolol. In this study of 24 patients, all techniques were satisfactory, no deaths occurred, and major organ morbidity was avoided.

Surgeons at some medical centers have performed cesarean section and tumor resection separately.[62, 63] A report of elective cesarean delivery followed by resection of pheochromocytoma[64] illustrates the concerns related to obstetric and anesthetic management of a joint procedure. These concerns were

1. Preoperative antihypertensive therapy with adrenergic blockers
2. Control of intraoperative blood pressure before delivery with short-acting vasoactive agents and adrenergic blockers, because once the tumor is removed serum catecholamines decrease rapidly
3. Avoidance of the depressant effects of large doses of opioids and benzodiazepines on the fetus before delivery.[64]

Preoperative use of a long-acting α-adrenergic blocker as a primary agent should possibly be avoided.

A report has appeared of an epinephrine infusion being needed to support blood pressure for 24 hours postoperatively, after a long-acting β-blocker had been given.[62] Magnesium sulfate (2–2.5 g/min) has been clinically helpful in maintaining cardiovascular stability during pheochromocytoma resection.[62, 65] Magnesium sulfate reduces systemic vascular resistance, slightly reduces mean arterial pressure in patients with severe pre-eclampsia,[66] and inhibits release of catecholamines from the adrenal medulla[67, 68] and peripheral adrenergic nerve terminals.[69] Magnesium sulfate also blocks catecholamine receptors and has a direct vasodilator effect.[70] Magnesium has the additional benefit of being familiar to obstetricians and obstetric anesthesiologists.

In the case described by James,[65] the patient was hypertensive immediately preoperatively, despite prior evidence of adequate α-adrenergic blockade. Treatment with additional α-blockers and propranolol did not control the blood pressure, but initiation of a magnesium sulfate infusion was successful. In one report, epidural anesthesia, combined with light general anesthesia and controlled ventilation, was associated with a stable operative course and minimal increase in circulating catecholamine levels.[61] In a similar case,[71] deafferentation was accomplished with a T1 sensory level; however, tumor retraction produced an abrupt increase in blood pressure (240/130), which was rapidly controlled with intravenous phentolamine in 1-mg increments (total dose 5 mg). No ECG abnormalities were seen intraoperatively, and vasopressors were not required after removal of the tumor. Sensory level on awakening was T5, and there was complete wound analgesia. The postoperative course was uneventful.[71] This case illustrates that, in the presence of sympathetic blockade with epidural anesthesia, postsynaptic receptors can still respond to the direct effects of a sudden increase in the circulating levels of catecholamines. Other possible problems with this technique include hypotension due to reduced sympathetic nervous system activity associated with ligation of the veins of the tumor and inadequate anesthesia if high abdominal exploration is required.

Autosomal Dominant Disease and Thyroid Nodule

When one endocrine adenoma has been identified, the question of MEA type-1 adenomatosis (Wermer's syndrome,* includes parathyroid adenoma or hyperplasia, pancreatic β-cell islet adenoma, pituitary adenoma, carcinoid syndrome, and adrenal cortical ade-

noma resulting in Cushing syndrome or hyperaldosteronism) or MEA type-2 adenomatosis (Sipple's syndrome) must be considered (Table 22–7). Fine-needle aspiration of a solitary thyroid nodule is recommended to rule out malignancy, because radionuclide scanning is contraindicated during pregnancy. About 50% of these women have a malignancy for which surgery is indicated.

Illustrative to these rare and complex endocrine disorders is the case history of a 25-year-old primigravida with a 34-week intrauterine pregnancy complicated by hypertension (blood pressure 170/100 mm Hg). Examination following admission revealed a single thyroid nodule and intermittent hypertension. Laboratory test findings confirmed elevated urinary VMA and plasma catecholamine and calcitonin levels. MRI revealed bilateral adrenal tumors (pheochromocytomas). After cesarean delivery, adrenalectomy was performed and subsequent medullary thyroid carcinoma was treated by total thyroidectomy.[64]

VON HIPPEL-LINDAU DISEASE

This familial disease is transmitted by an autosomal dominant gene and is characterized by hemangioblastomas of the retina, central nervous system (CNS), and viscera. It is associated with pheochromocytomas, renal cysts and renal cell carcinomas, pancreatic cysts, and epididymal cystadenomas. The possibility of spinal cord hemangioblastomas has discouraged administration of regional anesthesia in these patients.[72]

OTHER RARE ADRENAL GLAND DISORDERS

The incidence of Addison disease complicating pregnancy is unknown, and Cushing syndrome and pheochromocytomas are rare.

Addison Disease

Primary adrenal insufficiency is known as Addison disease. The patient excretes excessive amounts of sodium in the urine but retains potassium, leading to hyponatremia and hyperkalemia. Adrenal insufficiency may also occur as a result of pituitary failure or adrenal destruction, such as from adrenal tuberculosis or surgical removal of the adrenal glands.[73] Interestingly, there is one report of a woman with congenital 21-hydroxylase deficiency in whom pregnancy was further complicated by combined adrenal insufficiency and pre-eclampsia.[74]

---

*Editor's note: Not to be confused with *Werner* syndrome (premature aging), which has been described in pregnancy. (Ogawa M, Nagata H, Koyanagi T. Pregnancy complicated by Werner syndrome. Obstet Gynecol 1996;88:722).

Pathophysiology and Diagnosis

Plasma cortisol levels and cortisol-binding globulin levels are increased during normal pregnancy, but patients with Addison disease fail to show the expected rise in cortisol following adrenocorticotropic hormone (ACTH) stimulation.[75] Cortisol deficiency is accompanied by hyperpigmentation, weakness, fatigue, nausea, hypotension, and hypoglycemia. Hyponatremia, hyperkalemia, and volume depletion typify aldosterone insufficiency. Because nausea, vomiting, fatigue, weakness, and hyperpigmentation are common symptoms of pregnancy, the diagnosis of adrenal insufficiency is made more difficult. Clinical and laboratory features of adrenal insufficiency indicate deficiencies in cortisol and aldosterone.[75]

Many disorders of aldosterone biosynthesis and action occur, causing mineralocorticoid deficiency or excess.[76] Primary adrenal insufficiency in the neonatal period may result from intrapartum hemorrhage and traumatic breech delivery, or fulminating sepsis.[77] Autoimmune adrenal insufficiency occurs in older children and adults (2–3 in 100,000) as an isolated abnormality or as part of an autoimmune polyglandular deficiency syndrome (types I and II). In type II, women aged 20 to 40 years have chronic immune thyroiditis and insulin-dependent diabetes mellitus. The 21-hydroxylase enzyme is identified as a major adrenal autoantigen in these patients.[78] Hypoaldosteronism also occurs as a complication of the acquired immunodeficiency syndrome.[79] Whether the virus causes the adrenal insufficiency itself or whether other pathogens such as cytomegalovirus contribute is unclear. The antifungal drug ketoconazole may cause adrenal insufficiency because it inhibits mitochondrial cytochrome P450 enzymes such as cholesterol desmolase, 11β-hydroxylase, and aldosterone synthase.

Autosomal dominant or recessive forms of Addison disease are recognized in patients with pseudohypoaldosteronism,[76] which is defined as resistance to the action of aldosterone. Patients present shortly after birth with signs of mineralocorticoid deficiency, but they have markedly elevated plasma levels of aldosterone and renin. These elevated levels may be due to a lack of functional receptors, or the elevated plasma concentrations of aldosterone may downregulate normal receptors with a defect existing elsewhere in the pathway of aldosterone action.

Effect on Pregnancy

With adequate steroid replacement, pregnancy should be essentially uncomplicated with minimal risk.[76] Because acute adrenal insufficiency is a life-threatening condition that may be unmasked by the stress of labor and delivery, infection, and surgery, it is important to remain alert to this possibility in the undiagnosed patient with Addison disease. Overall prognosis for the fetus and newborn is good, although there are some reports of intrauterine growth restriction.[75]

Treatment

Essential therapy with glucocorticoids and mineralocorticoids is similar in women with Addison disease, whether pregnant or nonpregnant.

Anesthetic Management

With adequate replacement therapy, most women tolerate labor well. In addition, fluid balance and electrolytes levels should be normalized. Current techniques of epidural analgesia and regional or general anesthesia should be used when appropriate. Certain modifications are recommended for general anesthesia. For emergency surgery, infusion of hydrocortisone and fluid administration with careful invasive hemodynamic monitoring is indicated. Glucocorticoid deficiency can occur with autoimmune diseases, which results in primary hypothyroidism and hypoadrenalism, from an enzyme defect in cortisol synthesis, or from secondary causes of adrenal insufficiency, such as surgery or irradiation for pituitary or hypothalamic tumor. Circulatory collapse[80, 81] in addisonian patients under stress has several possible mechanisms[81] (e.g., loss of an enhanced response to catecholamines linked to steroids, altered receptor affinity, increased catecholamine metabolism, increased calcium uptake and altered electrolyte milieu, loss of cardiac glycogen, and decreased adenosine triphosphatase [ATPase] activity). Administration of incremental or low doses of anesthetic agents is recommended to avoid the risk of drug-induced myocardial depression. A peripheral nerve stimulator allows monitoring of neuromuscular blockade and titration of muscle relaxants, because skeletal muscle weakness is a typical feature of the disease. Whatever the etiology of onset of the adrenal insufficiency, there is potential for hypotension and circulatory collapse.

Cushing Syndrome

Pregnancy in patients with Cushing syndrome is rare, which is probably related to the fact that many affected women are infertile because of anovulation.[82–85] Cushing syndrome has been separated into two categories: (1) corticotropin-dependent, which is associated with excessive plasma corticotropin concentrations, stimulating the adrenal cortex to produce markedly elevated cortisol levels; and (2) corticotropin-independent, which is associated with excessive production of cortisol by abnormal adrenocortical tissue that suppresses the secretion of both corticotropin-releasing hormone (CRH) and corticotropin.[86] A review of the literature[82] in 1986 reported 33 women with Cushing syndrome in pregnancy; an adrenal adenoma was present in 15 (46%), adrenal hyperplasia in 12 (36%), and carcinoma in 6 (19%).

Diagnosis

The typical clinical features include weakness, muscle atrophy, abdominal striae, and easy bruising, and there may be abnormal glucose tolerance.[84] Cortisol levels are elevated during normal pregnancy, and much of this is protein bound. Pregnant women with Cushing syndrome do not have normal diurnal variation in cortisol levels. Following dexamethasone suppression tests, they fail to demonstrate suppression of baseline 17-hydroxycorticosteroid levels. Ultrasonography, magnetic resonance imaging, or computed tomography may be helpful in ruling out adenoma.

Effects on Pregnancy

Cushing syndrome has significant morbidity for mother and fetus.[82] Seventeen (41%) had preterm births, 7 (17%) spontaneous abortions, and 4 (10%) stillbirths. One third of patients had term births. Of the 15 women with adrenal adenomas, 44% developed pulmonary edema, and all had hypertension.

Treatment

In Koerten and coworkers' series,[82] unilateral or bilateral adrenalectomy during pregnancy (12–20 weeks) was performed in 7 women, and 1 received pituitary irradiation at 24 weeks' gestation. In these eight cases there were five term births, two premature births, and one spontaneous abortion. Surgery appears to produce the most favorable outcome with regard to pregnancy, but there are reports of successful medical therapy with metyrapone (one case) and the 5-HT antagonist cyproheptadine (three cases).[84–87] Transsphenoidal adenectomy has been successful during pregnancy in a patient with Cushing syndrome.[88]

Anesthetic Management

It is essential to evaluate coagulation, cardiovascular function, plasma glucose and electrolyte levels, and acid-base parameters in these patients before initiating any form of anesthesia. The greatest hazard during labor and delivery is severe hypertension. Thus, blood pressure should be monitored frequently and appropriate treatment initiated promptly. Control of blood pressure with hydralazine or labetalol is recommended. Severe or malignant-phase hypertension may be associated with cardiac failure and necessitates invasive monitoring. Polyuria and diabetes mellitus are frequent complications of Cushing syndrome and should be treated appropriately. Other complications include fluid retention, hypokalemia, and alkalosis, which also require treatment.

If regional anesthesia is planned, there may be technical problems related to central obesity, muscle wasting, osteoporosis with the potential for vertebral body collapse, and thinning and bruising of the skin.[88a] Psychiatric disturbances in the patient with uncontrolled Cushing disease may preclude regional anesthesia, as may coagulation abnormalities. Indirect sonographic guidance may prove helpful in identifying the midline, leading to successful regional anesthesia.[88b] Hypotension should be avoided by careful positioning with uterine tilt to avoid aortocaval compression, adequate fluid administration, and incremental injection of local anesthetics, because there may be an increased response to vasopressors.

Many of these women require operative delivery. Regional anesthesia and general anesthesia are appropriate, with the recognition that the patient may behave in a similar fashion to the patient with severe preeclampsia. A study of patients with severe pre-eclampsia revealed that appropriate anesthetic management with either regional or general technique can result in a successful outcome.[89] Intraoperatively, invasive hemodynamic monitoring can assist in the management of serious complications, such as cardiac failure and increased bleeding.

If severe hypertension is present on the patient's arrival to the operating room, hydralazine is administered according to protocol[89] and blood pressure is controlled to a range of 140 to 150/90 to 100 mm Hg. Before induction of general anesthesia, hypertension should be controlled to a diastolic pressure of 90 to 100 mm Hg with 50-µg boluses of nitroglycerin (dose 50–200 µg).[89] Intravenous opioids after cord clamping control, but do not eliminate, release of cortisol resulting from surgical stimulation.

CONCLUSIONS

Rare endocrine disorders are often a manifestation of a multisystem disorder, and they result from altered regulation of circulating hormone levels (Fig. 22–2). In pregnancy there are increased circulating levels of hormones from placental production. The importance of the hormone receptor complex is demonstrated by a decrease or an increase in receptors being associated with an endocrine deficiency or excess disorder. Furthermore, coupling of a hormone to a receptor allows the signal to be greatly amplified (e.g., hormone-sensitive adenylate cyclase system).[90, 91] Etiologies of rare endocrine disorders involve altered secretion, transport, inactivation, and clearance from the body (see Fig. 22–2). Complex drug interactions may occur at multiple sites (e.g., at the hypothalamic-pituitary-thy-

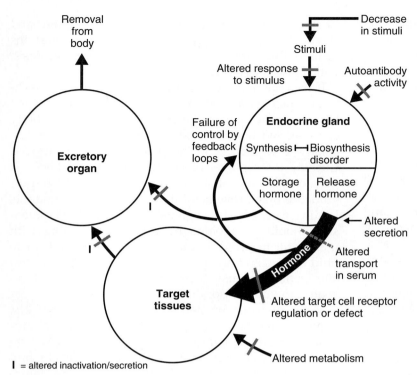

Figure 22–2. Steps in the pathways of endocrine disorders.

roid axis), and at extrathyroid pathways of thyroid hormone metabolism.[23, 92] Drugs may also alter hormone transport and production and clearance of hormone-binding proteins.[23]

Crises and emergencies typify the problems in diagnosis and management of rare and complex endocrine disorders. Life-threatening emergencies—for example, thyroid storm and diabetic ketoacidosis—need immediate and effective treatment, which is best managed by a team. Other examples of emergent management with high risk are found in patients with excessive circulating levels of hormones secreted by tumors or trophoblastic tissue (e.g., with a molar pregnancy).[93] We recommend a coordinated team approach, with early consultation of the anesthesiologist, to facilitate medical management.

References

1. American College of Obstetricians and Gynecologists. Thyroid disease in pregnancy. Technical Bull 181, June, 1993.
2. Mestman JH, Goodwin TM, Montoro MM. Thyroid disorders of pregnancy. Endocrinol Metab Clin North Am 1995;24:41.
3. Mastrogiannis DS, Whiteman VE, Mamopoulos M, Salameh WA: Acute endocrinopathies during pregnancy. Clin Obstet Gynecol 1994;37:78.
4. Davis LE, Lucas ML, Hankins GDV, et al. Thyrotoxicosis complicating pregnancy. Am J Obstet Gynecol 1989;160:63.
5. Clark SL, Cotton DB, Hankins GDV, Phelan JP. Thyroid storm in pregnancy. Handbook of Critical Care Obstetrics. Oxford, Blackwell, 1994, p 153.
6. Burrow GN. The management of thyrotoxicosis in pregnancy. N Engl J Med 1985;313:562.
7. Pugh S, Lalwani K, Awal A. Thyroid storm as a cause of loss of consciousness following anaesthesia for emergency Caesarean section. Anaesthesia 1994;49:35.
8. Burch HB, Wartofsky L. Life-threatening thyrotoxicosis. Endocrinol Metab Clin North Am 1993;22:263.
9. Kaplan JA, Cooperman LH. Alarming reactions to ketamine in patients taking thyroid medication: Treatment with propranolol. Anesthesiology 1971;35:229.
10. Maze M. Clinical implications of membrane receptor function in anesthesia. Anesthesiology 1981;55:160.
11. Halpern SH. Anaesthesia for Caesarean section in patients with uncontrolled hyperthyroidism. Can J Anaesth 1989;36:454.
12. Davis LE, Leveno KJ, Cunningham FG. Hypothyroidism complicating pregnancy. Obstet Gynecol 1988;72:108.
13. Burrow GN, Fisher DA, Larsen PR. Mechanisms of disease: Maternal and fetal thyroid function. N Engl J Med 1994;331:1072.
14. Glorieux J, Dussault JH, Morrissette J, et al. Follow-up at ages 5 and 7 years on mental development of children with hypothyroidism detected by Quebec screening program. J Pediatr 1985;107:915.
15. New England Congenital Hypothyroidism Collaborative. Neonatal hypothyroidism screening: Status of patients at 6 years of age. J Pediatr 1985;107:913.
16. Fisher DA, Foley BL. Early treatment of congenital hypothyroidism. Pediatrics 1989;83:785.
17. Rovet J, Ehrlick R, Sorbara D. Intellectual development in children with fetal hypothyroidism. J Pediatr 1987;110:700.
18. Glorieau J, Desjardins M, Lebarto M, et al. Useful parameters to predict the eventual mental development outcome of hypothyroid children. Pediatr Res 1988;24:6.
19. Fisher DA, Lehanan H, Lackey C. Placental transport of thyroxine. J Clin Endocrinol Metab 1964;24:393.
20. Abuid J, Klein AH, Foley TP Jr, Larsen PR. Total and free triiodothyronine and thyroxine in early infancy. J Clin Endocrinol Metab 1974;39:263.
21. Valsma T, Gons MH, deVijlder JJM. Maternal-fetal transfer of thyroxine in congenital hypothyroidism due to a total organification defect of thyroid agenesis. N Engl J Med 1989;321:13.
22. Fisher DA, Klein AH. Thyroid development and disorders of thyroid function in the newborn. N Engl J Med 1981;304:702.
23. Surks ML, Sievert R. Drugs and thyroid function. N Engl J Med 1995;333:1688.
24. Gupta A, Eggo MC, Utrecht JP, et al. Drug-induced hypothyroidism: The thyroid as a target organ in hypersensitivity reactions to anticonvulsants and sulphonamides. Clin Pharmacol Ther 1992;51:588.

25. Miller LR, Benumof JL, Alexander L, et al. Completely absent response to peripheral nerve stimulation in an acutely hypothyroid patient. Anesthesiology 1989;71:779.

26. American College of Obstetricians and Gynecologists. Diabetes and pregnancy. Technical Bull 200, Dec, 1994.

27. Hagay ZJ. Diabetic ketoacidosis in pregnancy: Etiology, pathophysiology, and management. Clin Obstet Gynecol 1994;37:39.

28. Montoro MN, Myers VP, Mestman JH, et al. Outcome in pregnancy in diabetic ketoacidosis. Am J Perinatol 1993;10:17.

29. Reece AE, Homko CH, Wiznitzer A. Hypoglycemia in pregnancies complicated by diabetes mellitus: Maternal and fetal considerations. Clin Obstet Gynecol 1994;37:50.

30. Kimmerle R, Heinemann L, Delecki A, Berger M. Severe hypoglycemia incidence and predisposing factors in 85 pregnancies in type I diabetic women. Diabetes Care 1992;15:1034.

31. Rayburn W, Piehl E, Jacober S, et al. Severe hypoglycemia during pregnancy: Its frequency and predisposing factors in diabetic women. Int J Gynaecol Obstet 1986;24:263.

32. Shnider SM, Abboud TK, Artal R, et al. Maternal catecholamines decrease during labor after lumbar epidural anesthesia. Am J Obstet Gynecol 1983;147:13.

33. Abboud TK, Artal R, Hendriksen EH, et al. Effects of spinal anesthesia on maternal circulating catecholamines. Am J Obstet Gynecol 1982;142:252.

34. D'Angelo RD, Anderion MT, Philip J, et al. Intrathecal sufentanil compared to epidural bupivacaine for labor analgesia. Anesthesiology 1994;80:1209.

35. Camann WR, Denney RA, Holby ED, Datta S. A comparison of intrathecal, epidural, and intravenous sufentanil for labor analgesia. Anesthesiology 1992;77:884.

36. Camann WR, Mintzer BH, Denney RA, Datta S. Intrathecal sufentanil for labor analgesia: Effects of added epinephrine. Anesthesiology 1993;78:870.

37. Arkoosh VA, Sharkey SJ, Norris MC, et al. Subarachnoid labor analgesia. Fentanyl and morphine versus sufentanil and morphine. Reg Anesth 1994;19:243.

38. Hays RL, Palmer CM: Respiratory depression after intrathecal sufentanil during labor. Anesthesiology 1994;81:511.

39. Stacey RGW, Watts SS, Kadim MY, et al. Single space combined spinal-epidural technique for analgesia in labour. Br J Anaesth 1993;71:499.

40. Datta S, Brown WU Jr. Acid-base status in diabetic mothers and their infants following general or spinal anesthesia for cesarean section. Anesthesiology 1977;47:272.

41. Datta S, Brown WU Jr, Ostheimer GW, et al. Epidural anesthesia for cesarean section in diabetic parturients: Maternal and neonatal acid base status and bupivacaine concentration. Anesth Analg 1981;60:574.

42. Kenepp NG, Shelley WC, Kumar S. Effects on newborn of hydration with glucose in patients undergoing Caesarean section with regional anaesthesia. Lancet 1980;1:645.

43. Kenepp NB, Kumar S, Shelley WC, et al. Fetal and neonatal hazards of maternal hydration with 5% dextrose solutions before Caesarean section. Lancet 1982;1:1150.

44. Moore DC, Batra MS. The components of an effective test done prior to epidural block. Anesthesiology 1981;55:693.

45. Cartwright PD, McCarroll SM, Antzaka C. Maternal heart rate changes with a plain epidural test dose. Anesthesiology 1986;65:226.

46. Leighton BL, Norris MC, Sos KM, et al. Limitations of epinephrine as a marker of intravascular injection in laboring women. Anesthesiology 1987;66:688.

47. Hood DD, Owen DM, Jones FM. Maternal and fetal effects of epinephrine in gravid ewes. Anesthesiology 1986;64:610.

48. Chestnut DH, Owen CL, Brown DK, et al. Does labor affect the variability of maternal heart rate during induction of epidural anesthesia? Anesthesiology 1988;68:622.

49. Marx GF, Elstein ID, Schuss M, et al. Effects of epidural block with lignocaine and lignocaine-adrenaline on umbilical artery velocity waveform ratios. Br J Obstet Gynecol 1990;97:517.

50. Cunningham FG, Gant NF, MacDonald PC, et al. Endocrine disorders. In Williams Obstetrics, 19th ed. Norwalk, CT, Appleton & Lange, 1993, p 1201.

51. Kaplan NM. Adrenal diseases: Pheochromocytoma. In Clinical Hypertension, 4th ed. Baltimore, Williams & Wilkins, 1986, p 375.

52. Botchan A, Hauser R, Kupferminc M, et al. Pheochromocytoma in pregnancy: Case report and review of literature. Obstet Gynecol Surv 1995;50:321.

53. Neumann HP, Berger DP, Sigmund G, et al. Pheochromocytomas, multiple endocrine neoplasia type 2, and von Hippel-Lindau disease. N Engl J Med 1993;329:1531.

54. Schenker JG, Chowers I. Pheochromocytoma and pregnancy. Review of 89 cases. Obstet Gynecol Surv 1971;26:739.

55. Schenker JG, Granat M. Pheochromocytoma and pregnancy: An updated appraisal. Aust N Z J Obstet Gynaecol 1982;22:1.

56. Bravo EL, Gifford REW. Pheochromocytoma: Diagnosis, localization, and management. N Engl J Med 1984;311:1298.

57. Stenstrom G, Swolin K. Pheochromocytoma in pregnancy: Experience of treatment with phenoxybenzamine in three patients. Acta Obstet Gynecol Scand 1985;64:357.

58. Smith RJ, Dluhy RG, Williams GH. Endocrinology. In Vandam LD (ed): To Make the Patient Ready for Anesthesia: Medical Care of the Surgical Patient, 2nd ed. Menlo Park, CA, Addison-Wesley, 1984, p 141.

59. Litt L, Roizen MF. Endocrine and renal function. In Brown DL (ed): Risk and Outcome in Anesthesia. Philadelphia, JB Lippincott, 1988, p 120.

60. Hunter JM. New neuromuscular blocking drugs. N Engl J Med 1995;332:1691.

61. Roizen MF, Horrigan M, Koike EI, et al. A prospective randomized trial of four anesthetic techniques for resection of pheochromocytoma. Anesthesiology 1982;57:A43.

62. James MFM. Use of magnesium sulphate in the anaesthetic management of pheochromocytoma: A review of 17 anaesthetics. Br J Anaesth 1989;62:616.

63. Stonham J, Wakefield C. Phaeochromocytoma in pregnancy. Anaesthesia 1983;38:654.

64. Van der Haart CH, Heringa MP, Dullaart RPF, Arnoudse JG. Multiple endocrine neoplasia presenting as phaeochromocytoma during pregnancy. Br J Obstet Gynaecol 1993;100:1144.

65. James MF. The use of magnesium sulphate in the anesthetic management of pheochromocytoma. Anesthesiology 1985;62:188.

66. Cotton DB, Gonik B, Dorik B, Dorman KF. Cardiovascular alterations in severe pregnancy-induced hypertension: Acute effects of magnesium sulphate. Am J Obstet Gynecol 1984;148:152.

67. Douglas WW, Rubin RP. The mechanism of catecholamine release from the adrenal medulla and the role of calcium in stimulus-secretion coupling. J Physiol 1963;167:288.

68. Lishajko F. Releasing effect of calcium and phosphate on catecholamines, ATP and protein from chromaffin granules. Acta Physiol Scand 1970;79:575.

69. Kirpekar SM, Misu Y. Release of noradrenaline by splenic nerve stimulation and its dependence on calcium. J Physiol 1967;188:219.

70. Altura BM, Altura BT. Magnesium ions and contraction of vascular smooth muscle in relationship to some vascular diseases. Fed Proc 1981;40:2674.

71. Cousins MJ, Rubin RB. The intraoperative management of phaeochromocytoma with total epidural sympathetic blockade. Br J Anaesth 1974;46:78.

72. Joffe D, Robbins R, Benjamin A. A Caesarean section and phaeochromocytoma resection in a patient with von Hippel-Lindau Disease. Can J Anaesth 1993;40:870.

73. Brent F. Addison's disease and pregnancy. Am J Surg 1950;79:645.

74. Yarnell RW, D'Alton ME, Steinbok VS. Pregnancy complicated by preeclampsia and adrenal insufficiency. Anesth Analg 1994;78:176.

75. O'Shaughnessy RW, Hackett KJ. Maternal Addison's disease and fetal growth retardation. J Reprod Med 1984;29:752.

76. White PC. Mechanisms of disease: Disorders of aldosterone biosynthesis and action. N Engl J Med 1994;331:250.

77. Migeon CJ, Lanes RL. Adrenal cortex: Hypo- and hyperfunction. In Lifshitz F (ed) Pediatric Endocrinology: A Clinical Guide, 2nd ed. New York, Marcel Dekker, 1990, p 333.

78. Winqvist O, Karlsson FA, Kampe O: 21-Hydroxylase, a major autoantigen in idiopathic Addison's disease. Lancet 1992;339:1559.

79. Brown LS Jr, Singer F, Killian P: Endocrine complications of AIDS and drug addiction. Endocrinol Metab Clin North Am 1991;20:1437.

80. Knudson L, Christiansen LA, Lorentzen JE: Hypotension during

and after operation in glucocorticoid-treated patients. Br J Anaesth 1981;53:295.

81. Deutschman CS: Anesthetic considerations in the use of corticosteroids and antibiotics. In Rogers MC (ed): Principles and Practice of Anesthesiology, vol 2. St. Louis, Mosby–Year Book, 1993.

82. Koerten JM, Morales WJ, Washington SR, et al. Cushing's syndrome in pregnancy: A case report and literature review. Am J Obstet Gynecol 1986;154:626.

83. Grimes EM, Gayez JA, Miller GL. Cushing's syndrome during pregnancy. Obstet Gynecol 1973;42:550.

84. Gormley MJ, Hadden DR, Kennedy TL, et al. Cushing's syndrome in pregnancy: Treatment with metyrapone. Clin Endocrinol 1982;16:283.

85. Kasperlik-Zaluska A, Migdalska B, Hartwig W, et al. Two pregnancies in a woman with Cushing's syndrome treated with cyproheptadine. Br J Obstet Gynaecol 1980;87:1171.

86. Orth DN. Cushing's syndrome. N Engl J Med 1995;332:791.

87. Montgomery DAD, Welbourne RB. Cushing's syndrome: 20 years after adrenalectomy. Br J Surg 1978;65:221.

88. Casson IF, Davis JC, Jeffreys RV, et al. Successful management of Cushing's disease during pregnancy by transsphenoidal adenectomy. Clin Endocrinol 1987;27:423.

88a. Glassford J, Eagle C, McMorland GH. Caesarean section in a patient with Cushing's syndrome. Can Anaesth Soc J 1984;31:447.

88b. Wallace DH, Currie JM, Santos R. Indirect sonographic guidance for epidural anesthesia in obese pregnant patients. Reg Anesth 1992;17:233.

89. Wallace DH, Leveno KJ, Cunningham FG, et al. Randomized comparison of general and regional anesthesia for cesarean delivery in pregnancies complicated by severe preeclampsia. Obstet Gynecol 1995;86:193.

90. Ross EM, Gilman A. Biochemical properties of hormone-sensitive adenylate cyclase (review). Annu Rev Biochem 1980;49:533.

91. Rodbell M. The role of hormone receptors, and GTP-regulatory proteins in membrane transduction. Nature 1980;284:17.

92. Bartalena L, Grasso L, Brogioni S, et al. Serum interleukin-6 in amiodarone-induced thyrotoxicosis. J Clin Endocrinol Metab 1994;78:423.

93. Solak M, Aturk G. Spinal anesthesia in a patient with hyperthyroidism and hydatidiform mole. Anesth Analg 1993;77:851.

HEMATOLOGIC DISORDERS
■ ■ ■ ■ ■ ■ ■

M. Joanne Douglas, M.D., and Penny J. Ballem, M.D.

BACKGROUND

Normal Hematologic Indices

During pregnancy there is a progressive increase in maternal blood volume that is largely the result of an increase in plasma volume (Table 23–1). This increase begins at the sixth week of gestation and plateaus at about 34 to 36 weeks' gestation.[1] The maximum is about 45 to 55% above baseline (1–1.5 l). Red blood cell (RBC) mass increases by 15 to 20% throughout pregnancy, with the hematocrit dropping to its low point at week 35 (physiologic anemia of pregnancy).[2, 3] The rise in RBC mass results in a high demand for iron and, as a result, total body iron stores decrease, reflected by the serum ferritin level, reaching a nadir at 28 to 32 weeks.[3] The anemia of pregnancy is accompanied by a rise in the mean corpuscular volume (range 90–102 fL), which is not accounted for by either vitamin B_{12} or folate deficiency. If iron stores are not maintained by the administration of iron supplements, iron deficiency results in a reduction in mean corpuscular volume (MCV). This lowering of MCV, however, is often still within the normal range for the nonpregnant state, and the diagnosis of iron deficiency can be missed. Combined iron and folate deficiency are common in

the setting of poor nutrition. The rise in the MCV (commonly pathognomonic of folate deficiency) may be negated by the low MCV associated with iron deficiency. Thus, clinicians must look for other signs of folate deficiency (hypersegmented polymorphonuclear leukocytes, reduced RBC folate levels).[1, 4]

During pregnancy, up to 25% of women show a mild to moderate leukocytosis (up to $15,000 \times 10^9/l$), which is due mainly to an increase in the number of neutrophils.[3, 5] Some debate continues as to whether the platelet count remains the same or has a progressive fall with increasing gestation.[6–10] Platelet volume appears constant, but there is an increase in the distribution of platelet size. As discussed later, approximately 8% of normal pregnant women sustain a fall in the platelet count to 90 to $150 \times 10^9/l$ during pregnancy. The underlying pathophysiology is unknown, but possible factors include a dilutional state due to the increase in plasma volume or due to the physiologic state in pregnancy of greater platelet turnover.[7, 11, 12]

The pregnant patient is considered to be "hypercoagulable," with most coagulation factors increasing during pregnancy. The most remarkable changes involve increases in factors VII, VIII (both F VIII:c and F VIII:von Willebrand [VWF]), X, XII, and fibrinogen.[13] As a result, there is a mild shortening of both the

TABLE 23–1. HEMATOLOGIC CHANGES OF NORMAL PREGNANCY

Parameter	Direction of Change	Time of Peak or Nadir
Blood volume	Increase (45–55%)	34–36 weeks
RBC mass	Increase (15–20%)	Term
Ferritin	Decrease	28–32 weeks
MCV	Increase	24–28 weeks
WBCs	Mild to moderate increase (25%)	Term
Platelet count	Same or decrease	32–36 weeks (nadir)
Factors VII,VIII,X,XII	Increase	
Fibrinogen	Increase	Term
Factor IX	Unchanged	
Factor XI	Decrease (62%)	Term
Protein C	Unchanged	
Protein S	Decrease (40–50%)	12 weeks
ATIII	Unchanged	

RBC = Red blood cell; WBC = white blood cell; MCV = mean cell volume; ATIII = antithrombin III

prothrombin time (PT), activated partial thromboplastin time (PTT), and thrombin time (TT). Concomitantly, there is a decrease in fibrinolytic activity, which rapidly returns to normal post partum. Proteins C and S are naturally occurring vitamin K–dependent physiologic inhibitors of thrombosis. Inherited deficiencies of these proteins lead to an increased tendency to thrombosis. Protein C levels do not change during pregnancy,[14] but there is an early (12-week) decrease in free and bound protein S levels[15] (40–50% of normal), which then remain stable to term. Antithrombin III (ATIII), one of the most powerful physiologic anticoagulants, remains stable throughout pregnancy in the absence of complications such as pre-eclampsia.

Hematologic Testing

A routine complete blood count (CBC) during early pregnancy (first trimester) is important to identify common, pre-existing hematologic disorders that may affect the pregnancy. The most common findings are iron deficiency anemias, thalassemic syndromes, and thrombocytopenias. Further studies and careful consideration of the impact of such abnormalities on both the mother and fetus should follow. In an uncomplicated pregnancy, a repeat blood count in the third trimester is done to assess the hematocrit in preparation for delivery.

Coagulation screening is generally performed only

- To investigate a significant bleeding history
- To follow factor levels in patients with established disorders
- During acute peripartum complications such as pre-eclampsia, massive hemorrhage, or disseminated intravascular coagulopathy (DIC)
- To monitor anticoagulation therapy.

Screening assays include platelets, PT, PTT, and fibrinogen levels. In the past, the bleeding time was used to predict the risk of bleeding as a consequence of thrombocytopenia or related platelet functional disorders. Its subjective nature as a measure of platelet function and its established lack of sensitivity and specificity[16, 17] as a predictor of clinical bleeding, however, have precluded its usefulness.[18] It does remain a helpful diagnostic test for patients with platelet function disorders.

Several centers are currently using thromboelastography to detect the risk of clinical bleeding[19, 20]; however, its sensitivity and specificity remain unproved. Thus, the ability of this test to predict the risk of bleeding into the epidural space during regional anesthesia is unknown.

Transfusion

The indications for transfusion of blood products during pregnancy are relatively few. In most instances, the need for blood products arises in preparation for delivery in patients with pre-existing disorders or in response to an acute peripartum complication such as acute abruption with DIC, severe pre-eclampsia, or postpartum hemorrhage.[21] Careful counseling of patients should be undertaken, even under emergent conditions, to alert them to the risks of blood products. In patients considered at high risk of hemorrhage, techniques used to attempt to decrease the need for homologous transfusion include autologous donation[21] and, at the time of operative delivery, acute hemodilution.[22]

Patients being prepared for surgery, in a setting where the use of blood products can be anticipated, should receive a full discussion in advance. Their wishes should be documented with regard to the blood products. Although now more than ever before, clinical and laboratory screening of blood donors are extremely rigorous, there are few blood products that carry no risk of transmissible diseases. At the current time, all donated blood products are tested for antibodies to hepatitis C, human immunodeficiency virus (HIV) I and II, HIV P24 Ag, human T cell lymphotropic virus (HTLV) I, and syphilis. All donated blood products are also tested for the hepatitis B virus (HBV) antigen. Awareness is growing for the existence of other agents (for example, the Creutzfeldt-Jakob agent) that as yet we are unable to detect.

Significant advances have been made in the inactivation of viruses in the manufacture of fractionated blood products (e.g., clotting factor preparations); however, it is critical that we continue to balance benefit with risk. Recombinant gene technology has enabled the development of some products, such as specific coagulation factors. The cost of these preparations is prohibitive, however, and we still remain largely dependent on plasma-derived products.

Apheresis

Apheresis involves separation of blood into its various components. Apheresis is a technique utilized during pregnancy to treat certain conditions. A complete review on this topic discusses the risks and potential benefits and outlines the reports in which it has been used in pregnancy.[23] Some of the conditions treated include myasthenia gravis; chronic myelogenous leukemia; thrombotic thrombocytopenic purpura (TTP); hemolytic uremic syndrome (HUS); and hemolysis, elevated liver enzymes, and low platelets (HELLP) syndrome. Apheresis also has been done in patients when there is a risk of fetal death. Such risks include antiphospholipid antibody syndrome, rare cell phenotypes, such as anti-P antibodies, causing complete congenital heart block, newborn Rh hemolytic disease, sickle cell disease, and alloimmune thrombocytopenia.

RED BLOOD CELL (RBC) ABNORMALITIES

Anemia

Anemia occurs commonly during pregnancy, as noted earlier, most frequently from hemodilution (physiologic anemia of pregnancy) or from poor nutrition due to inadequate intake of iron or folate. The broad spectrum of hemoglobinopathies, thalassemic syndromes, hemolytic anemias, and anemias related to primary bone marrow disorders can all occur in pregnancy. Furthermore, there is an increasing number of women with chronic disorders, such as renal failure, solid organ transplants, and rheumatologic conditions, which can be associated with anemias related to impaired erythropoiesis or drugs. The management throughout pregnancy of many of these patients is related to the potential effect of the anemia on both maternal and fetal well-being. A clear understanding of the pathophysiology of the anemia, inheritance patterns, and other mechanisms of involvement of the fetus is essential.

Transfusion of RBCs is only one potential intervention, which may or may not be necessary, and other therapeutic maneuvers should be weighed against the risks associated with transfusion. In most patients, particularly those with longstanding anemia, there is good physiologic compensation in the mother, and expectant management is appropriate. Erythropoietin in pregnancy is still experimental, but with the licensing of this product in Canada, there will be more opportunities to explore its usefulness.

Parturients with Anemia

Patients with compensated anemia tolerate anesthesia well. The choice of anesthetic technique and specific drugs is determined by the underlying disease. With regard to RBC transfusion, a careful assessment of the mother's hemodynamic status should be undertaken. There is no clear hemoglobin level threshold below which transfusion is essential. In a patient well compensated to the anemia (e.g., with chronic iron deficiency), a cesarean section can safely be undertaken with a hemoglobin level below 80 g/l. Unless there is evidence of ongoing hemolysis, active bleeding, or severe symptoms, compensated anemia should not be treated with transfusion. If transfusion is required, proper counseling of the patient should be undertaken with regard to the risks. Supplemental oxygen should be administered to women with a hemoglobin level less than 80 g/l.

Regional techniques are not contraindicated unless there is a concomitant hemostatic defect due to dysfunctional platelets (uremia) or thrombocytopenia (aplastic anemia). The temperature of the environment should be controlled for patients with temperature-sensitive hemolysis. In patients with combined cytopenias (thrombocytopenia and neutropenia), consideration should be given to appropriate interventions, such as antibiotics, and transfusion of specific products, such as platelets.

Hemoglobinopathies and the Thalassemias

Inherited abnormalities of hemoglobin structure (hemoglobinopathies) or synthesis (thalassemias) are important from the perspective of both the fetus and mother. Only 3% of maternal anemia occurs as a result of inherited abnormalities of hemoglobin structure or synthesis.[24] These abnormalities may produce asymptomatic maternal anemia or may lead to severe complications with increased perinatal morbidity and mortality. For those practitioners caring for women in the early stages of pregnancy, discussing a need or desire for prenatal diagnosis is very important, especially for women with sickle cell anemia and thalassemia.[25] Furthermore, in patients with ongoing chronic extravascular hemolysis and ineffective erythropoiesis, iron overload is an important, usually avoidable (in the carrier states), complication. Thus, iron supplementation in pregnancy should be withheld pending review of the serum ferritin level. Supplemental folic acid is essential to all patients with these syndromes due to the extra demands placed on the marrow in pregnancy.

Thalassemia

Many different forms of thalassemia are known, but alpha- and beta-thalassemic syndromes are most commonly seen in North America. The majority of patients with thalassemia have a benign carrier state (heterozygous beta-thalassemia and the two-gene deletion of alpha-thalassemia). Patients have mild anemia in early pregnancy and most follow a pattern similar to their nonthalassemic counterparts, with the physiologic anemia of pregnancy causing a drop in hemoglobin level. The drop in hemoglobin level is progressive until the middle of the last trimester, but the nadir of the hemoglobin level is significantly below the normal range for pregnancy. More clinically relevant is the fact that these patients usually compensate well for the degree of anemia.

The three-gene deletion state of alpha-thalassemia (hemoglobin H disease) is usually a mild to moderate hemolytic anemia in the nonpregnant state, which is associated with splenomegaly and chronic anemia. By the third trimester, some patients with this disorder may be symptomatic from the anemia. Fetal well-being and growth should be followed carefully, and evidence of compromise of fetal growth or significant symptoms in the mother may be an indication for transfusion.

Limited experience has been reported with patients

who have the most severe form (homozygous state) of beta-thalassemia in pregnancy. Most of the affected young women have symptomatic hemosiderosis by the time they reach the childbearing years, with associated endocrinopathy and cardiomyopathy. Fourteen pregnancies in nine patients with homozygous beta-thalassemia are reported in the literature.[26] Their obstetric management was complicated by severe anemia, chronic hypoxia, and myocardial hemosiderosis from iron overload. Cardiac dysrhythmias and congestive heart failure are common, and these complications are aggravated by the physiologic changes of pregnancy. Fetal problems included fetal loss, preterm labor, and intrauterine growth retardation. Another rare reported complication that is of interest to anesthesiologists is spinal cord compression by extramedullary hematopoiesis in a pregnant patient with thalassemia.[27] This condition was treated with blood transfusion with complete recovery.

Hemoglobinopathies

Patients with the homozygous states for hemoglobin C, D, and E present clinically with chronic hemolysis. Such patients behave in pregnancy the same as any patient with chronic hemolytic anemia, with increased demand for the nutritional building blocks used for erythropoiesis. They are susceptible to a number of acute crises—megaloblastic (from inadequate folate supplementation) and aplastic and hypersplenic (both often follow acute viral illness); however, these are unusual complications in pregnancy. Patients may present with combined abnormalities, particularly in association with the thalassemias. Some combinations are beneficial in terms of the severity of anemia (e.g., patients with β-chain hemoglobinopathies generally do better than those with alpha-thalassemia traits) and others are detrimental, with a more severe clinical course.

Anesthesia in the Thalassemias and Hemoglobinopathies

Anesthetic concerns are related to the underlying cardiac status in the setting of severe forms of thalassemia and, more commonly, to the degree of hemodynamic compensation with regard to the chronic anemia, its relative oxygen-carrying capacity, and its relationship to anesthesia. These clinical risks in anemic patients have to be balanced against the risks, both short-term and long-term, of transfusion when considering preparation for delivery. There are no specific contraindications to a particular anesthetic technique. In the severely anemic patient, however, opioid analgesia is probably relatively contraindicated. If opioids are used, oxygen saturation should be monitored and oxygen supplementation provided, if required. Risks and benefits are inherent in both general and regional anesthesia

for cesarean section. Careful attention must be paid to fluid balance.

Sickling Syndromes

Of the clinical sickling disorders, Hb SS and Hb SC forms of the disease have the most impact in pregnancy. Anemia is common and, because there is an increased risk of infection and vaso-occlusive crises,[28, 29] frequent assessment is required throughout pregnancy.[4, 24] There is an increased incidence of intrauterine growth retardation due to vaso-occlusion of placental vessels. Prophylactic RBC transfusion to maintain HbA levels above 20% to minimize sickling is controversial owing to the risk of transfusion-transmitted infection.[24, 30, 31] Some recommend transfusions only in those patients who develop complications during pregnancy.[31] Evidence suggests that in patients who receive transfusions, leukodepleted RBCs reduce the risk of transfusion-associated infection. The technique, however, is not fail-safe. Maternal mortality is generally a result of septicemia, thromboembolism, or cardiac failure after a hemolytic crisis.[28] Chronic lung disease resulting from obliteration of pulmonary arterioles and interstitial fibrosis has been reported. The lung disease may ultimately lead to pulmonary hypertension and right heart failure.[32]

Other sickling syndromes are much milder, with improved maternal and fetal outcome. Hb SD disease is rarer than Hb SS, but maternal and fetal outcomes are generally better. The combination of Hb S and Hb F does not generally produce clinical problems. Hb E, when combined with Hb S, produces mild disease. Sickle cell trait is the heterozygous form of sickle cell disease with a hemoglobin phenotype AS. Sickle cell trait is benign, with most patients being asymptomatic. Such patients still have increased demands for erythropoiesis in pregnancy, and supplemental folic acid is essential.

Anesthesia and the Sickling Syndromes

Anesthetic management aims to prevent sickling. Because sickling tends to occur under conditions of stasis, hypothermia, acidosis, and hypoxemia, anesthetic management should attempt to avoid them.[33-35] Areas of anesthetic controversy in sickle cell disease include use of direct intra-arterial pressure monitoring in preeclamptic patients (stasis from a noninvasive BP cuff versus risk of vaso-occlusion), regional or general anesthesia (generally accepted that regional is best but a study suggests that this belief may not be true),[35] and prophylactic blood transfusion (possible improved outcome versus risk of disease).

Epidural analgesia has been given for labor analgesia as well as for control of the pain during sickle cell crisis.[36] Shivering increases oxygen consumption and may be detrimental to the patient with sickle cell disease. Because shivering is a common occurrence with epidural anesthesia, efforts should be made to limit it by using warm intravenous fluids and keeping the environmental temperature warm. Measurement of oxygen saturation during labor and delivery should ensure adequate oxygenation. If the saturation level falls, supplemental oxygen should be provided.

Regional and general anesthesia are acceptable for cesarean section,[37, 38] although a review of surgery in sickle cell disease found that sickle cell disease–related postoperative complications were more frequent in patients with type Hb SS who received regional anesthesia.[35] The investigators questioned whether the increased rate of complications was related to the nature of the surgery rather than to the anesthetic technique. They postulated that cesarean section may be associated with more complications than other surgery and, because more of these procedures were performed using regional anesthesia, the increased use of regional anesthesia could have affected the results.

Principles of anesthetic management include maintenance of intravascular volume (crystalloid), administration of supplemental oxygen to avoid sickling from hypoxia, avoidance of acidosis, maintenance of adequate left uterine displacement, maintenance of normothermia, and prevention of peripheral venous stasis. These principles of treatment apply to all patients with any capacity for sickling, including those with the heterozygous Hb S carrier state. In more severe disorders, especially Hb SS, transfusion of warmed RBCs to maintain oxygen-carrying capacity and to increase the blood content of Hb A, when appropriate, is the other parameter to be considered. Furthermore, because these patients are at risk of high-output cardiac failure, some may require more invasive monitoring. Oxygen saturation monitoring should be continued during the postoperative period because hypoxia may occur, and supplemental oxygen should be provided as required.

Complications from anesthesia in patients with sickle cell trait are rare. One case has been reported of an intraoperative death during cesarean section in a patient with sickle cell trait.[39] Death was attributed to severe, concealed aorto-caval compression, such that once it was relieved a large volume of hypoxemic, acidotic blood was returned to the circulation, causing cardiac arrest.[39]

Hemolytic Anemias

Hemolytic anemias are best classified as *inherited* or *acquired* (Table 23–2).

Of the inherited group the most common are consequences of

- *Membrane disorders* making the RBC less flexible in the microcirculation and, thus, susceptible to hemolysis

TABLE 23–2. COMMON HEMOLYTIC ANEMIAS IN PREGNANCY

Inherited	
Membrane disorders	Hereditary spherocytosis
Metabolic disorders	Glucose-6-phosphate dehydrogenase deficiency
	Pyruvate kinase deficiency

Acquired	
	Autoimmune hemolytic anemia
	Idiopathic
	Associated with underlying connective tissue disease
	Miscellaneous
	Microangiopathic anemia (HELLP, PE, DIC)

HELLP = syndrome of hemolysis, elevated liver enzymes, low platelets; PE = pre-eclampsia; DIC = disseminated intravascular coagulopathy

- *Metabolic abnormalities*, which increase the sensitivity to oxidant stress.

Abnormal hemoglobins may also make the RBC susceptible to hemolysis; this subject was discussed earlier.

Acquired disorders causing RBC hemolysis are of two main groups:

- Those related to immune-mediated hemolysis
- Those associated with mechanical hemolysis due to microangiopathy or other uncommon mechanical stresses (mechanical hemolysis related to artificial heart valves).

Hemolysis can occur in the intravascular space, causing release of free hemoglobin with resulting hemoglobinuria and hemosiderinuria, or more commonly in the extravascular space, in the reticuloendothelial (RE) system primarily in the liver and spleen. Common laboratory parameters of ongoing chronic hemolysis include increased reticulocyte count, increased lactic dehydrogenase (LDH) level, increased unconjugated bilirubin level, and, in specific disorders, morphologic abnormalities on the peripheral smear.

Inherited Hemolytic Disorders

Hereditary Spherocytosis

This autosomal dominant disorder has an incidence of 200 to 300 in 1 million. It is the most common membrane disorder. The pathognomonic feature is the presence of spherocytes in the peripheral blood, associated with increased osmotic fragility of the RBCs on special testing in the laboratory. As a result of increased destruction of the abnormal cells in the RE system, patients commonly present with anemia, splenomegaly, and jaundice. Splenectomy is essentially curative, but because of the usually mild nature of this disorder, many patients have not undergone this surgery. The diagnosis may be made during pregnancy,[40] and although there are reports of hemolytic crises during pregnancy, most patients tolerate pregnancy well.[41, 42] Routine supplementation with folic acid and, if indicated (following assessment of serum ferritin), iron is necessary to ensure effective erythopoiesis. In the rare event of severe anemia, splenectomy may be required. Because anemia may worsen during episodes of infection (owing to increased hemolysis and possibly suppressed hematopoiesis), patients require frequent monitoring.

Other membrane abnormalities include hereditary elliptocytosis and hereditary stomatocytosis— but neither of these is improved by splenectomy. Most patients have a mild chronic hemolytic anemia that is unaffected by pregnancy. They, too, should have supplementation with folate and, if necessary, iron.

Red Blood Cell Enzyme Deficiencies

The most common hereditary deficiencies are those of glucose-6-phosphate dehydrogenase and pyruvate kinase. Both of these enzyme deficiencies make the RBC susceptible to oxidant stress, leading to greater susceptibility to hemolysis. The degree of hemolysis varies, with more severe episodes often triggered by oxidant drugs, including some of the antibiotics and nonopioid analgesics. These medications should be avoided (Table 23–3).

Acquired Disorders of the RBC Leading to Hemolysis

Autoimmune Hemolytic Anemias

Autoimmune hemolytic anemias result from the development of warm- (IgG) or cold- (IgM) reactive RBC autoantibodies. These disorders can occur at all ages but are more common in adults, particularly women. Autoimmune hemolytic anemia is usually idiopathic but may occur as a result of drugs, such as alpha-methyldopa, or in association with an underlying disease (about 25% of patients), such as systemic lupus erythematosus (SLE), rheumatoid arthritis, inflammatory bowel disease, or lymphoproliferative disease (chronic lymphocytic leukemia, non-Hodgkin's lymphoma).

Patients with IgG autoantibodies (warm-reactive) are more common, and they present with anemia, mild icterus, and splenomegaly. Laboratory findings include reticulocytosis and spherocytes on the peripheral

TABLE 23–3. DRUGS USED IN PREGNANCY THAT MAY INDUCE HEMOLYSIS

Autoimmune hemolytic anemia	Cephalosporins Penicillin Methyldopa
Oxidant hemolysis	Mephenamic acid p-aminosalicylic acid Sulfonamides

smear. If immune thrombocytopenia is present, the condition is known as Evans syndrome. In the blood bank there is a positive direct and indirect antiglobulin test for IgG. Specificity of the autoantibody may be determined but, in most cases, it is pan-reactive. Patients with idiopathic, immune hemolytic anemia usually respond well to corticosteroid therapy at a dose of prednisone, 1 mg/kg. These IgG autoantibodies have the potential to cross the placenta and cause fetal anemia. Serial amniocentesis is sometimes indicated in the antenatal period. Transfusion should be avoided unless the patient's symptoms are marked or the fetus is compromised by severe maternal anemia. Crossmatching of blood may be difficult owing to the presence of the pan-reactive autoantibody. It is particularly important to search for any information that indicates the presence of other *alloantibodies*, which makes the serologic work-up more complex.

In patients with immune hemolysis due to cold-reactive antibodies (IgM), the pathophysiology of hemolysis is different, resulting largely from the fixation of complement on the RBC membrane, with resultant hemolysis in the intravascular space. Thus, these patients may not have splenomegaly. They do not have spherocytes on their peripheral smear but have reticulocytosis, raised LDH and bilirubin levels, and increased hemosiderin in the urine. The diagnosis is made when cold-reactive antibodies with a broad thermal range are encountered.

This condition is rare in pregnancy and does not respond well to corticosteroids. Transfusion can be problematic; the use of a blood warmer and the maintenance of a warm environment are critical. Because IgM antibodies do not cross the placenta, fetal involvement does not occur.

Miscellaneous Causes of Hemolysis

Hemolysis may occur in patients with normal RBCs as a result of trauma from prosthetic heart valves or fibrin deposition in the microvasculature (microangiopathic anemia). In the case of trauma, chronic hemolysis during pregnancy is associated with a raised LDH level, possibly mild icterus, reticulocytosis, and hemosiderinuria with decreased plasma haptoglobin. Supplementation with both folic acid and iron is usually necessary to allow the bone marrow to compensate for ongoing loss. Microangiopathic hemolytic anemia is usually associated with acute DIC, pre-eclampsia, or acute vasculitis. Treatment of the underlying disorder is the most essential aspect of care. (See later under disorders of platelets.)

Abnormalities of Marrow

Aplastic Anemia

Aplastic anemia is a primary bone marrow disorder caused by hypocellularity of the marrow with resulting pancytopenia in the peripheral blood. The etiology of the marrow hypoplasia is varied. Aplastic anemia has been associated with exposure to radiation, organic solvents, various drugs, immune lesions, and viral diseases, particularly hepatitis. Other more unusual defects may involve only one cell line such as anemia due to RBC aplasia or neutropenia due to white blood cell aplasia.

Approximately 50% of cases of aplastic anemia are idiopathic in origin. Sporadic case reports of refractory hypoplastic anemia appear to be related to pregnancy; the condition regresses post partum.[43-48] The majority of pregnant women with aplastic anemia, however, had chronic aplastic anemia.[49]

The major risks during pregnancy are severe anemia, hemorrhage due to thrombocytopenia, and infection associated with neutropenia.[50] In the past, women with this condition were advised not to become pregnant or, if they did, to terminate the pregnancy. With the advent of better transfusion support, particularly with regard to platelets, this is no longer appropriate advice, particularly for those with mild to moderate disease.[49, 51]

Congenital Red Blood Cell Aplasias

Fanconi anemia is a rare congenital RBC aplasia that is inherited as an autosomal recessive trait. One case is reported of pregnancy in a patient with Fanconi anemia.[52] She had received "washed" RBCs during pregnancy. Labor was induced at term for pre-eclampsia, and eventually delivery was accomplished by cesarean section. The postpartum period was complicated by anemia, thrombocytopenia, epistaxis, and superficial wound hemorrhage.

Diamond-Blackfan anemia is a congenital RBC aplasia resulting from failure of a single hematopoietic cell line. Treatment generally consists of RBC transfusion with iron chelation and oral corticosteroids.[53] Bone marrow transplantation is also successful. Isolated reports are found of pregnancies in patients with this disorder.[54]

Anesthesia for Parturients With Aplastic Anemia

The principles of management for these patients are related primarily to ensuring adequate oxygen-carrying capacity and, more importantly, adequate hemostasis.[55] Of particular importance is planning in advance for delivery. Patients who have received previous transfusions or had previous pregnancies are at particular risk for being refractory to platelet transfusions because of the presence of human leukocyte antigen (HLA) antibodies. In this situation, HLA typing of the patient in advance (if not already done) and collection of HLA-matched platelets for support during delivery are necessary. With at least a 3-hour collection time, a 6-hour testing time, and a shelf-life of only 5 days for platelet concentrate, careful coordination with the

obstetrician is essential to facilitate delivery during the time that platelets are available. Similarly, patients who have received previous RBC transfusion may have RBC alloantibodies, which makes the finding of compatible RBCs difficult. Thus, advance warning to the hospital blood bank helps ensure the availability of these RBCs. In those patients who have never had exposure to blood products and are potential candidates for marrow transplants, careful consultation with the hematologist and transplantation team is essential to ensure that the appropriate products are utilized in order not to compromise chances for successful transplants.

A platelet count greater than 50×10^9/l is adequate for an uncomplicated vaginal delivery; however, in our opinion, for any form of regional anesthesia, episiotomy, or cesarean section, a count of 75 to 80×10^9/l is required for adequate hemostasis. In patients requiring transfusion of platelets to achieve these levels, a 1-hour post-transfusion platelet count is essential to ensure that the target range has been reached. Failure to achieve a rise in the platelet count of 5 to 10×10^9 platelets/l per random donor unit of platelets transfused is suggestive of immune refractoriness, which is related to HLA antibodies. The level of hemoglobin that is appropriate varies and depends to a certain extent on the degree of maternal compensation and fetal well-being and the projected amount of blood loss.

Providing adequate analgesia is important during labor because pain-induced hypertension can lead to intracranial hemorrhage in patients with severe thrombocytopenia. Because regional anesthesia is contraindicated in the severely thrombocytopenic patient, intravenous, patient-controlled analgesia with fentanyl is an acceptable option. The neutropenia associated with marrow hypoplasia places the patient at increased risk of infection. Special attention should be paid to the potential for infection at the time of invasive procedures, including surgery. Patients who have received a bone marrow transplant have special considerations, which are noted later in this chapter.

Paroxysmal Nocturnal Hemoglobinuria

Paroxysmal nocturnal hemoglobinuria is a rare, acquired clonal disorder of the bone marrow that may affect young adults. An abnormal clone at the stem cell level produces RBCs, platelets, and granulocytes that have an abnormal sensitivity to complement.[4] This condition leads to episodes of acute and chronic intravascular hemolysis, intermittent hemoglobinuria, and thrombotic tendency. Thrombocytopenia often occurs, whereas granulocytopenia, causing an increased sensitivity to infection, is less common. Some patients present with a clinical picture indistinguishable from that of aplastic anemia.

Venous thrombosis is frequent and is attributed to intravascular hemolysis with inappropriate activation of thrombin and subsequent thrombosis. Patients who have had episodes of thrombosis may be on long-term oral anticoagulation treatment, which, in pregnancy, is changed to subcutaneous heparin. Limited experience is reported with this disorder in pregnancy; however, several case reports describe severe thrombotic complications in unusual sites (maternal hepatic vein, cerebral venous sinus) and fetal loss.[56–58]

Washed RBCs should be given when transfusion is needed to correct anemia or when episodes of hemolysis occur.[57] Some evidence indicates that prophylactic transfusions may decrease the incidence of thrombotic complications, but this observation remains speculative because of the small number of patients with this condition and the inability to undertake properly structured research trials to address the question.

Sideroblastic Anemia

Sideroblastic anemia is a descriptive term for a variety of disorders that have in common a defect in heme biosynthesis and a defect in iron use. The disorders are inherited in either an autosomal recessive or a sex-linked pattern or are acquired in association with certain diseases (myelodysplastic syndromes, malignancy), drugs, or toxins. Ringed sideroblasts in the bone marrow are diagnostic. Medical management during pregnancy or at the time of delivery does not differ from that for a patient with hypoplastic anemia. Because this is a disorder associated with significant dyserythropoiesis, administration of exogenous iron is contraindicated unless the serum ferritin level suggests iron deficiency, which is highly unlikely. A single case report of pregnancy in a patient with sideroblastic anemia has appeared, in which the management consisted of maintenance of hematocrit through periodic transfusion of washed RBCs.[59]

PRIMARY MARROW MALIGNANT DISORDERS

The myeloproliferative disorders include, in order of appearance in the obstetric population, essential thrombocythemia (ET, also known as essential thrombocytosis), polycythemia rubra vera (PRV), chronic myelogenous (or granulocytic) leukemia (CML/CGL), and myelofibrosis with myeloid metaplasia. All arise from clonal stem cell defects, and these disorders are characterized by autonomous proliferation of the stem cell lines.

Essential Thrombocythemia

ET is the most common of the myeloproliferative disorders seen in pregnancy. Patients present with thrombocytosis that is often asymptomatic, particularly in the range below $1000 \times 10^9/l$. At presentation only 50% have splenomegaly and sustained elevation of platelet count usually greater than $1000 \times 10^9/l$. The platelet smear may be completely normal, or it may reveal the presence of giant platelets and hypogranular platelets. Anemia is rare unless there has been hemorrhage or iron deficiency. The major causes of morbidity and mortality are thrombosis (both arterial and venous) and hemorrhage.[60] Stroke and transient ischemic attacks are common and are related to inappropriate platelet activation in the microvasculature. Symptoms indicating that therapy is needed are erythromelalgia (burning pain in the fingertips), headaches, easy bruising, and mucous membrane hemorrhage. Interestingly, both thrombotic and hemorrhagic complications are usually controlled by lowering the platelet count. Studies of platelet function have failed to uncover a consistent pattern, and there is no laboratory assay that predicts predisposition of the patients to either bleeding or thrombosis. Some patients have spontaneous in vitro platelet aggregation or platelet "hyperaggregability," whereas others may lose platelet responsiveness to epinephrine.[61]

Other platelet function abnormalities include platelet membrane abnormalities, acquired storage pool deficiency, and metabolic abnormalities.

In patients with evidence of platelet-associated thrombosis without impaired hemostasis, and a platelet count in the range of $1500 \times 10^9/l$ or less, low-dose aspirin is often sufficient to control symptoms. The other two major therapeutic options for ET are to lower the platelet count by antiproliferative agents such as hydroxyurea or busulfan or, in the more acute situation, by plateletpheresis. No consensus exists on the use of hydroxyurea or busulfan during pregnancy.[61, 62]

Patients presenting with ET in pregnancy, along with their already existing risk for thrombosis, have a higher incidence of recurrent abortion, fetal growth retardation, premature delivery, and abruptio placentae. Randi and coworkers[63] reported on six normal pregnancies in five untreated patients. They believe that many patients do not warrant therapy during pregnancy. Probably because of the autonomous thrombopoiesis characteristic of this disorder, the platelet count actually decreases gradually during pregnancy in our experience, usually reaching its nadir at about 32 to 36 weeks, coinciding with the completion of plasma volume expansion (Fig. 23–1). Low-dose aspirin (80 mg daily) to minimize placental compromise from platelet thrombosis in the microvasculature has been reported with good results. At the present time there is no indication for routine heparin prophylaxis unless there is a history of venous thrombosis.

Polycythemia Rubra Vera

Polycythemia rubra vera (PRV), a chronic myeloproliferative disorder with an estimated incidence of 1 in

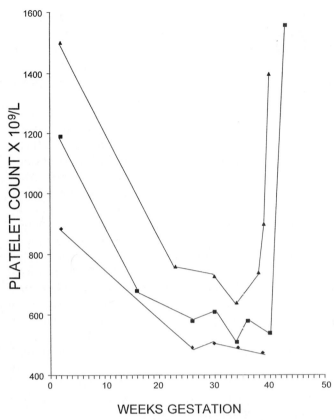

Figure 23–1. Platelet count of three patients with essential thrombocythemia demonstrating the physiologic decrease in platelet count that occurred during pregnancy.

50,000 within the general population, is occasionally seen in pregnancy.[64] It is characterized by an increase in RBC mass, which is usually associated with pancytosis and splenomegaly.[64–66] Symptoms are related primarily to the increased blood volume and viscosity. Like patients with ET, these patients are also at risk from both bleeding and hemorrhage. Through much of the natural history of the disease, these problems, as well as associated problems stemming from an increased blood volume, are well controlled with phlebotomy.[67]

In pregnancy, patients are at risk for poor obstetric outcome because of placental compromise. Because of the autonomous nature of erythropoiesis in this disorder, the plasma volume expansion of pregnancy results in a fall of the hematocrit throughout the first 34 weeks with a nadir late in the last trimester. Phlebotomy is safe during pregnancy and can be used to further reduce the hematocrit to minimize both maternal and fetal risk. Iron stores are diminished, and carefully limited supplementation may be necessary to ensure adequate iron delivery to the fetus. Iron supplementation must be done cautiously because it is through iron depletion that phlebotomy has its long-term dampening effect on erythropoiesis. An increased risk of cardiac failure is present owing to the increased cardiac output associated with PRV and pregnancy.

Leukemia

The majority of cases that occur during pregnancy are diagnosed during routine prenatal care. The incidence of acute leukemia is estimated at 1 in 100,000 pregnancies, and there is no evidence that pregnancy alters the incidence or prognosis of acute or chronic leukemia. Seventy-two cases of newly diagnosed leukemia during pregnancy were reported from 1975 to 1988.[68] Forty-four had acute myelogenous leukemia, 20 had acute lymphocytic, and 8 had chronic leukemia. Standard antileukemic chemotherapy can be administered safely during the second and third trimesters,[68, 69] but potential complications include a risk of hemorrhage and sepsis.[70] Breast-feeding is contraindicated when the mother is being treated with cytotoxic drugs.[71]

Lymphoma

Hodgkin's disease is the most common lymphoproliferative disorder in young people. Overall, lymphoma is the fourth most frequent cancer diagnosis among pregnant women.[72] The prevalence of non-Hodgkin's lymphoma is unknown. Pregnancy does not appear to affect the natural history of Hodgkin's disease,[73] nor does Hodgkin's disease affect the pregnancy. The high-grade lymphomas, including Burkitt's lymphoma, however, are rapidly progressive and require aggressive intervention and treatment in the pregnant woman.

Multiple Myeloma

This hematologic malignancy results from proliferation of a single clone of neoplastic plasma cells and is rare in pregnancy, with only seven documented cases reported to date.[74–76] Clinically, patients may present with a spectrum of problems, including mild unresponsive anemia, bone pain, pathologic fracture, neurologic deficit, and recurrent infection. Recurrent infection results from suppression of normal B cell function by the malignant clone. Spinal cord compression resulting from vertebral collapse with paraplegia occurs in approximately 14% of nonpregnant patients. Anemia occurs as a result of marrow infiltration and, in the latter stages of the disease, renal failure. An increased bleeding tendency may be found as a consequence of thrombocytopenia or through interference with platelet function or coagulation factors by monoclonal proteins. Patients can also develop a hyperviscosity syndrome with stroke, myocardial compromise, and skin infarction.

The cases reported in pregnancy have had diverse presentations. One woman presented with anemia during a routine antenatal visit,[76] whereas another presented 3 days post partum with bilateral leg weakness and back pain.[74] The offspring appear unaffected.[74]

Waldenström Macroglobulinemia

Waldenström macroglobulinemia is characterized by an IgM monoclonal gammopathy and recurring purpura. Patients with Waldenström macroglobulinemia have hepatosplenomegaly, frequently mild anemia, and usually some degree of renal insufficiency. Waldenström macroglobulinemia is very rare in pregnancy, with only one reported case.[77] That pregnancy was complicated by fetal growth restriction and fetal distress, and the patient underwent cesarean section using general anesthesia. Patients usually have normal coagulation studies and a normal platelet count and, in the absence of any obvious purpura, a low bleeding risk. They may be at increased risk for thrombosis, as a result of hyperviscosity related to the level of their monoclonal IgM protein.

Anesthesia for Patients with Malignant Marrow Disorders

No reports are found of anesthesia in parturients with essential thrombocythemia. Theoretically, regional and general anesthesia can be administered unless there is evidence of platelet dysfunction or ongoing hemorrhage, in which case regional anesthesia is contraindicated. In a patient presenting in the last trimester with a platelet count greater than $1500 \times 10^9/l$, consideration can be given to urgent plateletpheresis to reduce the platelet count, minimizing the risk of both thrombosis and bleeding. In the postpartum state, rebound, severe thrombocytosis occurs often; this should be anticipated, and intervention with chemotherapy and/or plateletpheresis, as well as low-dose aspirin, may be necessary to minimize the risk of thrombosis.

To date, there are no reports of the anesthetic management of a pregnant patient with PRV. In general, PRV patients have a high risk of hemorrhagic and thrombotic complications related to surgery.[67,78] These complications are best controlled by maintaining the hematocrit in the range of 0.4 to 0.45 through phlebotomy. In the event of emergency cesarean section, attention should be paid to positioning (to prevent venous stasis). Hemodilution should be performed, preferably with associated phlebotomy, if the hematocrit is greater than 0.45. Normotension should be maintained and supplemental oxygen provided.[79]

Although the advantages of vasodilatation, improved regional blood flow, and hemodilution occurring with regional blockade and intravenous fluid preload are significant, regional anesthesia should be avoided if the hematocrit is poorly controlled because of unpredictable bleeding risk. Fluids should be monitored carefully to prevent circulatory system overload, inducing cardiac failure. A report in the obstetric literature concerns a parturient who had an epidural procedure for a repeat cesarean section. No other details of the anesthetic management were given.[64]

The anesthetic management of patients with acute leukemia shares principles similar to those of aplastic anemia (discussed earlier). The complications of anesthesia and surgery most commonly are related to the pancytopenia associated with these disorders and/or their treatment. In patients with acute leukemia, aggressive large cell lymphoma, or chronic granulocytic leukemia (CGL) who remain untreated at the time of delivery, special attention must be given to the level of the blast cell count or, in the case of CGL, the total white blood cell count. Significantly increased blast cell counts place the patient at risk for hyperviscosity syndrome, including renal compromise, cerebral infarction, and other complications. Leukopheresis or rapid reduction of the white blood cell count with chemotherapy may be necessary to reduce the risk of anesthesia or even labor. Vigorous hydration is essential in these situations, with close monitoring required of urine output and renal function.

Bone Marrow Transplantation

Pregnancy has been reported following bone marrow transplantation for aplastic anemia and hematologic malignancies,[80] but it is relatively uncommon when total body irradiation (TBI) has been done before transplantation.

Anesthetic management should focus on the patient's current clinical status because multiple sequelae may result from the procedure. The technique of choice for analgesia and anesthesia is based on the patient's current hematologic and clinical condition.[81] TBI and/or chemotherapy can produce pulmonary fibrosis, and thus pulmonary function should be assessed. Attention should be directed to ensuring strict aseptic technique because patients are frequently prone to infections. Generally, there should be no contraindication to general or regional anesthesia. The patients have usually received multiple transfusions and are at risk for both transfusion-associated infection and alloimmunization to RBCs and platelets.

BLEEDING DISORDERS

In the past, regional anesthesia was considered contraindicated in any patient with a bleeding abnormality, even if there was no evidence of overt bleeding or bruising. This principle applied to parturients with platelet counts less than $100 \times 10^9/l$, those with mild von Willebrand disease, and those treated with heparin and/or aspirin. With better understanding of the pathophysiology of these disorders and the changes that occur with pregnancy, anesthesiologists are becoming more liberal in their use of regional anesthesia. Within certain limitations it is unlikely that this change will be accompanied by an increase in anesthetic-related complications.

The major concern with regional anesthesia is related to the development of spinal or epidural hematoma with resulting permanent neurologic damage. The incidence of neurologic damage in parturients is very low,[82, 83] and it is difficult to determine the relationship among epidural hematoma, regional anesthesia, and coagulopathy. Vandermeulen and coworkers[84] reviewed the literature on anticoagulants and central axial blockade. They emphasize the need to not be dogmatic but to individualize treatment to the patient, being aware of the relative risk. Another prospective study in nonparturients concluded that there was no correlation between antiplatelet medications and blood in the needle or catheter.[85] In situations in which regional anesthesia is contraindicated, intramuscular injections and pudendal blocks are similarly contraindicated (Table 23–4).

For many of the coagulation disorders, there is no literature as to the most appropriate anesthetic management. It is obvious from the obstetric literature that patients with many of these unusual conditions have received anesthetic care because they frequently undergo cesarean section. One assumes that general anesthesia was the technique used, but the technique rarely is stated. Specific anesthetic considerations for the bleeding disorders are outlined below following discussion of each particular disorder, but some general principles are outlined in Table 23–5.

THROMBOCYTOPENIA AND PLATELET FUNCTIONAL DISORDERS

Thrombocytopenia is the most common hematologic complication in pregnancy. The etiology varies from an apparent physiologic condition (gestational thrombocytopenia) to disorders associated with significant underlying pathology. The implications of a low platelet count with regard to anesthetic considerations in the pregnant woman vary according to the underlying pathophysiology of the thrombocytopenia (Table 23–6).

Several conflicting reports are found as to the natural

TABLE 23–4. **AVOID THE FOLLOWING IN PATIENTS WITH BLEEDING DISORDERS**

Intramuscular injections
Regional blocks including pudendal
Aspirin
NSAIDs (e.g., diclofenac, ibuprofen, naproxen)

TABLE 23–5. **PRINCIPLES OF ANESTHETIC MANAGEMENT**

1. Take a thorough history: Emphasis on family history of bleeding, bruising (especially during surgery, dental work)
2. Do a thorough physical examination: Bruising, bleeding, petechiae (blood pressure cuff, IV sites)
3. Lab work: CBC, platelet count, specific testing dependent on history, clinical course
4. Involve hematologist, if appropriate
5. Assess airway, feasibility of other techniques
6. Discuss risks/benefits of proposed procedure and what is known about risk
7. Discuss risks/benefits of blood products
8. Document discussion of 6 and 7
9. Proceed with regional anesthesia, if appropriate
10. Remember, if regional technique is contraindicated, so are pudendal block, intramuscular injections, NSAIDs, aspirin

history of the platelet count during pregnancy.[5, 7–12] If there is a change up to 36 weeks' gestation, it appears as a progressive decrease associated with a consistent increase in the mean plasma platelet volume. This observation suggests an increase in platelet consumption (younger platelets being larger), but limited kinetic studies have failed to confirm a shortened platelet life span in pregnancy. A study of platelet behavior demonstrates an increase in platelet reactivity in the third trimester of pregnancy.[86] This observation is consistent with our clinical experience in mild platelet functional disorders, which often improve in pregnancy. In general, platelet activation is the first stage of in-vivo hemostasis. In patients with hypoplastic thrombocytopenia and platelet counts less than $100 \times 10^9/l$, there is an indirect relationship between the platelet count

TABLE 23–6. **DISORDERS OF PLATELETS DURING PREGNANCY**

Disorder	Thrombocytopenia	Abnormal Platelet Function
Gestational thrombocytopenia	Yes	No
ITP	Yes	No
May-Hegglin anomaly	Yes	Possibly
Antiphospholipid syndrome	Yes	Very unusual
Cocaine	Yes	No
HIV	Yes	No
Microangiopathic syndromes	Yes	Only if significant decrease in fibrinogen
Bernard-Soulier syndrome	Yes	Yes
Chédiak-Higashi syndrome	No	Yes
Platelet storage pool deficiency	No	Yes
Glanzmann thrombasthenia	No	Yes
von Willebrand disease	No except with variant type IIB	Yes

ITP = idiopathic thrombocytopenic purpura; HIV = human immunodeficiency virus

TABLE 23–7. **DIAGNOSIS OF GESTATIONAL THROMBOCYTOPENIA**

History	Occurs late in pregnancy—3rd trimester
	No history bleeding or bruising
	Generally mild
	May have occurred in previous pregnancy, but not between pregnancies
Physical	Normotensive
	Normal physical exam, no bruising, bleeding
Laboratory	Platelet count >90 × 10^9/l
	Platelets may appear larger than normal
	No other cytopenias
	Normal UA, LFTs
	Normal coagulation indices

UA = uric acid; LFTs = liver function tests

and the bleeding time.[87] In conditions such as ITP, the relationship is shifted to the left, and in patients with platelet dysfunction, it is shifted to the right. Aspirin or nonsteroidal anti-inflammatory drugs (NSAIDs) in patients with any of these disorders can dramatically shift the relationship between platelet count and platelet function; therefore, these drugs should not be used in these conditions.

Gestational Thrombocytopenia

Gestational thrombocytopenia occurs in approximately 8% of all pregnant women.[88] It is generally mild with a platelet count greater than 90 × 10^9/l (Table 23–7). The patients and their neonates are not at increased risk of bleeding, and the platelet count, in the majority of patients, returns to normal 3 to 5 days post partum (Table 23–8). This pattern may be repeated in subsequent pregnancies.[89]

The diagnosis is usually one of exclusion. Particular emphasis should be placed on a normal platelet count in early pregnancy, no previously documented thrombocytopenia prior to pregnancy, and absence of any clinical evidence for impending pre-eclampsia. Thrombocytopenia that occurs before pregnancy or within the first trimester of pregnancy is generally idiopathic or immune thrombocytopenic purpura (ITP) (Table 23–9). Parturients with uncomplicated gestational thrombocytopenia can undergo regional anesthesia safely.[90, 91]

Idiopathic Thrombocytopenic Purpura

This is a common disease in young women and has an incidence of approximately 0.01 to 0.02% of

TABLE 23–8. **MANAGEMENT OF GESTATIONAL THROMBOCYTOPENIA**

Benign, no intervention
No contraindication to regional anesthesia
May be difficult to distinguish from mild ITP
Document platelet count in baby at birth

ITP = idiopathic thrombocytopenia

deliveries.[92] Studies of its pathophysiology have revealed the presence of platelet-specific autoantibodies (usually IgG) that recognize immunogenic glycoproteins on the platelet membrane. Generally speaking, the thrombocytopenia is related to increased destruction of sensitized platelets in the reticuloendothelial (RE) system; however, there also is evidence for antibody-mediated impaired thrombopoiesis.[93] Laboratory findings usually include isolated thrombocytopenia (antedating pregnancy or present early in pregnancy) with large well-granulated platelets and often normal hemostasis in spite of a significantly reduced platelet count. Not infrequently, there is a family history of other autoimmune disease (see Table 23–9). The most common conditions in the differential diagnosis include thrombocytopenia associated with SLE, HIV infections, and antiphospholipid antibodies. No specific laboratory test is available; however, the finding of glycoprotein-specific, platelet-associated antibodies is helpful. Rarely, there is a concomitant platelet functional abnormality.

Little data recommend treatment of an asymptomatic patient with a maternal platelet count above 20 to 30 × 10^9/l during the antenatal period (Table 23–10). At our institution, treatment (prednisone or intravenous immune globulin [IVIG]) is administered only for evidence of impaired hemostasis during pregnancy or to elevate the platelet count before the delivery or invasive procedure.[6] To date, using this approach, there have been no bleeding complications, and no patients have required transfusions. Those patients who require therapy usually respond to either prednisone 1 mg/kg or IVIG 2 g/kg over 2 to 5 days. Those who fail to respond to either may have a response to a combination of the two. Rarely, splenectomy is required during pregnancy and is best done during the second trimester.

Infants born to mothers with this disease may be thrombocytopenic because the antibody crosses the placenta.[94, 95] Our experience and the literature suggest that approximately 5% of neonates born to mothers with ITP have significant thrombocytopenia (<50 ×

TABLE 23–9. **DIAGNOSIS OF IDIOPATHIC THROMBOCYTOPENIA**

History	Usually history of thrombocytopenia, or
	Appears early in pregnancy
	Chronic course, low spontaneous remission
	Often normal hemostasis, in spite of significantly reduced platelet count
	Family history of autoimmune disease
Physical	Bruising, bleeding, petechiae
Laboratory	Large, well-granulated platelets (not giant platelets)
	Normal RBC, WBC indices
	Reduced platelet count
	Normal megakaryocytes in marrow
	Circulating or platelet-bound autoantibody

RBC = red blood cell count; WBC = white blood cell count

TABLE 23–10. MANAGEMENT OF ITP IN PREGNANCY

Follow maternal platelet count and clinical hemostasis
Antenatally: If clinical bleeding and platelets drop markedly, treat with IVIG, prednisone
Preparation for delivery: If platelet count <30 to 50 × 10⁹/l, treat with IVIG, prednisone
Response should occur in 24–48 hours
Regional anesthesia is appropriate if good clinical hemostasis is observed

IVIG = intravenous immunoglobulin

10⁹/l) at birth. Over the few days following birth, however, approximately 30 to 40% of neonates with a normal or near-normal count at delivery may become significantly thrombocytopenic. In a small number of patients who are considered at high risk to deliver a severely affected infant, assessment of fetal platelets before delivery may be appropriate.[96–98] This is achieved by percutaneous umbilical cord sampling (PUBS) or fetal scalp vein sampling.[99] Fetuses at high risk who may be appropriate for sampling include those of women who have previously undergone splenectomy for treatment of ITP (regardless of the platelet count), those women with previously affected infants, and women with significant thrombocytopenia during pregnancy (platelet count <50 × 10⁹/l).[100] If the fetus has a platelet count less than 50 × 10⁹/l, consideration should be given to delivery by cesarean section. The neonates of ITP mothers should be followed daily for 72 hours until their platelet count has stabilized. Formerly, many ITP patients underwent cesarean section, but further practice guidelines no longer recommend routine cesarean delivery.[101]

In preparation for delivery, it is often appropriate to administer a short course of steroids or IVIG near term (37–38 weeks) to elevate the platelet count, ensuring a full range of options for analgesia in these patients. No role exists for platelet transfusion unless there is life-threatening bleeding. As noted earlier, aspirin and NSAIDs are contraindicated.

Anesthetic management of women with ITP is usually straightforward. In most instances platelet function is excellent, and a platelet count of greater than 75 × 10⁹/l is more than adequate for regional anesthesia. A history of a lack of bleeding problems at a given platelet count often helps to reassure the anesthesiologist. A careful examination of the patient should be undertaken to assess hemostasis. In special situations, such as fetal distress and difficult airway, platelet counts as low as 40 to 50 × 10⁹/l may well be safe for spinal anesthesia (risk of bleeding in spinal space is less than the risk of general anesthesia).

Bernard-Soulier Syndrome

Bernard-Soulier syndrome is a rare, autosomal recessive bleeding disorder characterized by low-normal or diminished platelet count, giant platelets, and platelet dysfunction. Clinically, patients with this disorder have moderate to severe bleeding of the purpuric type. Very few pregnancies have been reported in women with this disorder.[102, 103] Platelets from these patients have a deficiency of platelet glycoproteins (GP) Ib, IX and V. GPIb:IX is an important functional binding site on the platelet membrane for von Willebrand factor. Thus, GPIb–deficient platelets cannot bind to the subendothelium of the injured vessel in vivo. In the laboratory, a prolonged bleeding time is characteristic of the disorder. Platelet studies reveal normal aggregation to ADP, collagen, and epinephrine but none to ristocetin. Complications that occur during pregnancy include both intrapartum and postpartum (2–3 weeks) hemorrhage.[102, 103] Platelet transfusions are ineffective if a previous transfusion has resulted in alloimmunization to GPIb:IX. Furthermore, in the presence of this type of platelet-specific antibody, the fetus may be at risk for immune-mediated thrombocytopenia, which is indistinguishable from neonatal alloimmune thrombocytopenia (NAIT). One report has appeared of treatment with intravenous gamma globulin resulting in a successful pregnancy.[102]

Close involvement with a hematologist is important, particularly in the care of an alloimmunized patient. Principles of anesthetic management include avoidance of invasive procedures, such as intramuscular injections and regional anesthesia including pudendal block. Platelet transfusion may be necessary if the patient is not alloimmunized. Intravenous opioid analgesia and nitrous oxide and oxygen in a 50:50 mixture for labor analgesia, and general anesthesia for cesarean section are reasonable options. Aspirin and NSAIDs are contraindicated.

May-Hegglin Anomaly

May-Hegglin anomaly is a rare hereditary disorder characterized by giant platelets and blue inclusions in the cytoplasm of leukocytes. It is inherited as an autosomal dominant trait with variable penetrance. These patients have both thrombocytopenia and platelet dysfunction. Platelet levels range from 10 × 10⁹/l to normal levels, and there may be a bleeding diathesis. Generally, patients are asymptomatic, but occasionally they have severe bleeding episodes that are related to thrombocytopenia.

Several reports are found of pregnancy in patients with the May-Hegglin anomaly.[104–109] Most have undergone cesarean section because the fetus, if affected, is at risk of intracranial hemorrhage. One case report documented a vaginal delivery after percutaneous umbilical blood sampling demonstrated a fetus with the May-Hegglin anomaly but adequate platelet count. [109]

A report documents general anesthesia for two cesar-

clinical picture. If the platelet count has been stable at $80 \times 10^9/l$ and there is no evidence of bleeding, regional anesthesia may be considered. If, however, the platelet count was $120 \times 10^9/l$, 1 hour previously and then becomes $80 \times 10^9/l$, regional anesthesia is probably inappropriate.

In the past, concern was raised about platelet function in this disorder because of results of studies comparing platelet count with bleeding time. Because these studies found no correlation between bleeding time and platelet count,[128, 129] regional anesthesia was considered contraindicated in patients with a platelet count less than $100 \times 10^9/l$. Most now agree that the bleeding time is not an accurate measure of the risk of bleeding (in the epidural space or elsewhere). Thromboelastography (TEG) is being used in some centers and has been found a helpful technique.[130] Epidural hematoma is a rare complication, and considerable experience has to be gained with TEG to demonstrate its efficacy in predicting the risk of this complication. Because regional anesthesia has definite advantages in patients with pre-eclampsia (improved intervillous blood flow, avoidance of potential difficult intubation), the risks and benefits of the procedure have to be weighed in each patient with HELLP syndrome.[131, 132]

Thrombotic Thrombocytopenic Purpura

This rare disorder (1:100,000) tends to occur primarily in young women, which increases the chance of its concurrence with pregnancy.[133] Fifty-eight percent of patients with TTP in pregnancy present before 24 weeks' gestation.[120] The pathognomonic features of TTP are fever, neurologic signs, microangiopathic hemolytic anemia, thrombocytopenia, and renal dysfunction. Pathologically, there are thrombi in the microvasculature. TTP probably has multiple pathogenic mechanisms.[134] Because both HELLP syndrome and TTP share significant clinical and laboratory features, it is important to differentiate between the two; the treatment is vastly different. The primary treatment of HELLP is delivery and possibly platelet or plasma transfusion. In contrast, continuation of the pregnancy and aggressive treatment of the mother with TTP is advocated, employing plasma exchange with frozen plasma.[135, 136] Platelet transfusions in TTP may actually result in a worsening of the condition.

Thrombocytopenia in TTP may be severe, and in a small number of patients there may be a history of previous episodes. Before the use of plasma exchange, maternal and fetal mortality were very high.[137] Hayward and coworkers[133] reviewed all cases of TTP in pregnancy at their hospital. Nine treated patients were found, of whom one died from "brain death," despite hematologic remission. The others had a complete remission of TTP, but most developed long-term complications. One was lost to long-term follow-up, and of the remaining seven, only one was completely well. The others suffered mild renal impairment, persistent hypertension, persistent memory loss and hemiparesis, subsequent relapse, optic nerve infarct, persistent myalgia, and arthralgia.[133]

TTP may occur post partum,[138] and there also appears to be a familiar form of relapsing TTP.[139, 140] Although the disease may have been successfully treated and in remission, it may also recur during pregnancy.[141] The overall prognosis has improved since the introduction of plasma exchange therapy.[142] Antiplatelet drugs appear to be helpful during pregnancy to reduce the risk of a severe relapse.[142]

Postpartum Hemolytic Uremic Syndrome

In the adult, HUS shares many similarities with TTP, with the distinguishing features being severe renal impairment, moderate thrombocytopenia, and less significant central nervous system manifestations. In contrast to TTP, HUS associated with pregnancy occurs in the postpartum period, and it is characterized by acute renal failure in association with microangiopathic hemolytic anemia. It is rare, with only 40 cases reported up to 1987.[120] The platelet count may be above $100 \times 10^9/l$, but most patients have more significant thrombocytopenia.

Management of Analgesia and Anesthesia for TTP/HUS

To date, there have been no reports of anesthetic management of the parturient with TTP. An excellent review of the principles involved is available, however.[143] Although it is normally optimal to stabilize a woman with TTP before delivery, parturients with TTP that is active at delivery may have severe thrombocytopenia and significant bleeding diathesis. Regional anesthesia and intramuscular injections should be avoided. Neurologic function is often tentative, and sedatives should be avoided or given with caution. Patients are prone to seizures, and appropriate precautions should be taken. Platelet transfusions should be avoided, and packed RBCs and frozen plasma should be administered through a large-bore catheter. Patients who have received multiple plasma exchanges may have a shunt, and the shunt should be managed appropriately. Careful management of intravascular volume and sustaining a good urine output are important to avoid further renal insult.

Intravenous patient-controlled or nurse-administered opioid analgesia, and a nitrous oxide and oxygen mixture are useful techniques for labor analgesia. For cesarean section, general anesthesia with special attention to gentle manipulation of the airway is advisable, especially if the patient's platelet count is less than 50 $\times$ 10^9/l. Rebound hypertension on intubation should be avoided, if possible, in patients with low platelet counts owing to the risk of intracranial hemorrhage. Hypotension must be avoided because of the potential for renal involvement.

Acute Fatty Liver

Acute fatty liver of pregnancy is a relatively rare disease of unknown etiology. Patients may present with malaise, nausea, vomiting, and upper abdominal pain. Rapid progression occurs over a 1- to 2-week period culminating in overt liver failure with jaundice and bleeding. Further deterioration may lead to seizures, coma, and death.[144, 145] Studies of liver function point to signs of hepatic failure (hypoglycemia; markedly elevated direct bilirubin, alanine aminotransferase, and blood ammonia levels; and often rising blood urea nitrogen and creatinine levels). Appearance of the peripheral smear is similar to that of other microangiopathic disorders; however, there are decreased ATIII levels, marked prolongation of PT and PTT,[6] and hypofibrinogenemia. Treatment should consist of aggressive support to address the hypoglycemia and coagulopathy, careful fluid and electrolyte management, and treatment of associated seizures.

Neonatal Alloimmune Thrombocytopenia (NAIT)

NAIT is caused by transplacental passage of maternal platelet-specific alloantibodies directed against specific antigens present on fetal but not maternal platelets. As a result, the fetus or neonate may be affected with severe thrombocytopenia, which may be associated with massive intracranial hemorrhage leading to significant morbidity and mortality. NAIT is the platelet equivalent of Rh disease; however, unlike erythroblastosis fetalis, NAIT can occur in the first pregnancy. The incidence of neonatal intracranial hemorrhage is 15 to 20%, with half of these cases occurring antenatally. Diagnosis in a pregnancy at risk is confirmed by cordocentesis.[146] Early diagnosis and treatment of the mother with weekly high dose–IVIG from approximately 20 weeks' gestation has dramatically improved the fetal and neonatal rate of mortality and morbidity associated with this disorder.

Because this disease affects the fetus and not the mother, analgesia and anesthesia for delivery are dependent on her wishes and overall clinical condition. Preparation of compatible maternal or homologous platelets is important to ensure their availability for the infant at delivery. Careful screening of the maternal blood for the transmissible diseases associated with blood transfusion (HIV, HBV, HCV, HTLV-I, syphilis, and cytomegalovirus) is also important before transfusing the neonate with maternal platelets.

VESSEL WALL DISORDERS

Bleeding from disorders of the vessel wall is usually mild and superficial. Vessel wall disorders are unusual and are generally classified as either inherited or acquired. The acquired disorders are much more common. For the most part, they fall into the category of vascular purpura, which arises from damage to the endothelium or its supporting matrix. Very little literature exists on the anesthetic implications in pregnancy. The hereditary vessel disorders are very uncommon, and limited information is available about these so-affected patients during pregnancy. A careful history and in some cases, as indicated, a careful assessment, preferably before pregnancy and at least well in advance of delivery, are necessary to fully understand the extent of the disease and its implications for anesthesia. In the acquired disorders, a careful physical examination to assess the presence of active purpura provides the best determination of bleeding risk.

Hereditary Hemorrhagic Telangiectasia (Osler-Weber-Rendu)

This is inherited as an autosomal dominant disease and is characterized by abnormal small blood vessels and arteriovenous (AV) fistulas involving almost all organs. The telangiectasia often appears as small blush areas on the skin, and mucous membrane involvement commonly appears as epistaxis or gastrointestinal hemorrhage. The physiologic changes of pregnancy accentuate the AV shunts owing to dilatation of the systemic vascular bed and increased blood volume and cardiac output, whereas hormonal changes may weaken the vessel walls.[147, 148] Hemothorax has been reported during pregnancy as a result of lung involvement,[148] and arterial hypoxemia and paradoxical embolism may reflect pulmonary shunts.[149] Congestive cardiac failure due to hepatic AV shunts and portal hypertension have occurred during pregnancy.[150] Fistulas have been reported in the epidural space and in the spinal cord.

Pseudoxanthoma Elasticum

Pseudoxanthoma elasticum (PXE) is an inherited connective tissue disorder with biosynthesis of abnormal collagen and elastin fibers, which may result in hemorrhage and thrombosis. Some investigators question whether PXE worsens during pregnancy.[151-153] Gastrointestinal hemorrhage may occur, and there is an increased incidence of cardiac dysrhythmias.

Allergic Purpura (Henoch-Schönlein Purpura)

This is mainly a disease of children, although several cases have been reported in pregnant women.[154-156] The clinical syndrome of purpura, hematuria, proteinuria, abdominal pain, gastrointestinal bleeding, and arthralgia is the consequence of a generalized vasculitis. The disease appears to be allergic in origin, but often an etiologic agent is not identified. The effect of pregnancy on Henoch-Schönlein purpura has yet to be determined. Plasmapheresis has been used to treat severe relapses during pregnancy, resulting in a successful outcome for mother and fetus.[154]

Anesthesia for Patients with Vessel Wall Abnormalities

In all of these disorders, anesthetic management is dependent on the status of the patient. No specific contraindications to regional anesthesia exist, but if there is ongoing hemorrhage, regional anesthesia is contraindicated. In many of these disorders there is the possibility of abnormal spinal and epidural vessels, increasing the chance of venipuncture with subsequent bleeding into the epidural space. In each situation, the risk-benefit analysis of the procedure determines whether, following appropriate informed consent, regional or general anesthesia should be administered. If regional anesthesia is chosen, patients should be followed closely for possible neurologic sequelae. To decrease risk associated with the procedure, the most experienced person should perform the block and it should be done in the midline position. The patient should understand that there may be an increased risk from a regional technique. The risks and benefits of the alternatives should be considered on a patient-by-patient basis.

One case report describes uneventful epidural anesthesia in a parturient in labor with hereditary hemorrhagic telangiectasia.[147] Relief of pain with subsequent decrease in catecholamines, attenuating the increased cardiac output from labor,[147] was considered important in reducing the distension of existing AV fistulas. Because there is the potential for paradoxical embolism through pulmonary fistulas, the epidural space should be identified through loss of resistance to saline rather than to air.

No reports of anesthesia in parturients with PXE appear in the literature. The major risk during pregnancy appears to be related to gastrointestinal hemorrhage, but most reports indicate an uneventful labor and delivery. One case report describes a difficult intubation in a nonpregnant patient with PXE.[157] The investigators suggested that the problem was the consequence of calcification and aggregation of the elastic fibers in the laryngeal ligaments and cartilage.

FACTOR DEFICIENCIES

Von Willebrand Disease

Von Willebrand disease (VWD) is the most common inherited bleeding disorder with a prevalence in the general population of 1%.[158] It has an autosomal dominant pattern of inheritance and therefore is seen equally in both males and females. Unlike hemophilia, phenotypic expression of the disorder varies within families. Approximately 90% of patients are classified as having as type I disease, which is characterized by a simple decrease in the level of plasma FVIII:VWF antigen and activity.[159] The other subtypes of VWD (IIa, IIb, III) involve abnormal configurations of the multimer and varying abnormalities of plasma- and platelet-associated von Willebrand factor. The majority of those patients who do not have type I disease have type II variants. Type III disease has prevalence of 1 in 1 million. If the clinical history is strongly suggestive of this disorder, testing for abnormalities of von Willebrand factor (VWF) and factor VIII complex should be done on at least two separate occasions if initial results are inconclusive.

Thrombocytopenia may accompany variant type IIb and is thought to result from binding of the abnormal VWF to platelets, with subsequent platelet aggregate formation and clearance.[160] It may prove difficult to distinguish between the thrombocytopenia of preeclampsia and variant VWD.

VWF is synthesized in the endothelial cell. It has been recognized for many years that, in pregnancy, plasma levels of VWF rise.[161] Thus, many patients achieve a clinical and laboratory remission in pregnancy. For those patients who require treatment, DDAVP at a dose of 0.3 μg/kg (to a maximum of 20 μg) is the treatment of choice, with the exception of patients with types IIb and III disease.[162] Infusion of DDAVP results in an instantaneous release of VWF from the endothelium and an immediate two- to threefold rise in plasma levels for both factor VIII:c and VWF. Repeated infusions, however, can cause hyponatremia and, on occasion, seizures, as well as a tachyphylactic response. Thus, in practice, DDAVP infusions are usually repeated only once or twice at 12-hour intervals after the initial infusion. Patients with type IIb VWD are at risk with infusion of DDAVP for worsening of the thrombocytopenia. For these patients and those with type III disease (severe form of VWD), Humate-C, a viral inactivated plasma-derived product containing both factors VIII:c and active VWF, is the treatment of choice.

Factor VIII Deficiency

This deficiency, also called hemophilia A, is an X-linked recessive trait that results in deficiency (activity level of 35% or less) of factor VIII. As a result, affected females are very rare. The clinical severity of bleeding varies from family to family but is generally constant within a particular family (Table 23–11). Thus, if the father has mild disease, his grandsons with the disorder are likely to have mild disease.

Because of lyonization of the X chromosome (inactivation of the X chromosome), 10 to 30% of nonpregnant carriers may have low levels of factor VIII activity and thereby are at risk for bleeding complications (usually at surgery).[163] Fortunately, factor VIII:c increases in pregnancy and, therefore, in the small number of carriers with symptomatic disease, remission usually occurs. Occasionally the levels remain low, and thus these patients are at risk of hemorrhage.

Factor IX Deficiency

This disease, also called hemophilia B and Christmas disease, is an X-linked recessive bleeding disorder that is indistinguishable from factor VIII:c deficiency (hemophilia A) in clinical spectrum and heredity. Fifty percent of the sons of heterozygous maternal carriers are hemizygous and affected, and 50% of the daughters of affected fathers or maternal carriers are heterozygous carriers. As is seen in hemophilia A, women may be significantly affected because of extreme lyonization. Those with very low factor levels are at risk of bleeding. Unlike hemophilia A, however, factor IX levels do not rise during pregnancy.[164]

Five cases of factor IX deficiency during pregnancy are reported in the obstetric literature to 1991.[165] Four patients were followed throughout gestation with monthly monitoring of factor IX levels, and three of four had intrapartum plasma or factor IX prophylaxis. The fourth patient reported at 28 weeks' gestation with thrombocytopenia and retrochorionic hemorrhage. She was treated with factor IX and eventually had a spontaneous vaginal delivery at 36 weeks' gestation. No mention is made of anesthetic or analgesic management.

Factor X Deficiency

Factor X is a vitamin K–dependent clotting factor. Its deficiency is one of the rarest, occurring less than 1 in 500,000 of the general population. It is inherited as an autosomal recessive trait. In pregnancy, factor X levels generally rise to 163% of normal activity at 30 weeks and return to normal 6 weeks post partum. Only two cases of factor X deficiency in pregnancy have been reported.[166, 167] In one, the factor X levels did not increase, and the patient required factor concentrate owing to placental abruption.[167] This patient eventually had an uneventful cesarean section with no mention made of anesthesia.

Factor XI Deficiency

This deficiency is transmitted as an autosomal recessive trait and is reported to occur in between 0.1 and 0.53% of Ashkenazi Jews. An increased frequency is also seen in families of Italian and German heritage. Unlike the classic hemophilias, the bleeding tendency does not correlate well with the level of factor XI, and assessment of the patient's risk is best achieved through a detailed patient and family history. Treatment is with replacement factor. These patients may present with a prolonged PTT and normal PT. Factor XI levels normally decrease during pregnancy, in contrast to other factors, which increase. At 28 weeks, factor XI level is 81% and at term 62% of nonpregnant levels. Depending on the level of factor XI at term, patients may require administration of the specific factor. Occasionally, patients develop an inhibitor that may require an anti-inhibitor complex to correct coagulation.[168] Generally, clinicians should treat a patient with a bleeding history and not treat a patient if there is no bleeding history.

Anesthesia for Parturients with Congenital Coagulopathies

All patients with a diagnosis of a congenital coagulopathy benefit from an early consultation with a hematologist and an anesthesiologist. These consultations allow an assessment of specific factor levels, their response during pregnancy, and anticipated management for labor and delivery.

Patients with VWD are frequently denied regional anesthesia despite the fact that most have an improvement in their coagulation status during pregnancy, because of an increase in antihemophilic factor and VWF. Many respond to the use of DDAVP.[169] Because VWF levels decrease rapidly post partum, it is necessary to continue to monitor patients' coagulation status and possibly administer DDAVP in the postpartum period.

Depending on the type of VWD and its status in pregnancy, regional anesthesia may safely be offered. Reports of successful epidural anesthesia in patients with type I disease are available.[170, 171] For cesarean section, spinal anesthesia may be preferred because of the smaller size of needle. Because the levels of VWF

TABLE 23–11. **SEVERITY OF HEMOPHILIA BASED ON FACTOR ACTIVITY LEVEL**

Clinical Severity	Clinical Sequelae	Clotting Factor Activity Level (%)
Severe	Spontaneous musculoskeletal and internal bleeding	<1
Moderate	Occasional, spontaneous musculoskeletal bleeding	1–5
Mild	Delayed-onset bleeding after trauma, surgery, and dental extraction	5–35

decrease post partum, patients should be followed closely when regional anesthesia is administered.

Hemophilia A and B are inherited as X-linked recessive genes. As a result, males are mainly affected. Because of lyonization of the gene, however, female carriers may exhibit coagulation abnormalities. This observation is important from the anesthetic perspective.

Inwood and Meltzer[172] have pointed out the potential anesthetic problems. A balance must be struck with regard to the benefits and risks of appropriate replacement therapy versus the benefits and risks of the anesthetic technique. If there is an overt coagulopathy, regional anesthesia is contraindicated, and an alternative technique should be chosen for labor analgesia. In patients with a deficiency of factor VIII:c, a good response to DDAVP can be anticipated and may normalize the factor VIII:c level. This technique is safe with none of the risks of factor concentrate. Consideration for factor replacement is based on the factor levels and their associated risk of delayed hemorrhage. Normalization of factor levels to minimize bleeding risk before surgery allows a broader spectrum of anesthetic options.

Patients should be identified early in pregnancy and a consultation with an anesthesiologist and hematologist arranged so that methods of management can be discussed. General anesthesia for cesarean section is the technique of choice if there is evidence of a coagulopathy.

CONGENITAL DISORDERS OF FIBRINOGEN

Three congenital abnormalities of fibrinogen are identified. These are afibrinogenemia, dysfibrinogenemia, and hypofibrinogenemia. The major problem with all of these is the risk of hemorrhage.[173, 174] Regional anesthesia is contraindicated.

A review documents 250 case reports of congenital dysfibrinogenemia.[175] Of these, 55% of patients were asymptomatic, 25% had a bleeding tendency, and 20% had a thrombotic tendency. The prevalence of dysfibrinogenemia in patients with a history of thrombosis is low, 0.8%. In pregnancy, severe bleeding is rare and is usually limited to the postpartum period. Women with a thrombotic tendency have a high incidence of spontaneous abortion and postpartum thrombosis. Two postulates are suggested for the dysfunction of the fibrinogen, as follows: (1) defective binding of thrombin to abnormal fibrin causes increased thrombin levels; and (2) defective stimulation of abnormal fibrin occurs during fibrinolysis.[175]

The primary problem is that of hemorrhage.[173, 174] Periodic transfusions of fibrinogen may be necessary during pregnancy to prevent miscarriage. In patients with evidence of thrombophilia, low-dose heparin may be required for prophylaxis. It is important that patients be identified early in pregnancy and a plan of management devised by the hematologist, obstetrician, and anesthesiologist. Regional anesthesia is contraindicated.

HYPERCOAGULABLE STATES

Pregnancy is defined as a hypercoagulable state, and parturients are therefore at greater risk of thrombosis. Parturients who have a hereditary predisposition to thrombosis (protein C, S, and ATIII deficiencies or hereditary resistance to activated protein C) or those who have antiphospholipid antibodies (lupus anticoagulant, anticardiolipin antibody) are at even greater risk.[176-178] ATIII deficiency is inherited as an autosomal dominant condition with a prevalence of 1 in 2000. Protein S is a cofactor for the anticoagulant effect of protein C. Because of the increased risks of thromboembolism and pregnancy loss, patients are generally treated with anticoagulation. Provided that there is not a recent history of thromboembolic disease (TED), treatment may consist of prophylactic heparin (low-dose, subcutaneous) and/or aspirin, in the setting of antiphospholipid antibodies. If there is a recent history of TED, the patient may undergo full anticoagulation with therapeutic subcutaneous heparin.

Anesthesia and Analgesia

Several case reports of the anesthetic management of these conditions now exist.[179] In cases when the patient is on full anticoagulant doses of intravenous heparin, analgesia can be managed with intravenous opioids, either as a nurse-administered bolus or a patient-controlled device. Patients who have been on low-dose, prophylactic heparin and whose last dose was administered 4 hours before the request for analgesia can receive epidural analgesia, provided that the PTT is normal and there is no evidence of a bleeding tendency. If cesarean section is required, spinal anesthesia provides a reasonable alternative, because the small needle is less likely to produce a venipuncture. Patients who are fully anticoagulated require general anesthesia.[180, 181]

ASPIRIN AND HEPARIN

Aspirin (low-dose, 80 mg daily) and heparin have been given for a number of conditions during pregnancy. Uses include treatment of patients with antiphospholipid antibodies, prophylaxis for pre-eclampsia or intrauterine growth retardation, or treatment of women with a history of thrombosis.[182-194]

Prophylactic heparin is designed to inhibit spontaneous activation of procoagulation mechanisms, namely spontaneous conversion of factor X to its activated form Xa. Used this way, it does not interfere significantly with platelet function or with activation of normal hemostasis at the site of injury. In Europe, in pregnant patients and in nonpregnant patients, low-molecular-weight heparin is being administered with increased frequency, but it is not yet approved for use in pregnant patients in North America. Early reports suggest that it is safe during pregnancy.[193, 194]

Although concerns have been raised about spinal and epidural techniques in parturients on prophylactic heparin and/or aspirin, experience with regional anesthesia has shown it to be safe.[82, 195–197] The regimen for prophylactic heparin administration maintains the PTT within the normal range. The PTT can be verified before regional anesthesia, in situations other than those of the patient with a positive test result for lupus anticoagulant. Obviously, if there is evidence of a bleeding diathesis (excess bruising or bleeding), regional anesthesia is contraindicated. When prophylactic subcutaneous heparin is given, neuraxial block is best delayed until 4 hours following the last dose.[181] In patients on therapeutic heparin, regional anesthesia is contraindicated,[181] unless the heparin is discontinued and a normal PTT is obtained. This approach, however, is associated with an increased risk of thrombosis. After the epidural catheter is inserted, heparin can be restarted. Removal of the epidural catheter should be delayed until the PTT is normal. In these situations, it is important to obtain informed consent, recognizing that the risk of the combination of epidural space catheterization and therapeutic anticoagulation cannot be estimated. In most patients, the risk of rethrombosis during labor and delivery outweighs the benefits of regional anesthesia, and, thus, care should be taken to ensure that the appropriate rationale is given.

MATERNAL HYDROPS

Rarely, fetal and/or placental hydrops is accompanied by maternal hydrops.[198–210] This syndrome has variously been called Ballantyne syndrome, mirror syndrome (hydrops), triple edema, and pseudotoxemia. Isoimmunization (Rh disease, anti-Kell, anti-Duffy antibodies), infection (various viruses such as parvovirus), alpha-thalassemia, sacrococcygeal teratoma, aneurysm of the vein of Galen in the fetus, and placental tumor have been implicated as the origin of hydrops in the fetus and placenta. The precise etiology of maternal hydrops is unknown.

Clinically, there are some similarities to pre-eclampsia, with massive edema, mild or moderate proteinuria, and mild hypertension—hence, the name *pseudotoxemia*. Other well-documented cases have no proteinuria or hypertension, however. The edema generally is severe, mainly involving the extremities. Clinically, the patient may complain of shortness of breath due to pulmonary edema and/or polyhydramnios, with upward pressure on the diaphragm, and ascites. An associated anemia and an elevated plasma uric acid level may be present. In some of the early reports, Rh isoimmunization was diagnosed on the basis of severe edema in the mother.

Because of the underlying fetal hydrops, this condition is associated with a high incidence of perinatal mortality. Delivery of the hydropic fetus and placenta generally leads to rapid devolution of the maternal syndrome. Until such time as delivery occurs, maternal morbidity resulting from pre-eclampsia, pulmonary edema, and renal failure can be significant.

Anesthetic involvement with these patients may include provision of analgesia for labor, resuscitation measures, and insertion of arterial and central catheters. If epidural analgesia is administered, a cautious approach to fluid loading and slow incremental injection of local anesthetic are essential.

SUMMARY

When a parturient presents with a hematologic abnormality (as a result of either pre-existing disease or pregnancy), the anesthesiologist must be aware of the ramifications of that disorder on management. Of particular importance is the need to fully inform the patient of the possible need for blood products and of the possible limitations of anesthetic technique, based on the underlying condition. Early consultation with the anesthesiologist and hematologist is essential, so that a coordinated approach to patient care can begin.

References

1. Hytten F. Blood volume changes in normal pregnancy. Clin Haematol 1985;14:601.
2. Bentley DP. Iron metabolism and anemia in pregnancy. Clin Haematol 1985;14:613.
3. Lockitch G. Hardbook of Diagnostic Biochemistry and Hematology in Normal Pregnancy. CRC Press. Boca Raton, FL, 1993.
4. Letzky E. Hematologic Disorders. In Barron WM, Lindheimer MD (eds): Medical Disorders During Pregnancy, 2nd ed. St. Louis, Mosby-Year Book, 1995.
5. Pitkin RM, Witte DL. Platelet and leukocyte counts in pregnancy. JAMA 1979;242:2696.
6. Ballem PJ. Diagnosis and management of thrombocytopenia in obstetrical syndromes. In Sacher RA, Brecher M (eds): Obstetrical Transfusion Practice. Bethesda, MD, American Association of Blood Banks, 1993, p 49.
7. Tygart SG, McRoyan DK, Spinnato JA, et al. Longitudinal study of platelet indices during normal pregnancy. Am J Obstet Gynecol 1986;154:883.
8. Sejeny SA, Eastham RD, Baker SR. Platelet counts during pregnancy. J Clin Pathol 1975;28:812.
9. Sill PR, Lind T, Walker W. Platelet values during normal pregnancy. Br J Obstet Gynecol 1985;92:480.
10. Singer CRJ, Walker JJ, Cameron A, et al. Platelet studies in normal pregnancy and pregnancy-induced hypertension. Clin Lab Haematol 1986;8:27.

11. Fay RA, Hughes AO, Farron NT. Platelets in pregnancy; Hyper-destruction in pregnancy. Obstet Gynecol 1983;61;238.

12. Gerbasi FR, Bottoms S, Farag A, et al. Increased intravascular coagulation associated with pregnancy. Obstet Gynecol 1990;75:385.

13. Stirling Y, Woolf L, North WR, et al. Haemostasis in normal pregnancy. Thromb Haemost 1984;52:176.

14. Faught W, Garner P, Jones G, Ivey B. Changes in protein C and protein S levels in normal pregnancy. Am J Obstet Gynecol 1995;172:147.

15. Comp PC, Thurnau GR, Welsh J, et al. Functional and immuno-logic protein S levels are decreased during pregnancy. Blood 1986;68:881.

16. Rodgers CRP, Levin J. A critical reappraisal of the bleeding time. Semin Thromb Hemost 1990;16:1.

17. Lind SE. The bleeding time does not predict surgical bleeding. Blood 1991;77:2547.

18. Ditto FF III, Gibbons JJ. Factitious prolongation of bleeding time associated with patient movement. Anesth Analg 1991;72:710.

19. Mallett SV, Cox DJA. Thromboelastography. Br J Anaesth 1992;69:307.

20. Orlikowski CEP, Payne AJ, Moodley J, et al. Thromboelastogra-phy after aspirin ingestion in pregnant and non-pregnant subjects. Br J Anaesth 1992;69:159.

21. Pepkowitz SH. Autologous blood donation and obstetric trans-fusion practice. In Sacher RA, Brecher ME (eds): Obstetric Trans-fusion Practice. Bethesda, MD, American Association of Blood Banks, 1993, p 77.

22. Grange C, Douglas MJ, Adams TJ, et al. Haemodilution for caesarean section. Can J Anaesth 1996;43:A59.

23. Owen HG, Brecher ME. Therapeutic apheresis of the pregnant patient. In Sacher RA, Brecher ME (eds): Obstetric Transfusion Practice. Bethesda, MD, American Association of Blood Banks, 1993, p 95.

24. ACOG Technical Bulletin. Hemoglobinopathies in pregnancy. Int J Gynaecol Obstet 1993;43:333.

25. Fischel-Ghodsian N. Prenatal diagnosis of hemoglobinopathies. Clin Perinatol 1990;17:811.

26. Savona-Ventura C, Bonello F. Beta-Thalassemia syndromes and pregnancy. Obstet Gynecol Surv 1994;49:129.

27. Singounas EG, Sakas DE, Hadley DM, et al. Paraplegia in a pregnant thalassemic woman due to extramedullary hematopoi-esis: Successful management with transfusions. Surg Neurol 1991;36:210.

28. El-Shafei AM, Dhaliwal JK, Sandhu AK. Pregnancy in sickle cell disease in Bahrain. Br J Obstet Gynaecol 1992;99:101.

29. Tuck SM, Studd JW, White JM. Pregnancy in sickle cell disease in the UK. Br J Obstet Gynaecol 1983;90:112.

30. Vichinsky EP, Haberkern CM, Neumayr L, et al. A comparison of conservative and aggressive transfusion regimens in the peri-operative management of sickle cell disease. N Engl J Med 1995;333:206.

31. Koshy M, Burd L. Management of pregnancy in sickle cell syndromes. Hematol Oncol Clin North Am 1991;5:585.

32. Van Enk A, Visschers G, Jansen W, et al. Maternal death due to sickle cell chronic lung disease. Br J Obstet Gynaecol 1992;99:162.

33. Searle JF. Anaesthesia in sickle cell states. A review. Anaesthesia 1973;28:48.

34. Esseltine DW, Baxter MRN, Bevan JC. Sickle cell states and the anaesthetist. Can J Anaesth 1988;35:385.

35. Koshy M, Weiner SJ, Miller ST, et al. Surgery and anesthesia in sickle cell disease. Blood 1995;86:3676.

36. Finer P, Blair J, Rowe P. Epidural analgesia in the management of labor pain and sickle cell crisis—a case report. Anesthesiol-ogy 1988;68:799.

37. Pattison J, Harrop-Griffiths AW, Whitlock JE, et al. Caesarean section in a patient with haemoglobin SC disease and a phaeochromocytoma. Anaesthesia 1990;45:958.

38. Edwards R. Anaesthesia for caesarean section in haemoglobin SC disease complicated by eclampsia. A case report. Br J An-aesth 1973;45:757.

39. The Anaesthesia Advisory Committee to the Chief Coroner of Ontario. Intraoperative death during caesarean section in a pa-tient with sickle-cell trait. Can J Anaesth 1987;34:67.

40. Ho-Yen DO. Hereditary spherocytosis presenting in pregnancy. Acta Haematol 1984;72:29.

41. Pajor A, Lehoczky D, Szakacs Z. Pregnancy and hereditary spherocytosis. Report of 8 patients and a review. Arch Gynecol Obstet 1993;253:37.

42. Maberry MC, Mason RA, Cunningham FG, et al. Pregnancy complicated by hereditary spherocytosis. Obstet Gynecol 1992;79:735.

43. Baker RI, Manoharan A, De Luca E, et al. Pure red cell aplasia of pregnancy: A distinct clinical entity. Br J Haematol 1993;85:619.

44. Perry CP, Harris RE. Successful management of pregnancy-induced pancytopenia. Obstet Gynecol 1977;50:732.

45. Fleming AF. Hypoplastic anemia in pregnancy. J Obstet Gynae-col Br Commonw 1968;75:138.

46. Collins DJ, Rosenthal DS, Goldstein DP, et al. Aplastic anemia in pregnancy. Obstet Gynecol 1972;39:884.

47. Cohen E, Ilan Y, Gillis S, et al. Recurrent transient bone marrow hypoplasia associated with pregnancy. Acta Haematol 1993;89:32.

48. Aggio MC, Zunini C. Reversible pure red-cell aplasia in preg-nancy (letter). N Engl J Med 1977;297:221.

49. Leong KW, Teh A, Bosco JJ, et al. Successful pregnancy follow-ing aplastic anemia. Post Grad Med J 1995;71:625.

50. Knispel JW, Lynch VA, Viele BD. Aplastic anemia in pregnancy: A case report, review of the literature, and a re-evaluation of management. Obstet Gynecol Surv 1976;31:523.

51. Aitchison RGM, Marsh JCW, Hows JM, et al. Pregnancy associ-ated aplastic anemia: A report of five cases and review of current management. Br J Haematol 1989;73:541.

52. Seaward PGR, Setzen R, Guidozzi F. Fanconi's anemia in preg-nancy. A case report. S Afr Med J 1990;78:691.

53. Halperin DS, Freedman MH. Diamond-Blackfan anemia: Etiol-ogy, pathophysiology, and treatment. Am J Pediatr Hematol Oncol 1989;11:380.

54. Rijhsinghani A, Wiechert RJ. Diamond-Blackfan anemia in preg-nancy. Obstet Gynecol 1994;83:827.

55. Bruce DL, Koepke JA. Anesthetic management of patients with bone-marrow failure. Anesth Analg 1972;51:597.

56. Frakes JT, Burmeister RE, Giliberti JJ. Pregnancy in a patient with paroxysmal nocturnal hemoglobinuria. Obstet Gynecol 1976;47:22S.

57. Hurd WW, Miodovnik M, Stys SJ. Pregnancy associated with paroxysmal nocturnal hemoglobinuria. Obstet Gynecol 1982;60:742.

58. Spencer JAD. Paroxysmal nocturnal haemoglobinuria in preg-nancy: Case report. Br J Obstet Gynaecol 1980;87:246.

59. Barton JR, Shaver DC, Sibai BM. Successive pregnancies compli-cated by idiopathic sideroblastic anemia. Am J Obstet Gynecol 1992;166:576.

60. Vadher BD, Machin SJ, Patterson KG, et al. Life-threatening thrombotic and haemorrhagic problems associated with silent myeloproliferative disorders. Br J Haematol 1993;85:213.

61. Schafer AI. Essential thrombocythemia. Prog Hemost Thromb 1991;10:69.

62. Katz LE, Goyert GL, Bloom RE, et al. Essential thrombocytosis in pregnancy: Is pharmacologic therapy indicated? (letter). J Maternal Fetal Med 1994;3:193.

63. Randi ML, Barbone E, Rossi C, et al. Essential thrombocythemia and pregnancy: A report of six normal pregnancies in five untreated patients. Obstet Gynecol 1994;83:915.

64. Ferguson TE II, Ueland K, Aronson WJ. Polycythemia rubra vera and pregnancy. Obstet Gynecol 1983;62:16S.

65. Wasserman LR. Polycythemia vera study group: A historical perspective. Semin Hematol 1986;23:183.

66. Hoffman R, Wasserman LR. Natural history and management of polycythemia vera. Adv Intern Med 1979;24:255.

67. Hocking WG, Golde DW. Polycythemia: Evaluation and man-agement. Blood Rev 1989;3:59.

68. Caligiuri MA, Mayer RJ. Pregnancy and leukemia. Semin Oncol 1989;16:388.

69. Zuazu J, Julia A, Sierra J, et al. Pregnancy outcome in hemato-logic malignancies. Cancer 1991;67:703.

70. Celo JS, Kim HC, Houlihan C, et al. Acute promyelocytic leuke-mia in pregnancy: All-trans retinoic acid as a newer therapeutic option. Obstet Gynecol 1994;83:808.

71. Doll DC, Ringenberg QS, Yarbro JW. Management of cancer during pregnancy. Arch Intern Med 1988;148:2058.

72. Ward FT, Weiss RB. Lymphoma and pregnancy. Semin Oncol 1989;16:397.

73. Gobbi PG, Attardo-Parrinello G, Danesino M, et al. Hodgkin's Disease and pregnancy. Haematologica 1984;69:336.

74. Malee MP. Multiple myeloma in pregnancy: A case report. Obstet Gynecol 1990;75:513.

75. Caudle MR, Dodd S, Solomon A. Multiple myeloma in pregnancy: A case report. Obstet Gynecol 1990;75:516.

76. Pajor A, Kelemen E, Mohos Z, et al. Multiple myeloma in pregnancy. Int J Gynaecol Obstet 1991;35:341.

77. Cheung VYT, Bocking AD, Hollomby D, et al. Waldenström hypergammaglobulinemic purpura and pregnancy. Obstet Gynecol 1993;82:685.

78. Ciliberti BJ, Mazzia VDB, Mark LC, et al. Polycythemia vera and anesthesia. N Y State J Med 1962; Feb 1:400.

79. Coleman AJ, Sliom CM. Polycythaemic hypoxaemia and general anaesthesia. A case report. Br J Anaesth 1966;38:653.

80. Lipton JH, Derzko C, Fyles G, et al. Pregnancy after BMT: Three case reports. Bone Marrow Transplant 1993;11:415.

81. Stein RA, Messino MJ, Hessel EA II. Anaesthetic implications for bone marrow transplant recipients. Can J Anaesth 1990;37:571.

82. Scott DB, Hibberd BM. Serious non-fatal complications associated with extradural block in obstetric practice. Br J Anaesth 1990;64:537.

83. Crawford JS. Some maternal complications of epidural analgesia for labour. Anaesthesia 1985;40:1219.

84. Vandermeulen EP, Van Aken H, Vermylen J. Anticoagulants and spinal-epidural anesthesia. Anesth Analg 1994;79:1165.

85. Horlocker TT, Wedel DJ, Schroeder DR, et al. Preoperative anti-platelet therapy does not increase the risk of spinal hematoma associated with regional anesthesia. Anesth Analg 1995;80:303.

86. Louden KA, Broughton Pipkin F, Heptinstall S, et al. A longitudinal study of platelet behaviour and thromboxane production in whole blood in normal pregnancy and the puerperium. Br J Obstet Gynaecol 1990;97:1108.

87. Harker LA, Slichter SJ. The bleeding time as a screening test for evaluation of platelet function. N Engl J Med 1972;287:155.

88. Burrows RF, Kelton JG. Incidentally detected thrombocytopenia in healthy mothers and their infants. N Engl J Med 1988;319:142.

89. Anteby E, Shalev O. Clinical relevance of gestational thrombocytopenia of < 100,000/μl. Am J Hematol 1994;47:118.

90. Rolbin SH, Abbot D, Musclow E, et al. Epidural anesthesia in pregnant patients with low platelet counts. Obstet Gynecol 1988;71:918.

91. Rasmus KT, Rottman, RL, Kotelko DM, et al. Unrecognized thrombocytopenia and regional anesthesia in parturients: A retrospective review. Obstet Gynecol 1989;73:943.

92. Burrows RF, Kelton JG. Thrombocytopenia at delivery. A prospective survey of 6715 deliveries. Am J Obstet Gynecol 1990;162:731.

93. Ballem PJ, Segal GM, Stratton JR, et al. Mechanisms of thrombocytopenia in chronic autoimmune thrombocytopenic purpura. Evidence of both impaired platelet production and increased platelet clearance. J Clin Invest 1987;80:33.

94. Paidas MJ, Haut MJ, Lockwood CJ. Platelet disorders in pregnancy: Implications for mother and fetus. Mt Sinai J Med 1994;61:389.

95. Cines DB, Dusak B, Tomaski A, et al. Immune thrombocytopenic purpura and pregnancy. N Engl J Med 1982;306:826.

96. Burrows RF, Kelton JG. Low fetal risks in pregnancies associated with idiopathic thrombocytopenic purpura. Am J Obstet Gynecol 1990;163:1147.

97. Cook RL, Miller RC, Katz VL, et al. Immune thrombocytopenic purpura in pregnancy: A reappraisal of management. Obstet Gynecol 1991;78:578.

98. Samuels P, Bussel JB, Braitman LE, et al. Estimation of the risk of thrombocytopenia in the offspring of pregnant women with presumed immune thrombocytopenic purpura. N Engl J Med 1990;323:229.

99. Moise KJ. Autoimmune thrombocytopenic purpura in pregnancy. Clin Obstet Gynecol 1991;34:51.

100. Yamada H, Fujimoto S. Perinatal management of idiopathic thrombocytopenic purpura in pregnancy: Risk factors for passive immune thrombocytopenia. Ann Hematol 1994;68:39.

101. George JN, Woolf SH, Raskob GE, et al. Idiopathic thrombocytopenic purpura: A practice guideline developed by explicit methods for the American Society of Hematology. Blood 1996;88:3.

102. Peng TC, Kickler TS, Bell WR, et al. Obstetric complications in a patient with Bernard-Soulier syndrome. Am J Obstet Gynecol 1991;165:425.

103. Saade G, Homsi R, Seoud M. Bernard-Soulier syndrome in pregnancy: A report of four pregnancies in one patient, and review of the Lterature. Eur J Obstet Gynecol Reprod Biol 1991;40:149.

104. Nelson LH, Dewan DM, Mandell GL. Obstetric and anesthetic considerations in the May-Hegglin anomaly. A case report. J Reprod Med 1993;38:311.

105. Kotelko DM. Anaesthesia for caesarean delivery in a patient with May-Hegglin anomaly. Can J Anaesth 1989;36:328.

106. Duff P, Jackson MT. Pregnancy complicated by rhesus sensitization and the May-Hegglin anomaly. Obstet Gynecol 1985;65:7S.

107. Siddiqui T, Lammert N, Danier P, et al. Immune thrombocytopenia and May-Hegglin anomaly during pregnancy. J Fla Med Assoc 1991;78:88.

108. Chatwani A, Bruder N, Shapiro T, et al. May-Hegglin anomaly: A rare case of maternal thrombocytopenia in pregnancy. Am J Obstet Gynecol 1992;166:143.

109. Takashima T, Maeda H, Koyanagi T, et al. Prenatal diagnosis and obstetrical management of May-Hegglin anomaly: A case report. Fetal Diagn Ther 1992;7:186.

110. Price FV, Legro RS, Watt-Morse M, et al. Chédiak-Higashi syndrome in pregnancy. Obstet Gynecol 1992;79:804.

111. Ito K, Yoshida H, Hatoyama H, et al. Antibody removal therapy used successfully at delivery of a pregnant patient with Glanzmann's thrombasthenia and multiple anti-platelet antibodies. Vox Sang 1991;61:40.

112. Edozien LC, Jip J, Mayers FN. Platelet storage pool deficiency in pregnancy. Br J Clin Pract 1995;49:220.

113. Abramowicz JS, Sherer DM, Woods JR. Acute transient thrombocytopenia associated with cocaine abuse in pregnancy. Obstet Gynecol 1991;78:499.

114. Birnbach DJ, Stein DJ, Fogelberg R, et al. Thrombocytopenia in the cocaine abusing parturient. Anesthesiology 1994;81:A1181.

115. Kain ZN, Mayes LC, Pakes J, et al. Thrombocytopenia in pregnant women who use cocaine. Am J Obstet Gynecol 1995;173:885.

116. Gershon RY, Fisher AJ, Graves WL. The cocaine-abusing parturient is not at an increased risk for thrombocytopenia. Anesth Analg 1996;82:865.

117. Ballem PJ, Belzberg A, Devine DV, et al. Kinetic studies of the mechanism of thrombocytopenia in patients with human immunodeficiency virus infection. N Engl J Med 1992;327:1779.

118. Glantz JC, Roberts DJ. Pregnancy complicated by thrombocytopenia secondary to human immunodeficiency virus infection. Obstet Gynecol 1994;83:825.

119. Mandelbrot L, Schlienger I, Bongain A, et al. Thrombocytopenia in pregnant women infected with human immunodeficiency virus: Maternal and neonatal outcome. Am J Obstet Gynecol 1994;171:252.

120. Weiner CP. Thrombotic microangiopathy in pregnancy and the postpartum period. Semin Hematol 1987;24:119.

121. Weinstein L. Preeclampsia/eclampsia with hemolysis, elevated liver enzymes, and thrombocytopenia. Obstet Gynecol 1985;66:657.

122. Sibai BM, Taslimi MM, El-Nazer A, et al. Maternal-perinatal outcome associated with the syndrome of hemolysis, elevated liver enzymes, and low platelets in severe preeclampsia-eclampsia. Am J Obstet Gynecol 1986;155:501.

123. Sibai BM, Ramadan MK, Usta I, et al. Maternal morbidity and mortality in 442 pregnancies with hemolysis, elevated liver enzymes, and low platelets (HELLP syndrome). Am J Obstet Gynecol 1993;159:1000.

124. Sibai BM, Ramadan MK, Chari RS, et al. Pregnancies complicated by HELLP syndrome (hemolysis, elevated liver enzymes, and low platelets): Subsequent pregnancy outcome and long-term prognosis. Am J Obstet Gynecol 1995;172:125.

125. Martin JN, Blake PG, Perry KG, et al. The natural history of

HELLP syndrome: Patterns of disease progression and regression. Am J Obstet Gynecol 1991;164:1500.

126. Martin JN, Blake PG, Lowry SL, et al. Pregnancy complicated by preeclampsia-eclampsia with the syndrome of hemolysis, elevated liver enzymes, and low platelet count: How rapid is postpartum recovery? Obstet Gynecol 1990;76:737.

127. Roberts WE, Perry KG, Woods JB, et al. The intrapartum platelet count in patients with HELLP (hemolysis, elevated liver enzymes, and low platelets) syndrome: Is it predictive of later hemorrhagic complications? Am J Obstet Gynecol 1994;171:799.

128. Ramanathan J, Sibai BM, Vu T, et al. Correlation between bleeding times and platelet counts in women with preeclampsia undergoing cesarean section. Anesthesiology 1989;71:188.

129. Schindler M, Gatt S, Isert P, et al. Thrombocytopenia and platelet functional defects in pre-eclampsia: Implications for regional anaesthesia. Anaesth Intensive Care 1990;18:169.

130. Whitta RKS, Cox DJA, Mallett SV. Thromboelastography reveals two causes of haemorrhage in HELLP syndrome. Br J Anaesth 1995;74:464.

131. Ramanathan J, Khalil M, Sibai BM, et al. Anesthetic management of the syndrome of hemolysis, elevated liver enzymes, and low platelet count (HELLP) in severe preeclampsia. A retrospective study. Reg Anesth 1988;13:20.

132. Crosby ET. Obstetrical anaesthesia for patients with the syndrome of haemolysis, elevated liver enzymes and low platelets. Can J Anaesth 1991;38:227.

133. Hayward CPM, Sutton DM, Carter WH, et al. Treatment outcomes in patients with adult thrombotic thrombocytopenic purpura-hemolytic uremic syndrome. Arch Intern Med 1994; 154:982.

134. Lian ECY. Pathogenesis of thrombotic thrombocytopenic purpura. Semin Hematol 1987;24:82.

135. Ambrose A, Welham RT, Cefalo RC. Thrombotic thrombocytopenic purpura in early pregnancy. Obstet Gynecol 1985;66:267.

136. Permezel M, Lee N, Corry J. Thrombotic thrombocytopenic purpura in pregnancy. Aust N Z J Obstet Gynaecol 1992;32:278.

137. Moon EC, Kitay DZ. Hematologic problems in pregnancy: II. Thrombotic (thrombohemolytic) thrombocytopenic purpura. J Reprod Med 1972;9:212.

138. Olenich M, Schattner E. Postpartum thrombotic thrombocytopenic purpura (TTP) complicating pregnancy-associated immune thrombocytopenic purpura (ITP). Ann Intern Med 1994;120:845.

139. Wiznitzer A, Mazor M, Leiberman JR, et al. Familial occurrence of thrombotic thrombocytopenic purpura in two sisters during pregnancy. Am J Obstet Gynecol 1992:166:20.

140. Uslu M, Guzelmeric K, Asut I. Familial thrombotic thrombocytopenic purpura imitating HELLP syndrome (hemolysis, elevated liver enzymes, and low platelets) in two sisters during pregnancy (letter). Am J Obstet Gynecol 1994;170:699.

141. Vianelli N, Gugliotta L, Catani L, et al. Thrombotic thrombocytopenic purpura; relapse and pregnancy (letter). Haematologica 1993;78:259.

142. Ezra Y, Rose M, Eldor A. Therapy and prevention of thrombotic thrombocytopenic purpura during pregnancy: A clinical study of 16 pregnancies. Am J Hematol 1996;51:1.

143. Pivalizza EG. Anesthetic management of a patient with thrombotic thrombocytopenic purpura. Anesth Analg 1994;79:1203.

144. Anday EK, Cohen A. Liver disease associated with pregnancy. Ann Clin Lab Sci 1990:20:233.

145. Samuels P, Cohen AW. Pregnancies complicated by liver disease and liver dysfunction. Obstet Gynecol Clin North Am 1992;19:745.

146. Daffos F, Forestier F, Kaplan C, et al. Prenatal diagnosis and management of bleeding disorders with fetal blood sampling. Am J Obstet Gynecol 1988;158:939.

147. Swinburne AJ, Fedullo AJ, Gangemi R, et al. Hereditary telangiectasia and multiple pulmonary arteriovenous fistulas: Clinical deterioration during pregnancy. Chest 1986;89:459.

148. Bevelaqua FA, Ordorica SA, Lefleur R, et al. Osler-Weber-Rendu disease. Diagnosis and management of spontaneous hemothorax during pregnancy. NY State J Med 1992;12:551.

149. Waring PH, Shaw DB, Brumfield CG. Anesthetic management of a parturient with Osler-Weber-Rendu syndrome and rheumatic heart disease. Anesth Analg 1990;71:96.

150. Livneh A, Langevitz P, Morag B, et al. Functionally reversible

151. Berde C, Willis DC, Sandberg EC. Pregnancy in women with pseudoxanthoma elasticum. Obstet Gynecol Surv 1983;38:339.

152. Lao TT, Walters BNJ, De Swiet M. Pseudoxanthoma elasticum and pregnancy. Two case reports. Br J Obstet Gynaecol 1984;91:1049.

153. Viljoen DL, Beatty S, Beighton P. The obstetric and gynaecological implications of pseudoxanthoma elasticum. Br J Obstet Gynaecol 1987;94:884.

154. Ray M, Posen GA. Henoch-Schönlein purpura in pregnancy. Can Med Assoc J 1985;132:1385.

155. Joseph G, Holtman JS, Kosfeld RE, et al. Pregnancy in Henoch-Schönlein purpura. Am J Obstet Gynecol 1987;157:911.

156. Merrill J, Lahita RG. Henoch-Schönlein purpura remitting in pregnancy and during sex steroid therapy. Br J Rheumatol 1994;33:586.

157. Levitt MWD, Collison JM. Difficult endotracheal intubation in a patient with pseudoxanthoma elasticum. Anaesth Intensive Care 1982;10:62.

158. Bloom AL. Von Willebrand factor: Clinical features of inherited and acquired disorders. Mayo Clin Proc 1991;66:743.

159. Ruggeri ZM. Structure and function of von Willebrand factor: Relationship to von Willebrand's disease. Mayo Clin Proc 1991;66:847.

160. Rick ME, Williams SB, Sacher RA, et al. Thrombocytopenia associated with pregnancy in a patient with type IIB von Willebrand's disease. Blood 1987;69:786.

161. Greer IA, Lowe GDO, Walker JJ, et al. Haemorrhagic problems in obstetrics and gynaecology in patients with congenital coagulopathies. Br J Obstet Gynaecol 1991;98:909.

162. Aledort LM. Treatment of von Willebrand's disease. Mayo Clin Proc 1991;66:841.

163. Furie B, Limentani SA, Rosenfield CG. A practical guide to the evaluation and treatment of hemophilia. Blood 1994;84:3.

164. Briet E, Reisner HM, Blatt PM. Factor IX levels during pregnancy in a woman with hemophilia B. Haemostasis 1982;11:87.

165. Guy GP, Baxi LV, Hurlet-Jensen A, et al. An unusual complication in a gravida with factor IX deficiency: Case report with review of the literature. Obstet Gynecol 1992;80:502.

166. Brody JI, Finch SC. Improvement of factor X deficiency during pregnancy. N Engl J Med 1960;263:996.

167. Konje JC, Murphy P, De Chazal R, et al. Severe factor X deficiency and successful pregnancy. Br J Obstet Gynaecol 1994;101:910.

168. Connelly NR, Brull SJ. Anesthetic management of a patient with factor XI deficiency and factor XI inhibitor undergoing a cesarean section. Anesth Analg 1993;76:1365.

169. Cameron CB, Kobrinsky N. Perioperative management of patients with von Willebrand's disease. Can J Anaesth 1990;37:341.

170. Cohen S, Daitch JS, Amar D, et al. Epidural analgesia for labor and delivery in a patient with von Willebrand's disease. Reg Anesth 1989;14:95.

171. Milaskiewicz RM, Holdcroft A, Letsky E. Epidural anaesthesia and von Willebrand's disease. Anaesthesia 1990;45:462.

172. Inwood MJ, Meltzer DB. The female carrier of haemophilia—a problem for the anaesthetist. Can Anaesth Soc J 1978;25:266.

173. Inamoto Y, Terao T. First report of case of congenital afibrinogenemia with successful delivery. Am J Obstet Gynecol 1985;153:803.

174. Goodwin TM. Congenital hypofibrinogenemia in pregnancy. Obstet Gynecol Surv 1989;44:157.

175. Haverkate F, Samama M. Familial dysfibrinogenemia and thrombophilia. Report on a study of the SSC subcommittee on fibrinogen. Thromb Haemost 1995;73:151.

176. Morrison AE, Walker ID, Black WP. Protein C deficiency presenting as deep venous thrombosis in pregnancy. Case report. Br J Obstet Gynaecol 1988;95:1077.

177. Trauscht-Van Horn JJ, Capeless EL, Easterling TR, et al. Pregnancy loss and thrombosis with protein C deficiency. Am J Obstet Gynecol 1992;167:968.

178. Owen J. Antithrombin III replacement therapy in pregnancy. Semin Hematol 1991;28:46.

179. Wetzel RC, Marsh BR, Yaster M, et al. Anesthetic implications of protein C deficiency. Anesth Analg 1986;65:982.

180. Rowbottom SJ. Epidural caesarean section in a patient with

congenital antithrombin III deficiency. Anaesth Intensive Care 1995;23:493.

181. Pattee CL, Penning DH. Obstetrical analgesia in a parturient with antithrombin III deficiency. Can J Anaesth 1993;40:507.

182. Schiff E, Peleg E, Goldenberg M, et al. The use of aspirin to prevent pregnancy-induced hypertension and lower the ratio of thromboxane A_2 to prostacyclin in relatively high risk pregnancies. N Engl J Med 1989;321:351.

183. Benigni A, Gregorini G, Frusca T, et al. Effect of low-dose aspirin on fetal and maternal generation of thromboxane by platelets in women at risk for pregnancy-induced hypertension. N Engl J Med 1989;321:357.

184. Walsh SW, Wang Y, Kay HH, et al. Low-dose aspirin inhibits lipid peroxides and thromboxane but not prostacyclin in pregnant women. Am J Obstet Gynecol 1992;167:926.

185. Sibai BM, Caritis SN, Thom E, et al. Prevention of preeclampsia with low-dose aspirin in healthy, nulliparous pregnant women. N Engl J Med 1993;329:1213.

186. CLASP (Collaborative Low-dose Aspirin Study in Pregnancy) Collaborative Group. CLASP: A randomized trial of low-dose aspirin for the prevention and treatment of pre-eclampsia among 9364 pregnant women. Lancet 1994;343:619.

187. Kaaja R, Julkunen H, Viinikka L, et al. Production of prostacyclin and thromboxane in lupus pregnancies: Effect of small dose of aspirin. Obstet Gynecol 1993;81:327.

188. Uzan S, Beaufils M, Breart G, et al. Prevention of fetal growth retardation with low-dose aspirin: Findings of the EPREDA trial. Lancet 1991;337:1427.

189. Trudinger BJ, Cook CM, Thompson RS, et al. Low-dose aspirin therapy improves fetal weight in umbilical placental insufficiency. Am J Obstet Gynecol 1988;159:681.

190. Nelson-Piercy C, De Swiet M. The place of low-dose aspirin in pregnancy. Int J Obstet Anesth 1994;3:3.

191. Greer IA, De Swiet M. Thrombosis prophylaxis in obstetrics and gynaecology. Br J Obstet Gynaecol 1993;100:37.

192. Sturridge F, De Swiet M, Letsky E. The use of low molecular weight heparin for thromboprophylaxis in pregnancy. Br J Obstet Gynaecol 1994;101:69.

193. Nelson-Piercy C. Low molecular weight heparin for obstetric thromboprophylaxis. Br J Obstet Gynaecol 1994;101:6.

194. Dulitzki M, Pauzner R, Langevitz P, et al. Low-molecular weight heparin during pregnancy and delivery: Preliminary experience with 41 pregnancies. Obstet Gynecol 1996;87:380.

195. Odoom JA, Sih IL. Epidural analgesia and anticoagulant therapy. Experience with one thousand cases of continuous epidurals. Anaesthesia 1983;38:154.

196. Wille-Jørgensen P, Jørgensen LN, Rasmussen LS. Lumbar regional anaesthesia and prophylactic anticoagulant therapy. Is the combination safe? Anaesthesia 1991;46:623.

197. Berqvist D, Lindblad B, Mätzsch T. Low molecular weight heparin for thromboprophylaxis and epidural/spinal anaesthesia—is there a risk? Acta Anaesth Scand 1992;36:605.

198. van Selm M, Kanhai HHH, Bennebroek Gravenhorst J. Maternal hydrops syndrome: A review. Obstet Gynecol Surv 1991;46:785.

199. Kaiser IH. Ballantyne and triple edema. Am J Obstet Gynecol 1971;110:115.

200. Quagliarello JR, Passalaqua AM, Greco MA, et al. Ballantyne's triple edema syndrome: Prenatal diagnosis with ultrasound and maternal renal biopsy findings. Am J Obstet Gynecol 1978;132:580.

201. O'Driscoll DT. A fluid retention syndrome associated with severe iso-immunization to the Rhesus factor. J Obstet Gynaecol Br Commonw 1956;63:372.

202. Rigsby WC, Vorys N, Copeland WE, et al. Antenatal diagnosis of the Rh erythroblastotic fetus. Obstet Gynecol 1961;18:579.

203. Nicolay KS, Gainey HL. Pseudotoxemic state associated with severe Rh isoimmunization. Am J Obstet Gynecol 1964;89:41.

204. Scott JS. Pregnancy toxaemia associated with hydrops foetalis, hydatidiform mole and hydramnios. J Obstet Gynaecol Br Empire 1958;65:689.

205. Goodlin RC. Impending fetal death in utero due to isoimmunization. The maternal syndrome; report of three cases. Obstet Gynecol 1957;10:299.

206. Howard John A, Duncan AS. The maternal syndrome associated with hydrops foetalis. J Obstet Gynaecol Br Commonw 1964;37:61.

207. Cohen A. Maternal syndrome in Rh iso-immunization. Report of a case. J Obstet Gynaecol Br Commonw 1960;67:325.

208. Ville Y, de Gayffier A, Brivet F, et al. Fetal-maternal hydrops syndrome in human parvovirus infection. Fetal Diagn Ther 1995;10:204.

209. Ordorica SA, Marks F, Frieden FJ, et al. Aneurysm of the vein of Galen: A new cause for Ballantyne syndrome. Am J Obstet Gynecol 1990;162:1166.

210. Dorman SL, Cardwell MS. Ballantyne syndrome caused by a large placental chorioangioma. Am J Obstet Gynecol 1995;173:1632.

. . .

24

INFECTIOUS DISEASES

. . . . . .

Gabriela R. Lauretti, M.D.

Many pregnancies are complicated by relatively trivial infections of the skin and the genitourinary and respiratory systems that have little impact on the administration of pain relief or anesthesia. Occasionally, however, we must manage a parturient who is profoundly septic from a number of possible etiologies, or one who is infected with an uncommon agent. This chapter describes the different classes of infection that can occur during pregnancy and their importance to the obstetric anesthesiologist.

BACTERIAL INFECTIONS

Bacterial infections of the skin and respiratory and genitourinary tracts can evolve into a systemic illness with bacteremia, leading to pregnancy-related complications such as preterm labor, premature rupture of membranes, miscarriage, pelvic inflammatory disease, chorioamnionitis, neonatal infection, cervicitis, urethritis, ectopic pregnancy, low birth weight, stillbirth, pneumonia, ARDS, and septic shock.[1–4] Antibiotic treatment during pregnancy is beneficial in reducing neonatal and maternal morbidity and mortality, and most bacterial infections are preventable and treatable.[3, 5–10] Vaginal bacterial diseases are often asymptomatic[11–13] and have little impact on the management by the obstetric anesthesiologist, although bacterial vaginosis may predispose the patient to preterm labor.[3, 10]

The incidence of maternal infection during labor is 3.1%.[14] Septicemia has been reported to complicate 0.07 to 0.8% of pregnancies.[15] The obstetric population has a high morbidity when severe sepsis develops.[16] The high rate may be due to blunting of specific cell-mediated immune responses during pregnancy and production by the fetus and placenta of various immunosuppressants.[17] Most extracellular bacterial infections are cleared by humoral immunity, and thus infections, such as pneumococcal or meningococcal meningitis, are no more common or serious during pregnancy. Intracellular organisms, however, such as *Mycobacterium tuberculosis* and *Listeria monocytogenes*, pose increased risks during pregnancy.[17]

The diagnosis of septicemia in the parturient can be confounded by the physiologic changes that accompany pregnancy.[4] Complications of sepsis include pneumonia, adult respiratory distress syndrome, disseminated intravascular coagulation, pulmonary edema, septic pulmonary edema, septic pulmonary embolus, septic shock, decreased left ventricular function, and cardiac arrest.[18, 19] Septic shock in the obstetric population is caused by gram-negative organisms in 95% of cases and gram-positive bacteria in the other 5%.[18] The diagnosis is made from the history, physical examination, and laboratory findings (Table 24–1). The most common vaginal bacterial infections of interest are listed in Table 24–2.

Anesthetic Management in the Presence of Bacterial Infection

In parturients with remote localized infections, there is probably no increased risk from epidural analgesia.[20]

TABLE 24–1. MATERNAL SEPSIS

Risk Factors	Previous history of recent upper respiratory or urinary tract infection, premature rupture of the membranes[14, 26]; >24 hours prolonged fasting[14]; bimanual examination of parturient with asymptomatic bacteria, prior to rupture of membranes[27]
Clinical Findings*	Minor—increased fetal tachycardia, shivering, hyperthermia, meconium-stained amniotic fluid, dystocia[14]
	Absolute—body temperature >38° C or <36° C, a white blood cell count >12,000 × 10⁹/l, <4,000 × 10⁹/l, or >10% immature (band) forms[26]
	Metabolic acidosis, altered mental status and oliguria are all signs of hypoperfusion and severe sepsis
Procedures	Continuous fetal heart monitoring; fetal scalp pH sampling[4]
	Extracorporeal carbon dioxide removal combined with low-frequency positive-pressure ventilation may be lifesaving for gravidas with adult respiratory distress syndrome unresponsive to traditional ventilatory therapy (PaO_2 less than 50 mm Hg on 100% oxygen)[28]

*At least two minor clinical findings must be present in the absence of any risk factors for 95% confidence interval to diagnose sepsis[14]

TABLE 24–2. **BACTERIAL INFECTIONS**

Etiologic Agent	Clinical Issues
Bacterial vaginosis (*Gardnerella vaginalis, Ureoplasma urealyticum, Mycoplasma hominis, Mobiluncus* species, *Bacteroides bivius*)	Polymicrobial condition; increased incidence during pregnancy; 3–95% incidence of endometritis after cesarean section, despite use of prophylactic antibiotics[29] Bacterial vaginosis may lead to preterm labor.
Neisseria gonorrhoeae	Increased in women with lowered immunity, commonly associated with HIV[30]; increased in women on birth control pills; systemic sepsis[31], endocarditis[32] and arthritis[13] are rare; pharyngitis from oral sex is possible; alters the inflammatory responses elicited in human infection[33]
Chlamydia trachomatis	Neonatal blindness; recurrent abortions[34]
Listeria monocytogenes	Mother: mild flu-like symptoms; infant: sepsis, pneumonia; placenta: macroabscesses[1]
Treponema pallidum	Clinical manifestations depend on chronologic state of the disease, the second phase associated with splenomegaly, lymphadenopathy, and widespread mucocutaneous lesions; tertiary phase characterized by cardiovascular and central and peripheral nervous systems lesions; linked to low socioeconomic status[35]; perinatal mortality of 60.2/1000 deliveries of newborns >1000 g[36]
Streptococcus species (Group A beta-hemolytic; Group B streptococci)	*Group A*—symptomatology varies from mild flu-like illness to tachypnea/cyanosis with poor peripheral circulation; associated with puerperal sepsis[37]; maternal postpartum meningitis after use of epidural catheter[38] and maternal death following epidural anesthesia[4] *Group B*—causes postpartum meningitis[39, 40]; vaginal exam prior to rupture of membranes may lead to bacteremia and meningitis before onset of labor[27] Possible role of nonsteroidal anti-inflammatory drugs in the progression of streptococcal infections to toxic shock syndrome[41]
Escherichia coli	Bacteriuria and pyelonephritis in pregnancy, hypertension, pre-eclampsia, anemia[42]; predisposition to ulcerative colitis?
Staphylococcus species (*S. aureus, S. haemolyticus, S. epidermidis*)	Vertical transmission extradural abscess formation occurs with[21] or without extradural analgesia[43]; systemic sepsis (multi-organ system involvement; adult respiratory distress syndrome)[28]; possible role of nonsteroidal anti-inflammatory drugs in the progression of staphylococcal infections to toxic shock syndrome[41]
Campylobacter species (*C. coli*)	Diarrhea, maternal dehydration, and electrolyte disturbances; bacteremia in pregnancy[44]; 90% prematurity, 80% neonatal mortality rate[45]
Actinomyces israelii	Right flank pain, clinically confused with appendicitis[46]
Clostridium botulinum	Anaerobe producing potent food-related toxin; maternal GI upset, dehydration, lethargy, muscle weakness, ↓ FRC; preterm labor, abruption; toxin does not cross placenta[47]

Cases of epidural abscess and meningitis, however, have been reported in association with epidural, subarachnoid, and combined spinal-epidural anesthesia in obstetrics.[21–23] Because these are serious complications, and because there are no absolutes in clinical medicine, the benefits of regional anesthesia in an infected parturient must be weighed carefully against the risks.[24, 25] These considerations are especially pertinent if the parturient abuses drugs or is immunocompromised (see later in the section on regional anesthesia and systemic infection).

Septicemia associated with hypovolemia, hypotension, and multi-organ hypoperfusion and failure is known as *septic shock* and is a contraindication to regional anesthesia. Thus, a thorough assessment of the intravascular volume status with a central venous pressure line (or pulmonary artery catheter in severe cases) is mandatory before anesthetic intervention. The need for urgent operative delivery must be balanced against the need for preoperative fluid resuscitation of the mother. Sympathetic blockade from epidural or spinal anesthesia may be disastrous in a septic hypovolemic parturient. If an emergency operative delivery is required, a general anesthetic technique is preferable, with a rapid-sequence induction of intravenous (IV)

ketamine 1 to 2 mg/kg and succinylcholine 1.5 mg/kg, with concomitant fluid resuscitation and antibiotic therapy. Anesthesia can be maintained with IV ketamine 2 to 4 $mg \cdot kg^{-1} \cdot hr^{-1}$, an oxygen and nitrous oxide (O_2/N_2O) mixture, and IV opioid. Epidural anesthesia and analgesia can be titrated carefully for nonurgent cesarean section or labor, provided that intravascular volume has been optimized and antibiotic therapy started.

VIRAL INFECTIONS

Viral infections in pregnancy constitute an area of concern to the obstetric anesthesiologist. Viruses of clinical interest include human immunodeficiency virus; hepatitis viruses; herpes simplex virus; cytomegalovirus; papillomavirus; viruses causing chickenpox, measles, rubella, and influenza; parvovirus; and others, all of which are associated with an increased risk for adverse perinatal outcome.

Human Immunodeficiency Virus

Epidemiology

In 1991 it was estimated that 1 in 250 people in the US tested positive for human immunodeficiency virus

(HIV) and that by 1995 the number of individuals with HIV infections, but without a diagnosis of acquired immunodeficiency syndrome (AIDS), was expected to increase by 40% or more.[48] Based on current levels of HIV and CD4+ testing, the Centers of Disease Control and Prevention estimated that the expanded definition would produce increased numbers of case reports. HIV appears more frequently in socioeconomically disadvantaged patients.[49] Risk factors include

- Homosexuality
- Intravenous drug use
- Sex with an IV drug abuser
- Crack cocaine use
- Blood or blood product transfusion
- Sexually transmitted disease
- Multiple sexual partners
- Tattoo of body surfaces.[49–51]

In a series of 16,868 pregnant women, 7.2 in 1000 tested positive for HIV infection.[51] Screening only those women with risk factors for infection detects 57% of HIV-seropositive patients, but if screening is done for all parturients, regardless of the presence of risk factors, the detection rate rises to 87%.[52] Similar results were demonstrated in a Brazilian study (55.6% versus 84.6%),[51] and these findings support routine HIV testing in all pregnant women. The enzyme-linked immunoabsorbent assay (ELISA) and the Western blot test remain the mainstays for the initial diagnosis of AIDS infection. Measures of CD4+ T-lymphocytes are utilized to guide clinical and therapeutic management of HIV-infected individuals.[53] Unfortunately, universal obstetric screening may be not feasible. The cost alone is prohibitive in poorer countries.[54] It is more prudent to apply universal precautions by wearing gloves, using eye protection, and taking care when handling blood and body fluids.[55]

Impact of HIV on Pregnancy and the Fetus

The risk of maternal HIV transmission to the fetus ranges from 9.1%[56] to 73%.[57] To date, it appears that clinical indicators alone are not adequate to identify a subset of women who are at risk of transmitting HIV to their offspring.[58]

(Editors' note: A substantial percentage of perinatally acquired HIV-1 infections occurs near, or at, delivery, suggesting that obstetric factors influence viral transmission. A study showed that the risk of transmission of HIV-1 from mother to infant increases when fetal membranes are ruptured more than 4 hours before delivery. This study, however, did not explore the influence of labor analgesia as a risk factor.[58a])

Asymptomatic HIV-positive women with a CD4+ count below 500/mm[3] or with p24 antigenemia were 10 times more likely to transmit the virus to their offspring.[59] Knowledge of a low CD4+ lymphocyte count, early in pregnancy, may help women decide whether to continue the pregnancy.

Ninety percent of the children who are infected with HIV contract the virus from their mother in utero, during delivery, or post partum. Breast-feeding is believed to add a 26% risk of vertical infection over and above the risk of transmission at delivery or in utero.[60] Transplacental transmission is the main route,[61] and the rate of perinatal transmission is the same for both sexes.[62] Whether there is an increased risk for adverse perinatal outcomes such as preterm labor, low birth weight, and postpartum endometritis is still controversial.[63, 64] To define the HIV status of a child born from a HIV-positive mother, 12 months of follow-up are necessary.[57]

A craniofacial HIV embryopathy has been described,[65] but subsequent investigations have not confirmed it. Studies reveal a similar frequency of congenital abnormalities in the noninfected population and no consistent pattern of defects.[56, 57, 66] This pattern suggests that transmission of virus occurs late in pregnancy or at the time of delivery.[66] Precautions to reduce the risk of transmission include removal of all maternal blood- and fluid-contaminated items immediately after delivery, avoidance of percutaneous umbilical cord sampling, and delivery techniques such as vacuum and forceps.[67] HIV infection of the infant is reduced by zidovudine therapy to HIV-infected mothers. Preliminary results of a randomized, controlled trial suggest that the rate of HIV transmission is significantly lower when HIV-positive pregnant women are treated with zidovudine, compared with placebo (8.3% versus 25.5%).[68] An effective vaccine to interrupt maternal-fetal transmission of the HIV virus is still under investigation.[69, 70]

Mode of Delivery in HIV-Infected Parturients

Cesarean section, if performed once labor has begun, does not provide any protective effect against intrapartum transmission of HIV-1.[71] Isolation of human T-cell lymphotrophic virus III (HTLV-III)/lymphadenopathy-associated virus (LAV) from cervical secretions of women at risk has been described previously.[72] The cervical mucous plug has antimicrobial properties and presents a physical and chemical barrier against bacterial invasion.[73] Duration of rupture of membranes for 4 hours or more is also a factor of risk.[74] Studies that include operative delivery before the onset of labor are necessary to determine the effect of parturition and cesarean section on vertical transmission of HIV-1 to the fetus. The risk of infection in the first-born twin is 2.8-fold greater than that of the second-born,[75] perhaps as a result of a longer contact with the mother's blood.

Herpes Simplex Virus

Herpes simplex virus (HSV) infection occurs in approximately 1 in 7500 births in the US.[121] Seventy-eight to 97% of patients with HSV-2 antibodies have no historical, clinical, or virologic evidence for HSV-2 infection. They are identified as HSV-2 carriers on the basis of results of HSV-2 screening.[122] HSV-1 has been isolated from the genitourinary tract or anal canal in 3.5% of women with HSV-1 antibodies,[123] of whom 66% were symptomatic.

Among patients with primary infection, dysuria is the most common complaint, which is present in 80% of patients. On examination, 71% have vulvar ulceration, 66% have tender inguinal lymph nodes, and 46% have a cervical ulcer. In cases of recurrent genital infection, only two thirds have vulvar ulceration.[123] Serologic tests for HSV-2 are highly reliable for detecting recurrent genital infections, whereas culture appears to be the most effective diagnostic technique for primary infections.[124]

Women with asymptomatic or unrecognized HSV-2 infections are at risk for delivering babies who will develop neonatal herpes. Neonatal herpes infection is associated with significant morbidity and mortality, despite antiviral therapy.[122] The majority of fetal complications result from ascending infection after rupture of membranes or after passage of the neonate through an infected birth canal. Cesarean section is recommended if genital herpes lesions are present at the time of the delivery.[125]

Evidence exists for HSV-1 reactivation in patients after the use of epidural morphine[126] and sustained-release morphine followed by epidural fentanyl.[127] The mechanism is unclear and speculative. The investigators suggest that opioid activity within the spinal nucleus of the trigeminal nerve may be responsible.[126] These findings make some practitioners cautious about the use of epidural morphine in immunocompromised parturients (e.g., those infected with HIV).

Cytomegalovirus

Cytomegalovirus (CMV) seroprevalence ranges from 30 to 100%.[128] The virus is frequently recovered from the cervix and urine of pregnant women.[129] Its incidence in the lower female genital tract has been reported at between 4 and 12%.[130] Clinically overt manifestations of virus replication are seldom seen, except in the immunologically compromised individual. The target organs in an adult are the liver, kidney, hematopoietic system, and endocervix.

After primary infection, the rate of transmission to the fetus is about 40%. More than 90% of the approximately 40,000 infants with congenital CMV infection born in the US each year appear normal at birth, however.[131] Recurrence of infection during pregnancy is due mainly to reactivation,[132] with reinfection more likely in the offspring of low-income nonwhite women. A high proportion of congenital CMV infection is due to recent maternal infection and not to reactivation of infection.[131] Screening the saliva for CMV appears to be a reliable, sensitive method for detection.[133] The virus can also be recovered from amniotic fluid.[134] To date, without an effective vaccine or therapy for CMV infection, there is no universal screening method. Cesarean section is preferable in infected individuals because cervical contamination is usually responsible for neonatal infection.[129, 135]

Papillomavirus

Condyloma acuminatum, a papillomavirus-induced disease, is a frequently occurring sexually transmitted disease.[136] Pregnant women represent a special group for papillomavirus screening, which reflects an increased expression of the virus as a consequence of hormonal depression of the immune system.[137]

The incubation period can extend up to 8 months. Diagnosis requires the use of molecular biologic techniques that identify the viral genome in cellular material from the lower genital tract.[138] The disease begins as small, verrucous growths usually on the vulva or genital area, and dysplasia is associated in 72.7% of the cases.[139] A tendency is present for the lesions to become more prominent during pregnancy and coalesce to form cauliflower-like masses, which are occasionally so extensive as to cause mechanical obstruction of the birth canal. Massive vulvar lesions may expose the gravida to lacerations, sepsis, and significant bleeding during normal delivery. Cesarean section using spinal or general anesthesia may be the safest option in these cases.

A possible relationship between maternal condyloma acuminatum and laryngeal papillomatosis in the newborn is controversial[140, 141] and appears not to be related to the mode of delivery.[142] Therapy during pregnancy may affect mode of delivery, however, because a study of 96 pregnant women revealed that cesarean section was required in 80% of untreated women compared with 18% of treated women.[142]

Varicella-zoster Virus

Varicella-zoster virus (VZV), which is the causative organism for chickenpox, is highly contagious with secondary attack rates of 80 to 90% and seroprevalence rates greater than 90% in most regions of the world.[143] Approximately 7000 pregnancies annually are complicated by varicella infection,[144] whereas about 6000 pregnant women annually have herpes zoster infection.[145]

The average varicella incubation period is 14 days, occurring more frequently during late winter and early spring. Within a day after fever, a nonsynchronous maculopapular rash appears on the skin and mucosa. The lesions rapidly appear as pruritic superficial thin-walled vesicles, disposed in crops.

Although the incidence of VZV is no higher in pregnant than in nonpregnant women, chickenpox during pregnancy appears to be associated with increased morbidity and mortality. Whether pregnancy and associated hormones have an effect on VZV replication is not known. Pregnant women are more likely to develop hypoglycemia,[146] pneumonia, encephalitis, hepatitis, pancreatitis, and nephritis after chickenpox infection. Most cases of varicella pneumonia in pregnancy occur in the third trimester, within a few days of the eruption of cutaneous lesions. In one report of 17 cases of varicella pneumonia during pregnancy, the mortality rate was 41%, compared with 17% in nonpregnant varicella pneumonia.[147] In-utero infection can be manifested as the congenital varicella syndrome, postnatal herpes zoster without a history of chickenpox in an infant, or positive immunity without clinical signs in the fetus or newborn.[148] Maternal viremia leads to transplacental infection in 25% of fetuses. The literature suggests that varicella syndrome can occur during the first half of pregnancy with an incidence of 2%.[149] It is the usual practice to give varicella-zoster immune globulin to VZV-seronegative pregnant patients and to consider those with a chickenpox history or positive VZV serology test result to be immune.[150] Low response of specific immunity or amnestic serologic responses after infection[150, 151] together with an immature or incomplete cellular immunity, however, are related to the failure to maintain virus latency, and repeated attacks can occur.

Measles

Between January 1988 and December 1991, approximately 50,000 cases of measles were reported in the general population in the US.[152] Nearly half of the cases were in previously vaccinated persons. Latinos accounted for 62% of the cases.

The clinical picture of measles includes generalized rash, which occurs simultaneously with the onset of the effector phase of the antiviral immune response,[153] cough, coryza, conjunctivitis, and temperature greater than 101° F for 3 or more days. Antibody status may be determined by ELISA[154]; however, the technical ease in performing syncytium inhibition assay will allow its widespread use.[155] A retrospective study of 58 women with measles during pregnancy revealed that they were nearly twice as likely to be admitted to a hospital, nearly three times as likely to be diagnosed with pneumonia, and more than six times as likely to die from measles complications.[156] This increase in morbidity and mortality is a result of the immune suppression from measles[157] and pregnancy. Thirty-one percent of pregnancies ended in spontaneous abortion (5 cases) or preterm delivery (13 cases). The preterm deliveries included two fetal deaths and three neonatal deaths. Fifty percent of pregnancies ended within 14 days of the onset of measles rash. No newborns were diagnosed with congenital measles.[156] A case of fetal death at 25 weeks' gestation revealed measles virus infection in the placenta. Neither inflammatory change nor measles virus antigen was found in any organ of the fetus.[158]

The prevention of measles in pregnancy will occur with more efficient vaccination coverage.[159] Susceptible pregnant women exposed to measles should receive immunoglobulin within 6 days of exposure, as should their newborn infants. Vaccination of measles-immune individuals is not harmful.[156]

Influenza Virus

Influenza is a major cause of respiratory disease in adults.[160] A characteristic feature is its striking contagiousness. Pregnancy alters maternal respiratory physiology, producing dyspnea and mucosal capillary engorgement that can mimic symptoms of upper respiratory tract infection and laryngitis. These changes may be exacerbated by a mild respiratory tract infection from influenza virus. This infection may not be innocuous in that there is a strong epidemiologic association between influenza A virus epidemics and meningococcal outbreaks.[161]

Regular and prior immunization is recommended to ensure protection against influenza illness.[162] Nowadays, live attenuated intranasal influenza vaccines offer the prospect of inducing broader and more durable immunity than that provided by current inactivated vaccines.[162] The live intranasal vaccines probably increase the appeal for a routine immunization strategy. Cold-adapted and inactivated vaccines are also safe and effective for preventing influenza A disease.[163]

Parvovirus B19

Human parvovirus B19 (fifth disease) was identified in 1975[164] and has been associated with hydrops fetalis since 1984.[165] Approximately 35 to 50% of the general population is susceptible to the virus, whereas 20% becomes infected after exposure.[166] The risk of fetal death ranges from 1 to 15%.[167] Diagnosis is confirmed by counterimmunoelectrophoresis or radioimmunoassay for immunoglobulin M to parvovirus B19 in the maternal serum, direct vision of blood viral particles through electron microscopy, or deoxyribonucleic acid

(DNA) test findings. Maternal symptoms include a flu-like illness; maculopapular rash; and symmetric polyarthralgia involving feet, hands, and knees that resolve spontaneously and are not correlated consistently with the presence or severity of fetal infection.[168] The infection may have no effect on the fetus or may result in aplastic anemia, nonimmunologic hydrops, and increased perinatal mortality. Ultrasonographic signs of fetal infection include ascites, effusion, skin edema, polyhydramnios, cardiomegaly, placentomegaly, and decreased fetal movement.[169] Maternal serum α-fetoprotein elevation may be the result of hepatic or placental damage and predicts poor fetal outcome.[170] Treatments have included in-utero fetal transfusion,[171] digitalization,[172] and serial thoracoabdominocenteses,[173] or a conservative approach.[168] A few cases in the literature have suggested that minimal fetal manifestations of infection usually resolve spontaneously within 5 weeks of diagnosis.[168]

Rubella

Rubella is a self-limiting low-risk maternal viral infection[174] with the potential to cause the serious fetal congenital rubella syndrome (CRS). Efforts are still necessary to achieve the goal to eradicate rubella and CRS in the US.[175]

The disease is unlikely to be acquired as a result of casual or brief contact. Seronegative patients are at greater risk of acquiring infection when they have been exposed more closely over a long period. Maternal postauricular adenopathy may be detectable a week before the development of a characteristic maculopapular rash and may persist for 1 to 2 weeks after disappearance of the rash. A high incidence of arthritis among young women has also been described.[176]

The risk of congenital rubella infection in seropositive pregnant women appears to be relatively low. The intrauterine infection rates were 10%, 11.8%, 2.9%, and 6.5% after maternal infection at 1 to 10, 11 to 14, 15 to 19, and 20 to 29 gestational weeks, respectively. Six among 95 fetuses from rubella-infected mothers had serologic evidence of congenital infections. Among the six fetuses, one had CRS, two were terminated during the second trimester, two were normal, and one was lost to follow-up. No evidence of rubella defects was found in the other 81 children during a 2- to 4-year follow-up period.[174]

Hantavirus Pulmonary Syndrome

A North American hantavirus was first identified in 1993 as a causative agent of a novel syndrome of acute pulmonary edema and shock, with more than 50% mortality due to respiratory failure and shock. The disease starts with a febrile prodrome accompanied by myalgia, dyspnea, and hypoxia, which may quickly progress to adult respiratory distress syndrome. The pathogenesis is related to the presence of virus antigens in the pulmonary capillaries. Proteinuria, mild elevations of creatinine levels, leukocytosis, and thrombocytopenia may be present.[177]

Puumala Virus

This epidemic virus has been known since 1983 and has been detected in Scandinavia, Russia, Germany, and France. The disease is manifested as high fever, myalgia, posterior and frontal headaches, photophobia, and vomiting, and a mild form of hemorrhagic fever with renal syndrome, known as nephropathia epidemica, which can deteriorate to acute renal failure. Treatment is supportive and may include dialysis.[178]

REGIONAL ANESTHESIA AND SYSTEMIC INFECTION

The incidence of meningitis after lumbar puncture appears to be similar to the incidence of spontaneous meningitis in bacteremic patients,[179, 180] although it is controversial.[181] The incidence of epidural abscess after lumbar epidural catheterization in obstetric patients is estimated to be 1 in 505,000,[182] as opposed to the rate of spontaneous epidural abscess formation in the general hospital population, which is estimated to be 0.2 to 1.2 per 10,000.[183] Because most cases of meningitis and abscess occur spontaneously, clinicians cannot be certain of differentiating spontaneous from lumbar puncture–induced complications.[179] Epidural abscess can also develop spontaneously in the postpartum period after general anesthesia.[184] Of interest, a disproportionate number of epidural abscesses follow thoracic epidural block, probably because of more difficult technique.[20] Patients receiving systemic or epidural steroids are at increased risk.[21] Epidural abscess may have a highly variable presentation, which can make diagnosis difficult. Early diagnosis should be considered in any patient who demonstrates signs of infection, significant back pain, post-spinal headache, radicular pain, weakness, paralysis, or bladder dysfunction.[21, 22]

It is not known how bacteria or viruses cross from the blood stream into the spinal fluid. Opioid analgesia,[120, 121] integrity of the immunologic system, blood-circulating bacterial and viral count, and virulence and survival in blood stream and spinal fluid are important factors in the development of meningitis. In rats, dural puncture is associated with the development of meningitis, provided that the animals are bacteremic at the time of the puncture. Antibiotic treatment before the puncture appears to eliminate this risk.[188] Antibiotic therapy was also protective in eight bacteremic obstetric patients (seven had placental pathology consistent with chorioamnionitis) submitted to regional anesthetic technique, and none of the patients had infectious complications such as epidural abscess or meningitis.[189] Nevertheless, there are published cases of meningitis and epidural abscess after spinal anesthesia, despite preoperative administration of antibiotics.[190, 191]

In the absence of guidelines, the anesthesiologist must consider the risk for regional versus general anesthesia individually, because no risk is acceptable unless there is a clear benefit. As stated earlier, the use of an epidural catheter appears to be relatively safe in parturients with localized infections, such as chorioamnionitis.[20, 189, 192] For patients with evidence of systemic infection, general anesthesia is recommended in emergency situations, if antibiotic therapy has not been started. Provided that intravascular volume has been replaced, antibiotic therapy has begun, and the patient has shown a positive response to therapy, regional anesthesia may be appropriate. Subarachnoid anesthesia should probably be avoided in patients during the acute (viremic) phase of a viral infection.

TROPICAL DISEASES

Tropical infectious diseases involve a diverse spectrum of infective agents that cause various symptoms as a result of targeting different organ systems. As a consequence of the diversified clinical picture, there is no strict rule to be dictated for anesthesia. Anesthesiologists need to be familiar with these infections to manage them. Choice of anesthetic depends on maternal and fetal status. Dural puncture is best avoided during an acute infection. Regional anesthesia is contraindicated in patients with coagulation disorders, which are common in some tropical diseases.

Dengue Virus

Dengue fever is a tropical mosquito-transmitted disease caused by infection with the dengue virus 1, 2, 3, or 4, but mainly type 1. The disease is endemic over a large part of Southeast Asia, South Pacific, Brazil, Africa, and Central America.[193, 194] One case has been reported in Italy.[195] The number of female mosquito *Aedes aegypti* per person appears to be a significant household risk factor.[196]

An epidemiologic investigation of a dengue outbreak that produced an 80% attack rate showed no change in rates of miscarriages, fetal deaths, or birth defects compared with a nonepidemic period.[197] Five confirmed cases of congenital dengue-3 infection have been reported, probably after placental infection following maternal exposure. This infection resulted in dengue hemorrhagic fever–dengue shock syndrome (DHF-DSS) in the neonatal period.[198] Live attenuated dengue vaccines are under investigation.[199] Clinical manifestations, laboratory signs, and treatment are described in Table 24–5. Life-threatening clinical conditions require effective utilization of blood bank technology and preventive measures during delivery to minimize blood loss.

TABLE 24–5. DENGUE DISEASE

	Clinical Manifestations	Hematology	Treatment
Dengue Fever (self-limited viruses)	(a) 4–5 day incubation period; sudden fever (103–105.8°F); intense headache, generalized muscular pain, periorbicular and joint pain, lymphadenopathy and anorexia (5–7 days) (b) In two thirds of cases, a maculopapular rash may appear on the third day, with petechiae in the axilla and on hands or feet. There is a pulse/temperature dissociation (i.e., high fever and low pulse rate). Depression and fatigue generally persist after resolution of acute symptoms[200]	Leucopenia, relative lymphocytosis and mild thrombocytopenia	Symptomatic treatment; avoid nonsteroidal anti-inflammatory drugs, which may impair coagulation
Dengue Hemorrhagic Fever–Dengue Shock Syndrome (DHF-DSS)	Most cases occur during a second DV infection; severity varies from insignificant to life-threatening bleeding with death within 12–24 hours, in the absence of adequate symptomatic treatment.[200, 201] Depression and fatigue generally persist after resolution of acute symptoms.[200] Antibody-dependent enhancement of DV growth in mononuclear phagocytes is thought to be the mechanism whereby pre-existing dengue antibodies confer excess risk for DHF-DSS.[202] Interleukin-1[233] and plasminogen crossreactive antibodies[204] may play an important role in the etiology of DHF-DSS	Leucopenia, lymphocytosis, and thrombocytopenia	As above; there is no way to prevent hemorrhagic sequelae

Yellow Fever Virus

Yellow fever (YF) was first recorded in Barbados in 1647. It is transmitted from person to person by infected mosquitos of *Aedes* and *Haemagogus* species and others,[205] and the fatality-to-case rate can be as high as 57%.[206] Clinical findings, laboratory findings, and treatments are described in Table 24–6. Diagnostic serology testing involves capture ELISA or neutralizing antibodies.

The increased number of women in military services who are routinely given YF immunization, the increased volume of international travelers, and the renewed interest in mass immunization have led to a growing number of women receiving YF vaccine during pregnancy in nonendemic areas.[207] The offspring appear to be particularly susceptible to neurologic infection. The high risk of natural infection plus maternal death during YF epidemics, however, outweighs the theoretical contraindications to vaccination.[208] In endemic countries, the best solution is replacing mass-emergency vaccination with routine vaccination. Maternal active immunity lasts at least 10 years, and newborn passive immunity lasts about 6 months.[209]

Leptospiroses

The pathogenic spirochetes are classified into various serogroups and serotypes like *fortbragg, hardjo, interrogans (icterohaemorrhagiae), autumnalis, bataviae, canicola, pomona, grippotyphosa, javanica, mankarso, djasmani, cynopteri,* and others. They infect a wide variety of domestic and wild animals. Each serotype tends to be associated with a particular vertebrate that acts as their natural reservoir. Infection is acquired through mucosal or skin contact with a contaminated environment such as urine or feces.[210] The infection has a seasonal prevalence for warm, wet weather. For the last 25 years, the number of leptospirosis infections has steadily increased among teenagers and people 20 to 30 years old. Patients are mainly sanitation workers,[211] farmers, butchers, coal miners, people involved in water sports, and hospital laboratory workers.[212] The clinical manifestations and treatment are described in Table 24–7. The diagnosis can be established by serologic investigation and by isolation of the pathogen.

Plasmodium Malaria

Malaria is a tropical blood parasitemia transmitted by the mosquito *Anopheles* species infected with *Plasmodium* species (*vivax, falciparum, malariae,* or *ovale*). The disease is more common in the rainy season and near infested water sources. Infectivity can be measured by the numbers of parasites in peripheral blood, through conventional Giemsa-stained blood smear. The sequestration of erythrocytes containing mature forms of *P. falciparum* in the microvasculature of vital organs, however, may cause large discrepancies between the peripheral blood parasite count and the total body parasite burden.[214] Clinical manifestations and treatment are described in Table 24–8. The malaria antigen ELISA is highly specific and sensitive for *P. falciparum* infections.[215]

Pregnancy is associated with increased susceptibility to *P. falciparum* malaria, especially in the primigravida.[216] In a series of 1358 pregnant women, 37.2% developed malaria, and the incidence of malaria declined from week 20 of gestation (12%) toward term (4.4%).[217] This decline may be due to low ring-surface antigen antibody levels[216] or changes in hormonal level.[218] Maternal death has been reported, but severe malaria during pregnancy is now rare. In Africa, the main adverse effect is low birth weight.[217] The placenta appears to be a site of preferential parasite sequestration and development. Indeed, the placenta may be black from depo-

TABLE 24–6. YELLOW FEVER (YF) VIRUS INFECTION

Clinical Findings	(a) First stage—after 3- to 6-day incubation period → fever, rigors, headache, backache, myalgia, and prostration, which improves in 2–3 days (b) After 1 day of apparent cure, a flushed face, swollen lips, bright red tongue, nausea, bradycardia, vomiting, tendency to bleed (black vomit, melena, bleeding gums, ecchymoses); may result in hepatorenal failure and death. The disease can progress from prodrome to death in 7–10 days.[209]
Laboratory Findings	First stage—lymphocytosis Albuminuria, oliguria, anuria, electrolytic imbalance, thrombocytopenia (signs of hepatic and renal failure)
Treatment	Symptomatic, best in a hospital setting (antiemetics, acetaminophen, avoid nonsteroidal anti-inflammatories that can impair coagulation). Serum electrolytes and acid-base balance should be estimated daily. A few cases may require hemodialysis, cardiotonic drugs, or monitoring of respiratory function.[209]

TABLE 24–7. LEPTOSPIROSES

Clinical Findings	Vary greatly following 1- to 2-week incubation period. After penetrating the skin or mucosa the leptospiretes invade the bloodstream and spread throughout the body causing hepatomegaly, meningitis, pancreatitis, diarrhea, hemorrhage, and hypotension. Clinically, varies from influenza-like illness to a severe fatal form of hepatorenal failure. Abdominal pain and vomiting (71.4%) are major presenting symptoms in the severe form.
Treatment	IV penicillin made a dramatic improvement in 21 of 24 patients in 24–72 hours, with no deaths.[213]

TABLE 24–8. MALARIA

Clinical Manifestations	(a) 85–90% of parasitemic episodes are asymptomatic. An estimated 3 to 4 48-hour cycles of schizogony may occur without eliciting either fever or macrophage activation. Fever develops, followed a day later by a spike in urinary neopterin, a product of monocytes/macrophages[220]
	(b) If symptomatic: recurrent episodes of fever and shivering are related to the cycles of intraerythrocytic schizogony; vomiting, anemia; splenomegaly. Headache, convulsions and mental slowness in cerebral malaria, icterus or acute renal failure may occur.[221, 222] Hemoglobin <8 g/dl is associated with intrauterine growth retardation in primigravidae.[223] The mother may develop pulmonary edema and hypoglycemia[224] in the third trimester. Hypoglycemia is possibly due to inhibition of gluconeogenesis caused by failure of hepatic lactate uptake.[225] There is a 50% reduction in serum vitamin A, due in part to impaired hepatic function[226]
Treatment	Traditional 7-day course of quinine therapy is associated with a 50% failure rate in pregnant women.[227] Serial thick-film parasite counts are a reliable method for identifying patients at risk of recrudescence.[228] Pregnant patients may require multidrug therapy[227] or larger dose of mefloquine, to achieve comparable blood levels, due to increased volume of distribution.[229] The combination of pyrimethamine/chloroquine appears to be highly effective.[230] Chemoprophylaxis[231] and avoidance of exposure are the only measures likely to protect both mother and baby[217]

sition of malarial pigment, even when the mother is asymptomatic.[219]

Theoretical concern exists about infection of the cerebrospinal fluid by infected erythrocytes during a dural puncture. Hypotension may exacerbate hepatic dysfunction, and excessive preanesthetic hydration may accentuate maternal anemia.

Mycobacterium Tuberculosis

Worldwide, tuberculosis (TB) remains the leading cause of death from a single infectious disease. Cases of active TB are increasing among pregnant women in epidemic communities and are also associated with HIV infections. Pregnancy itself does not contribute to the acquisition of TB[232] or its activation in HIV-infected women, however.[233] Incidence rates vary from 103 to 104 per 100,000 among black women.[233] Clinical manifestations and treatment are described in Table 24–9. Detection of *Mycobacterium tuberculosis* by culture re-

quires 6 to 8 weeks.[234] Diagnostic procedures include polymerase chain reaction assays (excellent specificity and sensitivity for bacilli detection) and direct identification of the pathogen from clinical specimens.[235]

Maternal clinical condition and effect of the treatment dictate the best anesthetic technique and anesthetic drugs. Adverse effects of rifampicin include renal failure, anemia, leukopenia, and thrombocytopenia. The major toxicities of isoniazid are on the peripheral nervous system, liver, and kidneys. Hepatitis seems more common in rapid acetylators, owing to a greater production of hydrazine, the potentially hepatotoxic isoniazid metabolite, which can also increase volatile anesthetic defluorination.[236]

Schistosomiasis

This parasitic disease is caused mainly by *Schistosoma mansoni, S. haematobium,*[239] or *S. japonicum.*[240] The infection occurs during immersion in infected river or lake water, where the larvae actively penetrate the skin and migrate predominantly to the bowel veins. Characteristic pruritus appears after larval penetration. The vermae grow and liberate numerous eggs that are evacuated through the bowel (or from the urine, if *S. haematobium*[241]). Contaminated feces can then restart the cycle, which involves snails[242] or cabbage mollusks as the definitive host. Clinical manifestations and treatment are described in Table 24–10. The disease affects mainly children or childbearing women who cook, wash clothes, or work near contaminated lakes or rivers. It is popularly known as *water belly* in Brazil and can appear as pseudopregnancy because of the ascites.

Pregnant women from endemic regions may have chronic or acute forms of the disease. Preoperative laboratory evaluation includes measurement of hepatic enzymes, coagulation parameters, albumin levels, hemoglobin, and renal function.[243] Hepatic ultrasonography permits a dynamic study of schistosomiasis morbidity with some precision.[244] A purified fraction of *S.*

TABLE 24–9. TUBERCULOSIS (TB)

Clinical Manifestations	The highest rate of TB in pregnant women was reported by Margono and coworkers. Clinical manifestations included 10 cases of pulmonary and 6 cases of extrapulmonary tuberculosis (2 meningeal, 1 mediastinal, 1 renal, 1 gastrointestinal, and 1 pleural)[233]
Treatment	13% of new cases are resistant to at least one antituberculous drug and 3.2% to both isoniazid and rifampicin. Multidrug-resistant TB is highly common in prisons.[237] New recommendations on TB therapy will likely include isoniazid, rifampicin, pyrazinamide, and ethambutol or streptomycin for initial therapy[238]

TABLE 24–10. **SCHISTOSOMIASIS**

Clinical Manifestations	Katayama fever (20–60 days after contamination, fever, diarrhea, coughing, abdominal pain, sudoresis, anorexia); periportal thickening, liver parenchymal lesions, melena, compensated or decompensated hepatosplenic syndrome, associated with grade II or III fibrosis and esophageal varices, hemorrhage,[244] nephropathy, and anemia. Rare associations include ischemic necrotizing colitis[247] and carcinoma of liver.[240] Eosinophilia is a major finding in parasitic infections[247]
Treatment	Oral praziquantel (a second dose 9 days later is required to kill all eggs[248]). Retaining a small number of *S. mansoni* may be advantageous to people in endemic areas, to constantly prime the immune response

mansoni eggs by ELISA may be of use in monitoring the effectiveness of control programs.[245] Antischistosomal vaccines are under investigation.[246]

Bubonic and Pneumonic Pestis

This infection occurs mostly after the bite of an infected flea. The disease is rapidly progressive and is characterized by bacteremia, high fever, delirium, and coma with a mortality rate as high as 90% if not treated. The bubonic form is caused by *Yersinia pestis* and can progress to septicemia; it may involve all organs. The pneumonic form is transmitted by *Pneumonia pestis* and is easily spread through aspiration of aerosol particles.

Pestivirus

This disease is produced by a primary viral infection early in gestation, usually a mild illness. The pestivirus, a zoonoses border disease virus, and bovine viral diarrhea virus cause a variety of congenital defects in sheep and cattle, including cerebellar hypoplasia, microcephaly, and myelin dysgenesis. Viral infection during pregnancy can result in abortion or the birth of an infected offspring. The newborn can have teratogenic defects and excretes virus in urine, amniotic fluid, white-blood cells, saliva, and feces.[249] The patient is treated symptomatically.

Vibrio cholerae

Epidemic and pandemic cholerae have been associated with the O1 and non-O1 serogroup of *Vibrio cholerae*.[250, 251] Cholera-like illness has a low morbidity and is associated with eating unwashed fruits and vegetables or drinking nonpasteurized milk and untreated water.[252] After an incubation period of a few hours to 3 days, there is a severe acute diarrheal syndrome, with vomiting and dehydration equivalent to a loss of 1 liter per hour. These organisms are oddly sensitive to acid gastric fluid. Interestingly, consumption of a drink made from the citrus fruit toronja was protective against illness in Peru. Acid fruits such as toronja (pH 4.1) inhibit *Vibrio* growth and may make contaminated water safer.[253]

The reservoirs are not known. Natural aquatic plants, environment, and phytoplankton may serve as effective reservoirs.[254] The virulence of *V. cholerae* strains is, in general, ascribed to enterotoxin production. Transmission normally occurs via infected human excreta and may be seasonal. After ingestion and passage through the human gut, the composition of the outer membrane protein of *V. cholerae* can be altered from environmental adaptation.[252]

Prompt diagnosis is important for quick medical intervention. The Cholera Screen is a highly specific monoclonal antibody-based coagglutination test, with the availability of results in less than 5 minutes.[255, 256] The infectious agents are sensitive to ampicillin, chloramphenicol, gentamicin, kanamycin, tetracycline, sulfamethoxazole, streptomycin, and other antibiotics.[252] Newer generations of cholera vaccine have been characterized in laboratories.[257]

Preoperative care involves intense rehydration and correction of electrolyte disturbances and poor nutritional status. The pregnant patient should be hospitalized during the acute phase. Anesthetic considerations in the acute phase are related to the management of clinical shock. General anesthesia following induction with IV ketamine, benzodiazepines, and succinylcholine and maintenance with halothane was used successfully for gynecologic surgery during a cholera epidemic.[258]

Chagas Disease

Transmission of *Trypanosoma cruzi* to humans is via the bite from an infected reduviid bug. Acute Chagas disease is usually a mild illness (lymphadenopathy and unilateral periorbital edema, known as *Romaña* sign). When the acute illness resolves, the patient enters the indeterminate phase, where life-long parasitemia may follow, and 10 to 30% of infected persons develop chronic Chagas disease years later. Characteristically, chronic disease presents as impairment of the cardiac conducting system (mainly left anterior hemiblock or anterior fascicular block), megacolon, and/or megaesophagus. Clinical manifestations include constipation, gastroesophageal reflux, and dysphagia. Serologic tests include Chagas immunoglobulin G ELISA, complement fixation, and indirect immunofluorescence.

Congenital disease occurs in 2 to 10% of infants born to infected mothers[259, 260] and may result in spontaneous abortion, fetal hydrops, stillbirth, and premature birth. Diagnosis is suggested by histologic evidence of placental villitis. No satisfactory drug treatments are available, nor is the means to prevent transmission of the parasite to the offspring. Patients who develop chronic Chagas disease tolerate regional or general anesthetic techniques well. Patients with the chronic form of Chagas disease also appear to complain of less pain postoperatively than healthy patients.

Psittacosis

Psittacosis is a pulmonary and systemic disease contracted from inhalation of dried psittacine bird or sheep excreta or handling of contaminated plumage. After replication in mononuclear phagocytes of the liver and spleen, the *Chlamydia psittaci* parasite spreads hematogenously to the lungs and other organs. The incubation period varies from 1 to 2 weeks. Infection typically causes a mild influenza-like illness. The infection may be associated with myocarditis, encephalitis, seizures, and focal neurologic lesions. Disseminated intravascular coagulation may occur in advanced cases. During pregnancy, patients with psittacosis may present with severe headache, atypical pneumonia (mainly in dependent lobes), hypoxemia, thrombocytopenia, anemia, hepatic dysfunction, and disseminated intravascular coagulation, culminating in death.[261] Chest radiographs usually show patchy reticular infiltrates radiating out from the hilar area or involving the basilar lung segments. Massive placental infection with impaired perfusion may ensue. Tetracyclines have been given after failure of erythromycin treatment. With persistent disease, early delivery of the fetus may provide good maternal and fetal outcomes.[262]

Typhoid Fever

Typhoid is predominantly a gastrointestinal gram-negative bacterial disease caused by *Salmonella typhi* and *S. paratyphi*. Ingestion of contaminated food is followed in 6 to 48 hours by abdominal cramps, sustained bacteremia, high fever, vomiting, and diarrhea. Associated dysfunction of multiple organs may be present, such as renal failure, hepatitis, meningitis, diffuse cerebral edema, brain abscess, and epidural abscess.[263, 264] Either a 14-day course of chloramphenicol or a 3-day course of ceftriaxone is effective,[265] in addition to supportive treatment. The possibility of developing meningitis or epidural and cerebral abscesses during the acute phase of the disease limits the use of epidural and spinal anesthesia.

Toxoplasmosis

Toxoplasma gondii is a cosmopolitan protozoan parasite of importance as a primary infection during pregnancy because of the risk of transmission to the newborn.[266] Immunocompromised women (e.g., HIV-positive mothers) are at increased risk. Lymphadenopathy, fever, and prostration are present in most cases, and less common signs include myalgia, hepatitis, maculopapular lesions, and pharyngitis.

Leishmaniasis

Leishmania panamensis, L. mexicana,[267] *L. tropica,* and *L. braziliensis* are the etiologic agents for mucocutaneous leishmaniasis. The *mucocutaneous form* is usually self-limiting. Destructive lesions of nasal, pharyngeal, and laryngeal mucosa can occur in the advanced stages of the disease and may lead to distortion of the face and difficult tracheal intubation (Fig. 24–2).

The *L. infantum*[268] and *L. donovani* varieties produce the *visceral form,* kala-azar.[269] Persistent transmission to humans is thought to require the presence of the sandfly vector. The incubation period varies from 9 days to 9 years. Kala-azar is characterized by insidious fever, shivering, anorexia, nausea and vomiting, hepatosplenomegaly, cutaneous lesions, anemia, and leukopenia. Most anti-leishmanial drugs in use are renal- and cardiac-toxic.[268, 269]

Q Fever

Coxiella burnetii during pregnancy may manifest clinically as flu-like symptoms or pneumonia (similar to *Mycoplasma pneumoniae* pneumonia). Organisms are airborne from infected feces, not by injection from tick bites. No rash occurs, but abnormal liver function and endocarditis can develop. The role of this rickettsial

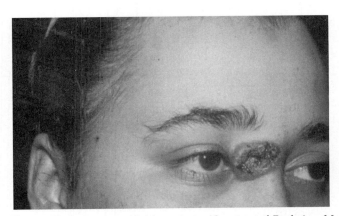

Figure 24–2. Cutaneous leishmaniasis. (Courtesy of Prof. Ana M. F. Roselino, Faculty of Medicine, Ribeirão Preto, University of São Paulo, São Paulo, Brazil.)

disease in pregnancy is controversial. Fetal death has been reported at 24 weeks of gestation in association with chronic maternal infection. The obstetrician in this case presented with pneumonia shortly after a dilatation and curettage procedure, possibly as a result of aerosolization of organisms from the infected placenta. The mother was treated with cotrimoxazole and the obstetrician with doxycycline.[270]

Viral Hemorrhagic Fever

Four viruses cause viral hemorrhagic fever (VHF): Ebola, Lassa, Marburg, and Congo-Crimean hemorrhagic fever viruses. Although the mode for nosocomial transmission differs for each of them, limited data do not permit clear distinctions.[271] The mortality rate of the Ebola VHF is 79%. Frequent symptoms include fever (94%), diarrhea (80%), and severe weakness (74%). Other symptoms include dysphagia (41%) and hiccough (15%).[272] The incubation period ranges from 2 days to 8 weeks, depending on the etiology. The risk for person-to-person transmission of VHF is highest during the latter stages of illness, which are characterized by vomiting, diarrhea, shock, and often hemorrhage. Risk factors include travel to specific locations where VHF has recently occurred and direct contact with body fluids or contaminated equipment. The virus can be detected by ELISA. Care must be taken in the handling of infected people and body fluids, as recommended by the Centers for Disease Control and Prevention.[271]

SUMMARY

Infections in the parturient can range from the mundane (head cold) to the exotic (Q fever). They can have minimal impact on the mother, fetus, and their attendants, or severe effects. Knowledge of route of transmission, incubation period, and clinical sequelae is important to the anesthesiologist. Certain infective agents cause CNS disease, which can confound both anesthetic management issues and diagnosis of postanesthetic neurologic complications. This chapter highlights the problems facing the anesthesiologist caring for the parturient who is HIV positive and provides the reader with useful information about uncommon infections in pregnancy.

References

1. Topalovski M, Yang SS, Boonpasat Y. Listeriosis of the placenta: Clinicopathologic study of seven cases. Am J Obstet Gynecol 1993;169:616.
2. Gibbs RS. Chorioamnionitis and bacterial vaginosis. Am J Obstet Gynecol 1993;169:460.
3. McGregor JA, French JI, Jones W, et al. Bacterial vaginosis is associated with prematurity and vaginal fluid mucinase and sialidase: Results of a controlled trial of topical clindamycin cream. Am J Obstet Gynecol 1994;170:1048.
4. Morgan P. Maternal death following epidural anaesthesia for Caesarean section delivery in a patient with unsuspected sepsis. Can J Anaesth 1995;42:330.
5. Rouse DJ, Goldenberg RL, Cliver SP, et al. Strategies for the prevention of early-onset neonatal group B streptococcal sepsis: A decision analysis. Obstet Gynecol 1994;83:483.
6. Mercer BM, Arheart KA. Antimicrobial therapy in expectant management of preterm premature rupture of membranes. Lancet 1995;346:1271.
7. Weir S, Feldblum PJ, Roddy RE. The use of nonoxynol-9 for protection against cervical gonorrhea. Am J Public Health 1994;84:910.
8. Thompson ME, Shaughnessy AF. Oral cephalosporins: Newer agents and their place in therapy. Am Fam Physician 1994;50:401.
9. Livengood CH III, McGregor JA, Soper DE, et al. Bacterial vaginosis: Efficacy and safety of intravaginal metronidazole treatment. Am J Obstet Gynecol 1994;170:759.
10. Mazor M, Chaim W, Bar-David J, et al. Prenatal diagnosis of microbial invasion of the amniotic cavity with Campylobacter coli in preterm labour. Br J Obstet Gynaecol 1995;102:71.
11. Livengood CH III, Thomason JL, Hill GB. Bacterial vaginosis: Diagnosis and pathogenic findings during topical clindamycin therapy. Am J Obstet Gynecol 1990;163:515.
12. Hillier SL. Diagnostic microbiology of bacterial vaginosis. Am J Obstet Gynecol 1993;169;455.
13. Muralidhar B, Rumore PM, Steinman CR. Use of the polymerase chain reaction to study arthritis due to Neisseria gonorrhoeae. Arthritis Rheum 1994;37:710.
14. Ducloy AS, Buy E, Ducloy JC, et al. Prediction of maternal infection before performing epidural analgesia of labor. Anesthesiology 1993;100:A194.
15. Blanco JD, Gibbs RS, Castaneda YS. Bacteremia in obstetrics: Clinical course. Obstet Gynecol 1981;58:21.
16. Ledger WJ. Bacterial infections complicating pregnancy. Clin Obstet Gynecol 1978;21:455.
17. Johnson RT. Infections during pregnancy. In Devinsky O, Feldmann E, Hainline B (eds). Neurological Complications of Pregnancy. New York, Raven Press, 1994, p 153.
18. Lee W, Clark SL, Cotton DB, et al. Septic shock during pregnancy. Am J Obstet Gynecol 1988;159:410.
19. Malhotra M, Gupto HL, Mondal A. Pulmonary complications of septicaemia in women. J Indian Med Assoc 1990;88:131.
20. Jakobsen KB, Christensen M-K, Carlsson PS. Extradural anaesthesia for repeated surgical treatment in the presence of infection. Br J Anaesth 1995;75:536.
21. Ngan Kee WD, Jones MR, Thomas P, Worth RJ. Extradural abscess complicating extradural anaesthesia for Caesarean section. Br J Anaesth 1992;69:647.
22. Lee JJ, Perry H. Bacterial meningitis following spinal anaesthesia for Caesarean section. Br J Anaesth 1991;66:383.
23. Harding SA, Collier RE, Morgan BM. Meningitis after combined spinal-extradural anaesthesia in obstetrics. Br J Anaesth 1994;73:545.
24. Carson D, Wildsmith JAW. The risk of extradural abscess. Br J Anaesth 1995;75:520.
25. Davies JM, Thistlewood JM, Rolbin SH, Douglas MJ. Infections and the parturient: Anaesthetic considerations. Can J Anaesth 1988;35:270
26. American College of Chest Physicians/Society of Critical Care Medicine Consensus Conference: Definitions for sepsis and organ failure and guidelines for the use of innovative therapies in sepsis. Crit Care Med 1992;20:864.
27. Braun TI, Pinover W, Sih P. Group B streptococcal meningitis in a pregnant woman before the onset of labor. Clin Infect Dis 1995;21:1042.
28. Greenberg LR, Moore TR. Staphylococcal septicemia and adult respiratory distress syndrome in pregnancy treated with extracorporeal carbon dioxide removal. Obstet Gynecol 1995;86:657.
29. Soper DE. Bacterial vaginosis and postoperative infections. Am J Obst Gynecol 1993;169:467.
30. Augenbraun MH, McCornmack WM. Sexually transmitted dis-

eases in HIV infected persons. Infect Dis Clin North Am 1994;8:439.

31. Smith LG, Summers PR, Miles RW, et al. Gonococcal chorioamnionitis associated with sepsis. Am J Obstet Gynecol 1989;160:153.

32. Holmes KK, Counts CW, Beaty HN. Disseminated gonococcal infection. Ann Intern Med 1971;74:979.

33. Rice PA, Mcquillen DP, Gulati S, et al. Serum resistance of Neisseria gonorrhoeae. Does it thwart the inflammatory response and facilitate the transmission of infection? Ann N Y Acad Sci 1994;730:7.

34. Witkin SS, Ledger WJ. Antibodies to Chlamydia trachomatis in sera of women with recurrent spontaneous abortions. Am J Obstet Gynecol 1992;167:135.

35. Bam RH, Cronjé HS, Griessel DJ, et al. Syphilis in pregnant patients and their offspring. Int J Gynecol Obstet 1994;44:113.

36. Nathan L, Twickler DM, Peters MT, et al. Fetal syphilis: Correlation of sonographic findings and rabbit infectivity testing of amniotic fluid. J Ultrasound Med 1993;2:97.

37. Martens PR, Mullie A, Goessens L. A near-fatal case of puerperal sepsis. Anaesth Intensive Care 1991;19:108.

38. Davis L, Hargreaves C, Robinson PN. Postpartum meningitis. Anaesthesia 1993;48:788.

39. Aharoni A, Potasman I, Levitan Z, et al. Postpartum maternal group B streptococcal meningitis. Rev Infect Dis 1990;12:273.

40. Fox BC. Delayed-onset postpartum meningitis due to group B streptococcus (letter). Clin Infect Dis 1994;19:350.

41. Stevens DL. Could nonsteroidal antiinflammatory drugs (NSAIDs) enhance the progression of bacterial infections to toxic shock syndrome? (Hypothesis). Clin Infect Dis 1995;21:977.

42. Schieve LA, Handler A, Hershow R, et al. Urinary tract infection during pregnancy: Its association with maternal morbidity and perinatal outcome. Am J Public Health 1994;84:405.

43. Kitching AJ, Rice AS. Extradural abscess in the postpartum period (letter). Br J Anaesth 1993;70:703.

44. Wong S, Yat-Cheung T, Yen K. Campylobacter infection in the neonate: Case report and review of the literature. Pediatr Infect Dis 1990;9:665.

45. Simor AE, Karmali MA, Jadavji K, et al. Abortion and perinatal sepsis associated with Campylobacter infection. Rev Infect Dis 1986;8:397.

46. Hickey K, McKenna P, O'Connell PR, et al. Actinomycosis presenting as appendicitis in pregnancy. Br J Obstet Gynaecol 1993;100:595.

47. Robin L, Herman D, Redett R. Botulism in a pregnant woman (letter). N Engl J Med 1996;335:823.

48. Farizo KM, Buehler JW, Chamberland ME, et al. Spectrum of disease in persons with human immunodeficiency virus infection in the United States. JAMA 1992;267:1798.

49. Lindsay MK. A protocol for routine voluntary antepartum human immunodeficiency virus antibody screening. Am J Obstet Gynecol 1993;168:476.

50. D'Angelo LJ. Epidemiology of acquired immunodeficiency syndrome and human immunodeficiency virus infection in adolescents. Ped Infect Dis J 1991;10:322.

51. Duarte G, Mussi-Pinhata M, Del-Lama J, et al. Valor de questionario especifíco na identificação de parturients de risco para infecção pelo vírus da imunodeficiência humana (HIV). J Bras Ginecol 1991;101:169.

52. Barbacci M, Repke JT, Chaisson RE. Routine prenatal screening for HIV infection. Lancet 1991;337:709.

53. National Institute of Health. State-of-the-art conference on azidothymidine therapy for early HIV infection. Am J Med 1990;89:335.

54. Bergsjf P. African plight. The hidden face of the AIDS epidemic. Acta Obstet Gynecol Scand 1994;73:669.

55. Hughes SC. AIDS: the focus turns to women (editorial). Int J Obstet Anesth 1993;2:1.

56. Quin TC, Kline RL, Halsey N, et al. Early diagnosis of perinatal HIV infection by detection of viral-specific Ig-A antibodies. JAMA 1991;266:3439.

57. Lindgren S. Clinical consequences of HIV and hepatitis during pregnancy. Can J Obstet Gynaecol 1994;66:SP87.

58. Viscarello RR, DeGennaro NJ, Cullen MT, et al. Perinatal AIDS: A decade of experience (SPO Abstracts). Am J Obstet Gynecol 1993;312:59.

58a. Landesman SH, Kalish LA, Burns DN, et al. Obstetrical factors and the transmission of human immunodeficiency virus type I from mother to child. N Engl J Med 1996;334:1617.

59. Tibaldi C, Ziarati N, Salassa B, et al. Asymptomatic women at high risk of vertical HIV-1 transmission to their fetuses. Br J Obstet Gynaecol 1993;100:334.

60. Perre PV. Postnatal transmission of human immunodeficiency virus type-1: The breast feeding dilemma. Am J Obstet Gynecol 1995;173:483.

61. Sprecher S, Soumen Koff G, Puissant F, et al. Vertical transmission of HIV in 15-week fetus. Lancet 1986;2:288.

62. AIDS—Brazil, Boletim Epidemiológico. July, 1994;7:6.

63. Geary F, Lindsay M, Graves W, et al. HIV infection as a risk for adverse perinatal outcome. Am J Obstet Gynecol 1994;170:227.

64. Temmerman M, Chomba EN, Ndiya-Achola J, et al. Maternal human immunodeficiency virus-1 infection and pregnancy outcome. Obstet Gynecol 1994;83:495.

65. Marion RW, Wiznia AA, Hutcheon G, et al. Human T cell lymphotrophic virus type III (HTLV-III) embryopathy: A new dysmorphic syndrome associated with intrauterine HTLV-III infections. Am J Dis Child 1986;140:638.

66. The European Collaborative Study. Perinatal findings in children born to HIV-infected mothers. Br J Obstet Gynaecol 1994;101:136.

67. Minkoff HL, Henderson C, Mendez H, et al. Pregnancy outcomes among mothers infected with human immunodeficiency virus and uninfected control subjects. Am J Obstet Gynecol 1990;163:1598.

68. National Institutes of Health, National Institute of Allergy and Infectious Diseases. AIDS Clinical Trial Group (ACTG 076). Clinical alert: Important information on the benefit of zidovudine (AZT) for the prevention of the transmission of HIV from mother to infant. Bethesda, National Institutes of Health, 1994, Feb 21.

69. Hansen JES. Initial events of human immunodeficiency virus infection. Role of carbohydrates and possibilities for intervention. Acta Obstet Scand 1994;73:91.

70. Burton DR, Pyati J, Koduri R, et al. Efficient neutralization of primary isolates of HIV-1 by a recombinant human monoclonal antibody. Science 1994;266:1024.

71. Viscarello RR, DeGennaro NJ, Andiman WA. Does mode of delivery affect the rate of perinatal transmission of HIV-1? (abstract). Am J Obstet Gynecol 1993;312:60.

72. Vogt MW, Witt DJ, Craven DE, et al. Isolation of HTLV-III/LAV from cervical secretions of women at risk for AIDS. Lancet 1986;1:525.

73. Romero R, Gomez R, Araneda H, et al. Cervical mucus inhibits microbial growth: A host defense mechanism to prevent ascending infection in pregnant and non-pregnant women (SPO abstract). Am J Obstet Gynecol 1993;312:57.

74. Minkoff H, Burns DN, Landesman S, et al. The relationship of ruptured membranes to vertical transmission of human immunodeficiency virus. Am J Obstet Gynecol 1995;173:585.

75. Goedert JJ, Duliegge AM, Amos CI, et al. High risk of HIV-1 infection for first-born twins. Lancet 1991;338:1471.

76. Report of a working group: Nomenclature and research case definitions for neurologic manifestations of human immunodeficiency virus-type 1 (HIV-1) infection. Neurology 1991;41:778.

77. Leger JM, Bouche P, Bolgert F, et al. The spectrum of polyneuropathies in patients infected with HIV. J Neurol Neurosurg Psych 1989;52:1369.

78. Applemann ME, Marshall DW, Brey RL, et al. Cerebrospinal fluid abnormalities in patients without AIDS who are seropositive for the human immunodeficiency virus. J Infect Dis 1988;158:193.

79. Marshall DW, Brey RL, Butzin CA, et al. CSF changes in a longitudinal study of 124 neurologically normal HIV-infected U.S. Air Force personnel. J Acquir Immune Defic Syndr 1991;4:777.

80. Dubois-Dalcq ME, Jordon CA, Kelly WB, et al. Understanding HIV-1 infection in the brain: A challenge for neurobiologists. AIDS 1990;4:S67.

81. Shapiro HM, Grant I, Weinger MB. AIDS and the central nervous system. Anesthesiology 1994;80:187.

82. Tom DJ, Gulevich SJ, Shapiro HM, et al. Epidural blood patch in the HIV-positive patient. Anesthesiology 1992;76:943.

83. Schwartz DM, Schwartz T, Cooper E. Anaesthesia and the child with HIV infection. Can J Anaesth 1991;38:626.

84. Stevenson GW, Hall SC, Rudnick S, et al. The effect of anesthetic agents on the human immune response. Anesthesiology 1990;72:542.

85. Markovic SN, Knight PR, Murasko DM. Inhibition of interferon stimulation of natural killer cell activity in mice anesthetized with halothane or isoflurane. Anesthesiology 1993;78:700.

86. Kepes ER, Andrews IC, Radnay PA, et al. Conduct for anesthesia for delivery with grossly raised cerebrospinal fluid pressure. N Y State J Med 1972;72:1155.

87. Goroszeniuk T, Howard RS, Wright JT. The management of labour using continuous lumbar epidural analgesia in a patient with a malignant cerebral tumour. Anaesthesia 1986;41:1128.

88. Finfer SR. Management of labour and delivery in patients with intracranial neoplasms. Br J Anaesth 1991;67:784.

89. Hilt H, Gramm HJ, Link J. Changes in intracranial pressure associated with extradural anaesthesia. Br J Anaesth 1986;58:676.

90. Wildsmith JAW. Extradural blockade and intracranial pressure. Br J Anaesth 1986;58:579.

91. Richards PG, Towu-Aghantse E. Dangers of lumbar puncture. Br Med J 1986;292:605.

92. Hughes SC, Dailey PA, Landers D, et al. Parturients infected with human immunodeficiency virus and regional anesthesia. Anesthesiology 1995;82:32.

93. Birnbach DJ, Bourlier RA, Choi R, Thys DM. Anaesthetic management of Caesarean section in a patient with active recurrent genital herpes and AIDS-related dementia. Br J Anaesth 1995;75:639.

94. Miller LG, Galpern WR, Dunlap K, et al. Interleukin-1 augments gamma-aminobutyric acid-A receptor function in brain. Mol Pharmacol 1991;39:105.

95. Fassoulaki A, Desmonts JM. Prolonged neuromuscular blockade after a single bolus dose of vecuronium in patients with acquired immunodeficiency syndrome. Anesthesiology 1994; 80:457.

96. Parry GJ. Peripheral neuropathies associated with human immunodeficiency virus infection. Ann Neurol 1988;23:S49.

97. Till M, MacDonnell KB. Myopathy with human immunodeficiency virus type 1 (HIV-1) infection: HIV-1 or zidovudine? Ann Intern Med 1990;113:492.

98. Shelton MJ, O'Donnell AM, Morse GD. Didanosine. Ann Pharmacol Ther 1992;26:660.

99. Squinto SP, Mondal D, Bolck AL, et al. Morphine-induced transactivation of HIV-1 LTR in human neuroblastoma cells. AIDS Res Hum Retroviruses 1990;6:1163.

100. Bayer BM, Daussin S, Hernandez M, et al. Morphine inhibition of lymphocyte activity is mediated by an opioid-dependent mechanism. Neuropharmacology 1990;29:369.

101. Pruett SB, Han YC, Fuchs BA. Morphine suppresses primary humoral immune responses by a predominantly indirect mechanism. J Pharmacol Exp Ther 1992;262:923.

102. Rolbin SH, Cohen MM, Levinton CM, et al. The premature infant: Anesthesia for cesarean delivery. Anesth Analg 1994;78:912.

103. Deseda CC, Sweeney PA, Woodruff BA, et al. Prevalence of hepatitis B, hepatitis C and human immunodeficiency virus infection among women attending prenatal clinics in San Juan, Puerto Rico, from 1989–1990. Obstet Gynecol 1995;85:75.

104. Zambon MC, Lockwood MJD. Hepatitis C seroconversion in pregnancy. Br J Obstet Gynaecol 1994;101:722.

105. Fong TS, Valinluck B, Govindarajan S, et al. Marked improvement in sensitivity of second-generation tests for acute hepatitis C virus infection. J Infect Dis 1993;168:519.

106. Niu MT, Polish LB, Robertson BH, et al. Multistate outbreak of hepatitis A associated with frozen strawberries. J Infect Dis 1992;166:518.

107. Badur S, Lazizi Y, Ugurlu M, et al. Transplacental passage of hepatitis B virus DNA from hepatitis B e antigen-negative mothers and delayed immune response in newborns. J Infect Dis 1994;169:704.

108. Reinus JF, Leikin EL, Alter HJ, et al. Failure to detect vertical transmission of hepatitis C virus. Ann Intern Med 1992;117:881.

109. Wejstal R, Widell A, Persson AS, et al. Mother-to-infant transmission of hepatitis C. Ann Intern Med 1992;117:887.

110. Murphy D, Willems B, Delage G. Use of the 5′ noncoding region for genotyping hepatitis C virus. J Infect Dis 1994;169:473.

111. Kelen GD, Green GB, Purcell RH, et al. Hepatitis B and hepatitis C in emergency department patients. N Engl J Med 1992;326:1399.

112. Andreone P, Gramenzi A, Curssaro C, et al. Familial cluster of hepatitis C virus type 1. J Infect Dis 1994;170:1042.

113. Dusheiko GM. Progress in hepatitis C research. Lancet 1994;344:605.

114. Lam JP, McOmish F, Burns SM, et al. Infrequent vertical transmission of hepatitis C virus. J Infect Dis 1993;167:572.

115. Cenac A, Pedroso ML, Djibo A, et al. Hepatitis B, C, and D virus infections in patients with chronic hepatitis, cirrhosis, and hepatocellular carcinoma: A comparative study in Niger. Am Trop Med Hyg 1995;52:293.

116. Paul DA, Knigge MF, Ritter A, et al. Determination of hepatitis E virus seroprevalence by using recombinant fusion proteins and synthetic peptides. J Infect Dis 1994;169:801.

117. Wang JT, Lin JT, Sheu JC, et al. Hepatitis E virus and posttransfusion hepatitis. J Infect Dis 1994;169:229.

118. Bradley DW. Enterically transmitted non-A, non-B hepatitis. Br Med Bull 1990;46:442.

119. Male CG, Martin R. Puerperal spinal epidural abscess. Lancet 1973;1:608.

120. Nicolini U, Guarnieri D, Gianott GA, et al. Maternal platelet activation in normal pregnancy. Obstet Gynecol 1994;83:65.

121. Brown J, Corey L. Maternal genital herpes and gender of offspring. Am J Obstet Gynecol 1991;165:84.

122. Frenkel LM, Garratty EM, Shen JP, et al. Clinical reactivation of herpes simplex type 2 infection in seropositive pregnant women with no history of genital herpes. Ann Intern Med 1993;118:414.

123. Koutsky LA, Stevens CE, Holmes KK, et al. Underdiagnosis of genital herpes by current clinical and viral-isolation procedures. N Engl J Med 1992;326:1533.

124. Cunningham AL, Lee FK, Ho DWT, et al. Herpes simplex virus type 2 antibody in patients attending antenatal or STD clinics. Med J Aust 1993;158:525.

125. Roberts SW, Cox SM, Dax J, et al. Genital herpes during pregnancy: No lesions, no cesarean. Obstet Gynecol 1995;85:261.

126. Crone LA, Conly JM, Clark KM, et al. Recurrent herpes simplex virus labialis and the use of epidural morphine in obstetric patients. Anesth Analg 1988;67:318.

127. Valley MA, Bourke DL, McKenzie AM. Recurrence of thoracic and labial herpes simplex virus infection in a patient receiving epidural fentanyl. Anesthesiology 1992;76:1056.

128. Smith MA, Singer C. Sexually transmitted viruses other than HIV and papillomaviruses. Urol Clin North Am 1992;19:47.

129. Shen C-Y, Chang SF, Yen MS, et al. Cytomegalovirus excretion in pregnant and non-pregnant women. J Clin Microbiol 1993;31:1635.

130. Byard RW, Mikhael NZ, Orlando G, et al. The clinicopathological significance of cytomegalic inclusions demonstrated by endocervical biopsy. Pathology 1991;23:318.

131. Fowler KB, Stagno S, Pass RF, et al. The outcome of congenital cytomegalovirus infection in relation to maternal antibody status. N Engl J Med 1992;326:663.

132. Huang ES, Alford CA, Reynolds DW, et al. Molecular epidemiology of cytomegalovirus infection in women and their infants. N Engl J Med 1980;303:958.

133. Balcarek KB, Warren W, Smith RJ, et al. Neonatal screening for congenital cytomegalovirus infection by detection of virus in saliva. J Infect Dis 1993;167:1433.

134. Grose C, Meehan T, Weiner CP. Prenatal diagnosis of congenital cytomegalovirus infection by virus isolation after amniocentesis. Pediatr Infect Dis J 1992;11:605.

135. Abulafia O, DuBeshter B, Dawson AE, et al. Presence of cytomegalovirus inclusion bodies in a recurrent ulcerative vaginal lesion. Am J Obstet Gynecol 1993;4:1179.

136. Gonzalez MI. Papillomavirus in the cervix. Its relationship with dysplasias and other sexually transmitted diseases. Acta Obstet Gynecol Scand 1993;72:502.

137. Czeglédy J, Rylander E, Evander M, et al. Relation between the presence of human papillomavirus type 16 deoxyribonucleic acid in cervicovaginal cells and general health condition. Am J Obstet Gynecol 1993;169:386.

138. Morrison EAB, Goldberg GL, Hagan RJ, et al. Self-administered

home cervicovaginal lavage: A novel tool for the clinical-epidemiologic investigation of genital human papillomavirus infections. Am J Obstet Gynecol 1992;167:104.

139. Ho GY, Burk RD, Klein S, et al. Persistent genital human papillomavirus infection as a risk factor for persistent cervical dysplasia. J Nat Canc Inst 1995;87:1365.

140. Cook TA, Cohn AM, Brunschwig P, et al. Wart-viruses and laryngeal papillomas. Lancet 1983;1:782.

141. Medeiros SF. Codiloma—um inquérito. Femina 1985;13:1092.

142. Duarte G. Doenças sexualmente transmissíveis durante o ciclo grávido-puerperal. In: Temas de Obstetrícia Edson Nunes de Morais (ed), Editora Roca, São Paulo, 1992;29:385.

143. Straus SE, Osrtove JM, Inchauspe G, et al. Varicella-zoster virus infections. Ann Intern Med 1988;108:221.

144. Balducci J, Rodis JF, Rosengren S, et al. Pregnancy outcome following first-trimester varicella infection. Obstet Gynecol 1992;79:5.

145. Brazin SA, Simkovich JW, Johnsos WT. Herpes zoster during pregnancy. Obstet Gynecol 1979;53:175.

146. Balraj V, John TJ. An epidemic of varicella in rural southern India. J Trop Med Hyg 1994;97:113.

147. Harris RE, Rhoades ER. Varicella pneumonia complicating pregnancy: Report of a case and review of literature. Obstet Gynecol 1965;25:734.

148. Brunell PA. Varicella in pregnancy. The fetus, and the newborn: Problems in management. J Infect Dis 1992;166:S42.

149. Preblud SR. Varicella. Complications and costs. Pediatrics 1986;78:728.

150. Martin KA, Junker AK, Thomas EE, et al. Occurrence of chickenpox during pregnancy in women seropositive for varicella-zoster virus. J Infect Dis 1994;170:991.

151. Terada K, Kawano S, Yoshihiro K, et al. Varicella-zoster virus (VZV) reactivation is related to the low response of VZV-specific immunity after chickenpox in infancy. J Infect Dis 1994;169:650.

152. Center for Disease Control and Prevention. Measles surveillance—United States. MMWR CDC Surveill Summ 1992;41(SS-6):1.

153. Griffin DF, Ward BJ, Esolen LM. Pathogenesis of measles virus infection: A hypothesis for altered immune responses. J Infect Dis 1994;170:S24.

154. Smoak BL, Novakoski WL, Mason CJ, et al. Evidence for a recent decrease in measles susceptibility among young American adults. J Infec Dis 1994;170:216.

155. Forthal DN, Landucci G, Habis A, et al. Measles virus-specific functional antibody responses and viremia during acute measles. J Infect Dis 1994;169:1377.

156. Ebehart-Phillips JE, Frederick PD, Baron RC, et al. Measles in pregnancy: A descriptive study of 58 cases. Obstet Gynecol 1993;82:797.

157. Esolen LM, Ward BJ, Moench TR, et al. Infection of monocytes during measles. J Infect Dis 1993;168:47.

158. Moroi K, Saito S, Kurata T, et al. Fetal death associated with measles virus infection of the placenta. Am J Obstet Gynecol 1991;164:1107.

159. Tamin A, Rota PA, Wang Z, et al. Antigenic analysis of current wild type and vaccine strains of measles virus. J Infect Dis 1994;170:795.

160. Shortridge KF. The next pandemic influenza virus. Lancet 1995;346:1210.

161. Hubert B, Watier L, Garnerin P, et al. Meningococcal disease and influenza-like syndrome: A new approach to an old question. J Infect Dis 1992;166:542.

162. Gruber WC, Hinson HP, Holland KL, et al. Comparative trial of large-particle aerosol and nose drop administration of live attenuated influenza vaccines. J Infect Dis 1993;168:1282.

163. Edwards KM, Dupont WD, Westrich MK, et al. A randomized controlled trial of cold-adapted and inactive vaccines for the prevention of influenza A disease. J Infect Dis 1994;169:68.

164. Woernle CH, Anderson LJ, Tattersall P. Human parvovirus B19 infection during pregnancy. J Infect Dis 1987;156:17.

165. Brown T, Anand A, Ritchie LD, et al. Intrauterine parvovirus infection associated with hydrops fetalis. Lancet 1984;2:1033.

166. Rodis JF, Quinn DL, Gary GW, et al. Management and outcomes of pregnancies complicated by human B19 parvovirus infection: A prospective study. Am J Obstet Gynecol 1990;163:1168.

167. Mead BP. Parvovirus B19 infection and pregnancy. Contemp Obstet Gynecol 1989;9:56.

168. Sheikh AU, Ernest JM, O'Shea M. Long-term outcome in fetal hydrops from parvovirus B19 infection. Am J Obstet Gynecol 1992;167:337.

169. Carlson DE, Platt LD, Medearis AL, et al. Prognostic indicators of the resolution of nonimmune hydrops fetalis and survival of the fetus. Am J Obstet Gynecol 1990;163:1785.

170. Simpson JL, Elias S, Morgan CD, et al. Does unexplained second-trimester (15 to 20 weeks gestation) maternal serum α-fetoprotein elevation presage adverse perinatal outcome? Pitfalls and preliminary studies with late second- and third-trimester maternal serum α-fetoprotein. Am J Obstet Gynecol 1991;164:829.

171. Peters M, Nicolaides K. Cordocentesis for the diagnosis and treatment of human fetal parvovirus infection. Obstet Gynecol 1990;75:501.

172. Naides SJ, Weiner CP. Antenatal diagnosis and palliative treatment of nonimmune hydrops fetalis secondary to fetal parvovirus B19 infection. Prenat Diagn 1989;9:105.

173. Humphrey W, Magoon M, O'Shaughnessy R. Severe non-immune hydrops secondary to parvovirus B19 infection: Spontaneous reversal in utero and survival of a term infant. Obstet Gynecol 1991;78:900.

174. Hwa HL, Shyu MK, Lee CN, et al. Prenatal diagnosis of congenital rubella in Taiwan. Obstet Gynecol 1994;84:415.

175. Rubella and congenital rubella syndrome—United States, January 1, 1991–May 7, 1994. MMWR 1994;43:391.

176. Ueno Y. Rubella arthritis. An outbreak in Kyoto. J Rheumatol 1994;21:874.

177. Ksiazek TG, Peters CJ, Rollin PE, et al. Identification of a new North American hantavirus that causes acute pulmonary insufficiency. Am J Trop Med Hyg 1995;52:117.

178. Rollin PE, Bowen MD, Kariwa H, et al. Short report: Isolation and partial characterization of a puumala virus from a human case of nephropathia epidemica in France. Am J Trop Med Hyg 1995;52:577.

179. Eng RHK, Seligman SJ. Lumbar puncture-induced meningitis. JAMA 1981;245:1456.

180. Smith KM, Deddish RB, Ogata ES. Meningitis associated with serial lumbar punctures and posthemorrhagic hydrocephalus. J Pediatrics 1986;109:1057.

181. Teele DW, Dashefsky B, Rakusan T, et al. Meningitis after lumbar puncture in children with bacteremia. N Engl J Med 1981;305:1079.

182. Scott DB, Hibbard BM. Serious non-fatal complications associated with extradural block in obstetric practice. Br J Anaesth 1990;64:537.

183. Hlavin ML. Kaminski HJ, Ross JS, et al. Spinal epidural abscess: A ten-year perspective. Neurosurgery 1990;27:177.

184. Schreiner EJ, Lipson SF, Bromage PR, et al. Neurological complications following general anaesthesia. Three cases of major paralysis. Anaesthesia 1983;38:226.

185. Jakobsen KB, Christensen M-K, Carlsson PS. Extradural anaesthesia for repeated surgical treatment in the presence of infection. Br J Anaesth 1995;75:536.

186. Ngan Kee WD, Jones MR, Thomas P, et al. Extradural abscess complicating extradural anaesthesia for Caesarean section. Br J Anaesth 1992;69:647.

187. Lee JJ, Parry H. Bacterial meningitis following spinal anaesthesia for Caesarean section. Br J Anaesth 1991;66:383.

188. Carp H, Bailey S. The association between meningitis and dural puncture in bacteremic rats. Anesthesiology 1992;76:739.

189. Bader AM, Gilbertson L, Kirz L, et al. Regional anesthesia in women with chorioamnionitis. Reg Anesth 1992;17:84.

190. Berman RS, Eisele JH. Bacteremia, spinal anesthesia, and development of meningitis. Anesthesiology 1978;48:376.

191. Loarie DJ, Fairley HB. Epidural abscess following spinal anesthesia. Anesthesiology 1978;57:351.

192. Goodman EJ, de Horta E, Taquiam JM. Safety of spinal and epidural anesthesia in parturients with chorioamnionitis. Reg Anesth 1996;21:436.

193. Center for Disease Control and Prevention. Dengue type 3 infection—Nicaragua and Panama, October–November 1994. JAMA 1995;273:840.

194. Sharp TW, Wallace MR, Hayes CG, et al. Dengue fever in US

troops during Operation Restore Hope, Somalia, 1992–1993. Am J Trop Med Hyg 1995;53:89.

195. Nuti M, Messa M, Mioni G, et al. Presumed first case of hemorrhagic fever with renal syndrome in north-eastern Italy. Trans Royal Soc Trop Med Hyg 1991;85:789.

196. Rodriguez-Figueroa L, Rigau-Perez JG, Suarez EL, et al. Risk factors for dengue infection during an outbreak in Yanes, Puerto Rico in 1991. Am J Trop Med Hyg 1995;52:496.

197. Mirovsky J, Holub J, Nguyen BC. Influence de la dengue sur la grossesse et le foetus. Gynecol Obstet (Paris) 1965;65:673.

198. Poli L, Chungue E, Soulignac O, et al. Dengue materno-foetale, à propos de 5 cas observés pendant l'épidemie de Tahiti (1989). Bull Soc Pathol Exot 1991;84:513.

199. Dharakul T, Kurane I, Bhamarapravati N, et al. Dengue virus-specific memory T cell responses in human volunteers receiving a live attenuated dengue virus type 2 candidate vaccine. J Infect Dis 1994;170:27.

200. Secretaria do Estado da Saúde—Centro de Vigilância Epidemiológica Prof. Alexandre Vranjac. Manual Sobre Dengue, 1994.

201. Liam CK, Yap BH, Lam SK. Dengue fever complicated by pulmonary haemorrhage manifesting as haemoptysis. J Trop Med Hyg 1993;96:197.

202. Halstead SB, Porterfield JS, O'Rourke EJ. Enhancement of dengue virus infection in monocytes by flavivirus antisera. Am J Trop Med Hyg 1980;29:638.

203. Chang DM, Shaio MF. Production of interleukin-1 (IL-1) and IL-1 inhibitor by human monocytes exposed to dengue virus. J Infect Dis 1994;170:811.

204. Chungue E, Burucoa C, Boutin JP, et al. Dengue 1 epidemic in French Polynesia, 1988–1989: Surveillance and clinical, epidemiological, virological and serological findings in 1752 documented clinical cases. Trans Royal Soc Trop Med Hyg 1992;86:193.

205. Rawlins SC, Hull B, Chadee DD, et al. Sylvatic yellow fever activity in Trinidad, 1988–1989. Trans Royal Soc Trop Med Hyg 1990;84:142.

206. De Cock KM. Epidemic yellow fever in eastern Nigeria. Lancet 1986;19:630.

207. Tsai TF, Paul R, Lynberg MC, et al. Congenital yellow fever infections after immunization in pregnancy. J Infect Dis 1993;168:1520.

208. Nasidi A, Monath TP, Vandenberg J, et al. Yellow fever vaccine and pregnancy: A four year prospective study. Trans R Soc Trop Med Hyg 1993;87:337.

209. Secretaria do Estado da Saúde—Manual de Vigilância Epidemiológica—Febre Amarela. São Paulo (atualizado de 1986), 1994.

210. Secretaria do Estado da Saúde—Manual de Vigilância Epidemiológica—Leptospirose. São Paulo, 1994.

211. Ratnam S, Everard COR, Alex JC. Prevalence of leptospiral agglutinins among conservancy workers in Madras City, India. J Trop Med Hyg 1993;96:41.

212. Onyemelukwe NF. A serological survey for leptospirosis in the Enegu area of eastern Nigeria among people at occupational risk. J Trop Med Hyg 1993;96:301.

213. Kuriakose M, Eapen CK, Punnoose E, et al. Leptospirosis—clinical spectrum and correlation with seven simple laboratory tests for early diagnosis in the Third World. Trans Royal Soc Trop Med Hyg 1990;84:419.

214. White NJ, Chapman D, Watt G. The effects of multiplication and synchronicity on the vascular distribution of parasites in falciparum malaria. Trans R Soc Trop Med Hyg 1992;86:590.

215. Voller A, Bidwell DE, Chiodini PL. Evaluation of a malaria antigen ELISA. Trans Royal Soc Trop Med Hyg 1994;88:188.

216. Mvondo JL, Mark MA, Sulzer AJ, et al. Malaria and pregnancy in Cameroonian women. Naturally acquired antibody responses to asexual blood-stage antigens and the circumsporozoite protein of Plasmodium falciparum. Trans R Soc Trop Med Hyg 1992;86:486.

217. Nosten F, Ter Kuile F, Maelankirri M, et al. Malaria in pregnancy in an area of unstable endemicity. Trans R Soc Trop Med Hyg 1991;85:424.

218. Landgraf B, Kollaritsch H, Wiedermann G. Parasite density of Plasmodium falciparum malaria in Ghanaian schoolchildren: Evidence for influence of sex hormones? Trans R Soc Trop Med Hyg 1994;88:73.

219. Steketee RW, Breman JG, Paluku KM, et al. Malaria infection in pregnant women in Zaire: The effects and potential for intervention. Ann Trop Med Parasitol 1988;82:113.

220. Brown AE, Herrington DA, Webster HK, et al. Urinary neopterin in volunteers experimentally infected with Plasmodium falciparum. Trans R Soc Trop Med Hyg 1992;86:134.

221. Taylor WRJ, Prosser DI. Acute renal failure, acute rhabdomyolysis and falciparum malaria. Trans R Soc Trop Med Hyg 1992;86:361.

222. Wattanagoon Y, Srivilairit S, Looareesuwan S, et al. Convulsions in childhood malaria. Trans R Soc Trop Med Hyg 1994;88:426.

223. Brabin BJ, Ginny M, Sapau J, et al. Consequences of maternal anaemia on outcome of pregnancy in a malaria endemic area in Papua New Guinea. Ann Trop Med Parasitol 1990;84:11.

224. White NJ, Warrel DA, Chanthavanish P, et al. Severe hypoglycemia and hyperinsulinemia in falciparum malaria. N Engl J Med 1983;309:61.

225. Saeed BO, Atabani GS, Nawwaf A, et al. Hypoglycaemia in pregnant women with malaria. Trans R Soc Trop Med Hyg 1990;84:349.

226. Davis TME, Garcia-Weeb P, Fu LC, et al. Antioxidant vitamins in acute malaria. Trans R Soc Trop Med Hyg 1994;88:596.

227. Nosten F, Ter Kuile F, Thwai KL, et al. Spiramycin does not potentiate quinine treatment of falciparum malaria in pregnancy. Trans R Soc Trop Med Hyg 1993;87:305.

228. Long GW, Fries L, Hoffman SL. Polymerase chain reaction amplification from Plasmodium falciparum on dried blood spots. Am J Trop Med Hyg 1995;52:344.

229. Na Bangchang K, Davis TME, Looareesuwan S, et al. Mefloquine pharmacokinetics in pregnant women with acute falciparum malaria. Trans R Soc Trop Med Hyg 1994;88:321.

230. Okoyeh JN, Lege-Oguntoye L, Emembolu JO, et al. Sensitivity of Plasmodium falciparum to pyrimethamine in vivo and to sulphadoxine/pyrimethamine combination in vitro in pregnant women of northern Nigeria. J Trop Med Hyg 1993;96:56.

231. Greenwood AM, Menendez C, Tood J, et al. The distribution of birth weights in Gambian women who received malaria chemoprophylaxis during their first pregnancy and in control women. Trans R Soc Trop Med Hyg 1994;88:311.

232. Schaefer G, Zervoudakis IA, Fuchs F, et al. Pregnancy and pulmonary tuberculosis. Obstet Gynecol 1975;46:706.

233. Margono F, Mroueh J, Garely A, et al. Ressurgence of active tuberculosis among pregnant women. Obstet Gynecol 1994;83:911.

234. Huebner RE, Good RC, Tokars JI. Current practices in mycobacteriology: Result of a survey of state public health laboratories. J Clin Microbiol 1992;31:771.

235. Sugita Y, Sasaki T, Nakajima H. Practical use of polymerase chain reaction for the diagnosis of steroid induced tuberculous lymphadenitis. J Trop Med Hyg 1994;97:65.

236. Rich SA, Sbordone L, Mazze RI. Metabolism by rat hepatic microsomes of fluorinated ether anesthetics following isoniazid administration. Anesthesiology 1980;53:489.

237. Valway SE, Greifinger RB, Papania M, et al. Multidrug-resistance in the New York State prison system, 1990–1991. J Infect Dis 1994;170:151.

238. Ellner JJ, Hinman AR, Dooley SW, et al. Tuberculosis symposium: Emerging problems and promise. J Infect Dis 1993;168:537.

239. El-Sayed HF, Rizkalla NH, Mehanna S, et al. Prevalence and epidemiology of Schistosoma mansoni and S. haematobium infection in two areas of Egypt recently reclaimed from the desert. Am J Trop Hyg 1995;52:194.

240. Li Y, Yu D, Li Y, et al. A study and analysis of the deaths due to advanced Schistosoma japonicum infection in the Dongtong Lake area of China. J Trop Med Hyg 1993;96:128.

241. Braun-Munziger RA, Southgate BA. Egg viability in urinary schistosomiasis. III: Repeatability and reproducibility of new methods. J Trop Med Hyg 1993;96:179.

242. Idris MA, Ruppel A, Numrich P, et al. Schistosomiasis in the southern region of Oman: Vector snails and serological identification of patients in several locations. J Trop Med Hyg 1994;97:205.

243. Rabello ALT, Lambertucci JR, Freire MH, et al. Evaluation of proteinuria in an area of Brazil endemic for schistosomiasis using a single urine sample. Trans R Soc Trop Med Hyg 1994;87:187.

244. Domingues AL, Lima ARF, Dias HS, et al. An ultrasonographic study of liver fibrosis in patients infected with Schistosoma mansoni in north-east Brazil. Trans R Soc Trop Med Hyg 1993;87 555.

245. Doenhoff MJ, Butterworth AE, Hayes RJ, et al. Seroepidemiology and serodiagnosis of schistosomiasis in Kenya using crude and purified egg antigens of Schistosoma mansoni in ELISA. Trans R Soc Trop Med Hyg 1993;87:42.

246. Basch PF. Antischistosomal vaccines: Beyond the laboratory. Trans R Soc Trop Med Hyg 1993;87:589.

247. Neves J, Raso P, Pinto DM, et al. Ischaemic colitis (necrotizing colitis, pseudomembranous colitis) in acute schistosomiasis mansoni: Report of two cases. Trans R Soc Trop Med Hyg 1993;87:449.

248. Giboda M, Smith M. Schistosoma mansoni eggs as a target for praziquantel: Efficacy of oral application in mice. J Trop Med Hyg 1994;97:98.

249. Potts BJ, Berry LJ, Osburn BI, et al. Viral persistence and abnormalities of the central nervous system after congenital infection of sheep with border disease virus. J Infect Dis 1985;151:337.

250. Nair GB, Ramamurthy T, Bhattacharaya SK, et al. Spread of Vibrio cholerae O139 Bengal in India. J Infect Dis 1994;169:1029.

251. Echeverria P, Hoge CW, Bodhitta L, et al. Molecular characterization of Vibrio cholerae O139 isolates from Asia. Am J Trop Hyg 1995;52:124.

252. Huq A, Parveen S, Qadri F, et al. Comparison of Vibrio cholerae serotype O1 strains isolated from patients and the aquatic environment. J Trop Med Hyg 1993;96:86.

253. Mujica OJ, Quick RE, Palacios AM, et al. Epidemic cholera in the Amazon: The role of produce in disease risk and prevention. J Infect Dis 1994;169:1381.

254. Islam MS, Miah MA, Hasan K, et al. Detection of non-culturable Vibrio cholerae O1 associated with a cyanobacterium from an aquatic environment in Bangladesh. Trans R Soc Trop Med Hyg 1994;88:298.

255. Coldwell RR, Hasan JKA, Huq A, et al. Development and evaluation of a rapid, simple, sensitive, monoclonal antibody-based coagglutination test for direct detection of Vibrio cholerae O1. FEMS Microbiol Let 1992;97:215.

256. Islam MS, Hasan MK, Miah MA, et al. Specificity of Cholera Screen test during an epidemic of cholera-like disease due to Vibrio cholerae O 139 synonym Bengal. Trans R Soc Trop Med Hyg 1994;88:424.

257. Sack RB, Albert MJ. Cholera vaccine workshop. J Infect Dis 1994;170:256.

258. Ginosar Y, Shapira SC. The role of an anaesthetist in a field hospital during the cholera epidemic among Rwandan refugees in Goma. Br J Anaesth 1995;75:810.

259. Azogue E. Women and congenital Chagas disease in Santa Cruz, Bolivia: Epidemiological and sociocultural aspects. Soc Sci Med 1993;37:503.

260. Gilson GJ, Harner KA, Abrams J, et al. Chagas disease in pregnancy. Obstet Gynecol 1995;86:646.

261. Murray HW, Tuazon CU. Atypical pneumonias. Med Clin North Am 1980;64:507.

262. Ghermam RB, Leventis LL, Miller R. Chlamydial psittacosis during pregnancy: A case report. Obstet Gynecol 1995;86:648.

263. Rodriguez RE, Valero V, Watanakunakorn C. Salmonella focal intracranial infections: Review of the world literature (1884–1984) and report of an unusual case. Rev Infect Dis 1986;8:31.

264. Wetering JV, Visser LG, Buchem MAV, et al. A case of typhoid fever complicated by unexpected cerebral edema. Clin Infect Dis 1995;21:1057.

265. Acharya G, Butler T, Ho M, et al. Treatment of typhoid fever: Randomized trial of a three-day course of ceftriaxone versus a fourteen-day course of chloramphenicol. Am J Trop Med Hyg 1995;52:162.

266. Doehring E, Reiter-Owana I, Bauer O, et al. Toxoplasma gondii antibodies in pregnant women and their newborns in Salaam, Tanzania. Am J Trop Med Hyg 1995;52:546.

267. Chable-Santos B, Van Wynsberghe NR, Canto-Lara SB, et al. Isolation of Leishmania(L) mexicana from wild rodents and their possible role in the transmission of localized cutaneous leishmaniasis in the state of Campache, Mexico. Am J Trop Med Hyg 1995;53:141.

268. Balzam M, Fenech F. Acute renal failure in visceral leishmaniasis treated with sodium stibogluconate. Trans R Soc Trop Med Hyg 1992;86:515.

269. Jha TK, Giri YN, Singh TK, Jha S. Use of amphotericin B in drug-resistant cases of visceral leishmaniasis in north Bihar, India. Am J Trop Med Hyg 1995;52:536.

270. Raoult D, Stein A. Q fever during pregnancy—a risk for women, fetuses, and obstetricians (letter). N Engl J Med 1994;330:71.

271. Update: Management of patients with suspected viral hemorrhagic fever—United States. JAMA 1995;274:374.

272. Update: Outbreak of Ebola viral hemorrhagic fever—Zaire, 1995. JAMA 1995;274:373.

25

DERMATOSES

Margaret Bunce Garahan, M.D., and Anita Licata, M.D.

THE SKIN AS AN ORGAN SYSTEM

As the largest organ of the human body, the skin plays various critical roles. It forms the water-resistant elastic barrier that protects internal organs from external infection and insult. It assists in temperature regulation with its secretory glands, fat, and rich, dynamic vascular system. Sunlight on the skin facilitates vitamin D production, whereas the melanin pigment found there protects the body from ultraviolet radiation. A sensitive sensory organ, the skin also reveals emotions.[1]

The epidermis, the outermost layer, contains melanocytes as well as tough keratin tissue. In the dermis, active sweat and sebaceous glands, nerve endings, blood vessels, and elastic fibers are found. The vascular hypodermis, or subcutaneous tissue, harbors fat cells and sensory fibers.

ANESTHETIC EFFECTS ON SKIN FUNCTION

Pain is often a warning signal of a body part in distress, demanding attention. General and regional anesthetics mask the pain, thereby increasing the likelihood of injury such as pressure sores, nerve impingement, and trauma. Invasive techniques violate the protective barrier, by definition, inviting bleeding and infection.

Thermoregulation is compromised by muscle paralysis and inability to shiver, as well as by the myriad vasoactive and anticholinergic drugs commonly administered. Hypercapnea and vasodilation associated with anesthesia increase blood flow to the affected areas. These anesthetic effects uncouple the body's centrally driven regulation of temperature from the usual primary reactions of vascular and sweat gland changes.

The anesthesiologist must consider these functions while establishing a perioperative care plan. Guidelines for skin preparation and needle use in the performance of invasive procedures, in patients with dermatologic problems,[2–5] are provided in Table 25–1.

NORMAL SKIN CHANGES OF PREGNANCY

Physical changes in the pregnant woman, along with hormonal influences, cause dermatologic variations. Most of these manifestations are benign, nonproblematic, and temporary, although some (such as striae gravidarum or "stretch marks") may persist long after the delivery. Although the rest of this chapter discusses pathologies of the skin in relation to pregnancy, Table 25–2 delineates those skin changes seen so often in the gravid population that they are considered normal.[6–8]

TABLE 25–1. SKIN PREPARATION AND NEEDLE GUIDELINES FOR INVASIVE PROCEDURES

Skin Preparation/Scrub

There is no universally accepted method for skin preparation

Three cutaneous antiseptics are in common use: 10% povidone-iodine solution, 70% alcohol, and 2% aqueous chlorhexidine (Hibiclens). Of these, only chlorhexidine, which binds most actively to the skin, has residual antimicrobial activity once the skin has dried. This lasts for hours. All three are comparable in providing protection from infection for the short period immediately after topical administration

Chlorhexidine is toxic to mucous membranes, and should not be used near eyelids, lips, or auditory canals

Blisters or bullae should not be vigorously scrubbed, because scrubbing can cause tissue damage and spread of some types of lesions. If such lesions are in the field of a scrub preparation, they should be gently yet generously treated with antiseptic, in a nonfrictional manner

Although topical antiseptics have not been shown to modify disease processes, they can dry skin temporarily, exacerbating eczematous lesions. Therefore, a treatment with petroleum jelly may be beneficial, following a procedure

Needle Instrumentation

When certain pathologic lesions such as psoriasis and sarcoid are traumatized, they are often reactivated

In general, avoid blistered, raw, and open skin when performing invasive procedures, because there is an increased risk of infection

Do not instrument actively infected skin, blisters or bullae, or the lesions of malignant melanoma

Inflammatory sites may be instrumented, with the caveat that the area may harbor *Staphylococcus aureus*

Eczematous patches are not clinically infected, but often are colonized with *S. aureus*. This skin is best left undisturbed

TABLE 25–2. **NORMAL SKIN CHANGES OF PREGNANCY**

Hyperpigmentation of scars, nevi, and areolae are seen, along with the midline abdominal linea nigra, and facial melasma or "mask of pregnancy"

Striae gravidarum or stretch marks can be found on the abdomen, breasts, arms, and thighs

Vascular changes include vessel proliferation, congestion, and vasomotor instability. Varicosities, telangiectasias, and spider angiomas are common, as well as palmar erythema, gingival swelling, and generalized edema

Hair growth modifications rarely include hirsutism. However, the growth cycle of scalp hair changes. The growth phase (anagen) is prolonged, resulting in a thick head of hair. Post partum, a high percentage of the follicles simultaneously enter the resting (telogen) phase, which results in the shedding of strands. This persists for several months.

NOMENCLATURE

The labeling of dermatoses in pregnant and nonpregnant patients has undergone numerous revisions over the years. Many named diseases were found to be identical histologically, representing various clinical manifestations of the same entity. Conversely, other entities looked alike clinically, but were later found to be pathophysiologically distinct. Attempts have been made in this chapter to use the most accurate and currently acceptable nomenclature. Unfortunately, a universally accepted system for naming these diverse dermatologic diseases has not yet evolved.

DERMATOLOGIC DISEASES SEEN ONLY IN PREGNANCY

Polymorphic Eruption of Pregnancy or Pruritic Urticarial Papules and Plaques of Pregnancy

This intensely pruritic eruption is the most common gestational dermatosis, classically manifesting as red papules and plaques (Table 25–3). In the US, the disorder was named descriptively *pruritic urticarial papules and plaques of pregnancy* (PUPPP) by Lawley and colleagues in 1979.[9] Because a few cases may develop vesicles, target lesions, or diffuse erythema, however,

TABLE 25–3. **DERMATOLOGIC DISEASES**

Dermatologic Diseases Seen Only in Pregnancy
Polymorphic eruption of pregnancy (pruritic urticarial papules and plaques of pregnancy)
Intrahepatic cholestasis of pregnancy (pruritus gravidarum)
Pemphigoid of pregnancy (herpes gestationis)
Pustular psoriasis of pregnancy (impetigo herpetiformis)

Other Dermatologic Diseases in Pregnancy

Ehlers-Danlos syndrome	Malignant melanoma
Epidermolysis bullosa	Neurofibromatosis
Erythema multiforme	Pruritic folliculitis
Erythema nodosum	Pyogenic granuloma

the British recommend the term *polymorphic eruption of pregnancy* (PEP),[10] which is gaining acceptance in the world literature. The same clinical entity has also been called Bourne's toxemic rash of pregnancy[11] and Nurse's late onset prurigo of pregnancy.[12]

The incidence of PEP is not clearly established because of the benign nature of the disease and probable underreporting, but is thought to be 1 in 120 to 240 pregnancies.[10, 11]

Clinical Features

The intense itch is accompanied by a skin eruption of erythematous urticarial papules, papulovesicles or plaques, sometimes surrounded by pale halos (Fig. 25–1). The abdomen, particularly the striae, is affected first, with spread to the back and extremities. Generally there is facial sparing.[13] The mucosa is never involved.

Nonspecific histologic findings include perivascular lymphocytes and eosinophils, along with keratosis, spongiosis, and acanthosis.[14] A negative direct immunofluorescent skin biopsy result differentiates the entity from pemphigoid of pregnancy, which can have a similar clinical appearance.[6] Most cases are diagnosed clinically. Consultation should be obtained, however, for atypical presentations and bullous or pustular lesions, or for a patient complaint of systemic symptoms.

Pregnancy and Medical Management

This disease is found only in pregnancy. Usually arising in the third trimester, or rarely, immediately post partum, the majority of cases present in primagravidas and do not recur. It is seen more often with twin gestations, excessive maternal weight gain, and male fetuses.[15, 16] The course of pregnancy is not altered, and there is no additional fetal risk.

Treatment is supportive with topical steroids and antipruritics such as diphenhydramine and hydroxyzine. Topical antipruritics such as calamine or menthol can be used, but phenol is contraindicated in pregnancy. Symptoms may improve within 72 hours with topical treatment, although occasionally systemic steroids are needed. Untreated lesions tend to disappear within a week of delivery.[15] No systemic manifestations of this disease occur.

Anesthetic Management

Anesthetic choices should consider the pre-existing pruritus. It is unknown if spinal or epidural opioids exacerbate the discomfort. It is prudent to avoid anesthetic agents that can release histamine (e.g., *d*-tubocurarine, morphine); see Table 25–4.

Lumbar administration of local anesthetics for spinal or epidural anesthesia is acceptable, avoiding affected areas of skin, if possible. Because this lesion is not

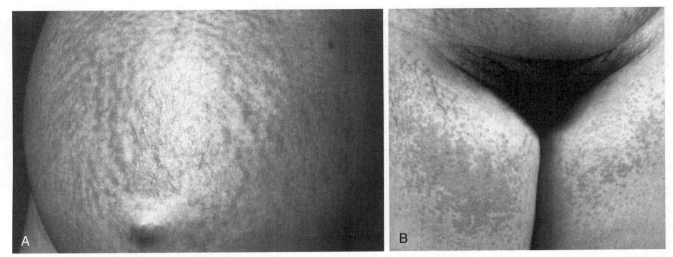

Figure 25–1. Polymorphic eruption of pregnancy (pruritic urticarial papules and plaques of pregnancy). *(A)* The earliest lesions are tiny erythematous papules frequently localized to the striae gravidarum. *(B)* Lesions coalesce to form erythematous plaques and spread to involve buttocks and thighs. (Courtesy of Klaus Wolff, M.D. From Fitzpatrick TB, Eisen AZ, Wolff K (eds). Dermatology in General Medicine, 4th ed., vol 2. New York, McGraw-Hill, 1993, p 2109.)

infected, however, needle instrumentation through it is not specifically contraindicated.

Intrahepatic Cholestasis of Pregnancy or Pruritus Gravidarum

Pruritus gravidarum, now called *intrahepatic cholestasis of pregnancy*, is characterized by a generalized itching that occurs in as many as 15 to 20% of pregnancies.[6, 16] Of these, 3% subsequently develop the severe form, which has fetal implications.[17] The clinical entity is also referred to as *prurigo gravidarum, recurrent cholestasis of pregnancy*, and *benign recurrent intrahepatic cholestasis*. The proposed etiology is hepatic cholestasis resulting from estrogen and progesterone effects on biliary metabolism.[8] A genetic predisposition is suggested by the observed familial tendency of this pruritus.[18]

Clinical Features

The large majority of patients present with an impressive generalized pruritus with an absence of skin lesions, except for excoriations caused by scratching.[18, 19] Troublesome areas are the abdomen and extremities. Cases considered severe are manifested by jaundice, nausea, emesis, right upper quadrant abdominal discomfort, and increased risk of cholelithiasis.[6]

Because there are no primary skin lesions, there is no histology to pursue. Liver biopsy shows dilated bile canaliculi, minimal inflammatory response, and nonspecific cholestasis in the more severe cases.[19] Plasma bile salt elevation is associated with itching, but there is no correlation between concentration of the bile salts and severity of the itch.[20] Laboratory findings include mildly to moderately increased levels of conjugated bilirubin, alkaline phosphatase, and lipids. Although transaminase levels may be slightly elevated, higher levels should raise the suspicion for a hepatocellular process such as viral hepatitis.[19, 21]

No coexisting diseases occur with this entity. Its diagnosis is suggested by pruritus with an absence of lesions and no other indications of systemic involvement save jaundice.[21] Other causes of pruritus must be ruled out, such as drug reaction, lymphoma, scabies, other liver diseases, renal failure, anemia, hyperthyroidism, and hypothyroidism.[18, 22]

Pregnancy and Medical Management

Patients with intrahepatic cholestasis usually present in the second half of pregnancy. Intrahepatic cholestasis

TABLE 25–4. ANESTHETIC MEDICATIONS AND HISTAMINE RELEASE

Agents That Cause Histamine Release	Agents That Do Not Cause Histamine Release
Opioids: morphine, codeine, meperidine	Opioids: fentanyl, alfentanil, sufentanil (these can cause pruritus, especially if given spinally)
Neuromuscular blocking agents: curare, gallamine, metocurine, mivacurium, atracurium	Neuromuscular blocking agents: vecuronium, pancuronium, rocuronium, pipecuronium, cisatracurium, succinylcholine*
Thiobarbiturates: thiopental, thiamylal	Barbiturates: methohexital, pentobarbital
Antibiotics: vancomycin	Intravenous induction agents: propofol, etomidate, ketamine
Anticholinergics: atropine	Benzodiazepines: midazolam, diazepam

*Histamine release occurs but is slight and clinically unimportant if the drug is injected slowly.

recurs in about half of subsequent pregnancies and with oral contraceptive use. The course of the pregnancy itself is not affected by the disease, but there are fetal implications. Fisk and Storey[23] found low birth weight and prematurity (44%) in the more severe cases, along with an increased incidence of meconium (45%) at birth. They also reported a perinatal mortality of 0.35%, but this is no different from the incidence in the general population. Postpartum symptoms resolve spontaneously.

Treatment is symptomatic. Unfortunately, resolution of symptoms can be elusive. Phototherapy with ultraviolet B (UVB) radiation; antihistamines; topical steroids; and cholestyramines, which bind bile acids, are all possibilities. Supplemental vitamin K before delivery may be needed if fat absorption is affected by the bile changes.[24]

Anesthetic Management

Significant liver pathology must be ruled out with laboratory tests (serum glutamic-oxaloacetic transaminase [SGOT], serum glutamic-pyruvic transminase [SGPT], alkaline phosphatase, bilirubin levels). Other causes of itching must be ruled out by checking complete blood count (CBC), blood urea nitrogen (BUN), serum creatinine, and, possibly, thyroid function. (See the differential diagnosis.) Results of the physical examination should be normal, with the exception of excoriation.

The airway is not affected. The choice of anesthetic need not be modified because of this disease, although narcotic use may exacerbate pruritus or lead to biliary spasm (rare). No special considerations exist for monitoring or postoperative care.

Pemphigoid of Pregnancy or Herpes Gestationis

The term *herpes gestationis* (HG) was initially used by Milton in 1872.[25] This autoimmune disease of pregnancy is nonviral, thereby bearing no relation to herpes simplex, other than the observable eruption of vesicles. The name *pemphigoid gestationis* or *pemphigoid of pregnancy* (PP) was assigned by the British because of immunopathologic similarities between the disease in pregnancy and bullous pemphigoid (BP). Although the two are closely related in antigen-antibody features, there are sufficient clinical dissimilarities to justify their distinction. Most notably, BP is a disease of the elderly with no known reaction to hormonal stimulation.[26]

PP is a rare disorder, with a reported incidence ranging from 1 in 3000 to 1 in 50,000. The latter estimate is thought to be more valid. PP is found primarily in whites, presumably because the subtypes of the specific associated human lymphocyte antigens (HLA) are seldom seen in the black population.[27] Incidence among other races is unknown.

Clinical Features

The lesions of PP are polymorphic, with erythematous urticarial plaques that migrate outward from the peripheral margins, often becoming ringed with vesicles and tense bullae. The eruption typically begins periumbilically, with spread to the abdomen, trunk, buttocks, and extremities (Fig. 25–2).[26] Facial and oral lesions are rare. The pruritus can be intense.

A skin biopsy sample examined by immunofluorescent microscopy shows a subepidermal blister with basement membrane deposits of C3 complement and occasionally IgG antibodies.[21] The antigenic target is a 180-kd hemidesmosomal protein, identical to one of the proteins recognized in bullous pemphigoid. Women with PP may develop additional autoantibodies, and there are sporadic reports of Graves disease, alopecia areata, and primary biliary cirrhosis.[27] One study of 75 patients with PP revealed that 11% subsequently developed Graves disease.[28]

The differential diagnosis includes dermatitis herpetiformis, PEP, erythema multiforme, and BP. The most likely diseases with this presentation are PEP and PP. Proper diagnosis is important, because only the latter recurs with subsequent pregnancies and has potential fetal effects. Skin biopsy for immunofluorescence is the diagnostic test of choice, allowing identification of the pathologic antibodies microscopically.[29]

Pregnancy and Medical Management

Patients with PP generally present during the second trimester, but the condition may occur later, even post partum. The disease usually flares immediately after

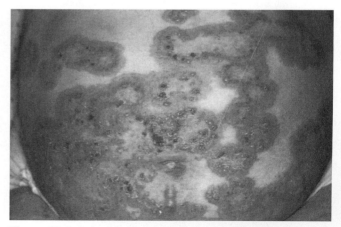

Figure 25–2. Pemphigoid of pregnancy (herpes gestationis). Eruption in a pregnant woman on day 10 demonstrates urticarial plaques with vesicles at the margins. Lesions migrate peripherally to become merged. (From Sams WM, Lynch PJ (eds). Principles and Practice of Dermatology, 2nd ed. New York, Churchill Livingstone, 1996, p 463.)

delivery and then slowly resolves over weeks to months post partum.[30] PP has also been associated with choriocarcinoma of pregnancy, hydatiform mole, and oral contraceptive use,[6] implicating hormonal influence and placental tissue[27] in the pathogenesis of this anti-epidermal antibody-mediated disease.

Lawley and coworkers[31] noted a 22% incidence of preterm delivery and 3 fetal deaths among 40 documented cases of PP. Holmes and Black[32] reported low birth weight in 26% of 50 studied births. Shornick and Black[33] subsequently confirmed these reports of a tendency to premature and small-for-gestational age babies, but found no increase in fetal mortality. Neonatal gestational herpes occurs in under 10% of children of affected mothers.[27] Passive transfer of IgG antibody is the probable mechanism resulting in mild, self-limiting skin lesions.[34]

The goal is to limit blister formation, secondary infection, and scarring.[26] Systemic steroids are the cornerstone of therapy. Less successful treatment modalities include pyridoxine and plasmapheresis.[27] Oral antihistamines are given to treat the impressive itch. Infants of mothers who were dependent on high-dose steroids should be assessed for adrenal insufficiency.[26]

Anesthetic Management

PP is an antibody reaction, not an infective process; therefore, invasive procedures can be used in mildly involved areas, if necessary. Utilizing the unaffected skin is best, however. Blisters should not be the sites for needles or frictional preparations. Stress-dose steroid should be employed if the patient is receiving daily steroid medication. Possible exacerbation of pruritus should be considered when using narcotics.

The airway is not involved. No specific recommendations are needed for anesthetic choices and postoperative care.

Pustular Psoriasis of Pregnancy or Impetigo Herpetiformis

This noninfectious pustular dermatosis was first described by Von Hebra in 1872.[35] It is extremely rare, with just over 100 cases cited in the world literature.[19] The term *impetigo herpetiformis* is a medical misnomer because the disease is related to neither bacterial impetigo nor viral herpes.[6] The term *pustular psoriasis of pregnancy (PPP)* is preferred, because the disease clinically and histologically resembles a variant of pustular psoriasis.[36, 37] The etiology remains elusive.

Clinical Features

The onset is usually acute, with a concomitant fever and eruption of erythematous plaques rimmed with sterile pustules. The lesions first appear in the skin folds of the groin and under the breasts. The pustules expand and migrate outward, and they may eventually cover a significant portion of the body, including mucous membranes and nails (Fig. 25–3). The face, hands, and feet are generally spared, although painful oral and esophageal erosions have been reported.[19] Secondary infections and vegetative lesions are complications of the more serious, persistent forms. The skin eventually becomes crusted while healing and may remain hyperpigmented.[7, 18, 35]

Remarkable systemic symptoms often accompany the skin lesions. These symptoms include fever, chills, nausea, vomiting, diarrhea, malaise, and arthralgia. Convulsions and tetany may occur from hypocalcemia. Pruritus is rare.[7, 18, 35]

Laboratory evaluation is needed to differentiate pustular psoriasis from an infectious process, a pustular drug reaction, or Sweet's syndrome (acute febrile neutrophilic dermatosis). Histologically, the findings in PPP are consistent with those of psoriasis, with characteristic subcorneal collections of neutrophils. Immunofluorescence test results are negative, differentiating it from PP. Unless there is a secondary infection, skin and blood culture results are negative. Abnormal laboratory findings include elevated sedimentation rate, leukocytosis with left shift, hypoalbuminemia, and hypocalcemia, occasionally associated with hypoparathyroidism.[6, 18]

Pregnancy and Medical Management

Patients with PPP present usually in the third trimester, although the condition has been described in the second trimester.[35] Before the advent of systemic steroid and antibiotic treatments, both fetal and maternal

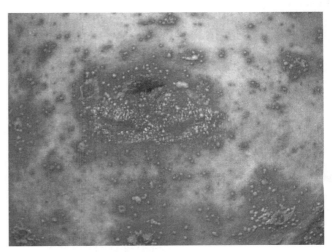

Figure 25–3. Pustular psoriasis of pregnancy (impetigo herpetiformis). Note erythematous patches that are studded with tiny superficial pustules. (Courtesy of Klaus Wolff, M.D. From Fitzpatrick TB, Eisen AZ, Wolff K (eds). Dermatology in General Medicine, 4th ed, vol 2. New York. McGraw-Hill, 1993, p 2109.)

demise were common. Winton and Lewis[19] reported in 1982 that "a large percentage of patients succumbed within days or weeks to hyperthermia, prostration, renal failure, or cardiac failure. Abortion, stillbirth, and neonatal death were frequent."

Placental insufficiency and stillbirth may still occur, despite apparent disease control with corticosteroids. Maternal mortality is now rare.[19] The disease clears spontaneously post partum, but it may recur earlier in the course of subsequent pregnancies.[38]

Hypocalcemia is treated medically, and antibiotics are administered for secondary infections. Prednisone is usually initiated at 1 mg·kg^{-1}·day^{-1} and then tapered as quickly as possible. The synthetic retinoids etretinate and isotretinoin, which are now the drugs of choice for pustular psoriasis treatment, are potent teratogens and are contraindicated in pregnancy.[6] Other approaches such as methotrexate and dapsone have had limited success,[35] and they should be given with caution in pregnancy.

Anesthetic Management

The need for steroids and supplemental doses should be assessed perioperatively. Because of the associated derangement in calcium metabolism, ionized serum calcium, phosphate, and magnesium levels should be measured preoperatively and postoperatively. Although severe calcium deficiency is rare, intravenous calcium gluconate should be given before surgery, if needed. Roizen recommends 10 to 20 ml of 10% calcium gluconate at an initial rate of 10 ml/min. Because the effect on serum calcium levels is short-lived, a further recommendation is to administer 10 ml of 10% calcium gluconate, diluted in 500 ml of solution, over about 6 hours.[39] If the hypocalcemia is chronic, it is reasonable to try to maintain serum calcium levels in the low-normal range. Respiratory alkalosis decreases serum levels of ionized calcium,[39] and thus normocarbia is recommended during controlled ventilation.

The electrocardiogram must be evaluated because changes reflect the calcium status. The QT interval may be prolonged owing to delays in ventricular repolarization, and it should be monitored intraoperatively.[39]

Patients in various states of "control" of this disease may also present with dehydration from nausea, emesis, and diarrhea; hypoalbuminemia; renal and cardiac compromise; and heightened potential for tetany and seizures. The anesthesiologist must remain vigilant in searching for signs of these derangements and must ensure that the mother's condition is stable before anesthetic intervention and birth.

The airway may be compromised with esophageal and oral mucosal lesions, especially during a peripartum flare. Because secondary skin infection is not uncommon with this disease, affected areas of skin should be avoided for invasive procedures. The choice of anes-

thetic techniques remains standard, with consideration of the earlier-mentioned complications.

OTHER DERMATOLOGIC DISEASES AND PREGNANCY

Ehlers-Danlos Syndrome

Clinical Features

The skin is fragile, thin, and easily torn in this genetic disease of collagen synthesis. Frequently, cutaneous hemorrhages are followed by cutaneous pseudotumors, which are a form of scarring. Surgical sutures hold poorly because skin margins are friable.[40]

Nine subtypes of this disease have been identified, with varying degrees of clinical severity. Typically there is hyperdistensible skin and hypermobile joints, with vascular fragility. The vascular fragility leads to varicose veins and excessive bleeding, despite normal clotting factors. An increased risk of aortic rupture, aortic regurgitation, mitral valve prolapse, and cardiac conduction abnormalities exists. Gastrointestinal and uterine collagen fibers are highly affected, which may result in bowel and uterine rupture. Pneumothorax risk is also increased in this population.[1, 41–43]

Pregnancy and Medical Management

Three inheritance patterns have been identified: autosomal dominant, recessive, and X-linked. Prevalence is 1 in 156,000.[40] Maternal or fetal disease leads to premature rupture of membranes and preterm delivery.[44] Maternal mortality is as high as 25%, primarily due to bleeding complications.[45] Diagnosis of this congenital disease is achieved by antenatal or neonatal tissue biopsy. Treatment is symptomatic; there is no cure. Genetic counseling is recommended before conception.[40]

Anesthetic Management

Because of the varied presentations of this disease, and probable multi-organ involvement, the following anesthetic recommendations are presented. Prophylactic antibiotics should be considered for patients with cardiac abnormalities, which predispose them to subacute bacterial endocarditis. Bleeding tendency complicates arterial and large-bore peripheral and central venous access; intravenous fluids may extravasate into distensible skin unnoticed. Intramuscular injections and instrumentation of the nose or esophagus should be avoided, also because of bleeding risk.[43]

Clinicians must carefully weigh the risks, benefits, and patients' wishes in considering the types of anesthesia. Spinal and epidural anesthesia have been used safely.[41] Anesthetic drug choices are as usual, with ability to treat hypertension aggressively if needed, to minimize blood loss. Sufficient crossmatched blood must be available, because there is risk of hemorrhage, postpartum bleeding, and wound dehiscence. General anesthesia requires delicate handling of the airway because of possible cervical spine involvement as well as tissue injury. Low airway pressures are needed because of the risk of pneumothorax.[43] Spontaneous ventilation is best, if possible. Elaborate padding of pressure points is necessary throughout the perioperative period.

Epidermolysis Bullosa

The disease entity known as *epidermolysis bullosa* (EB) was first described in 1886 by the German physician Koebner.[46] It is now known to include at least 23 clinical variants, all having three features in common: genetic transmission, fragile skin, and recurrent bullae or blister formation following minimal mechanical trauma. The true incidence of the three major subsets (simplex, junctional, and dystrophic) of this heterogeneous group of disorders is unknown. More than 2200 patients are enrolled in the National Epidermolysis Bullosa Registry, however.[30]

Clinical Features

The degree of disease manifestation and prognosis varies widely within and among subtypes. For example, EB simplex onset may be noted from birth to adulthood, with trivial to extensive blistering. Although rarely seen in the simplex group, oral and esophageal bullae resulting in microstomia, ankyloglossia, and esophageal strictures are noteworthy in the junctional and dystrophic disease categories. In the severe forms of EB, pervasive blistering with crusting and atrophic scarring of the skin and mucous membranes can lead to compromise of the gastrointestinal, genitourinary, ocular, and musculoskeletal systems (Fig. 25–4).[29]

Coexisting diseases that have been cited are pyloric atresia, amyloidosis, multiple myeloma, diabetes mellitus, and hypercoagulable states. Anemia of chronic disease and malnutrition, with electrolyte abnormalities, may also be seen.[47] Partridge and Phil[48] note that although reference is made to an increased incidence of porphyria in EB patients, those tested have been found to be negative.

Some variants of EB are autosomal dominant, and some recessive, all with variable expression, accounting for the broad ranges of life expectancy and clinical presentation. For those with severe cases of junctional and recessive dystrophic EB, the disease is often fatal within the first 2 years of life.[49] Those who survive infancy have lifelong exacerbations following minimal

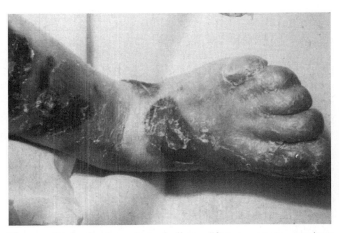

Figure 25–4. Epidermolysis bullosa. Blisters, crusts, erosions, atrophic scarring, and early web formation mark this severe, dystrophic form of the disease. (From Sams WM, Lynch PJ (eds). Principles and Practice of Dermatology, 2nd ed. New York, Churchill Livingstone, 1996, p 477.)

trauma. This course profoundly affects their lifestyles and capabilities. Fairly normal activity is tolerated by those with mild disease.

Classification of the three major groups (simplex, junctional, and dystrophic) is based on electron microscopic findings related to structure. Gene mutations leading to cleavages within and between the dermal and epidermal layers play a role in the pathogenesis.[29, 50] General diagnosis may be simple and obvious early in life, but subtype classification requires either immunofluorescent mapping or transmission electron microscopy. Gene sequencing ultimately will allow true subtype diagnosis.

Pregnancy and Medical Management

Although there is no evidence that pregnancy accelerates the disease process, or that the disease affects the course of the pregnancy, the fetus is clearly at risk for transmission of this inherited disease. Prepregnancy genetic counseling is therefore indicated. Prenatal diagnosis of the fetus is available via fetal skin biopsy.[49] Treatment consists of protective and supportive care. Because trivial trauma can lead to devastating skin lesions, utmost care is indicated in physical examinations and therapeutic interventions.

Anesthetic Management

Because of the extreme sensitivity of skin and mucous membranes, modifications in anesthetic monitoring must be made to avoid shearing or rubbing of the involved areas. The clinical importance of each perioperative monitor must be assessed in relation to the potential trauma it may cause the patient. Webroll can be placed under blood pressure cuffs, tourniquets, and stethoscopes. Electrocardiographic electrode adhesive should be cut away or left covered, and the electrodes attached to the skin with gauze banding or loose paper tape over the entire torso. Needle electrodes can be immobilized with gauze wrapping. Because adhesive tapes should be avoided completely, intravenous and arterial lines may be held in place with gauze or they may be sutured, as necessary.

If disease progression makes intravenous access impossible, a central venous catheter may be needed and a cutdown procedure performed, as noted by Berryhill and coworkers in 1978.[51] The eyes should be generously lubricated rather than taped for corneal protection. Invasive procedures may penetrate scar tissue but should not directly enter a bulla.

Regional anesthesia has been administered successfully for cesarean births. Broster and coworkers[47] presented cases of effective spinal and epidural management, including local skin infiltration at the site of epidural placement, without the subsequent formation of a bulla. The epidural catheter was used for labor analgesia and subsequently during cesarean birth for cephalopelvic disproportion. The investigators chose this regional technique to avoid the possible complications of trauma to the airway.

Airway management remains the primary concern in general anesthesia. Oral intubation is relatively safe in terms of avoiding new bullae formation and its hemorrhagic consequences. James and Wark[52] noted an increased incidence of difficult intubation due to scarring and restricted mouth opening, however, and they suggested that a vasoconstrictor-soaked gauze may prove helpful if an oral bulla ruptures. Berryhill and coworkers[51] advocate a laryngoscopic blade and a small endotracheal tube, "dripping" in lubricant and sterile ointment, if intubation of the trachea is necessary. Positive-pressure ventilation via a face mask may cause significant trauma. These same investigators describe the application of a thick coat of lubricant and hydrocortisone ointment to both the facial skin and anesthetic face mask, with no more than light nonshearing pressure applied. Artificial airways were avoided, and spontaneous ventilation was assisted intermittently. It is unknown if cricoid pressure was applied. Interestingly, their case involved emergency cesarean birth for a woman with significant lumbar lesions, precluding a regional technique.

The choice of anesthetic agents need not be affected by the disease unless the patient presents with significant systemic involvement. Although the association with porphyria is unproved, the clinician may choose among the readily available alternatives to sodium pentothal. In the parturient, ketamine is a recommended option. Deep paralysis with a nondepolarizing muscle relaxant eliminates the risk of succinylcholine-induced fasciculations and potential skin trauma. Deep paralysis also facilitates an atraumatic intubation. Rapid-sequence intubation protocol is necessary to guard against aspiration. Intramuscular injections should be avoided, if possible.[1]

Erythema Multiforme

Erythema multiforme (EM) is an acute, sometimes recurrent, inflammatory disease of the skin and mucous membranes. EM *minor* describes cases of typical target lesions, lacking mucosal involvement and constitutional symptoms of fever, malaise, and arthralgias. EM *major*, also known as *Stevens-Johnson syndrome*, is a far more serious, life-threatening disease with mucosal lesions and occasional multisystem involvement.[53] In half of reported cases the specific etiology is never identified. Precipitating factors are thought to include viral, bacterial, fungal, and parasitic infections, as well as drugs such as barbiturates, antibiotics, nonsteroidal anti-inflammatory agents, salicylates, anticonvulsants, and digitalis. Stevens-Johnson syndrome may also be a manifestation of a collagen-vascular or neoplastic disease.[48]

EM occurs primarily in young healthy persons. One third of cases are recurrent, and these are usually preceded by recurrent herpes simplex virus (HSV) infection. Prophylactic or suppressive therapy with acyclovir prevents attacks. Mortality in EM major is between 3 and 18%.[1, 53]

Clinical Features

Purpuric, vesiculobullous target lesions may accompany macules, papules, and urticarial-appearing areas on any part of the body. These lesions can arrive as a storm and may last 1 to 4 weeks. Patients with EM major may develop large bullae with ulcerated erosions of the nose, mouth, trachea, and bronchus. The conjunctiva, esophagus, and colon are at risk along with the genital mucosa, which may lead to vaginal stenosis. Nutrition is compromised because of the painful oral pathology.[48]

Bacterial secondary infection is not uncommon. Hepatitis, glomerulonephritis, cardiac involvement, and pneumonia are less common serious complications.[53] Fluid and electrolyte balance may be deranged, and the patient may be anemic.[48] Mortality is primarily due to secondary infections and pneumonia.[48]

Target lesions have an identifiable histopathology of necrotic keratinocytes, dermal endothelial swelling, and papillary edema. Diagnosis is based on histology, but underlying disease must be sought via screening laboratory tests and consideration of infectious etiologies. If target lesions are not present, the differential diagnosis process is lengthy.[53]

Pregnancy and Medical Management

Idiopathic EM is more common in pregnancy.[54] The most commonly associated infections are from HSV and mycoplasma. Drug reaction is a trigger as well. The effect of EM on the fetus and the course of pregnancy is not well documented. Underlying pathologies that are associated with this problem, however, may lead to complications of pregnancy.

Because the disease is often mild and self-limiting, treatment can be symptomatic. Controversial treatment for those with more serious disease includes steroids and skin débridement. Systemic support including respiratory therapy may be needed; associated conditions should be treated and suspect drugs discontinued. Unfortunately, more definitive treatment has not been identified.[53]

Anesthetic Management

Anesthetic considerations are similar to those for patients with epidermolysis bullosa. Considerations are extreme caution with an ulcerated airway and avoidance of friction on bullous lesions. Positive-pressure ventilation may increase the risk of pneumothorax in the presence of pulmonary bullae.[43] Ketamine has been used successfully in these patients,[1] but nitrous oxide should be avoided in the presence of pulmonary blebs.[43] Regional anesthesia may offer the least risk if the lumbar area is unaffected.

Erythema Nodosum

Erythema nodosum is characterized by tender red nodules usually first appearing on the extensor surfaces of the lower extremities. Skin changes are thought to be a hypersensitivity reaction to medication or infection at distant sites. Although 30% of cases are idiopathic, the most common triggering agents are drugs, particularly antibiotics, streptococcal infection, and sarcoidosis. Numerous other associations include malignancies such as Hodgkin's disease and leukemia; bacterial, fungal, viral, and protozoan infections; and inflammatory bowel disease.[55]

The incidence and etiology are thought to vary with different populations. The prevalence in Western countries is less than 1%.[56] The disease is most common in women aged 20 to 40 years. The disease is thought to be precipitated by pregnancy and oral contraceptives, thus suggesting estrogen involvement in its pathogenesis.[6]

Clinical Features

A prodrome of arthralgia, fever, chills, malaise, and rarely abdominal pain may herald the eruption of warm, tender, erythematous nodules. These nodules can become multiple, and plaques may appear on the trunk, arms, neck, and face. Nodules do not ulcerate, but they are transformed from red to a livid violet,

then turn yellow, as a bruise, during the usual 3- to 6-week course of the illness. A less common chronic form of the disease can last for years. Frequently, there is aseptic joint swelling with lower extremity edema, but the mucosal surfaces are not involved.[48, 53, 55]

A deep incisional biopsy containing subcutaneous fat is required for histopathologic diagnosis. Acutely, neutrophils are seen in the fat tissues, interlobular septa, and small vessels. This stage is followed by chronic lymphocytic septal infiltration and eventually noncaseating granuloma, which is rare. These findings are highly suggestive but not specific to erythema nodosum.[53] Bartelsmeyer[55] states, "The most likely conclusion is that erythema nodosum represents the end stage of an immunologic process that can be initiated by a wide variety of antigenic stimuli."

Classic skin findings along with the incisional biopsy results should yield a working diagnosis. Treatment consists of eliminating the causative substance or underlying disorder. Untreated, the disease is self-limiting within 5 to 6 weeks, but the patient is at risk from the underlying primary process.[48] Useful laboratory tests include CBC, pharyngeal culture, and chest radiograph for coccidioidomycosis, blastomycosis, and histoplasmosis, and intradermal skin test for tuberculosis.

A chest radiograph is indicated. The ionizing radiation from a chest radiograph is 5–10 mrads ($\sim$0.1 mGy), which is less than 5% of the maximal recommended exposure in pregnancy. Abdominal shielding minimizes exposure to the fetus.[57]

Pregnancy and Medical Management

Pregnancy is thought to be a stimulus leading to exacerbation of this rare disease, if not the primary inciting factor. It is generally seen in the first trimester.[58] The disease is not known to affect the course of pregnancy or the fetus.

As mentioned earlier, treatment is of the underlying disease, and there is a multitude of possible triggering conditions to be considered. Symptomatic relief with nonsteroidal anti-inflammatory agents is often successful. Systemic corticosteroids are generally avoided because of the probability of an ongoing infective process.[53] Topical steroids, emollients, and oral antihistamines have been employed.[6] Obstetric concerns are those dictated by the presentation and treatment of the underlying pathology.

Anesthetic Management

Elucidation of the etiology is important, and the involvement of other organ systems must be considered. A chest radiograph should be examined for evidence of sarcoid or other lesions. Pulmonary function tests may be indicated.[48]

Steroids should be avoided unless directly indicated.[48] Joint pain consistent with arthritis dictates careful airway assessment and patient positioning.[48] Antiseptic precautions are especially important because of possible infectious etiologies.[48] A needle may be placed through a reactive area, because the nodules are not infected. Regional or general anesthesia can be administered. There are no special postoperative considerations.

Malignant Melanoma

Cutaneous melanoma is a visible tumor arising from malignant melanocytic cells in the skin.[59] The incidence of this disease is rising faster than that of any other cancer in the US, and it is projected that by the year 2000 the prevalence will be 1 in 90.[60] Half of that population will be female, and one third of them will be of childbearing age.[61] Thus, melanoma during pregnancy will become increasingly common.

Risk factors are diverse and include a positive family history (10-fold increased risk),[62] white race, light complexion, increased numbers of nevi, and tendency to sunburn.[63] The role of UV sunlight remains highly suspect, along with depletion of the earth's ozone layer. UV light alone, however, does not induce melanoma in animals.[64]

Clinical Features

Some melanomas arise from pre-existing nevi, whereas others arise de novo. The characteristic ABCD markings differentiate the melanoma from the expected hyperpigmentation of nevi during pregnancy. The American Academy of Dermatology describes them as follows:

- A—asymmetry
- B—border irregularity
- C—color variation or dark black color
- D—diameter greater than 0.6 cm (the size of a pencil eraser).[64]

Diagnosis is by skin biopsy; prognosis is directly related to the level of thickness and depth of invasion. Lymph node involvement and distant metastases are grim findings. The current 5-year survival rate is 83%, but the overall population mortality rate has increased nearly 150% in the US over the past 40 years.[64]

Multiple organ systems can be affected by metastases. The primary targets are liver, lung, bone, and brain.[65] Once these distant visceral sites are involved, the prognosis is very poor, with a median survival interval of 6 months or less.[63]

Pregnancy and Medical Management

The prognosis for the woman diagnosed with melanoma during pregnancy is a subject of debate.[66] The prevailing thought is that pregnancy does not change the natural history of this disease.[67, 68] The 5-year survival rate for women with melanoma during pregnancy is similar to that of the nonpregnant population (86%).[69] Terminating a pregnancy does not extend or precipitate remission.[70] Although it is the most common malignancy to metastasize to the placenta and fetus, cases are extremely rare. Only 16 cases have been reported, with four fetal deaths. Therefore, termination of pregnancy to avoid this unhappy outcome is not recommended.[71]

Surgical excision is the treatment of choice for early stages of the disease, with or without lymph node sampling, depending on involvement. Palliative treatment is available for those with advanced metastatic disease. Palliative approach includes radiation, immunotherapy, corticosteroid therapy, and chemotherapy, all of which have a significant impact on the mother and fetus. Schwartz[71] recommends ". . . early delivery of the fetus in the third trimester once fetal lung maturation has been achieved . . . for (advanced) stage patients."

Several chemotherapeutic agents have been tried, with only 25% response rates. All antineoplastic agents have mutagenic, teratogenic, carcinogenic, and abortifacient potential. Obviously, it is best to avoid them in pregnant and nursing mothers, but some clinicians may believe that the benefits outweigh risks. Four drugs that have been used are listed next, with known organ effects.[72]

1. Bleomycin: renal, hepatic, pulmonary, and vascular involvement
2. Vincristine: autonomic dysfunction, uric acid neuropathy (joint and low back pain), neurotoxicity (blurred vision, cerebellar effects), distal extremity pain, and syndrome of inappropriate antidiuretic hormone (SIADH) secretion
3. CCNU (lomustine): blood dyscrasia, lung, liver, and renal pathology
4. DTIC (dacarbazine): blood dyscrasia; liver and renal compromise.

Anesthetic Management

The preoperative assessment of the parturient with malignant melanoma should focus on the history of the disease and the treatment protocols she has received. Review of systems includes clinical symptoms of organ involvement, from tumor metastases to the brain, liver, lungs, and bone, and from therapeutic measures mentioned earlier. Blood tests to evaluate the current status are CBC, BUN, serum creatinine, serum electrolytes, uric acid, and tests of liver function and coagulation. Lung spirometry should be reserved for patients with clinical symptoms of pulmonary compromise. It is unlikely that the airway will be affected unless radiation therapy has targeted this area.

Regional anesthesia is acceptable. Blood dyscrasias, including thrombocytopenia, must be considered as usual in anesthetic management. General anesthetic choices should reflect an awareness of any systemic pathology. These considerations are minimal in those with local disease only, but they may be important in parturients with advanced disease, such as those with pulmonary, hepatic, and neurologic compromise.

Neurofibromatosis

This autosomal dominant disease (also known as von Recklinghausen disease) is consistently, slowly progressive. Numerous nerve sheath–derived neurofibromas grow in the skin, along peripheral nerves and nerve roots, as well as on viscera innervated by the autonomic nervous system.[73] Ranging in size from a few millimeters to large masses weighing several kilograms, they can be discrete or can be interdigitating through surrounding tissue, causing functional compromise and cosmetic distress. The incidence is 1 in 3500,[73] with 100% genetic penetrance and variable phenotypic expression. Half of all clinical cases appear to be spontaneous mutations.

Clinical Features

Café-au-lait spots are a hallmark of the disease. The lesions are tan macules ranging in size from 1.5 cm to more than 15 cm. Histologic features consist of basilar hyperpigmentation of the epidermis with giant melanosomes.[73] These spots are often present at birth; they increase in number until about age 6 years and enlarge in proportion to the child's growth. Lesions are rarely seen on the scalp, palms of the hands, or soles of the feet.

Malignant neurofibrosarcomas develop in about 3% of patients with neurofibromatosis.[74] Seen also are optic glioma, pseudoarthrosis with tibial bowing, short stature, scoliosis, microcephaly, seizures, decreased mental capacity, pheochromocytoma, diffuse interstitial lung disease,[75] renal artery stenosis from mass effect, and vertebral changes from fibroma.[73] Neurofibromas rarely appear before adolesence and may first develop during pregnancy.

Definitive diagnostic criteria include two of seven clinical features, including (1) six or more café-au-lait spots, (2) inguinal or axillary freckling, (3) optic gliomas, (4) specific osseous lesions, (5) neurofibromas, (6) Lisch nodules of the iris (seen in 95% of cases by age 10), and (7) affected first-degree relative. Magnetic resonance imaging (MRI) is indicated for management decisions as the disease progresses. There is no cure. Surgical treatment is reserved for cosmetic debilitation and functional compromise. The carbon dioxide laser has been utilized to excise numerous small cutaneous lesions.[73]

Pregnancy and Medical Management

Neurofibromas often increase in size and number during pregnancy, which can lead to significant functional compromise particularly with spinal involvement. Luckily, there may be partial or complete regression post partum. This disease can be associated with hypertension during pregnancy. It is speculated that the vascular beds are fixed in size and unable to accommodate the increased fluid volumes of pregnancy, thus causing the hypertension. An unreplicated study describes an increased incidence of stillbirth.[76]

No medical treatment is available for neurofibromatosis. Symptomatic treatment may include anticonvulsants for seizure activity. Management during pregnancy requires vigilance for organ involvement with expected neurofibroma growth and surgical treatment, if necessary.

Anesthetic Management

Assessment should be made for pulmonary involvement, including implications of kyphoscoliosis and chronic lung disease. Preoperative spirometry, intraoperative blood gas analysis, and postoperative ventilatory support may be indicated. Signs of systemic pathology such as pheochromocytoma, renal artery stenosis, and seizures must be carefully considered. Clinicians must be prepared to treat hypertension quickly. Neurologic changes should be documented preoperatively. The airway examination may identify cervical spine compromise or laryngeal fibromas, necessitating fiberoptic intubation or other special considerations such as MRI for further assessment. Protection of pressure points is important because of the disease's natural history of neurologic abnormalities.[48]

Regional anesthesia is contraindicated only if there is evidence of elevated intracranial pressure from intracranial tumors. Otherwise, spinal and epidural techniques are preferred for labor and delivery, including cesarean birth.[77, 78] Needle placement should avoid areas of spinal neurofibromas. MRI confirmation is required before any invasive procedure is performed if there are clinical symptoms or signs of spinal cord compromise. The café-au-lait spots need not be avoided. No specific anesthetic agents are recommended for general anesthesia. Autonomic hyperreflexia should be expected in patients with spinal cord lesions above the mid-thorax. Succinylcholine should be limited if muscular atrophy is present. Sensitivity to nondepolarizing neuromuscular blocking agents (NMBA) has been noted.[48, 79]

Pruritic Folliculitis of Pregnancy

This erythematous, follicular, papular eruption was first described in 1981 in six patients in their second or third trimesters of pregnancy.[80] The lesions are distributed primarily on the trunk and resolve quickly post partum or with topical steroid cream.[21, 81] Incidence and etiology are unknown.[82] Laboratory values are normal. Histological examination shows amicrobial folliculitis with neutrophils.[81] Some investigators believe that this is a form of hormonally induced acne,[83, 84] and others believe that it is a variant of PEP.[21] No known maternal or fetal effects occur.[21, 82] Thus, anesthetic concerns are limited to avoiding affected sites, if possible, when performing invasive procedures. Because the lesions are not infected, however, this is not an absolute recommendation.

Pyogenic Granuloma

These "pregnancy tumors" are found on the gingiva of 2% of pregnant women. They are friable red nodules that bleed easily with mild trauma. A coexisting gingivitis is often present. Histologically, the granulation tissue is infiltrated with inflammatory cells and covered with a stratified epithelium. No link with infection has been established. Surgical treatment is sought in extreme cases. Otherwise, spontaneous involution occurs post partum.[7, 8, 22] Potential for difficult airway management is the only anesthetic consideration with this disorder.

BACTERIAL AND VIRAL DISEASES WITH DERMATOLOGIC MANIFESTATIONS
(Table 25–5)

Herpes Simplex Virus

Skin Lesion. Herpes simplex virus (HSV) is marked by collections of erythematous papules, vesicles, and pustules with eventual crusting by 7 to 10 days. Recurrences of the disease are less symptomatic and manifest less cutaneous involvement.[85]

Symptoms and Course. Primary infections often cause symptoms of fever, lymphadenopathy, malaise,

TABLE 25–5. BACTERIAL AND VIRAL DISEASES WITH DERMATOLOGIC MANIFESTATIONS

Herpes simplex virus	Parvovirus B19
HIV	Rubella
Human papillomavirus	Rubeola
Lyme disease	Varicella
Neisseria gonorrhoeae	

and myalgia associated with viremia. Latency periods can last years, and there is no cure.

Maternal-Fetal Transmission. The virus generally spreads from mother to fetus during close mucocutaneous contact at birth.

Newborn Pathology. This is a feared disease of the newborn, with 60% mortality. Fetuses are often born prematurely, and half of survivors suffer neurologic or ophthalmic morbidity.[86]

Medical Therapy and Effects. Acyclovir, the only known medical treatment, decreases symptoms but does not provide a cure. Its safety in pregnancy is unknown. Acyclovir is excreted via the kidney, with minimal maternal toxicity.

Anesthetic Implications. Epidural morphine has been shown to reactivate latent HSV after cesarean birth,[87, 88] and thus the risks and benefits should be carefully weighed. One investigator cautions against regional anesthesia in women with primary attacks of HSV at the time of birth, because of the risk of viremia.[89]

Human Immunodeficiency Virus

Skin Lesion. Dermatologic eruptions are common as a result of immunosuppression. Herpes simplex may be found on the oropharynx or vulva. Herpes zoster is usually seen in a dermatomal pattern on the face, torso, or extremities. Lesions of molluscum contagiosum, which are firm, translucent papules of viral etiology, may be widespread. Other lesions include oral and vulvar candidiasis; chronic acneiform staphylococcal folliculitis on the face, thorax, and back; and Kaposi's sarcoma of any region. Seborrheic dermatitis may be present on the face and chest.[90]

Symptoms and Course. Human immunodeficiency virus (HIV) causes irreversible immunosuppression with multiple complex constitutional symptoms. Quiescent periods occur, but there is no cure. Treatment is palliative and varies with opportunistic infection.

Maternal-Fetal Transmission. Transmission of the virus to the fetus occurs in 15 to 40% of cases, probably via the placenta.[91] The time of transmission remains unknown, and therefore it cannot be prevented.[86] Transmission can be decreased with maternal antiretroviral therapy, however.

Newborn Pathology. Affected babies appear disease-free until about 8 months of life. The median survival time is only 3 years.[86]

Medical Therapy and Effects. Acyclovir is often given. Oral ketoconazole has potential hepatotoxicity. Zidovudine (AZT), which so far is thought to be non-teratogenic, may cause maternal anemia, neutropenia, rash, and proximal myopathy.[92] Many new drugs are becoming available, with as yet unknown effects on pregnancy.

Anesthetic Implications. Strict transmission precautions must be used. Multi-organ pathology is possible. Regional anesthesia has not been found to be contraindicated.[93] (For further discussion, see Chapter 24.)

Human Papillomavirus

Skin Lesion. Genital papules and verrucous friable growths mark this entity.

Symptoms and Course. The warty protrusions are more likely to appear in pregnancy. Swelling, pain, itch, and mechanical obstruction can disturb the birth canal. The patient may be immunocompromised or may have coexisting genital infections.[85]

Maternal-Fetal Transmission. The virus is most likely transmitted at birth, transvaginally. It is unknown if transplacental or hematogenous spread may occur.[85]

Newborn Pathology. A low incidence of clinical disease occurs. Latency for associated laryngeal papillomatosis in childhood is up to 5 years.

Medical Therapy and Effects. The common medications podophyllin, fluorouracil cream, and alpha-interferon are contraindicated in pregnancy. Acceptable treatments are nonsystemic, such as laser vaporization and topical trichloroacetic acid.[85]

Anesthetic Implications. Cesarean birth may be needed because of mass effect. There are no specific anesthetic recommendations.

Lyme Disease

Skin Lesion. Erythema chronicum migrans, an expanding erythematous patch with central clearing, is the observed lesion marking infection by the spirochete *Borrelia burgdorferi*. The lesions are usually fairly large and asymptomatic. Lesions are most common in the thigh, groin, and axilla. Smaller, annular, secondary lesions may be seen as well.[94]

Symptoms and Course. Flu-like symptoms are common and may remain mild or develop into a chronic systemic syndrome. The syndrome is characterized by neurologic changes (meningitis, cranial nerve palsies), cardiac abnormalities (myocarditis and heart block), and arthritis.

Maternal-Fetal Transmission. The mechanism of transfer of this spirochete is transplacental. Adverse outcomes appear in 32% of affected pregnancies. Adverse outcomes include preterm labor, fetal demise, and cardiac abnormality. The placenta should be examined at birth for spirochetes.[95]

Newborn Pathology. Cardiac abnormality, syndactyly, cortical blindness, and rash in the newborn are potential sequelae of maternal-fetal transfer.[95]

Medical Therapy and Effects. Doxycycline is the usual therapy but is avoided during pregnancy because of potential fetal effects. Penicillin, amoxicillin, ceftriaxone, and erythromycin have been given. Some physicians use prophylactic treatment in pregnant mothers with tick bites.[95]

Anesthetic Implications. Multi-organ involvement must be considered in this syndrome.

Neisseria gonorrhoeae (Gonococcus)

Skin Lesion. Disseminated gonococcemia is characterized by small vesiculopustules and purpuric macules that may enlarge up to 2 cm in diameter. These lesions are common around joints and on the soles and palms. The clinical differential diagnosis includes meningococcemia, bacterial endocarditis, Rocky Mountain spotted fever, and vasculitis. Diagnosis of gonococcemia requires isolation of organisms from skin lesions or from blood cultures.

Symptoms and Course. The mother may be asymptomatic or may have fever, arthralgia, and malaise, with possible meningitis, myocarditis, and pericarditis.[90] Purulent cervical and urethral discharge is usual early in infection.

Maternal-Fetal Transmission. Transmission may occur during fetal passage through an infected birth canal[96] or by transplacental transmission.[97] Complications include preterm labor and fetal loss.[90]

Newborn Pathology. Untreated gonococcal ophthalmia can cause blindness. Urethritis is possible in males. Dissemination leads to meningitis and arthritis.[96]

Medical Therapy and Effects. Medical treatment consists of penicillin or ceftriaxone, with optional additional cefotetan, gentamicin, or ciprofloxacin.[98] The newborn is also treated with ophthalmic silver nitrate, tetracyline, or erythromycin.

Anesthetic Implications. Infection precautions are indicated.

Parvovirus B19 (Fifth Disease)

Skin Lesion. The most characteristic appearance, usually seen in young children, is a bright red "slapped cheeks" erythema. More common in adults is a pink, lacy, reticulate rash on the torso and extremities.

Symptoms and Course. The mother may present with concurrent upper respiratory symptoms, fever, and myalgia acutely. Arthritis of the hands, wrist, and knee may follow.[90]

Maternal-Fetal Transmission. Transmission is via placental transfer. Other than a single reported event of aplastic anemia and fatal hydrops fetalis,[99] no adverse outcomes have been seen in over 170 documented maternal cases.[99]

Newborn Pathology. No newborn pathology has

been reported, with the exception of the earlier mentioned case.

Medical Therapy and Effects. No known medical treatment is available. Intrauterine transfusions to the fetus suffering aplastic anemia are at the experimental stage.[90]

Anesthetic Implications. General recommendations listed at the end of the chapter should be reviewed.

Rubella (German Measles)

Skin Lesion. A generalized macular rash lasts 3 days.

Symptoms and Course. Fever and malaise are usually mild; arthralgia, neuritis, and thrombocytopenia are rare manifestations. Thirty percent of affected adults are asymptomatic.[100]

Maternal-Fetal Transmission. Transmission is transplacental. Infections in early pregnancy lead to more extensive pathologies and demise than those in later pregnancy.

Newborn Pathology. The effects of in-utero exposure run the spectrum from a normal neonate to one with multiple congenital anomalies to spontaneous abortion. "Virtually every organ may be involved, transiently, progressively, or permanently."[101]

Medical Therapy and Effects. No antiviral therapy is available. Treatment is symptomatic and is generally unnecessary for the mother. Immunization of women before a first pregnancy is strongly encouraged by departments of public health.

Anesthetic Implications. Given the extremely serious consequences of fetal exposure to this virus, it is essential that the anesthesiologist be vaccinated, if he or she has not already acquired immunity to the disease.

Rubeola (Measles)

Skin Lesion. Koplik spots on the buccal mucosa are the initial pathognomonic sign (1-mm white dot encircled by a rosy red ring). The subsequent total body maculopapular rash begins on the head and neck and spreads caudally.

Symptoms and Course. A prodrome of fever and malaise, precedes the dermatologic signs. Conjunctivitis and oral pharyngeal involvement ensue. A cough may persist 10 days, along with lymphadenopathy and splenomegaly. Infrequent but serious complications include bacterial pneumonia, viral laryngotracheobronchitis, myocarditis, encephalitis, and thrombocytopenic purpura.[102]

Maternal-Fetal Transmission. The mode of transmission is transplacental. Maternal infection may lead to preterm labor. No consensus exists on induction of

spontaneous abortion by this virus, and there are no known congenital malformations.[102, 103]

Newborn Pathology. Transplacental transmission within days of birth leads to congenital measles, which can range in severity from mild to fatal (32%). It is hoped that the fatality rate is decreasing with the advent of aggressive antibiotic treatment of secondary bacterial infections[103] and maternal immunization.

Medical Therapy and Effects. Treatment is symptomatic for uncomplicated disease; antibiotics are given as needed. Exposed pregnant women should receive immune serum globulin.[103]

Anesthetic Implications. The anesthesiologist should review and examine for involvement of the oral pharynx, respiratory system, and neurologic system. If the patient has been ill, she may be dehydrated with resultant electrolyte derangements.

Varicella

Skin Lesion. The primary infection is called chickenpox. It is manifested by an erythematous rash, followed by punctate vesicles that become purulent and eventually crust over. Itching is significant. Adult reactivation of this virus is known as herpes zoster or, more commonly, shingles, which consist of vesicular lesions in a dermatomal distribution.[103]

Symptoms and Course. The rash and constitutional symptoms can last a week. The period of infectivity begins 48 hours before the eruption of the rash and continues until the skin lesions crust over. The incidence of varicella is estimated at one to seven cases per 10,000 pregnancies. Compared with their nonpregnant counterparts, these women are at increased risk for severe presentations of the disease. They are more susceptible to pneumonia, which can be fulminant, requiring full respiratory support. Mortality from pneumonia has been reported.[104]

Maternal-Fetal Transmission. Transmission is transplacental. First-trimester maternal infection can lead to the congenital varicella syndrome, consisting of limb hypoplasia and psychomotor retardation. If infected at term, maternal antibody is protective to the fetus only if IgG crosses the placenta prior to birth. Maternal shingles is not only rare but nonproblematic because antibody formation follows the primary chickenpox and is readily available to the fetus.[103]

Newborn Pathology. If the mother becomes infected and the fetus is born before antibody formation, neonatal varicella infection is likely, with 30% neonatal fatality. If birth commences more than 5 days after the onset of maternal symptoms, infants either are unaffected or exhibit mild varicella. Immune globulin is recommended for newborns at risk for serious infection.[103]

Medical Therapy and Effects. Varicella zoster immune globulin (VZIG) can be given to pregnant women exposed to the virus. No resultant maternal systemic consequences or fetal changes occur.[103]

Anesthetic Implications. Because parturients with acute varicella are at risk for life-threatening pneumonia, elective instrumentation of the airway should be avoided if possible, and regional anesthesia should be administered. Any sign of wheezing, rales, or fever should heighten concern for acute pulmonary crisis, requiring appropriate respiratory support.

AUTOIMMUNE DISEASES WITH DERMATOLOGIC MANIFESTATIONS
(Table 25–6)

Dermatomyositis

Skin Lesion. The pathognomonic features of dermatomyositis are heliotrope rash and Gottron papules. *Heliotrope* refers to periorbital and eyelid violaceous erythema and edema that may involve the entire face. The same coloring is seen in Gottron papules commonly found on the metacarpophalangeal and more distal interphalangeal joints and extensor aspects of the knees and elbows.[105]

Symptoms and Course. This is a multisystem disease characterized by necrotizing inflammatory myopathy of striated muscle. The etiology is unknown, but immunologic mechanisms are thought to play a role in the development of this pathology.[106] Up to 20% of cases are associated with an underlying, usually occult, neoplasm.[43] Proximal symmetric muscle weakness is progressive, with elevated serum creatinine phosphokinase levels and abnormal electromyography findings. Weakness of swallowing musculature, of intercostal muscles, and of the diaphragm leads to problems with airway protection and ventilation. This may result in pneumonia. Myocardial fibrosis can cause heart block and left ventricular dysfunction.[43, 107] Mortality rates have improved with steroid use, from 33% to 8%, although mortality remains high in those patients with concurrent malignancy. Remissions and exacerbations are common.[105]

Maternal-Fetal Transmission. Although surviving neonates show no indication of congenital defect or acquired disease, there is a high rate of fetal loss (50%). Maternal disease is exacerbated by pregnancy and does not necessarily remit post partum.[108]

Newborn Pathology. If the fetus survives the pregnancy, there are no subsequent newborn complications directly related to the mother's disease.[108] Some genetic predisposition to expression of the disease as an adult, however, may be present.[107]

Medical Therapy Effects. During periods of activity of the disease, there is a negative nitrogen balance due to muscle destruction. Steroids are the mainstay of therapy. Alternatives include steroid-sparing immunosuppressants and antimalarial medications, but these carry risks to the fetus and are reserved for the most severe maternal symptoms.[107] Malignancy-associated dermatomyositis resolves with successful treatment of the underlying neoplasm.

Anesthetic Implications. Systemic manifestations should be evaluated, particularly lung function and cardiac status, if the patient is symptomatic. Airway compromise with increased risk of aspiration and need for postoperative ventilatory support must be considered. Vital capacity, blood gas analysis, and chest radiography may be valuable. Because of the muscular pathology, some recommend avoidance of malignant hyperthermia–triggering agents[43] and use of small incremental doses of both depolarizing and nondepolarizing NMBAs. Some have shown a normal response to NMBAs, however.[43, 109]

Pemphigus Vulgaris

Skin Lesion. Flaccid blisters and erosions are found on the skin and oral mucosa. They appear in the first or second trimester or post partum.[110] Immunofluorescence techniques demonstrate IgG autoantibodies against desmosomal proteins in the serum and epidermis.

Symptoms and Course. Fewer than 30 cases of this autoimmune bullous disease in pregnancy have been reported because it usually appears in those well beyond childbearing years.[110, 111] Before the advent of systemic corticosteroid treatment in the 1950s, there was a grim 5-year mortality rate of 100%. That has been reduced to 5%, with most deaths now caused by the complications of immunosuppressive therapy.[112]

Maternal-Fetal Transmission. The disease may be precipitated or aggravated by pregnancy. The antibodies do cross the placenta.

Newborn Pathology. Transient skin lesions can be seen in the newborn.[113] Reports indicate poor fetal outcome (preterm delivery or death) when mothers have severe disease.[110]

Medical Therapy and Effects. Systemic steroids are the mainstay of therapy. Supplementary immunosuppressive treatment with azathioprine, methotrexate, cyclophosphamide, or cyclosporin may be needed,[110] although adverse fetal effects may result. Remissions are rare, and patients may require medical treatment for life.[112]

Anesthetic Implications. The anesthetic plan for this rare disease must consider the maternal use of immu-

---

TABLE 25–6. AUTOIMMUNE DISEASES WITH DERMATOLOGIC MANIFESTATIONS

Dermatomyositis	Scleroderma
Pemphigus vulgaris	Systematic lupus erythematosus
Polyarteritis nodosa	

nosuppressive agents and the possibility of secondary infection. Some patients have coexistent myasthenia gravis and thymoma.[114, 115] Because the oral lesions can resemble those of epidermolysis bullosa, airway management is similar (see earlier). The need for an airway or endotracheal tube must be avoided, if possible.[1] Usual respect for bullae requires nonfrictional scrub technique and avoidance of invasive procedures through a bulla.

Polyarteritis Nodosa

Skin Lesion. Polyarteritis nodosa is a systemic vasculitis affecting medium-sized arteries of all organs, including the skin. Cutaneous involvement is identified in 23% of cases, including tender nodules, ulcerations, and erythemas.[116]

Symptoms and Course. Although the etiology of this immune-mediated disease is generally unknown, cases may occur following infection with hepatitis B or beta hemolytic streptococcus. The disease generally affects middle-aged adults. Commonly affected organs are kidney, liver, heart, and gastrointestinal tract. Central nervous system and musculoskeletal involvement occur less often. Five-year survival has improved to 96% with steroid and immunosuppressive treatment, although the disease can be fatal with renal, cardiac, and hepatic compromise.[109, 116]

Maternal-Fetal Transmission. Antibody transmission is a rare complication of pregnancy. The effect of pregnancy on the disease process is unknown, although deterioration and death have been noted.[117] Fetal outcomes have been variable from spontaneous abortion to near-term delivery.[118]

Medical Therapy and Effects. Steroid dose varies with symptoms. Cyclophosphamide and sulfapyridine have been tried, although neither is recommended in pregnancy. Cyclophosphamide causes bone marrow depression and blood dyscrasia, inhibits cholinesterase activity, induces hepatic enzymes, and decreases the immune response to infections. Long-term use is cardiotoxic and can lead to hemorrhagic cystitis, SIADH secretion, and pulmonary fibrosis.[72]

Anesthetic Implications. The anesthesiologist should consider multi-organ pathology, especially of the kidneys, heart, and liver. Hypertension may be acute or chronic, and maintaining the patient's baseline blood pressure is recommended.[109] This can be facilitated by the placement of an arterial line. Effects of medical therapy should be considered in the anesthetic plan.

Scleroderma

Skin Lesion. Excessive collagen production results in thick, taut, sclerotic skin, which is most prominent on the face and distal extremeties. Limited or localized scleroderma, also called the **CREST** syndrome, is characterized by **c**alcinosis, **R**aynaud phenomenon, **e**sophageal strictures, **s**clerosis, and **t**elangiectasias. Diffuse or systemic scleroderma is distinguished by additional serious and progressive internal organ involvement. In addition to thick, sclerotic, and occasionally extremely pruritic skin, "salt-and-pepper" hyperpigmentation and hypopigmentation may be seen. Cutaneous ulcers of fingertips and joints, often associated with calcinosis, are painful, and they may occur along with microstomia and retraction of the lips and mandible. Flexion contractures can be problematic as well.[119]

Symptoms and Course. This is a diffuse disease of fibrosis. Skin and internal organs (usually lung and kidney) are affected, resulting in pulmonary hypertension and fibrosis, renal failure with resistant hypertension, esophageal dysmotility, pericarditis, and cardiac fibrosis with conduction deficits. The disease is not necessarily, relentlessly progressive and fatal, although it may be.[107, 119]

Maternal-Fetal Transmission. No reports of systemic scleroderma in a newborn of a mother with scleroderma are found.[120] Fetal outcome is grim, however, because of maternal morbidity and mortality. Pregnancy exacerbates maternal disease in half the cases, and spontaneous abortion and stillbirth are not uncommon.[121]

Newborn Pathology. No specific disease pattern ensues, but there is increased mortality due to preterm delivery and other perinatal complications.[117]

Medical Therapy and Effects. Vasodilators are recommended for treatment of Raynaud phenomenon (nifedipine, alpha-methyldopa). Colchicine and griseofulvin may also provide some relief. No general agreement exists on a treatment regimen, and goals are often limited to symptomatic treatment.[119] Steroid use is controversial. Oral penacillamine and extracorporeal photopharesis have been tried.

Anesthetic Management. Multiple considerations remain for the anesthesiologist owing to the complex nature of this disease. The following precautions are recommended:

- Preoperative history and physical examination dictate which laboratory tests are needed to assess renal, cardiac, and pulmonary involvement.
- Chest radiographs and pulmonary and cardiac function tests can be done. Evidence of restrictive lung disease with decreased diffusion capacity is often noted.
- Vasoconstriction and skin changes can make intravenous and monitoring access difficult, necessitating central catheterization.
- Pulmonary artery cannulation or central venous pressure monitoring may be needed for patients with pulmonary hypertension and right or left heart failure.

- Gastrointestinal tract abnormalities can interfere with vitamin K absorption, resulting ultimately in clotting abnormalities.
- Airway compromise is expected from involved facies, and careful planning of endotracheal intubation is necessary. Decreased esophageal motility must be considered as well.
- General anesthesia is affected by decreased lung compliance and need for increased inspired oxygen concentration. Postoperative ventilatory support may be necessary, particularly with narcotic depression of respiratory drive.
- In cases of renal compromise, nondepolarizing NMBAs, such as atracurium and vecuronium, should be utilized because of their nonrenal mode of metabolism.[122]
- Warmth must be maintained.
- Positioning with meticulous padding is warranted.
- Regional anesthesia is acceptable, with the caveat that one may ultimately need to protect the airway if there is a complication during surgery.[121, 123]
- Successful management of labor and vaginal delivery with epidural anesthesia has been reported.[123]
- Stress-dose steroids should be given as needed.

Systemic Lupus Erythematosus (SLE)

Skin Lesion. Vascular reactivity to autoantibody stimuli causes this multisystem disorder. Facial butterfly-like malar rash or generalized morbiliform eruption with edema may be the first sign of or may signify exacerbation of the disease. Onset can be acute or chronic and progressive, worse with exposure to sunlight, leading to elevated plaques with dense scaling.[107] Facial swelling may be severe, with accompanying oral and nasopharyngeal ulceration. Epidermal necrosis is possible.[124] Severity of the disease ranges from isolated skin involvement (chronic cutaneous) to subacute to systemic SLE.

Symptoms and Course. The disease has a fluctuating course, with multi-organ involvement. Possible manifestations include nonerosive arthritis, Raynaud phenomenon, pericarditis, pleuritis, glomerulonephritis with proteinuria and eventual renal failure, seizure disorder, thrombocytopenia, leukopenia, and hemolytic anemia. Pregnancy may exacerbate the disease but does not appear to affect long-term outcome. Risk of maternal death is highest in the peripartum period, due to pulmonary hemorrhage or lupus pneumonitis. An increased risk of severe pre-eclampsia is present, which may be difficult to differentiate from lupus nephritis.[117, 125]

Maternal-Fetal Transmission. The incidence of spontaneous abortion is 40%, often seen up to week 28 of gestation. It is not related to the severity of the mother's disease. It does seem to be related to the presence of lupus anticoagulant and anticardiolipin antibodies, however, which cross the placenta. The exact mechanism of destruction is unknown, but the placenta may have infarcts with fetal growth retardation. In addition, there is an increased risk of late fetal demise due to its hypertension or renal failure.[117]

Newborn Pathology. Neonatal lupus syndrome consists of hematologic, dermatologic, and cardiologic abnormalities (complete heart block). Fortunately, two thirds of infants born to affected mothers are normal. Maternal steroid use rarely leads to hypoadrenal crisis in the newborn.[126]

Medical Therapy and Effects. Nonsteroidal anti-inflammatory drugs (NSAIDs) including aspirin are the mainstay of therapy. Steroids and heparin are used as needed. No teratogenic risk from NSAIDs has been shown, but increased neonatal hemorrhage with platelet malfunction is possible,[117] as well as premature closure of the ductus arteriosus. Azathioprine is a cytotoxic drug that can be given during pregnancy only with great caution. Azathioprine has no known fetal effects post partum, but it may impair the eventual reproductive capacity of females via chromosomal aberrations of the ova.[117] Maternal effects of azathioprine can include blood dyscrasias from bone marrow suppression, hepatitis or biliary stasis, and gastrointestinal sensitivity.[72]

Anesthetic Implications. In addition to considering systemic pathologies, compromise of the airway with lesions and edema should be of concern to the anesthesiologist. Raynaud phenomenon may preclude radial arterial line placement and interfere with pulse oximetry. Neuropathies must be documented preoperatively. Laboratory values that may be abnormal include CBC, clotting studies, and creatinine. PTT may be elevated in the presence of lupus anticoagulant (LA), in which case it is not associated with a bleeding tendency.[127] In fact, the blood in these patients clots easily. Patients are at risk for thromboses of blood vessels in the brain, placenta, and lower extremities. Thus, the LA status becomes important. Regional anesthesia must take into account the coagulation potential. Careful positioning, stress-dose steroids as needed, and early crossmatching of blood are recommended. Vigilance must be maintained for the occurrence of pre-eclampsia.[128]

SUMMARY

Skin lesions in the parturient may present the anesthesiologist with a clinical dilemma. Dermatoses may represent one manifestation of a systemic illness, from an autoimmune or infective origin, or may be a normal pregnancy finding. It is important to consult with a dermatologist if there is any doubt. This chapter is a guide for the obstetric anesthesiologist, allowing rational decisions to be made about skin preparation

TABLE 25–7. GENERAL GUIDELINES FOR ANESTHESIA IN THE PRESENCE OF DERMATOLOGIC DISEASE

Anesthetic management of pregnant patients with dermatologic diseases requires not only the standard concerns in caring for the parturient and the fetus, but also an understanding of the skin disorder, the possible involvement of other organ systems, and the effects of therapeutic drug treatments

A systematic approach should be used to identify organs affected by the disease process. Preoperative testing is dictated by symptoms as well as likelihood of specific organ involvement. Intraoperative monitoring and anesthetic choices are modified to include the same principles that govern anesthetic care in other patients with those coexisting diseases

Airway complication is more likely in patients with manifestations of restricted mouth opening and jaw movement, oral-pharyngeal lesions whether painful or not, the presence of bullae in the respiratory tract, and any infective process. Such presentations may lead to awake intubation of the trachea under fiberoptic guidance, or may pose such risk to the patient as to contraindicate endotracheal intubation in all but life-threatening situations

Regional anesthesia and other invasive procedures are acceptable when sites of entry are not affected. If lesions are present in the target field, however, the skin disease must be identified as infected or noninfected, with obvious care to avoid instrumentation and spread of the former

In patients with bullous diseases, avoid frictional rubbing and trauma during placement of monitors, tourniquets, and other interventional activities

Steroids are commonly used in this population. The need for perioperative stress doses should be considered

and needle puncture for regional anesthetic techniques and about anesthesia provision when dermatologic disease is present (Table 25–7).

References

1. Smith GB, Shribman AJ. Anaesthesia and severe skin disease. Anaesthesia 1984;39:443.
2. Maki DG, Ringer M, Alvarado CJ. Prospective randomised trial of povidone-iodine, alcohol, and chlorhexidine for prevention of infection associated with central venous and arterial catheters. Lancet 1991;338:339.
3. Kaul AF, Jewett JF. Agents and techniques for disinfection of the skin. Surg Gynecol Obstet 1981;152:677.
4. Aly R, Maibach HI. Comparative antibacterial efficacy of a 2-minute surgical scrub with chlorhexidine gluconate, povidone-iodine, and chloroxylenol sponge brushes. Am J Infect Control 1988;16:173.
5. Soulsby ME, Barnett JB, Maddox S. Brief Report: The antiseptic efficacy of chloroxylenol-containing vs. chlorhexidine gluconate-containing surgical scrub preparation. Infect Control 1986;7:223.
6. Rapini RP, Jordan RE. The skin and pregnancy. In Creasy RK, Resnick R (eds): Maternal-Fetal Medicine, 2nd ed. Philadelphia, WB Saunders, 1989, p 1114.
7. Errickson CV, Matus NR. Skin disorders of pregnancy. Am Fam Physician 1994;49:605.
8. Eudy SF, Baker GF. Dermatopathology for the obstetrician. Clin Obstet Gynecol 1990;33:728.
9. Lawley TJ, Hertz KC, Wade TR, et al. Pruritic urticarial papules and plaques of pregnancy. JAMA 1979;241:1696.
10. Holmes RC, Black MM. The specific dermatoses of pregnancy: A reappraisal with specific emphasis on a proposed simplified clinical classification. Clin Exp Dermatol 1982;7:65.
11. Bourne G. Toxemic rash of pregnancy. J Roy Soc Med 1962;55:462.
12. Nurse DS. Prurigo of pregnancy. Austral J Dermatol 1968;9:258.
13. Landon MB. Dermatologic disorders. In Gabbe SG, Niebyl JR, Simpson JL (eds): Obstetrics, 2nd ed. New York, Churchill Livingstone, 1991, p 1218.
14. Lever WF, Schaumburg-Lever G. Histopathology of the Skin, 7th ed. Philadelphia, JB Lippincott, 1990, p 153.
15. Catanzarite V, Quirk JG. Papular dermatoses of pregnancy. Clin Obstet Gynecol 1990;33:754.
16. Callen JP, Fabre VC. Cutaneous manifestations of systemic diseases. In Moschella SL, Hurley HJ (eds): Dermatology, 3rd ed. Philadelphia, WB Saunders, 1992, p 1686.
17. Habif TP. Clinical Dermatology, 3rd ed. St. Louis, CV Mosby, 1996, p 804.
18. Yancey KB, Lazarova Z. Dermatoses of pregnancy. In: Arndt KA, Leboit PE, Robinson JK, et al (eds): Cutaneous Medicine and Surgery, vol I. Philadelphia, WB Saunders, 1992, p 365.
19. Winton GB, Lewis CW. Dermatoses of pregnancy. J Am Acad Dermatol 1982;6:977.
20. Greaves MW. Pathophysiology and clinical aspects of pruritus. In Fitzpatrick TB, Eisen AZ, Wolff K, et al (eds): Dermatology in General Medicine, 4th ed, vol I. New York, McGraw-Hill, 1993, p 416.
21. Dacus JV. Pruritus in pregnancy. Clin Obstet Gynecol 1990;33:738.
22. Hanno R, Saleeby ER, Krull EA. Disorders of pregnancy. In Demis DJ (ed): Clinical Dermatology, 22nd rev, vol 4. Philadelphia, Lippincott-Raven, 1995, p 1.
23. Fisk NM, Storey GN. Fetal outcome in obstetric cholestasis. Br J Obstet Gynaecol 1988;95:1137.
24. Riley CA. Liver diseases in pregnancy. In Reece EA, Hobbins JC, Mahoney MJ, et al (eds): Medicine of the Fetus and Mother. Philadelphia, JB Lippincott, 1992, p 1077.
25. Milton JL. The Pathology and Treatment of Diseases of the Skin. London. Robert Hardwick, 1872, p 201.
26. Yancey KB. Herpes gestationis. Immunodermatology 1990;8:727.
27. Shornick JK. Herpes gestationis. J Am Acad Dermatol 1987;17:539.
28. Shornick JK. Herpes gestationis. Dermatol Clin 1993;11:527.
29. Fine J. Bullous diseases. In Moschella SL, Hurley HJ (eds): Dermatology, 3rd ed. Philadelphia, WB Saunders, 1992, p 685.
30. Fine J. Non-immunologic Bullous Disease. In Sams WM, Lynch PJ (eds): Principles and Practice of Dermatology, 2nd ed. New York, Churchill Livingstone, 1996, p 475.
31. Lawley TJ, Stingl G, Katz SI. Fetal and maternal risk factors in herpes gestationis. Arch Dermatol 1978;110:67.
32. Holmes RC, Black MM. The fetal prognosis in pemphigoid gestationis (herpes gestationis). Br J Dermatol 1984;110:67.
33. Shornick JK, Black MM. Fetal risks in herpes gestationis. J Am Acad Dermatol 1992;26:63.
34. Boh EE, Millikan LE. Vesiculobullous diseases with prominent immunologic features. JAMA 1992;268:2893.
35. Burgdorf WH. Impetigo herpetiformis. In Demis DJ (ed). Clinical Dermatology, 22nd rev, vol 2. Philadelphia, Lippincott-Raven, 1995, p 1.
36. Baker H, Ryan TJ. Generalized pustular psoriasis. A clinical and epidemiological study of 104 cases. Br J Dermatol 1968;80:771.
37. Oosterling RJ, Nobrega RE, Duboeuff JA, et al. Impetigo herpetiformis or generalized pustular psoriasis. Arch Dermatol 1978;114:1527.
38. Beveridge GW, Harkness RA, Livingston JR. Impetigo herpetiformis in two successive pregnancies. Br J Dermatol 1966;78:106.
39. Roizen MF. Diseases of the endocrine system. In Katz J, Benumof JL, Kadis LB (eds): Anesthesia and Uncommon Diseases, 3rd ed. Philadelphia, WB Saunders, 1990, p 254.
40. Nelder KH. Inherited elastic tissue malformations. In Arndt KA, Leboit PE, Robinson JK, et al (eds): Cutaneous Medicine and Surgery, vol I. Philadelphia, WB Saunders, 1996, p 1770.
41. Brighouse D, Guard B. Anaesthesia for Caesarean section in a patient with Ehlers-Danlos syndrome, type IV. Br J Anaesth 1992;69:517.
42. Millar WL. Other hereditary disorders. In Katz J, Benumof JL, Kadis LB (eds): Anesthesia and Uncommon Diseases, 3rd ed. Philadelphia, WB Saunders, 1990, p 146.
43. Stoelting RK, Dierdorf SF. Anesthesia and Coexisting Disease, 3rd ed. New York, Churchill Livingstone, 1993, p 427.
44. Romero R, Ghidini A, Bahado-Singh R. Premature rupture of the membranes. In Reece EA, Hobbins JC, Mahoney MJ, et